Nutrition and Disease Management for Veterinary Technicians and Nurses

Nutrition and Disease Management for Veterinary Technicians and Nurses

Third Edition

Ann Wortinger and Kara M. Burns

WILEY Blackwell

Published by John Wiley & Sons, Inc., Hoboken, New Jersey.
Published simultaneously in Canada.

For general information on our other products and services or for technical support, please contact our Customer Care Department within the United States at (800) 762-2974, outside the United States at (317) 572-3993 or fax (317) 572-4002.

Wiley also publishes its books in a variety of electronic formats. Some content that appears in print may not be available in electronic formats. For more information about Wiley products, visit our website at www.wiley.com.

Library of Congress Cataloging-in-Publication Data Applied for:

Paperback ISBN: 9781119861041
LCCN: 2024002544

ePDF: 9781119861065
epub: 9781119861058

Cover Design: Wiley
Cover Images: © Ann Wortinger and Kara M. Burns

Set in 9.5/12.5pt STIXTwoText by Straive, Chennai, India

SKY10066027_012924

Contents

Preface

Nutrition is an area of veterinary medicine that is very easy for the veterinary nurse/technician to have an active role. Many of the commercial food producers have even concentrated on educating veterinary nurses/technicians on nutrition through webinars, conference tracks, and self-paced courses.

As with any other area of education, you still need to know the fundamentals to understand what is being taught. Unfortunately, the nutrition fundamentals are often not taught in veterinary technology education. While chemistry, microbiology, and math are required at most schools, even these do not adequately address basic animal nutrition. We all are taught the basic nutrients in a diet: water, protein, fats, vitamins, minerals, and carbohydrates but what is lacking is, how do they work together, what happens to them inside the body, and what changes occur with aging or disease?

So where does this leave a veterinary technician or veterinary nurse who wants to know more about nutrition, who wants to really understand what is going on inside the animal and how nutrients play a role? Usually, they start by going through the available veterinary nutrition books if they are not overwhelmed and terrified by the first chapter, it is a miracle! These books are often more detailed than a technician needs or wants to know; one can get lost in these details and miss the basic points. If you go to human nutrition books, the unique nutritional needs of our most common species dogs, cats, horses, birds, and pocket pets, are not addressed, although basic nutrition may be presented in a less technical manner. Some people enroll in an online program, but the basics are still often missing from these, and referencing these, later on, can be challenging. We love having reference books available whenever we have a question or need clarification on a point of interest, and we often have questions and need clarification. Many commercial food producers also provide technical helplines, but you still need to understand the basics before you can ask for clarification!

We have plowed through nutrition books from the very basic pet owner books to the extremely technical veterinary books, and all of them have something to offer but will you read long enough to understand them? We were fortunate to have veterinarians willing to explain misunderstood points and concepts and encourage us to review specific tools and areas of interest. Without them, we would have had a much more difficult time understanding and utilizing nutrition in our day-to-day practice. After all, that is the ultimate goal of nutrition, is it not?

Ann Wortinger and Kara M. Burns, 2024

My goal in writing this book was to provide a book for a technician and nurse, that was both relevant and technical but understandable and usable. This is not a dummied-down version of a veterinary nutrition book, but one that focuses on the unique interests of technicians and nurses and how we use nutrition in practice and at home. For the third edition, I have asked my good friend and partner in nutrition, Kara M. Burns to provide her spin on disease management and alternate species nutrition. I am very excited to have Kara helping contribute to the third edition.

The book is organized into five sections. The first section addresses the basics of nutrition by looking at energy and nutrients; how the individual nutrients of water, carbohydrates, fats, proteins, vitamins, and minerals are utilized by the body; digestion; absorption of these nutrients; energy balance; the GI microbiome; and prebiotics, probiotics, and synbiotics, and finally those ever-popular, nutrition calculations!

Section II covers nutritional requirements for cats and dogs by going through the history and regulation of pet food, understanding how to read pet food labels, understanding nutrient content and types of foods and how they differ, and evaluating raw food diets, preservatives, and home-made diets, as well as offering resources for alternative diets.

Section III covers different feeding regimens and body condition scoring both definition and use and takes feeding from pregnancy and lactation through neonatal, growth, and adult maintenance feeding and into geriatrics. Section III will also cover feeding for performance animals, special feeding requirements for cats, nutrition myths, and how to calculate the cost of feeding.

Section IV covers the nutritional management of disease, looking at GI disease, critical care nutrition, assisted feeding techniques, hepatic disease, dermatology, the role of fatty acids in disease management, endocrine and metabolic diseases, cancer, trauma and infection, weight management, FLUTD, and others. This section includes a lot of new content on commonly seen diseases and newer areas of research.

The final section addresses the feeding management of other species, including horses, birds, and pocket pets. Each section will build on the information covered in previous sections, allowing for practical use of the information learned.

My cats and chickens are not thrilled when I start calculating caloric intake, nutrient distribution, or metabolizable energy. I am sure that Kara's varied pet population feels much the same way, but they too will ultimately benefit from our knowledge, as have innumerable clients, patients, coworkers, and students.

My hope is that through this edition of our nutrition book, you too will come to appreciate the important role nutrition plays in veterinary medicine, both through prevention and therapeutic use. You will have a better understanding of basic digestion, nutrient use by the body, and how food can affect our patients from the prenatal period through their death (hopefully many years down the line). And lastly that you will bring nutrition into your practice and use it to improve the quality of care that is provided to your patients. Nutrition is an ever-evolving field in veterinary medicine, and I hope this book serves as a stepping stone for future learning. Kara and I love veterinary nutrition, and we hope that you will come to love it too! #nutritionnerds!

Ann Wortinger, 2024

Acknowledgments

Working on this third edition has been challenging on many fronts. I changed jobs towards the final chapters, weathered a global pandemic, continued with my speaking schedule (virtually), became more comfortable with Zooming, and decided to add a sunroom on to our house! Enough activities to distract the hardiest of writers.

Kara and I have expanded the chapters and information provided, allowing both of us to further spread the nutrition word! As many of you know, Kara and I were on the organizing committee for the Academy of Veterinary Nutrition Technicians (AVNT) and are still on the Executive Committee for the VTS (Nutrition). We are very lucky that in 2022, the AVNT attained full recognition from the NAVTA CVTS. A labor of love for both of us!

My feline editorial staff has changed since the last edition; Dusty, our blind Detroit stray, remains in the chief lap warmer and contributor position, and Poppy, our TNR rescue, has stepped up to be my Zoom buddy. Jack, Millie, and BeeGee have the enviable job of seeing how much hair can be released on my desk, as well as making much use of our window cat-ledge. All of the cats had the unfailing ability to know exactly which book or article I was currently working on or would need next. You very kindly marked it with your furry bodies. Supervision was conducted from my lap, my desk, and the pet stairs. How does anyone work without a feline editorial staff?

And last but not least, my husband, Todd, who has had to undergo nightly discussions on new points of interest in nutrition, challenges with computers, and lots of late dinners! Thank you all for your continued support and for ensuring that I ate on a regular basis and knew I was appreciated and loved!

Ann Wortinger

I am honored to have again partnered with my good friend Ann Wortinger to write *Nutrition and Disease Management for Veterinary Technicians and Nurses, 3rd Edition*. We have seen this dream come to fruition, along with our other passion project: the Academy of Veterinary Nutrition Technicians. In 2022, the AVNT gained full recognition – a huge milestone which Ann and I are thrilled to see continue to grow. We both see the value of proper nutrition and the foundation for health that proper nutrition provides to veterinary patients.

Finding one's soul mate is a true gift from God. I am truly blessed to have been given the gift of Ellen Lowery, DVM, PhD, MBA, as my wife and best friend. You make my life complete and give me the courage to pursue all of my dreams. Thank you for your encouragement and support in this endeavor and for constantly supporting my desire to write this book! Thank you for being the love of my life!

Thank you to my parents, Bernard "Red" and Marilyn Burns who instilled in me a love of all of God's creatures.

I would like to thank the entire team at Wiley Blackwell for their support and expertise in making this third edition a reality!

I continue to have an expansive editorial staff that has contributed their supervisory abilities along this writing journey. Our cats O'Malley (our snowshoe) and Oliver Queen – "Ollie" (our Persian) have been consistently trying to help me with chapters by walking across my keyboard. Our French bulldogs Molly and Maggie, each trying to move their beds in my office to be the closest to me while I write. And Brees, our Border collie/Australian shepherd cross who has to put up with the Frenchies and keep them in line. Our Meyer's Parrot Bella, our Green Cheek Conure Loki, and our lovebirds Sookie, Stevie, and Mick. Thank you all for bringing such joy to my life.

Kara M. Burns

About the Companion Website

This book is accompanied by a companion website:

www.wiley.com/go/wortinger/3e

This website includes:
- Cases and the Keys.
- Review Questions with the Answers.

Section I

The Basics of Nutrition

1

Nutrients and Energy

Introduction

Animals, unlike plants, cannot generate their own energy and require a balanced diet to grow normally, maintain health once they are mature, reproduce and perform physical work.[1,2] Plants can convert solar energy from the sun into carbohydrates through photosynthesis, but they too require water, vitamins and minerals for optimal growth and production. Animals, in turn, either eat plants or eat other animals that eat plants to obtain their energy.[1,2]

Nutrients

For animals, energy is provided in the diet through nutrients. Nutrients are components of the diet with specific functions within the body and contribute to growth, tissue maintenance and optimal health.[1,2] Essential nutrients are those components that the body cannot synthesize at a rate adequate to meet its needs, so they must be included in the diet. These nutrients are used as structural components in bone and muscle, enhancing or being involved in metabolism, transporting substances such as oxygen and electrolytes, maintaining normal body temperature and supplying energy.[1,2] Nonessential nutrients can be synthesized by the body and obtained either through production by the body or through the diet.[1,2] Nutrients are further divided into six major categories: water,

carbohydrates, proteins, fats, vitamins and minerals.

Energy is not one of the major nutrients, but after water, it is the most critical component of the diet, energy needs always being the first requirement to be met in an animal's diet.[1,2] After energy needs have been met, nutrients become available for other metabolic functions.[1,2] Approximately 50–80% of the dry matter (DM) in a dog's or cat's diet is used for energy.[1,2] The body obtains energy from nutrients by oxidation of the chemical bonds found in proteins, carbohydrates and fats.[2]

Oxidation is the process of a substance combining with oxygen, resulting in the loss of electrons.[3] This oxidation occurs during digestion, absorption and transport of nutrients into the body's cells.[2] An essential energy-containing compound produced during this oxidative process is adenosine triphosphate (ATP), a common high-energy compound composed of a purine (adenosine), a sugar (ribose) and three phosphate groups.[2,3]

The biochemical reactions that occur within the body either use or release energy. Anabolic reactions require energy for completion, and catabolic reactions release energy upon completion.[2] ATP and other energy-trapping compounds pick up part of the energy released from one process and transfer it to other processes.[2] This energy is used for pumping ions, molecular synthesis and activating contractile proteins. These three processes essentially describe the total use of energy by the animal.[2] Without the energy supplied

Nutrition and Disease Management for Veterinary Technicians and Nurses, Third Edition. Ann Wortinger and Kara M. Burns.
© 2024 John Wiley & Sons, Inc. Published 2024 by John Wiley & Sons, Inc.
Companion Website: www.wiley.com/go/wortinger/3e

through the diet, these reactions would not occur, and death would follow.[2]

ATP is a usable form of energy for the body but not a good form of energy storage because it is used quickly after being produced.[2] Glycogen and triglycerides are longer-term storage forms of energy.[2] In fasting animals, when the body needs energy, it uses stored glycogen first, stored fat second, and finally, amino acids from body protein as a last resort.[2] The triglycerides found in fats cannot be converted into glucose. Only the glycerol backbone can be utilized for this purpose. For proteins/amino acids, they must undergo gluconeogenesis to be converted into usable glucose.[4]

Measures of Energy

Energy is the capacity to do work. This is measured most commonly in the United States as a calorie. A calorie is the amount of heat required to increase 1 g of water from 14.5 to 15.5 °C (or 1 °C) in a bomb calorimeter.[4,10] As this unit of measure is very small, we commonly use the term kilocalorie (1000 cal). When looking at food labels, this is the unit that is being referenced, a kilocalorie or kcal.

Although kcal is used in the United States, a joule is the International System of Units (abbreviated SI) unit measure of energy. 1 kcal = 4.184 J. As with calories, a joule is a small unit of measure, and megajoule (1,000,000 J, 10^6, abbreviated MJ) and kilojoule (1000 J, 10^3, abbreviated KJ) are the units most commonly used in animal nutrition.[4,10] For small animal nutrition, the kilojoule is used most. For large animal nutrition, the megajoule is used.

Gross Energy

The total amount of potential energy contained within a diet is called gross energy (GE). GE in food is determined by burning the food in a bomb calorimeter and measuring the total amount of heat produced. Unfortunately, animals are not able to use 100% of the energy contained in food. Some are lost during digestion and assimilation of nutrients and in urine, feces, respiration and heat production.[1,2]

Digestible Energy

Digestible energy (DE) refers to the energy available for absorption across the intestinal mucosa, the energy lost is found in the feces. Metabolizable energy (ME) is the amount of energy actually available to the tissue for use. The energy lost is that found in the feces and urine. ME is the value most often used to express the energy content in pet foods.[1,2]

When GE values are readjusted for digestibility and urinary losses, ME values of 3.5 kcal/g are assigned to proteins and carbohydrates and 8.5 kcal/g to fats. These values are called modified Atwater factors.[1,2] These were developed by American Association of Feed Control Officials (AAFCO) to produce an equation that would more accurately reflect the digestibility of commercial pet foods, which tend to have a lower digestibility than typical human foods.[4]

The ME of a diet or food ingredient depends on its nutrient composition and the animal consuming it.[1,2] If a dog and horse eat the same high-fiber diet, the horse will have a higher ME value due to its better fiber digestion ability than a dog. These differences in digestion can also be seen between dogs and cats, though not to the same extent as with an herbivore.

There are three methods to determine the ME in a diet: direct determination using feeding trials and total collection methods, calculation from analyzed protein levels, carbohydrates, and fats in the diet and extrapolating data collected from other species.[1,2]

Feeding Trials

Feeding trials using the species of concern are the most accurate method of determining a food's ME content. However, this can be time-consuming and expensive and requires access to large numbers of test animals.[1,2] The

AAFCO, the government body that oversees pet food production, has specific requirements for feeding trials; in general, they require a minimum of eight animals for a maintenance diet, at least 1 year of age, being fed the food in question for a minimum of 26 weeks. Food consumption is measured and recorded daily. Individual body weights should be recorded at the beginning, weekly and end, and a minimum database of blood work is required at the beginning and end of the study. A veterinarian must give all animals a complete physical exam at the beginning and end of the study; they are evaluated for general health, body and hair condition with comments recorded. Animals, not to exceed 25% (2 animals), may be removed for non-nutrition-related reasons only during the first two weeks of the study. A necropsy is conducted on any animal that dies during the study. There are additional conditions for foods used during pregnancy, lactation or growth.[5] Manufacturers of some of the premium pet foods routinely measure the ME of their formulated diets and ingredients through the use of controlled feeding trials.[1,2] Feeding trials are a time-consuming and expensive way to test ME in pet foods. Still, it is also the most accurate method and has the greatest potential to expose any deficiencies or excesses in a particular diet.

Calculation Method

ME values can also be determined using the calculation method. This involves using mathematical formulas to estimate a food's ME from its analyzed protein, carbohydrate and fat content. The formulas used for dog and cat diets have constants that account for fecal and urinary energy losses.[1,2] The method does not account for the digestibility or quality of ingredients. Therefore, excesses or deficiencies may not be apparent. ME is calculated using standard values for each nutrient. But each nutrient's actual energy may be different from the standard (see Table 1.1).

Table 1.1 Examples of AAFCO certification claims.

1. Animal feeding trials using AAFCO's procedures substantiate that … provides complete and balanced nutrition for maintenance.
2. This product is formulated to meet the nutritional levels established by the AAFCO dog food profile for adult dogs.
3. Animal feeding tests using AAFCO's procedures substantiate that … provides complete and balanced nutrition for all life stages of cats.
4. …is formulated to meet nutritional levels established by the AAFCO cat food nutrient profiles for growth and maintenance.[1,2]

Actual GE for triglycerides ranges from 6.5 to 9.5 kcal/g, proteins range from 4.0 to 8.3 kcal/g and carbohydrates range from 3.7 to 4.3 kcal/g. The standard values assigned to these nutrients are triglycerides 9.4 kcal/g, proteins 5.65 kcal/g and carbohydrates 4.15 kcal/g.[4] These values reflect GE rather than the modified Atwater numbers typically assigned when doing pet food calculations. GE does not account for fecal or urinary losses in a diet or the energy used during digestion.[4]

Data from other species can be used when direct data is not available for particular food ingredients in a particular species. This is especially common with cat food ingredients. The species most often used for comparison is the pig. Although this method of estimating ME is not as accurate as direct measurement, data collected from swine experiments have been reported to correlate well with values from other species with simple stomachs.[1,2]

The method used to attain AAFCO certification is required to be listed on the product label. Most companies that use feeding trials clearly state this; those using calculation methods or extrapolation methods may be a little vague in how the certification is obtained (see Table 1.2).[1,2]

Energy Density

The energy density of a pet food refers to the number of kilocalories provided in a given weight or volume. In the United States, energy density is expressed as kilocalories (kcal) of

Table 1.2 Example of nutrient density and nutrient distribution.

Nutrient density:
Protein 21 g/96.25 g/100 kcal
Fat 23.8 g/96.25 g/100 kcal
Carbs 51.45 g/96.25 g/100 kcal

Nutrient distribution:
Protein 21 g/96.25 g/100 kcal = 22%
$\quad$ (21 ÷ 96.25) × 100 = 22%
Fat 23.8 g/96.25 g/100 kcal = 25%
$\quad$ (23.8 ÷ 96.25) × 100 = 25%
Carbs 51.45 g/96.25 g/100 kcal = 53%
$\quad$ (51.45 ÷ 96.25) × 100 = 53%

Calorie calculation:
Protein 22% of 100 kcal = 22 kcal/96.25 g of food
Fat 25% of 100 kcal = 25 kcal/96.25 g of food
Carbs 53% of 100 kcal = 53 kcal/96.25 g of food

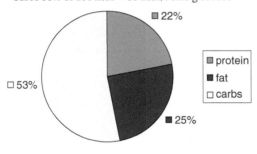

Table 1.3 Examples of nutrient density and caloric distribution.

Dog food for growth, dry:
Calories (ME): 4491 kcal/kg, 485 kcal/cup
Caloric distribution:
$\quad$ Protein 29%
$\quad$ Fat 46%
$\quad$ Carbohydrate 25%

Dog food for maintenance, canned:
Calories (ME): 1108 kcal/kg, 409 kcal/can
Caloric distribution:
$\quad$ Protein 34%
$\quad$ Fat 58%
$\quad$ Carbohydrate 8%

Cat food for maintenance, dry:
Calories (ME): 4490 kcal/kg, 459 kcal/cup
Caloric distribution:
$\quad$ Protein 29%
$\quad$ Fat 47%
$\quad$ Carbohydrate 24%

Cat food, hairball formula, dry:
Calories (ME): 3692 kcal/kg, 280 kcal/cup
Caloric distribution:
$\quad$ Protein 30%
$\quad$ Fat 29%
$\quad$ Carbohydrate 41%

Therapeutic recovery diet, canned:
Calories (ME): 2000 kcal/kg, 340 kcal/can
2.14 kcal/ml-canine
2.11 kcal/ml-feline
Caloric distribution:
$\quad$ Protein 29%
$\quad$ Fat 66%
$\quad$ Carbohydrate 5%

ME per kg or pound of food.[1,2] The energy density must be high enough for the animal to consume enough food to meet its daily energy requirements. Energy density will be the primary factor that determines the amount of food eaten each day.[1,2] The ability to maintain normal body weight and growth rate is the criteria used to determine the appropriate quantity of food fed.

Because energy intake determines total food intake, diets must be appropriately balanced so that requirements for all other nutrients are met at the same time that energy requirements are met.[1,2] For this reason, it is more appropriate to express nutrient energy levels in a diet in terms of ME than as a percentage of the food's weight or DM (see Table 1.3).[1,2]

Expressing nutrient content as units per 1000 kcal of ME is called nutrient density.[1,2]

Remember, fats contain almost three times the energy of proteins or carbohydrates and may only be a small portion of the weight of the diet but supply most of the calories. If looking only at weight, a diet may look low in fat, but be just the opposite.

When evaluating different diets, it is important to look at the caloric distribution and nutrient density rather than the percentage of the food's weight, typically expressed as DM. This will allow you to compare foods of differing moisture or energy contents. This method is somewhat limited compared to

Table 1.4 Calculating nutrients as a percentage of metabolizable energy.

Total calories in 100 g of food

Protein = 3.5 kcal/g × grams in food
Fat = 8.5 kcal/g × grams in food
Carbohydrate = 3.5 kcal/g × grams in food
Total calories/100 g = protein calorie + fat calorie + carbohydrate calorie

Percentage of ME contributed by each nutrient (caloric distribution)

Protein = (protein calories/100 g divided by total calories/100 g) × 100 = %ME
Fat = (fat calories/100 g divided by total calories/100 g) × 100 = %ME
Carbohydrate = (carbohydrate calories/100 g divided by total calories) × 100 = %ME

---

nutrient density because caloric distribution only considers the energy-containing nutrients of the food. The AAFCO requires that the energy value of a pet food be expressed in kcal of ME (see Table 1.4).[1,2]

Excess energy intake is much more common in dogs and cats than energy deficiency. The current estimates given by the American Veterinary Medical Association (AVMA) show that greater than 50% of dogs and cats are overweight (10–15% above their desired body weight) or obese (20–25% above their desired body weight)[6] Excessive energy intake has been shown to have several detrimental effects on dogs during growth, especially those of large and giant breeds. Feeding growing puppies to attain a maximal growth rate appears to be a significant contributing factor in developing skeletal disorders such as osteochondrosis and hip dysplasia (see Figures 1.1 and 1.2).[1,2]

Excessive energy intake during growth also affects the total number of fat cells the animal has. If the animals overconsume during their growth phase, this can contribute to obesity later in life. Once a fat cell has been formed, it will never go away, and research has shown that individual cells produce hormones that help them retain their stored fat.[1,2,7] Obesity has been linked to the development of orthopedic problems later in life and increased diabetes, hyperlipidemia, pancreatitis and heart failure. A study conducted by Nestle Purina demonstrated that by simply reducing the amount of food fed to a controlled group of Labradors by 25%, they, on average, lived 1.5 years longer than their pair mate, had less incidence of orthopedic problems, cancer and metabolic diseases (see Figure 1.3).[8]

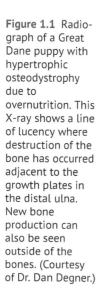

Figure 1.1 Radiograph of a Great Dane puppy with hypertrophic osteodystrophy due to overnutrition. This X-ray shows a line of lucency where destruction of the bone has occurred adjacent to the growth plates in the distal ulna. New bone production can also be seen outside of the bones. (Courtesy of Dr. Dan Degner.)

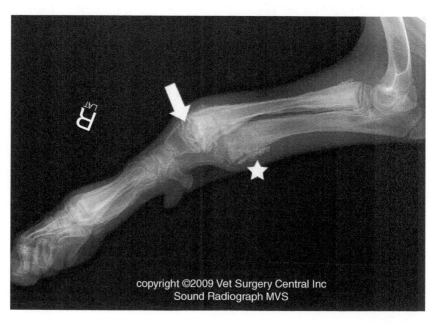

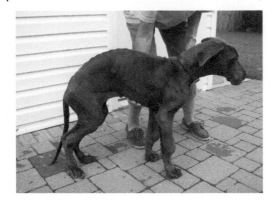

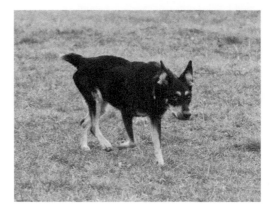

Figure 1.2 A Great Dane puppy showing the joint enlargement seen with hypertrophic osteodystrophy due to overnutrition. (Courtesy of Dr. Dan Degner, with permission.)

Figure 1.3 Weight loss secondary to diabetes mellitus. A common complication of this disease is weight loss due to lack of glucose utilization by the cells, causing protein catabolism of the muscle to meet the body's energy requirements with the decreased energy availability.

Inadequate energy intake results in reduced growth rate and compromised development in young dogs and cats and weight loss and muscle wasting in adult animals. In healthy animals, this is most commonly seen in hardworking dogs and pregnant or lactating females fed a diet too low in energy density.[1,2]

Weight loss is also seen in sick animals that are either unable or unwilling to eat adequate amounts of food or whose disease process causes energy loss or increased energy use.[9]

References

1 Case LP, Carey DP, Hirakawa DA et al. (2000) Energy and water. In Gross et al. (eds), Canine and Feline Nutrition (2nd edn), pp. 3–14, Mosby: St Louis MO.

2 Gross KL, Yamka RM, Khoo C et al. (2010) Macronutrients. In MS Hand, CD Thatcher, RL Remillard et al. (eds), Small Animal Clinical Nutrition (5th edn), pp. 49–66, Marceline MO Walsworth Publishing Mark Morris Institute.

3 Whitney E, Rolfes SR (2008) Glossary in Understanding Nutrition (11th edn), p. GL-12, Belmont CA: Thomson Wadsworth.

4 Delaney SJ, Fascetti AJ (2012) Basic nutrition overview. In AJ Fascetti, SJ Delaney (eds), Applied Veterinary Clinical Nutrition, pp. 9–21, Ames IO: Wiley-Blackwell.

5 Hand MS, Thatcher CD, Remillard RL, Roudebush P (2010) AAFCO Feeding Protocols for dog and cat foods. In MS Hand, CD Thatcher, RL Remillard et al. (eds), Small Animal Clinical Nutrition (5th edn), p. 8, Marceline MO Walsworth Publishing.

6 Study: Over half of pet dogs and cats were overweight in 2015. https://www.avma.org/javma-news/2016-06-15/study-over-half-pet-dogs-and-cats-were-overweight-2015. Accessed June 6, 2021.

7 Toll PW, Yamka RM, Schoenherr WD, Hand MS (2012) Obesity. In MS Hand, CD Thatcher, RL Remillard et al. (eds), Small Animal Clinical Nutrition (5th edn), p. 502, Marceline MO Walsworth Publishing Mark Morris Institute.

8 Kealy RD, Lawler DF, Ballam JM et al. (2002) Effects of diet restriction on life span and age-related changes in dogs. Journal of the American Veterinary Medical Association 220: 1315–20.

9 Donoghue S, Kronfeld DS, Case LP *et al.* (1994) Feeding hospitalized dogs and cats. In JM Wills, KW Simpson (eds), *The Waltham Book of Clinical Nutrition of the Dog and Cat*, p. 29, Oxford: Butterworth-Heinemann.

10 Hynd P (2019) Introduction to animal nutrition. In *Animal Nutrition from Theory to Practice*, pp. 14–7, Boston MA: CABI Publication.

2

Water

Introduction

Water is the single most important nutrient in terms of survivability. Animals can live for weeks without any food, using their body fat and muscle for energy production, but a loss of only 10% of their body water can result in death.[1–3] It is also one of three nutrients that do not contribute any calories to the diet.

Within the body, water functions as a solvent that facilitates cellular functions and as a transport medium for nutrients and the end products of cellular metabolism. Water can absorb much of the heat generated during metabolic reactions with a minimal increase in temperature. Water also helps to transport heat away from the working organs through the blood.[1,2]

Water is an essential component in normal digestion because it is necessary for hydrolysis, splitting larger molecules into smaller ones through the addition of water.[1,2] Examples of hydrolysis would include lipase, an enzyme that hydrolyzes fats; amylase, an enzyme that hydrolyzes amyloid; a complex carbohydrate and peptidase, an enzyme that hydrolyzes peptides, complex groups of amino acids.[4] Elimination of waste products through the kidneys also requires a large amount of water, which acts as both a solvent for the toxic metabolites and as a carrier medium.[1,2]

Water regulates oncotic pressure that helps the body maintain its shape; one manifestation of the loss of oncotic pressure is dehydration with loss of skin elasticity. Water is found in all body fluids, helps to lubricate the joints and eyes, provides protective cushioning for the nervous system and aids in gas exchange in respiration by keeping the alveoli moist and expanded.[2]

Water accounts for the most significant proportion of any of the nutrients in an animal's body, varying from 40–80% of the total amount. The percent of water varies with species, condition and age.[1,2] Generally, lean body mass (muscle) contains 70–80% water and 20–25% protein, with adipose tissue (fat) containing 10–15% water and 75–80% fat. The younger and leaner the animal is, the more water it contains. The fatter the animal, the lower the animal's water content.[2]

Water Quality

Because of water's role as a solvent, the potential exists that other substances can enter the animal's body that had not been planned for. Salinity (a water's salt content), nitrates, nitrites, inorganic chemicals and microbial contamination are examples of only a few contaminants found in water supplies.[5] Routine measurement of water quality looks at these dissolved solids with a reading of total parts per million (ppm) and is reported as "total dissolved solids" (TDS). Water containing less than 5000 ppm TDS is generally considered acceptable for consumption. A level above 7000 ppm of TDS is considered unsuitable for livestock and poultry consumption.[5] Human recommendations are less than 500 ppm of

TDS, which is considered a better recommendation for companion animals.

For anyone with access to city water, TDS testing is done through the local public health department. For those using well water or other sources of water, having a commercial analytical laboratory screen the water for TDS, pesticide residues and other chemicals would be recommended.[2]

Water Loss

Water is lost in several ways. Obligatory loss from the kidneys is the minimum amount of water required by the body to rid itself of the daily load of urinary waste products. Facultative loss is the remaining portion of the urine that is excreted in response to the normal water reabsorption rate of the kidneys and to mechanisms responsible for maintaining proper water balance in the body. Fecal water accounts for a much smaller portion of the water lost.[1] The third route of water loss is through evaporation from the lungs during respiration. Water can also be lost through perspiration, but accounts for only a small portion of water loss for most companion animals. In dogs and cats, evaporative and perspiration water loss is very important for regulating normal body temperature during hot weather.[1]

Water Gains

Daily water consumption must compensate for these continual losses. The total water intake comes from three possible sources: water present in food, metabolic water and drinking water.[1]

The amount of water found in the diet depends on the type of food being fed; dry food can have a moisture content as low as 7%, with some canned foods as high as 84%. Within limits, increasing the water content of food increases the diet's acceptability to the animal.[1]

Metabolic water is the water that is produced during the oxidation of energy-containing nutrients in the body. Oxygen combines with the hydrogen atoms removed from carbohydrates, proteins and fats during digestion to produce water molecules.[1,6] The metabolism of fat produces the greatest amount of metabolic water on a weight basis, and protein catabolism produces the smallest amount.[1] Metabolic water accounts for a relatively insignificant portion of the water intake, only 5–10% of the total daily intake.[1,5]

The most significant source of water intake is voluntary drinking. Numerous factors can affect an animal's voluntary oral intake, including ambient temperature, type of diet being fed, level of exercise, physiologic state and health.[1,6] Water intake increases with an increase in ambient temperature and increased exercise because of evaporative loss through the lungs due to panting to cool the body. The amount of food being fed can also affect water intake: as the calories increase, so does the amount of waste products that the body needs to get rid of, increasing the amount of urine produced. If this increase in calories results in weight gain, there will also be an increased loss due to panting to help with thermoregulation.[1,6]

Voluntary Oral Intake

The type of diet being fed and its composition can dramatically affect the voluntary oral intake of water. A study on dogs found that when the test animals were fed a diet containing 73% moisture, they obtained only 38% of their daily water needs from drinking water. When they were abruptly switched to a diet containing only 7% water, voluntary oral intake immediately increased to 95% or more of the total daily intake.[1] When cats are fed only canned food, their voluntary oral intake is likewise very low. When cats are fed food with very high water content, they can maintain a normal water balance with no additional drinking water.[6] This could be seen with liquid or gruel recovery diets and some commercial canned diets with a high amount of sauce.

Water requirements are related to maintaining appropriate water balance in the animal. Dogs and cats meet most of their water requirements through water included in food and voluntary oral intake. As a general guideline, the daily water requirement, expressed in ml/day for dogs and cats, is roughly equivalent to the daily energy requirement (DER) in kcal/day. For dogs, this is 1.6× the resting energy requirement (RER). For cats, 1.2 × RER.[2,5]

Domestic cats, descendants of desert animals, typically form more concentrated urine than dogs. Actual water requirements for cats may be less than those for dogs. Water needs can best be met through access to clean, fresh water at all times.[2,5,6] Dogs will show thirst and drink voluntarily when body water decreases by 4% or less. Cats do not voluntarily drink until they lose as much as 8% of their body water. In addition, cats fed dry food diets will typically consume less water per day than those fed canned food diets.[6]

If fresh, palatable, clean water is available and proper amounts of a balanced diet are fed, most dogs and cats can accurately self-regulate their water balance through voluntary oral intake.[1,2,6] Typically, thirst ensures that water intake meets or exceeds the body's requirements. Inadequate water intake can reduce appetite and reduce production on many levels, including growth, lactation, reproduction and physical activity.[2]

References

1 Case LP, Carey DP, Hirakawa DA, Daristotle L (2000) Energy and Water. In *Canine and Feline Nutrition* (2nd edn), pp. 3–14, Mosby: St Louis MO.

2 Gross KL, Wedekind KL, Cowell CS *et al.* (2000) Nutrients. In MS Hand, CD Thatcher, RL Remillard *et al.* (eds), *Small Animal Clinical Nutrition* (4th edn), pp. 21–36, Marceline, MO: Walsworth Publishing for Mark Morris Institute.

3 Wills JM (1996) Basic Principles of Nutrition and Feeding. In N Kelly, J Wills (eds), *Manual of Companion Animal Nutrition and Feeding*, pp. 14–5, Ames, IA: Iowa State Press.

4 Whitney E, Rolfes SR (2008) Digestion, absorption and transport. In *Understanding Nutrition* (11th edn), pp. 76–7, Belmont, CA: Thomson Wadsworth.

5 Gross KL, Jewell DE, Yamka RM *et al.* (2012) Macronutrients. In MS Hand, CD Thatcher, RL Remillard *et al.* (eds), *Small Animal Clinical Nutrition* (5th edn), pp. 51–3, Marceline, MO: Walsworth Publishing.

6 Case LP (2003) The Cat as an Obligate Carnivore. In *The Cat: Its behavior, nutrition and health*, pp. 295–7, Ames, IA: Iowa State Press.

3

Carbohydrates

Introduction

Carbohydrates are the major energy-containing part of plants, making up between 60% and 90% of their dry-matter weight.[1] This class of nutrients comprises the elements carbon, hydrogen and oxygen and is classified as monosaccharides, disaccharides, oligosaccharides or polysaccharides and has the general formula of $(CH_2O)_n$.[1,2] The hydrogen and oxygen are usually present in the same ratio as that found in water (H_2O), giving rise to the name carbohydrate or hydrated carbon.[3]

Carbohydrates are not essential nutrients but rather provide energy for the essential systems to do their jobs. In those species where fiber is not easily digested, the nondigestible carbohydrates found in fiber can be essential for normal gastrointestinal function and health.[4]

As a nutrient, carbohydrates act primarily as an energy source, allowing amino acids and fatty acids to build and maintain the body. When more carbohydrates are consumed than are needed by the body for energy, they may be converted into body fat and stored or serve as starting materials for the metabolism of other compounds.[3,4]

Monosaccharides

Monosaccharides are also called simple sugars and are the simplest form of carbohydrates, being composed of sugar units containing between 3 and 7 carbon atoms.[1,2] The chief monosaccharides are glucose, fructose (fruit sugar) and galactose (milk sugar).[1,2] Monosaccharides can combine to form polymers, and these can be enormous molecules containing many thousands of individual monosaccharide units.[3]

Glucose is a moderately sweet simple sugar found in commercially prepared corn syrup and sweet fruits such as grapes and berries. It is also the chief end product of starch digestion and glycogen hydrolysis in the body. Glucose is the form of carbohydrate found circulating in the bloodstream and is the primary carbohydrate used by the body's cells for energy.[1] Glucose is a 6-carbon ring in the shape of a hexagon, onto which the hydrogen and oxygen compounds are attached. This 6-carbon configuration gives the monosaccharides their other name of hexoses. Glucose is also known as dextrose (see Figure 3.1).[5]

Fructose, commonly called fruit sugar, is a very sweet sugar found in honey, ripe fruits and vegetables. It is also formed from the digestion or hydrolysis of the disaccharide sucrose.[1] Fructose is also a 6-carbon sugar, but the structure differs from glucose in that 2 of the carbons are outside of the ring structure, giving the molecule a pentagon shape (see Figure 3.2).[5]

Galactose is not found in a free form in foods. However, it makes up 50% of the disaccharide lactose, which is found in the milk of all mammals.[1] It has the same number and kinds of atoms as glucose, with only the

Nutrition and Disease Management for Veterinary Technicians and Nurses, Third Edition. Ann Wortinger and Kara M. Burns.
© 2024 John Wiley & Sons, Inc. Published 2024 by John Wiley & Sons, Inc.
Companion Website: www.wiley.com/go/wortinger/3e

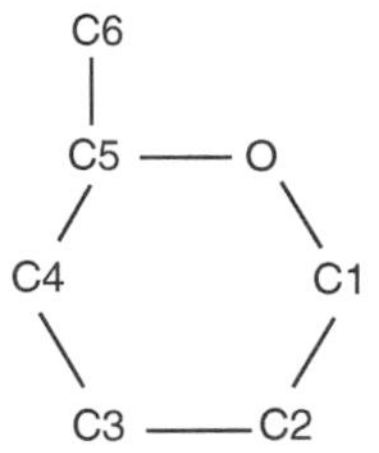

Figure 3.1 6-carbon hexagon glucose.

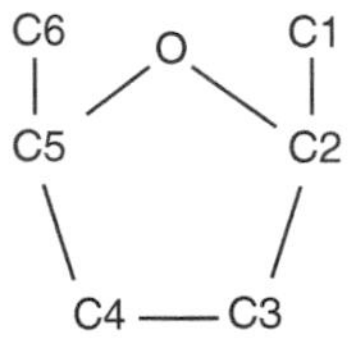

Figure 3.2 6-carbon pentagon fructose.

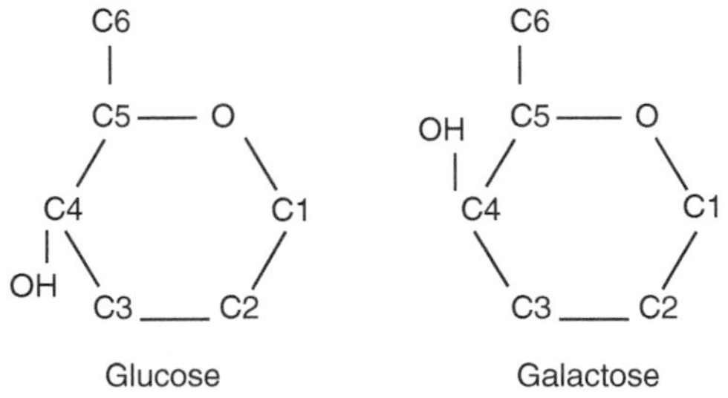

Glucose   Galactose

Figure 3.3 Glucose and galactose molecules.

position of 1 OH group being slightly different.[5] (see Figure 3.3).

Disaccharides

Disaccharides are made up of two monosaccharide units linked together. Lactose, the sugar found in mammalian milk, contains glucose and galactose. This is the only carbohydrate of animal origin.[1,2] Lactose intolerance, as seen in some adult animals, is caused by a deficiency of the enzyme beta-galactosidase. This deficiency prevents the glucose and galactose molecules from separating, making this a nondigestible carbohydrate.[3] Sucrose, commonly called table sugar, contains a molecule of glucose linked to a molecule of fructose. This

is the most common sugar found in plants.[1,2] Maltose is formed by linking two glucose molecules and is produced whenever a starch molecule is broken down. This can be seen during digestion or during the fermentation process that yields alcohol. Maltose is a minor constituent of only a few foods.[5]

Oligosaccharides

Oligosaccharides are carbohydrates made up of 3–10 monosaccharide units, making them polymers. These units may be the same or a mix of different monosaccharides. They are often difficult to digest, and if found in quantity as with some plant materials, may be associated with gastrointestinal disturbances or flatulence.[2,3] Those containing fructose are called fructooligosaccharides (FOS), but many other oligosaccharides are found in plants.[2] FOS's in the diet supply food for the microbiome in the intestine, increases nitrogen digestion and retention, improves stool quality and reduces fecal odors.[1]

This class of carbohydrates is used commonly for their prebiotic effects. A prebiotic is defined as "non-digestible food ingredients that selectively stimulate a limited number of bacteria in the colon to improve the host health."[6] This beneficial effect is seen because these fibers are resistant to the breakdown by enzymes in the host intestines, but can be broken down by certain gut bacteria helping to support the limited growth of these bacteria. Prebiotic fibers reduce fecal odor by modifying the fecal concentration of certain digestive by-products and improving immune function by influencing gut-associated immune cells.[6] More information on the intestinal microbiome can be found in Chapter 10 and prebiotics in Chapter 11.

Polysaccharides

Polysaccharides consist of many thousands of monosaccharide units. They are found widely in plants being used for cell wall material (cellulose) and energy storage (starch in the form of amyloid and amylopectin for plants and glycogen for animals).[1,3] Cereal grains, such as corn, wheat, sorghum, barley and rice, are the primary ingredients in pet foods that provide starch.[1] Complex carbohydrates of plant origin other than starch are dietary fiber or non-starch polysaccharides. These include cellulose, hemicellulose, pectin and the plant gums and mucilages.[1,3] Plant fibers differ from starches and glycogen in that their monosaccharide units have a different bonding configuration (beta bonds instead of alpha bonds). These bonds resist digestion by the gastrointestinal enzymes of most monogastrics, making their energy unavailable for absorption in the small intestine.[1] (see Figure 3.4).

Certain microbes found in the large intestine of dogs and cats can break down fiber to varying degrees, even though the animal themselves cannot break down the fiber.[1] This bacterial fermentation produces short-chain fatty acids (SCFAs) and other end products. The SCFAs that are produced in the most significant numbers are acetate, propionate and butyrate.[1] These SCFAs are a significant energy source for the small intestine's enterocytes and colonocytes of the large intestine.[1] Fiber in the diet also functions as an aid in the proper functioning of the gastrointestinal tract

Fiber type	Solubility	Fermentability
Beet pulp	Low	Moderate
Cellulose	Low	Low
Rice bran	Low	Moderate
Gum arabic	High	Moderate
Pectin	Low	High
Carboxy mellthy-cellulose	High	Low
Methylcellulose	High	Low
Cabbage fiber	Low	High
Guar gum	High	High
Locust bean gum	High	Low
Xanthan gum	High	Moderate

Figure 3.5 Dietary fiber fermentation in dogs. *Source*: Case et al.[1]/Scientific Research Publishing Inc.

and as a dietary diluent that decreases the total energy density of the diet.[1]

Glycosaminoglycans are complex polysaccharides associated with proteins. They form integral parts of the interstitial fluid, cartilage, skin and tendons. The primary glycosaminoglycans are chondroitin sulfate and hyaluronic acid (see Figure 3.5).[2]

Carbohydrate Types

Polysaccharides that the intestinal enzymes can digest are designated as starches, while those resistant to digestion and instead undergo fermentation, or bacterial digestion are designated as fibers.[6] For most starches, digestibility increases with the degree of gelatinization.

Gelatinization is when starch crystals are melted and hydrated (water added to the molecule) when heated or cooked. Extrusion cooking, a process used to produce dry pet foods, produces gelatinization through the application of heat, as does the canning process.[6]

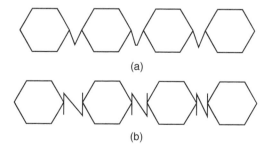

(a)

(b)

Figure 3.4 (a) Glucose molecules are connected with alpha bonding. Enzymatic hydrolysis occurs at these sites. The enzymes must be able to fit like a key in a lock for the break to occur. (b) Cellulose with beta bonding. Alpha enzymes cannot breakdown these molecules as they do not "fit" into the lock properly.

Table 3.1 Resistant starch classification.

RS1	Starch is physically trapped within the starch granule and is released during processing and chewing.
RS2	Starch granule structures, such as those found in raw potatoes, tapioca, and bananas.
RS3	Recrystallized starch forms after cooking when starch is cooled or dried, as seen with cooked rice.
RS4	Chemically modified starch resistant to enzymatic hydrolysis.

Resistant Starches

Resistant starch (RS) resists digestion in the small intestine. There are four classifications of RS based on how quickly glucose is released from the starch (see Table 3.1).

RS_1 and RS_2 starches represent residues of starches that digest slowly and incompletely in the small intestine. RS_3 starches are highly resistant to digestion by intestinal enzymes and are instead fermented by the colonic bacteria producing SCFAs.[2]

RS may have various functions related to their dietary fiber-like properties, including reducing food's glycemic index, decreasing the glucose and insulin responses in food and improving bowel health. RS can also be used as a fiber source for gluten-free and hypoallergenic foods.[2]

Carbohydrate Digestion

Carbohydrate digestion in dogs begins in the mouth with salivary amylase. On the other hand, cats lack salivary amylase, and carbohydrate digestion begins in the duodenum with pancreatic amylase. Amylase hydrolyses starches to maltose, maltotriose, dextran and glucose.[7] These products of digestion are absorbed across the intestinal villi by simple diffusion and active transport systems, primarily in the duodenum.[7]

Carbohydrate Functions

Carbohydrates have several functions in the body. The monosaccharide glucose is an important energy source for many tissues. A constant supply of glucose is necessary for the proper functioning of the central nervous system (CNS), and glycogen, the storage form of glucose within the body, is present in the heart muscle as an important emergency energy source for the heart.[1] Glycogen stored in the liver and muscle can be hydrolyzed to supply additional energy to the cells when circulating glucose is low. The CNS and red blood cells are wholly dependent on glucose for energy, while other tissues within the body can utilize other substances to obtain energy.[6] The amount of glycogen stored in the heart and the tissues is only enough to meet the basal requirements for ~24 h.

Carbohydrates also supply carbon skeletons for the formation of nonessential amino acids. They are needed to synthesize other essential body compounds, such as glucuronic acid, heparin, chondroitin sulfate, immunopolysaccharides, deoxyribonucleic acid (DNA) and ribonucleic acid (RNA).[1] When joined with proteins or lipids, some carbohydrates also become essential structural components in the body's tissues.[1] When metabolized for energy to carbon dioxide and water, they become a heat source for the body.[2] Finally, simple carbohydrates and starches consumed in excess of the body's needs are stored as glycogen or converted to fat.[2]

Not only do carbohydrates provide energy for the body, but digestible carbohydrates also have a protein-sparing effect. By providing enough carbohydrates for the body to meet its energy needs, protein is spared from being used for energy and is available for tissue repair and growth.[1,2] Conversely, if insufficient carbohydrates are available in the diet, protein will be used to meet energy needs decreasing the amount available for tissue repair and growth.[1]

Cats and Carbohydrates

Cats have a unique metabolism among companion animals that limit their ability to use large amounts of carbohydrates efficiently.

- Low activities of the intestinal enzymes sucrase and lactase.
- The sugar transport system in the intestinal tract is not able to adapt to varying levels of dietary carbohydrates.
- Lack hepatic glucokinase activity, limiting their ability to assimilate simple sugars.
- Pancreatic amylase is only 5% of what dogs produce.

- No salivary amylase is produced.
- Lack sweet receptors on the tongue.[7]

These differences support the classification of cats as obligate carnivores, but that does not mean that they cannot digest and utilize carbohydrates. If large amounts of carbohydrates are fed to cats (>40% dry matter), signs of maldigestion can be seen, such as diarrhea, bloating and flatulence.[6] Differences can also be seen among the different carbohydrate sources and their effects on blood glucose. Normal cats can maintain a normal blood glucose level when fed diets low in carbohydrates and high in protein by using a process called gluconeogenesis, where protein is used for energy instead of carbohydrates.[6]

References

1 Case LP, Carey DP, Hirakawa DA, Daristotle L (2000) Carbohydrates. In *Canine and Feline Nutrition* (2nd edn), pp. 15–8, St Louis, MO: Mosby.

2 Gross KL, Wedekind KL, Cowell CS *et al.* (2000) Nutrients. In MS Hand, CD Thatcher, RL Remillard *et al.* (eds), *Small Animal Clinical Nutrition* (4th edn), pp. 36–48, Marceline, MO: Walsworth Publishing for Mark Morris Institute.

3 Price CJ, Bedford PCG, Sutton JB (1993) Nutrients and the requirements of dog and cats. In JW Simpson, RS Anderson, PJ Markwell (eds), *Clinical Nutrition of the Dog and Cat*, pp. 20–2, Cambridge, MA: Blackwell.

4 Delaney SJ, Fascetti AJ (2012) Basic nutrition overview. In AJ Fascetti, SJ Delaney (eds), *Applied Veterinary Clinical Nutrition*, p. 13, Ames, IO: Wiley-Blackwell.

5 Whitney E, Rolfes SR (eds) (2008) The carbohydrates, sugars, starches, and fibers. In *Understanding Nutrition* (11th edn), pp. 101–8, Belmont, CA: Thomson Wadsworth.

6 Gross KL, Jewell DE, Yamka RM *et al.* (2012) Macronutrients. In MS Hand, CD Thatcher, RL Remillard *et al.* (eds), *Small Animal Clinical Nutrition* (5th edn), p. 77, Marceline, MO: Walsworth Publishing for Mark Morris Institute.

7 Philip H Dog and cat nutrition. In *Animal Nutrition from Theory to Practice*, pp. 279–84, Boston, MA: CABI Publication.

4

Fats

Introduction

Dietary fat is part of a group of compounds known as lipids that share the property of being insoluble in water (hydrophobic) but soluble in other organic solvents.[1,2] Lipids that are solid at room temperature are commonly called fats, and that liquid at room temperature are called oils.[2]

Lipids can be further categorized into simple lipids, compound lipids and derived lipids.[1] The simple lipids include triglycerides, the most common form of fat present in the diet and waxes.[1] Triglycerides are made up of three fatty acids linked to one molecule of glycerol; the waxes contain a greater number of fatty acids linked to a long-chain alcohol molecule.[1] (see Figure 4.1).

Compound lipids are composed of a lipid, such as a fatty acid, linked to a non-lipid compound. Lipoproteins, which carry fat in the bloodstream, are a type of compound lipid. The derived lipids, products of both compound and straightforward fats include sterol compounds, such as cholesterol and the fat-soluble vitamins A, D, E and K.[1]

Fat has numerous metabolic and structural functions. Fat provides insulation around myelinated nerve fibers and aids in the transmission of nerve impulses. Compound lipid molecules such as phospholipids and glycolipids serve as structural components for cell membranes and transport nutrients and metabolites across these membranes.[1]

Triglycerides

Triglyceride is the most important fat in the diet and can be differentiated in foods according to each triglyceride molecule's types of fatty acids.[1] Fatty acids vary in carbon-chain length and may be saturated, monounsaturated or polyunsaturated.[1] Saturated fatty acids contain no double bonds between the carbon atoms and are, therefore, "saturated" with hydrogen atoms.

Monounsaturated fatty acids have one double bond, and polyunsaturated fatty acids (PUFAs) contain two or more double bonds.[1] In general, the triglycerides found in animal fats contain a higher percentage of saturated fatty acids than vegetable fats.[1] The more double bonds a fatty acid has, the less stable the molecule is and the more susceptible to oxidation, resulting in rancidity.

Fats function in the body as a form of energy storage. Significant accumulated fat deposits can be found under the skin (subcutaneous fat), around the vital organs and in the intestines' membranes (omental fat).[1,2] The fat deposits also serve as insulators, protecting the body from heat loss and as a protective layer around the vital organs to guard against physical injury.[1] Although animals have a limited capacity to store carbohydrates in the form of glycogen, they have an almost unlimited capacity to store surplus energy in the form of fat.[1] Fats also provide the body with essential fatty acids (EFAs) and provide a carrier for the fat-soluble vitamins A, D, E and K.[1,2]

Nutrition and Disease Management for Veterinary Technicians and Nurses, Third Edition. Ann Wortinger and Kara M. Burns.
© 2024 John Wiley & Sons, Inc. Published 2024 by John Wiley & Sons, Inc.
Companion Website: www.wiley.com/go/wortinger/3e

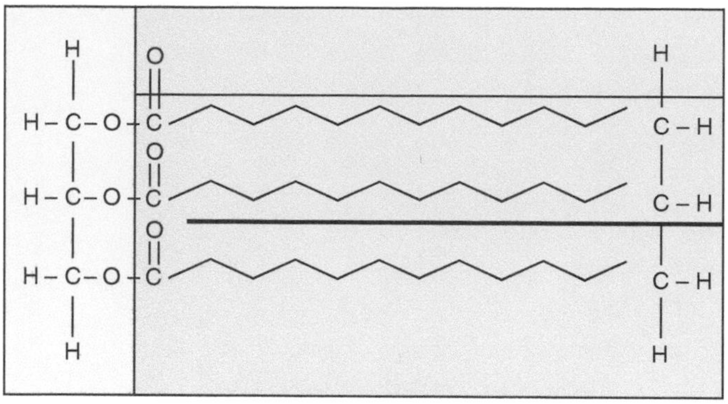

Figure 4.1 Triglyceride molecule.

Lipoproteins

Lipoproteins provide for the transport of fats through the bloodstream. Fats, by their nature, do not dissolve in the water-based bloodstream and must become incorporated in micelles which can carry them through the bloodstream to the various areas needed in the body.

A lipoprotein contains one hydrophobic end and a hydrophilic end. The hydrophilic end points to the outside of the molecule and allows the lipoprotein to be carried into the bloodstream. The hydrophilic end points inward and allows for the transport of molecules not soluble in water, such as fats. The percentage of triglycerides to cholesterol inside the lipoprotein molecules determines the density or weight of the molecule. (see Table 4.1).

Cholesterol

Cholesterol can be found in the diet in the form of cholesterol and converted from plant sterols. Cholesterol is also able to be synthesized by the liver.[2] Lipoproteins are used to transport cholesterol throughout the body. Cholesterol is used by the body to form the bile salts necessary for proper fat digestion and absorption. It is also a precursor for steroid hormones, including testosterone, estrogen, progesterone, cortisol and aldosterone.[1] Along with other lipids, cholesterol forms a protective layer in the skin that prevents excessive water loss and the invasion of foreign substances.[1]

Table 4.1 Lipoprotein classes.

Lipoprotein	Acronym	Protein: lipid ratio	Triglycerides / Cholesterol
Chylomicron	CM	1:99	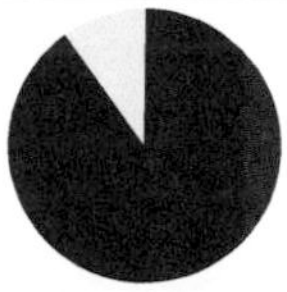
Very low-density lipoprotein	VLDL	10:90	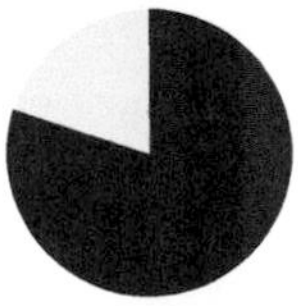
Low-density lipoprotein	LDL	25:75	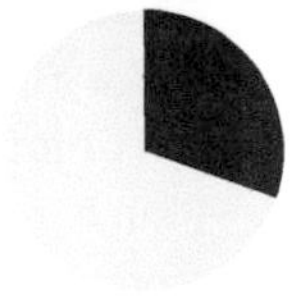
High-density lipoprotein	HDL	50:50	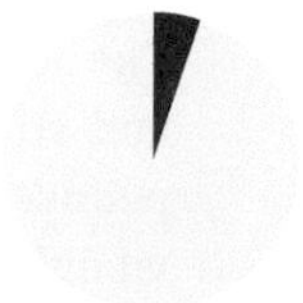

Source: Gross et al.[2]/Mark Morris Institute.

Nutrient Density

Of any nutrients, fat provides the most concentrated form of energy, almost three times that of carbohydrates and proteins. Each gram of fat provides 8.5 kcals (modified Atwater factors), as opposed to the 3.5 kcals provided by proteins or carbohydrates. The digestibility of fat is usually higher than that of carbohydrates and proteins.[1] This is especially important when increasing the caloric density of a food. By increasing the fat, the available calories and the digestibility of the food, increases substantially.

Fat Digestion

Unlike many other nutrients, instead of being broken down for digestion and use by the body, fats undergo elongation and desaturation (losing hydrogen atoms) for use in the body. Most fat digestion occurs in the duodenum, where pancreatic lipase and bile acids help transform triglycerides.[6] Monoglycerides, long-chain fatty acids, phospholipids, cholesterol and fat-soluble vitamins form micelles with the help of the emulsifying bile salts.[2] These micelles enter the enterocyte, where they will again be converted into triglycerides. The triglycerides will combine with protein, phospholipids and cholesterol to form chylomicrons.[6] The chylomicrons enter the intestinal lymphatics *via* the lacteals of the intestinal villi and are transported to the thoracic duct to enter the systemic circulation.

Essential Fatty Acids

Dietary fat provides a source of EFAs. The EFAs are generally recognized as linoleic acid, alpha-linolenic acid and arachidonic acid. These are either omega-3 EFAs (alpha-linolenic acid) or omega-6 EFAs (linoleic acid and arachidonic acid).[1,2] The omega-3 and omega-6 fatty acids are essential because the body cannot synthesize them. The body can synthesize the omega-9 fatty acids and higher and saturated fatty acids seen. Therefore, these are seen as nonessential fatty acids.[2] All of the

Table 4.2 Parent Class for EFAs and derivative compounds.

Omega-3 fatty acids	Omega-6 fatty acids
Stearadonic acid	Linoleic acid
Eicosatetroaenoic acid	γ-linoleic
Eicosapentaenoic acid (EPA)	Dihomo-γ-linoleic acid
Docosapentaenoic acid	Arachidonic acid
Docosahexaenoic acid (DHA)	

Source: Adapted from Hynd,[5] 2019.

EFAs are polyunsaturated fatty acids (PUFAs), with the position of the first double bond being denoted by the omega term when counting from the terminal (methyl) end of the chain.[1,2] For omega-3 FAs, the first double bond is located between the 3rd and 4th carbon from the end of the chain. For the omega-6 FAs, the first double bond is located between the 6th and 7th carbons from the end of the chain. (see Table 4.2).

In most animals, gamma-linolenic acid and arachidonic acid can be synthesized from linoleic acid. If adequate linoleic acid is provided in the diet, there would be no dietary requirement for gamma-linolenic acid or arachidonic acid. The exception to this would be the cat that requires a dietary source of arachidonic acid regardless of the amount of linoleic acid found in the diet. Cats lack the metabolic pathway necessary to perform the conversion of linoleic acid to arachidonic acid.[1,3] Research has also shown that dogs cannot effectively convert alpha-linoleic acid to docosahexaenoic acid (DHA). Hence, oils derived from fish rather than seed oils are better sources if long-chain omega-3 fatty acids are desired.[4] Unsaturated fatty acids cannot be converted between families such as the omega-3 or omega-6 families, and monounsaturated and saturated fatty acids cannot be converted to EFAs.[2] (see Table 4.3).

The first number is the number of carbon atoms. The *n* designation indicates the number

Table 4.3 Fatty acid structure.[1,2]

Saturated- Lauric acid (12:0)
$CH_3-CH_2-CH_2-CH_2-CH_2-CH_2-CH_2-CH_2-CH_2-CH_2-CH_2-COOH$
Monounsaturated-Palmitoleic acid (16:1n-7)
$CH_3-CH_2-CH_2-CH_2-CH_2-CH_2-CH=CH-CH_2-CH_2-CH_2-CH_2-CH_2-CH_2-CH_2-COOH$
Polyunsaturated
Linoleic acid (18:2n-6)
$CH_3-CH_2-CH_2-CH_2-CH_2-CH=CH-CH_2-CH=CH-CH_2-CH_2-CH_2-CH_2-CH_2-CH_2-CH_2-COOH$
Alpha-linolenic acid (18:3n-3)
$CH_3-CH_2-CH=CH-CH_2-CH=CH-CH_2-CH=CH-CH_2-CH_2-CH_2-CH_2-CH_2-CH_2-CH_2-COOH$
Arachidonic Acid (20:4n-6)
$CH_3-CH_2-CH_2-CH_2-CH_2-CH=CH-CH_2-CH=CH-CH_2-CH=CH-CH_2-CH=CH-CH_2-CH_2-CH_2-COOH$

of double bonds, and the last number is the location of that double bond from the terminal methyl (CH_3) end.

The best sources of linoleic acid (omega-6 family) are vegetable oils, such as corn, soybean and safflower oils. Pork fat and poultry fat contain appreciable amounts of linoleic acid, but beef and butterfat contain very little.[1] Arachidonic acid (omega-3 family) can be found only in animal fats. This is especially important in cat diets. Because of the essential requirement for arachidonic acid, cats cannot be fed a balanced vegetarian diet as the only source of arachidonic acid is in animal fats.[3] Some fish oils are rich in arachidonic acid and are also found in small amounts in poultry and pork fat.[1]

The EFAs have multiple functions within the body, including the synthesis of prostaglandins and leukotrienes.[4] Omega-6 fatty acids have functionally distinct effects compared with those of the omega-3 family.[2] Eicosanoids (a product of any omega EFAs families) produced from the omega-3 family are less immunologically stimulating than those from the omega-6 or 9 families. This means that they have less potential to produce an inflammatory reaction in the body.[2]

This is important in situations where decreasing the inflammatory response is desired, such as before and after surgery, after trauma, burns, injury, or some types of cancer or assisting in the control of dermatitis, arthritis, inflammatory bowel disease and colitis.[2] Adjusting the omega-3 to omega-6 fatty acid ratio in therapeutic diets can decrease these responses.

The skin contains a large store of arachidonic acid but cannot convert linoleic acid to arachidonic acid at this site.[4] Adding arachidonic acid to food previously absent increases food efficiency and enhances skin condition by reducing water loss through the skin.[2] This causes a shinier, glossier coat with less skin flaking.

Short-Chain Fatty Acids

Short-chain fatty acids (SCFA) are products of bacterial fermentation by the intestinal microbiome. These fatty acids have fewer than 6 carbons in length. The most important of these SCFAs produced by bacterial fermentation are acetic acid (acetate)$C_2H_4O_2$, propionic acid (propionate)$C_3H_6O_2$, and butyric acid (butyrate)$C_4H_8O_2$.

Acetate is used directly by peripheral tissues for energy. Propionate is converted to glucose after transportation to the liver. Butyrate is converted to ketone bodies by the colonocytes and used as energy directly by these cells.[5]

Lipid Functions

Lipids are essential for absorbing fat-soluble vitamins A, D, E and K. The type of fat required for this absorption is not specific.[2]

Most importantly to our animals, fats improve the palatability and texture of the diets being fed.[1,2] The problem with this would be as the fat content of the diet increases, so does the caloric density and palatability: this can easily lead to overconsumption of the diet, in turn leading to obesity.

Lipid Deficiencies

Fatty acid deficiencies in the diet impair wound healing, cause a dry, lusterless coat, scaly skin and change the lipid film on the skin, predisposing the animal to skin infections. With an inadequate amount of fats, fat-soluble vitamins are also not adequately absorbed, and deficiencies can be seen.[2] Decreased caloric density of the diet and decreased palatability can cause weight loss due to decreased food intake.

References

1 Case LP, Carey DP, Hirakawa DA, Daristotle L (2000) Fats. In *Canine and Feline Nutrition* (2nd edn), pp. 19–22, St Louis, MO: Mosby.

2 Gross, Kathy L; Wedekind, Karen L; Cowell, Christopher S et al. Nutrients. In *Small Animal Clinical Nutrition 4*, Hand, Michael S; Thatcher, Craig D; Remillard, Rebecca L, et al., eds. 2000; pp 59-66 Marceline, MO. Walsworth Publishing.

3 Case LP (2003) The cat as an obligate carnivore. In *The Cat: Its Behavior, Nutrition, and Health*, pp. 300–2, Ames, IA: Iowa State Press.

4 Outerbridge CA (2012) Nutritional management of skin diseases. In AJ Fascetti, SJ Delaney (eds), *Applied Veterinary Clinical Nutrition*, p. 158, Ames, IO: Wiley-Blackwell.

5 Hynd P (2019) Digestion in the mono-gastric animal. In *Animal Nutrition from Theory to Practice*, p. 57, Boston, MA: CABI Publication.

6 Hynd P (2019) Introduction to animal nutrition. In *Animal Nutrition from Theory to Practice*, p. 28, Boston, MA: CABI Publication.

5

Protein and Amino Acids

Introduction

Proteins are large, complex molecules composed of hundreds to thousands of amino acids. These amino acids are composed of carbon, hydrogen, oxygen, nitrogen and sometimes sulfur and phosphorus.[1-3] Although hundreds of amino acids exist in nature, only 20 are commonly found as protein components.[2] Proteins are linear polymers of amino acids. The amino group of one amino acid and the carboxyl group of another amino acid are joined together through a peptide bond. Amino acids joined together are called peptides. Two bonded together are a dipeptide, three a tripeptide and more than three a polypeptide.[2] Once hydrolysis begins in the body, simple proteins yield only amino acids or their derivatives.[1] Proteins can also bond to other molecules; this yields a valuable basis for simple classification.[4]

Simple proteins give rise to their basic amino acids units only. Examples would include:

- Albumins are globular proteins found in egg white, blood plasma and milk.
- Collagens are fibrous proteins present in connective tissue and are converted to gelatin on prolonged heating.
- Elastins are fibrous elastic proteins found in arterial walls and skin.[4]

Conjugated proteins give rise to other distinctive substances in addition to amino acids.

- Glycoproteins contain carbohydrates, as seen with mucus.
- Lipoproteins contain lipids and function to carry fat throughout the bloodstream as seen with LDL (low-density lipoproteins), HDL (high-density lipoproteins) and VLDL (very low-density lipoproteins).
- Phosphoproteins contain a phosphorus group such as casein in milk.
- Chromoproteins contain a pigment group such as heme in hemoglobin.
- Nucleoproteins combine proteins and nucleic acids, as with DNA and RNA[1,2,4]

Protein is required in the diet to provide a source of amino acids to build, repair and replace body proteins. They also supply nitrogen for the synthesis of nonessential amino acids and other nitrogen-containing compounds.[3] Amino acids are divided into two groups, nonessential and essential.[1] The distinction between these two groups is that the essential amino acids must be included in the diet. At the same time, the body can synthesize the nonessential amino acids from other precursors at a rate sufficient to meet physiologic needs.[1] (see Table 5.1).

Some proteins are conditionally essential in that they are required in amounts exceeding the body's ability to produce them at times, usually during certain physiologic or disease conditions.[2] Nitrogen, found in the side amine group on the protein, is essential for synthesizing the nonessential amino acids and is also required to synthesize other

Nutrition and Disease Management for Veterinary Technicians and Nurses, Third Edition. Ann Wortinger and Kara M. Burns.
© 2024 John Wiley & Sons, Inc. Published 2024 by John Wiley & Sons, Inc.
Companion Website: www.wiley.com/go/wortinger/3e

Table 5.1 Essential and nonessential amino acids for dogs and cats.

Essential amino acids	Nonessential amino acids
Arginine	Alanine
Histidine	Asparagine
Isoleucine	Aspartate
Leucine	Cysteine
Lysine	Glutamate
Methionine	Glutamine
Phenylalanine	Glycine
Taurine (cats only)	Hydroxylysine
Tryptophan	Hydroxyproline
Threonine	Proline
Valine	Serine
	Tyrosine

Source: Case et al.[1]/Scientific Research Publishing Inc.

nitrogen-containing molecules, including nucleic acids, purines, pyrimidines and certain neurotransmitter substances.[5]

Functions of Proteins

Proteins in the body have numerous functions. They are the major structural components of hair, feathers, skin, nails, tendons, ligaments and cartilage.[1] Contractile proteins such as myosin and actin are involved in regulating muscle action. The enzymes that catalyze the body's essential metabolic reactions and are essential for nutrient digestion and assimilation are also protein molecules.[1] Many hormones that control the homeostatic mechanisms of various body systems are composed of proteins such as insulin and glucagon, both involved in controlling normal blood sugar levels. Proteins found in the blood act as important carrier substances, including hemoglobin to carry oxygen between the lungs and the cells, lipoproteins which help transport fats throughout the body; and transferrin which carries iron through the blood.[1] Plasma proteins are also involved in maintaining the acid-base balance acting as the largest source of buffers in the blood. Finally, proteins are involved in the body's immune system in immunoglobulins to make the antibodies that provide disease resistance.[1]

Obligate carnivores, such as the cat, have the highest overall protein requirement compared to any other mammals, including the dog.[3] This is not due to a higher requirement for essential amino acids, but rather because of some nitrogen catabolic enzymes in the liver of the cat that is permanently set to handle a high level of dietary protein; their activity is not modified or down-regulated even when the cat is receiving a low protein diet.[4] Cats cannot conserve nitrogen from the body's general nitrogen pool. This inflexibility of liver enzyme activity and fixed high rate of catabolic activity obligates cats to consume a high-protein diet.[3]

All proteins in the body are in a constant state of renewal and degradation. Though tissues vary in their turnover rate, all protein molecules in the body are eventually catabolized and replaced.[1-4] During growth or reproduction, additional protein is needed to create new tissue. A regular supply of protein and nitrogen is necessary to maintain normal metabolic processes and provide for tissue maintenance and growth. The body can synthesize new proteins from amino acids, provided that all of the necessary amino acids required for that protein synthesis are available to the tissue cells.[1] A high rate of protein synthesis occurs in producing red and white blood cells, epithelial cells of the skin, and those lining the GI tract and the pancreas.[2] Muscle protein composes nearly 50% of the total body protein but only accounts for 30% of the new protein synthesized. Visceral and organ proteins compose a smaller portion of the total body protein but account for 50% of synthesized new proteins.[2] Rates of protein synthesis and degradation for any particular protein can change under different physiologic conditions.[2]

Protein consumed over what the animal requires is viewed as surplus. As amino acids cannot be stored in the body above the small amount found in each cell in the amino acid pool, surplus amino acids are either used directly for energy production (gluconeogenesis) or converted to glycogen and stored in the muscle or liver, or fat and stored in adipose tissue.[5]

Glucogenic and Ketogenic Amino Acids

Most amino acids, except lysine and leucine, are glucogenic and can be used to form glucose. These amino acids can be converted into glucose through gluconeogenesis. The process involves first converting the amino acids into alpha-keto acids and then into glucose. Both of these processes occur in the liver.[6]

Gluconeogenesis is a normal process in cats and occurs in dogs during periods of catabolism when insufficient carbohydrates are ingested to meet metabolic needs.[2,6] (see Table 5.2).

Only two amino acids are strictly ketogenic, lysine and leucine. These amino acids are degraded into precursors of ketone bodies (acetyl coenzyme A). The production of ketone bodies for energy is important when insufficient carbohydrates are in the diet or when carbohydrates cannot be accessed, as with diabetes mellitus.[6] When this process is excessive, ketosis is seen, as with diabetic ketoacidosis (DKA).

Dietary Protein

The body does not care where the amino acids come from for their use, whether the body synthesizes them, supplied in the diet as single amino acids or as intact proteins. Because of this, it can accurately be said that the body does not have a "protein requirement," but rather an amino acid requirement.[1] Absorbed amino acids and small di- and tripeptides are reassembled into "new" proteins by the liver and other tissues in the body.[2] After absorption, the amino acids go toward tissue

Table 5.2 Glucogenic and ketogenic amino acids.

Glucogenic	Ketogenic	Both
Alanine	Leucine	Isoleucine
Glycine	Lysine	Phenylalanine
Cystine		Tryptophan
Serine		Tyrosine
		Threonine

synthesis, especially muscles and liver, synthesis of enzymes, albumin, hormones and other nitrogen-containing compounds and deamination (removal of the amine group), and use of the remaining carbon skeletons for energy.[2]

Proteins in the diet serve several functions. They provide the essential amino acids (used to synthesize protein in the growth and repair of tissue) and are the body's primary nitrogen source.[1] Nitrogen is essential for synthesizing the nonessential amino acids and other nitrogen-containing compounds such as nucleic acids and certain neurotransmitter substances. Amino acids in the diet can also be metabolized for energy in a process called gluconeogenesis, or the making of glucose from noncarbohydrate compounds.[1] The gross energy of amino acids, once fecal and urinary losses are accounted for, are approximately the same as carbohydrates, 3.5 kcal/g.[1] A secondary function of proteins in dog and cat diets is to provide a source of flavor. Different flavors can be created when proteins in the diet are cooked in the presence of carbohydrates and fats. As the protein content in the diet increases, the food generally becomes more palatable, and the acceptability by the animal increases.[5]

Structural proteins in all tissues, especially in muscle, liver and serum albumin, can be considered amino acid stores. These stores are not the same as the fat and carbohydrate stores, representing active, functional tissue. The use of these stores by the body for amino acids will decrease the function and ability of the animal.[2] Muscle stores represent the largest reserve from which amino acids can be drawn in times of need, though too much body protein loss can impair muscle function, including decreased cardiac and respiratory function.[2]

The protein's digestibility and quality affect how a dog or cat can use the protein in the diet as a source of amino acids and nitrogen.[1] Proteins that are highly digestible and contain all essential amino acids in their proper proportions relative to the animal's needs are considered high-quality proteins. Those that are either low in digestibility or limiting in one or more essential amino acids are of lower quality.[1] The higher the protein quality in the diet, the less quantity will be needed by the animal to meet all of its essential amino acid needs.[1]

Protein Quality

The chemical score is an index that involves comparing the amino acid profile of a given protein with the amino acid profile of a reference of very high quality. Egg protein is typically used as the reference protein and is given a chemical score of 100. The essential amino acid that is in the largest deficit in the test protein is called the limiting amino acid because it will limit the body's ability to use that protein.[1] Using a visual concept called Liebig's barrel, if each amino acid is represented as a stave in the barrel, as a percentage length of the volume present, the limiting amino acid, found in the lowest quality, would be the shortest stave. The water level would never rise above this level, regardless of how many other amino acids are present. (see Figure 5.1).

The percentage of that amino acid present in the protein relative to the corresponding value in the reference protein determines the chemical score of the test protein.[1] The three amino acids in food proteins that are most often limiting are methionine, tryptophan

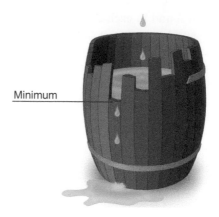

Figure 5.1 Liebig's barrel https://en.wikipedia.org/wiki/Liebig. *Source*: DooFi/Wikipedia Commons/Public Domain.

and lysine. Having a chemical score can be helpful information concerning the amino acid deficits of a protein source, but its value is based entirely on the level of the most limiting amino acid in the food and does not take into account the proportions of all of the remaining amino acids.[1]

Biologic value is defined as the percentage of absorbed protein that is retained by the body. It is a measure of the ability of the body to convert absorbed amino acids into body tissue.[1] One problem with using biological value to measure protein quality is that it does not account for protein digestibility. In theory, if a small portion of a very indigestible protein that is absorbed is used efficiently by the body, it could still have a very high biologic value.[1] Protein quality can only be determined through feeding trials, and digestibility is not usually listed on the product label. (see Table 5.3)[5]

Multiple protein sources are often combined together in pet foods to improve the overall quality and amino acid profile when foods are formulated. Food can be formulated with a higher-quality protein profile by combining proteins based on their relative amino acid excesses and deficiencies. This method of improving protein quality is called protein complementation.[2] Amino acid fortification is another method for improving the protein

Table 5.3 Protein quality of common pet food ingredients.

Ingredient	Percent protein	Chemical score	Biologic value
Egg (dried)	45–49%	100	94
Casein	80%	58	80
Beef, pork, lamb, chicken	29%	69	74
Soybean meal	48%	47	73
Whole corn	8%	41	59
White rice	7%	43	65
Wheat	14%	43	65
Collagen	88%	0	0

Source: Adapted from Gross et al.[2]

quality in foods. In this method, one or more amino acids are added to food when the primary source of protein may be limiting. This is seen most commonly with methionine and lysine.[2]

Taurine

Taurine is an essential amino acid in cats, which in most mammals can be synthesized from methionine and cysteine. It belongs to a separate group of amino acids, called amino-sulphonic acids, and does not form part of the polypeptide chains like the other amino acids.[3,4] Cats have a very limited ability to synthesize taurine from other sulfur-containing amino acids, and therefore have an increased dietary requirement for it.[3,4] Taurine is necessary for bile acid conjugation to aid in the digestion of fats and is necessary for normal retinal function, reproductive and myocardial function.[3] Taurine is present only in animal tissues. Consumption of a diet containing high levels of plant products and cereal grains may not provide sufficient taurine, even if meat-based products are included in the diet.[3]

Taurine requirements for cats consuming canned foods are substantially higher than those for cats consuming dry foods.[3,4] The heat used to process the canned foods can damage the protein in the diet and lead to the production of indigestible protein by-products. These products are less digestible than untreated protein and travel to the large intestine, where intestinal microbes ferment them. These bacterial populations responsible for the fermentation also degrade taurine.[3] This ultimately increases the fecal loss of taurine for cats fed canned food diets. As a substantial proportion of the taurine requirements of adult cats are to replace the taurine lost in the feces through bile loss, anything that increases this loss also increases their requirements.[3]

References

1 Case LP, Carey DP, Hirakawa DA, Daristotle L (2000) Protein and amino acids. In *Canine and Feline Nutrition* (2nd edn), pp. 23–8, St Louis, MO: Mosby.
2 Gross KL, Wedekind KL, Cowell CS *et al.* (2000) Nutrients. In MS Hand, CD Thatcher, RL Remillard *et al.* (eds), *Small Animal Clinical Nutrition* (4th edn), pp. 48–59, Marceline, MO: Walsworth Publishing.
3 Case LP (2003) The cat as an obligate carnivore. In *The Cat: Its Behavior, Nutrition, and Health*, pp. 303–8, Ames, IA: Iowa State Press.

4 Simpson JW, Anderson RS, Markwell PJ (1993) Nutrients and the requirements of dog and cats. In CJ Price, B PCG, JB Sutton (eds), *Clinical Nutrition of the Dog and Cat*, pp. 23–7, Cambridge, MA: Blackwell.

5 Case LP, Daristotle L, Hayek M, Raasch MF (2011) Protein and amino acids. In *Canine and Feline Nutrition* (3rd edn), pp. 21–5, St Louis, MO: Mosby.

6 Hynd P (2019) Introduction to animal nutrition. In *Animal Nutrition from Theory to Practice*, p. 39, Boston, MA: CABI Publication.

6

Vitamins

Introduction

Vitamins are defined by their physical and physiologic characteristics. For a substance to be classified as a vitamin, it must have five basic characteristics: (1) it must be an organic compound different from fat, protein and carbohydrate, (2) it must be a component of the diet, (3) it must be essential in minute amounts for normal physiologic function, (4) its absence must cause a deficiency syndrome and (5) it must not be synthesized in quantities sufficient to support normal physiologic function.[1] These definitions are important because not every vitamin is essential for every species.

Vitamins are needed in minute quantities to function as essential enzymes, enzyme precursors or coenzymes in many of the body's metabolic processes.[1,2] A general classification scheme for vitamins divides them into two groups: the fat-soluble vitamins—A, D, E and K, and the water-soluble vitamins—Vitamin C and the B-complex vitamin group.[2] Unlike carbohydrates, proteins or fats, vitamins do not supply any energy for the animal. However, they are essential in assisting the enzymes in releasing energy from these nutrients.[3]

For dogs and cats, the only essential water-soluble vitamins are the B-complex vitamins. Dogs and cats can synthesize vitamin C from glucose, unlike humans and guinea pigs, for which vitamin C is an essential vitamin.[4] The fat-soluble vitamins A, D and E are seen as essential. In contrast, vitamin K can typically be manufactured in adequate amounts by the intestinal microflora.[4]

Because of the differences in water solubility and chemical structure in vitamins, they are absorbed into the body through various means.[1] Fat-soluble vitamins require bile salts and fat to form micelles for absorption. They are then passively absorbed through the lacteals (usually in the duodenum and ileum) and transported with chylomicrons to the liver via the lymphatic system.[1] Water-soluble vitamins are absorbed by way of active transport. Some vitamins require a carrier protein, like B12 (cobalamin) and the protein, intrinsic factor, whereas others require a sodium-dependent, carrier-mediated absorption pump.[1]

Fat-soluble vitamins can be stored in the body's lipid deposits, making them more resistant to deficiency, but are also more likely to result in toxicity.[1,2] Water-soluble vitamins are depleted faster because of limited storage and are less likely to cause toxicity but more likely to become deficient.[1,2]

Vitamin requirements differ based on the life stage of the animal. Growing and reproducing animals make new tissues and require higher levels of vitamins, minerals, protein and energy for optimal performance.[1] As animals age, metabolic and physiologic changes may also increase the requirements for vitamins.[1]

Various disease conditions may affect vitamin status. Prolonged starvation deprives animals of vitamins and other nutrients and depletes the vitamin stores. Polyuric diseases

Nutrition and Disease Management for Veterinary Technicians and Nurses, Third Edition. Ann Wortinger and Kara M. Burns.
© 2024 John Wiley & Sons, Inc. Published 2024 by John Wiley & Sons, Inc.
Companion Website: www.wiley.com/go/wortinger/3e

such as diabetes mellitus and chronic renal failure may increase the excretion of water-soluble vitamins. Additionally, certain antibiotic drugs may decrease the intestinal microflora responsible for vitamin K synthesis, and diuretic drug therapy may increase the excretion of water-soluble vitamins.[1] Since vitamins are organic compounds, they can be destroyed by various means, rendering them unable to perform their duties.[3]

As the vitamins were named in the order that they were discovered, it is preferred to refer to them by their chemical names (niacin, thiamin), especially when various forms of each are available (D2, D3), with additional designations made based on the side-chain functional groups, such as methylation, adenylation and hydrogenation.[5]

Synthetic and naturally made vitamins are used by the body similarly, though they may have different availabilities.[1] All commercial pet foods contain vitamin supplementation. It is challenging to formulate a diet that meets all the vitamin requirements entirely from ingredient sources. Because of these vitamin additions, it is usually unnecessary and perhaps unwise to supplement commercial foods with additional vitamin supplements.[1] Supplementation may be necessary for certain diseases but should be part of a monitored long-term treatment plan directed by the veterinary team.[1] (see Table 6.1).

Fat-Soluble Vitamins

Vitamin A

Plants do not contain vitamin A per se but instead contain provitamins in the form of carotenes and carotenoids. Beta-carotene has the most significant vitamin A activity compared to the other carotenoids but has only half the potency of pure vitamin A.[1] The carotenoids are the dark red pigments in plants that provide the deep yellow/orange color.[2]

Vitamin A can also be found in some animal tissues, with the highest concentrations found in the liver and fish liver oils, as well as milk and egg yolks.[1,2]

Vitamin A is absorbed almost exclusively as retinol into the lymphatic system with low-density lipoproteins (LDL) and transported to the liver, mainly deposited in the hepatocytes and parenchymal cells.[1] A unique transport protein called retinol-binding protein is responsible for picking up vitamin A from the liver and transporting it throughout the body.[6]

Vitamin A is necessary for normal functioning in vision, bone growth, reproduction, tooth development and maintenance of epithelial tissue, including the mucous membranes lining the respiratory and gastrointestinal tracts.[1]

With vitamin A deficiencies, differentiation of new epithelial cells fails to occur, and normal epithelial cells are replaced with dysfunctional cells. Epithelial cells that do not function properly lead to lesions in the epithelium and increased susceptibility to infection.[1] Normal spermatogenesis in males and regular estrous cycles in females are also dependent on vitamin A.[2] Without vitamin A, the rods in the eyes become increasingly sensitive to light changes, which eventually leads to night blindness.[2]

Vitamin A toxicities can result in skeletal malformation, spontaneous fractures and internal hemorrhage.[1] Other signs may include anorexia, slow growth, weight loss, skin thickening, increased blood clotting time, enteritis, congenital abnormalities, conjunctivitis, fatty infiltration of the liver and reduced function of the liver and kidneys.[1]

Unlike dogs and most other animals, cats require preformed vitamin A or retinol. They lack the intestinal enzyme necessary to convert beta-carotene to active vitamin A.[1,2,4,7] Preformed vitamin A can only be found in animal tissues, further supporting the evidence that cats are obligate carnivores.[1,2,7]

Table 6.1 Essential vitamins for animals. Name, chemical forms and functions.

Vitamin lettering system	Chemical and biochemical forms	Functions
A	Retinoic acid	Epithelial maintenance
	Retinal	Keratinization
	Retinol	Vision
		Antioxidant
		Mutagenesis protection
D2 (plants)	Calciferol	Calcium absorption (intestinal)
D3 (animals)	1, 25 dihydroxycholecalciferol	Calcium resorption (renal)
	1, 24 dihydroxy vitamin D3	
	Ergocalciferol	
E	α-tocopherol	Antioxidant (with selenium)
	tocotrienols	Gene expression
		Signal transduction
K	Menaquinone (animals) K2	Blood clotting
	Phylloquinone (plants) K1	Synthesis of prothrombin
B1	Thiamine	Component of transketolase
	Thiamine pyrophosphate (TPP)	Component of decarboxylases
		Energy production
		Neural function
B2	Riboflavin	Energy production
	Flavin mononucleotide (FMN)	Blood cell synthesis
	Flavin adenine dinucleotide (FAD)	
B3	Niacin	Energy production
	Nicotinamide adenine dinucleotide (NAD)	
B5	Pantothenic acid	Component of acetyl coenzyme A
		Fatty acid utilization
		Carbohydrate utilization
		Protein utilization
		Energy production
B6	Pyridoxine	Component of 50 enzymes in carbohydrate and protein metabolism
		Skin maintenance
		Neural function
		Red blood cell formation
B7	Biotin	Protein and fatty acid metabolism

(Continued)

Table 6.1 (Continued)

Vitamin lettering system	Chemical and biochemical forms	Functions
B9	Folic acid	Methyl group transfers
		Protein metabolism
		Gene expression
B12	Cobalamin	Component of methylmalonyl coenzyme A
	Cyanocobalamin	Methyl group transfer
	Hydroxocobalamin	Folate metabolism
	Adenosylcobalamin	Methionine metabolism
		Red blood cell synthesis
		DNA synthesis
Choline		Component of acetylcholine neurotransmitter
		Component of phosphatidylcholine
		Methyl group transfer

Source: Hynd, Philip et al.[5]/Csiro Publishing.

Vitamin D

Vitamin D consists of a group of compounds that regulate calcium and phosphorus metabolism in the body. The two most important of these compounds are vitamin D2-ergocalciferol and vitamin D3-cholecalciferol. Vitamin D2 is found primarily in harvested or injured plants but not in living plant tissue. Because of this, it is only of importance to herbivores.[2] Vitamin D3 is synthesized in the skin of animals when its precursor 7-dehydrocholesterol is exposed to ultraviolet light from the sun.[2] The 7-dehydrocholesterol is made in the liver from the fatty acid, cholesterol.[6] This form of vitamin D can be obtained either through the synthesis in the skin or from consuming animal products containing cholecalciferol.[2] Cholecalciferol (D3) is most often associated with animal-sourced products, while ergocalciferol (D2) is associated with plant-sourced products.[6]

Both ingested and endogenous vitamin D3 are stored in the liver, muscle and fat tissue. Cholecalciferol is an inactive storage form of vitamin D. To become active, it must first be transported from the skin or intestines to the liver, where it is hydroxylated (an OH compound is added) to form 25-hydroxycholecalciferol. This compound is then transported to the kidneys, where the addition of another OH group further converts it to one of several metabolites, the most active form being called calcitriol.[1,2,6] Although inactive vitamin D is considered a vitamin, calcitriol (1,25-dihydroxycholecalciferol) is often classified as a hormone because it is produced by the body and its mechanism of action.[2,6]

The primary function of vitamin D is to enhance intestinal absorption, mobilization, retention and bone deposition of calcium and phosphorus.[1] In the intestines, vitamin D stimulates the synthesis of calcium-binding proteins, enhancing the absorption of dietary calcium and phosphorus.[2] Vitamin D also affects normal bone growth and calcification by acting with parathyroid hormone (PTH) to mobilize calcium from the bone and causing an increase in phosphate reabsorption in the kidneys. The net effect of vitamin D's actions in the intestines, bones and kidneys increases plasma calcium and phosphorus to the level necessary for normal mineralization and remodeling of the bone.[2] Other target cells for vitamin D outside of the bones include the immune system, brain, nervous systems, pancreas, skin, muscles, cartilage and reproductive organs.[6]

Signs of vitamin D deficiency are frequently seen with simultaneous deficiencies or imbalances of calcium and phosphorus. Clinical signs generally include rickets in young animals, enlarged costochondral junctions, osteomalacia, osteoporosis in adult animals and decreased plasma calcium and inorganic phosphorus concentrations.[1]

Vitamin D toxicity is usually associated with increases in vitamin D3 rather than vitamin D2. Excessive intake can result in hypercalcemia, soft tissue calcification and ultimately death.[2] Of the fat-soluble vitamins, this one is most likely to have toxic effects when consumed in excessive amounts.[6]

Marine fish and fish oils are the richest natural sources of vitamin D in foods but may pose a risk for toxicity. Researchers have found that moist foods generally contain higher vitamin D levels than dry foods, and some moist foods exceed the Association of American Feed Control Officials (AAFCO) maximal allowances.[1] Other dietary sources include freshwater fish and egg yolks. Beef, liver and dairy products contain smaller amounts of vitamin D. The most common synthetic source of vitamin D in pet foods includes deactivated animal sterol in sheep lanolin (cholecalciferol), vitamin D3 supplementation, deactivated plant sterol (ergocalciferol) and vitamin D2 supplementation.[1,4]

For most animals, exposure to direct sunlight for UV production of vitamin D is poor due to their living situations (primarily house pets), darkly pigmented skin, or thick hair coats.[2] It has been suggested that if the skin of dogs and cats were exposed to sunlight rather than shaded by their hair, they would be able to synthesize adequate amounts of vitamin D.

However, research done by Drs. Hazewinkel and Morris have not supported this theory.[4]

Vitamin E

Vitamin E is made up of a group of chemically related compounds called tocopherols and tocotrienols.[1,2] Alpha-tocopherol is the most active form of vitamin E in the body and is the compound most commonly found in pet foods. Unfortunately, this form is also the least potent in the form of an antioxidant in foodstuffs. Delta tocopherol is the most potent antioxidant for foods but is also the least biologically active form.[1] Because of this mix of activities, vitamin analyses of foodstuffs are not reliable for determining vitamin activity.[1] Most foods add mixed tocopherols to cover all the biological and antioxidant bases.

Within the body, vitamin E is found in at least small amounts in almost all tissues, with the liver able to store the most significant amounts.[2] Vitamin E is absorbed from the small intestine by non-saturable, passive diffusion into the intestinal lacteals and is transported via the lymphatics to the general circulation.[1] Absorption of vitamin E is enhanced by the simultaneous digestion and absorption of dietary fats. There is a very high correlation between tocopherol levels and the plasma's total lipid or cholesterol concentration.[1] The vitamin is found in the highest concentrations in membrane-rich cell fractions such as the mitochondria and microsomes.[1]

The need for vitamin E in the diet is markedly influenced by dietary composition, with increased need seen with increased levels of polyunsaturated fatty acids (PUFAs), oxidizing agents, vitamin A, carotenoids and trace minerals. A decreased need is seen with increased levels of fat-soluble antioxidants, sulfur-containing amino acids and selenium.[1]

The chief function of vitamin E in the diet is a potent antioxidant functioning to prevent free radicals' chain reaction, producing more free radicals.[6] PUFAs present in the foods and the lipid membranes of the body's cells are very vulnerable to oxidative damage. Vitamin E interrupts the oxidation of these fats by donating electrons to the free radicals that induce lipid peroxidation.[2] Vitamin E also protects vitamin A and sulfur-containing amino acids from oxidative damage.[2]

Vitamin E has a close relationship with the trace mineral selenium. Selenium is a cofactor for the enzyme glutathione peroxidase, which reduces the peroxides formed during fatty acid oxidation. The inactivation of these peroxides by glutathione peroxidase protects the cell membrane from further oxidative damage.[1,2,7] By preventing the oxidation of cell membrane fatty acids and the formation of peroxides, vitamin E spares selenium, while selenium creates a similar effect and can reduce the animal's vitamin E requirement.[1,2,7]

Deficiencies in vitamin E are seen primarily in the neuromuscular, vascular and reproductive systems. Most signs are attributed to membrane dysfunction, resulting from oxidative damage and disruption of critical cellular processes.[1] Clinical signs in dogs include degenerative skeletal muscle disease associated with muscle weakness, degeneration of testicular germinal epithelium, impaired spermatogenesis and gestation failure. In cats, deficiency signs include steatitis, focal interstitial myocarditis, focal myositis of skeletal muscle and periportal mononuclear infiltration of the liver.[1]

Vitamin E is one of the least toxic vitamins; animals can tolerate very high doses without adverse effects. However, at extremely high doses, antagonism with other fat-soluble vitamins may occur, resulting in impaired bone mineralization, reduced hepatic storage of vitamin A and coagulopathies as a result of decreasing absorption of vitamins D, A and K.[1]

Vitamin E is synthesized only by plants, the richest sources being vegetable oils and, to a lesser extent, seeds and cereal grains. Tocopherol concentrations are highest in green leaves. Animal tissues tend to be low in vitamin E, with the highest levels in fatty tissues.[1]

Vitamin K

Vitamin K comprises a group of compounds called quinones. Vitamin K1 (phylloquinone) occurs naturally in green leafy plants, and bacteria synthesize vitamin K2 (menaquinone) in the large intestine.[1,2,7] Vitamin K3 (menadione) is the most common form of synthetic vitamin K and has a vitamin activity two to three times higher than that of natural vitamin K1.

Vitamin K is required for normal blood clotting, as it is needed to produce normal prothrombin (factor II) and to synthesize clotting factors VII, IX and X in the liver.[1,2,7] Vitamin K is also involved in synthesizing osteocalcin, a protein that regulates the incorporation of calcium phosphates in growing bone.[1]

Vitamin K is found in green leafy vegetables such as spinach, kale and cabbage. Generally, animal sources contain lower amounts of vitamin K, though liver, egg, alfalfa, oilseed and certain fish meals are reasonably good sources.[1,2] The synthesis of vitamin K by intestinal bacteria of dogs and cats can contribute at least a portion, if not all, of the daily requirements for these species.[2] Coprophagy increases vitamin K absorption in dogs.[1]

Deficiency can occur with intestinal malabsorption diseases, ingestion of anticoagulants (mouse or rat poisons), destruction of the gut microflora by antibiotic therapy and congenital defects.[1] Vitamin K3 has lower lipid solubility and is the most effective form of vitamin K for cases of malabsorption, while vitamin K1 is the only form of vitamin K effective in anticoagulant poisonings.[1] Deficiency can also be seen in cats being fed certain commercial foods containing high levels of salmon or tuna.[1]

Toxicity was only reported once and occurred secondary to warfarin (rodenticide) ingestion when vitamin K1 was given intravenously instead of subcutaneously or orally, as recommended.[1]

Water-Soluble Vitamins

B-Complex Vitamins

The B-complex vitamins are all water-soluble vitamins initially grouped together because of similar metabolic functions and occurrences in foods.[2] These nine vitamins act as coenzymes for specific cellular enzymes involved in energy metabolism and tissue synthesis.[2] Coenzymes are small organic molecules that must be present with an enzyme for a specific reaction to occur, similar to a key being required for a lock to engage.[2] The vitamins thiamin (B1), riboflavin (B2), niacin (B3), pantothenic acid (B5), pyridoxine (B6) and biotin (B7) are all involved in the conversion of food to energy. Folic acid (B9), cobalamin (B12) and choline are essential for cell maintenance, growth and blood cell synthesis.[1,2]

Sources for the B-complex vitamins include organ meats and the germinal parts of grains and yeasts. Vitamin B12, cobalamin, is the exception, as it can only be obtained from animal sources.[4]

Thiamin

Thiamin, also called vitamin B1, is a component of the coenzyme thiamine pyrophosphate, playing an essential role in carbohydrate metabolism.[1–3,7] The thiamin requirement of an animal would be directly related to the carbohydrate content of the diet being fed.[2,7]

Thiamin is hydrolyzed to free thiamin by intestinal phosphatases before absorption by intestinal cells. Absorption takes place primarily in the jejunum by an active, carrier-mediated transport system. The absorbed thiamin is transported in red blood cells and plasma. The tissues then take up the thiamin. The heart, liver and kidneys have the highest concentrations of thiamin in the body.[1]

A deficiency of thiamin results in an impairment of carbohydrate metabolism with an accumulation of pyruvic and lactic acids within the body. This causes clinical signs related to the central nervous system because of the dependence of this system on a constant source of carbohydrates in the form of glucose for energy.[2,7]

Thiamin deficiencies can be seen with inadequate dietary intake or a high intake of thiamine antagonists. Thiaminases are found in high concentrations in raw fish, shellfish, bacteria, yeast and fungi. Thiaminases are destroyed by cooking.[1]

Thiamine can be readily found in many foods, with good sources being brewer's yeast, whole grain cereals, organ meats and egg yolk. Thiamine is heat-labile and is progressively destroyed by cooking.[1,2,7]

Riboflavin

Riboflavin, vitamin B2, is the precursor to a group of enzymatic cofactors called flavins. Flavins, when linked to proteins, are called flavoproteins.[1] It is named for its yellow color (flavin) and because it contains the simple sugar D-ribose (ribo).[2] It is relatively stable with heat processing but is easily destroyed by exposure to light and irradiation.[2]

Riboflavin functions in the body as a component of two different coenzymes, flavin mononucleotide and flavin adenine dinucleotide.[2] Both of these coenzymes are required in oxidative enzyme systems that function to release energy from carbohydrates, fats and proteins, as well as in several biosynthetic pathways.[2]

After absorption in the intestinal tract, about 50% of the riboflavin in the blood is bound to albumin, and the other half to globulins.[1] Additionally, microbial synthesis of riboflavin occurs in the large intestine of most species.[2] The amount synthesized is dependent on the carbohydrate content of the diet.[1,3]

Deficiency in dogs and cats is uncommon, but signs of dermatitis, erythema, weight loss, cataracts, impaired reproduction, neurologic changes and anorexia can be seen. Toxicity has not been reported in the dog or cat.[1,3]

Because there appears to be little storage of riboflavin in the body, daily intake of this vitamin is critical.[1] Good sources of riboflavin include dairy products, organ meats, muscle meats, eggs, green plants and yeast. Cereal grains are poor sources of riboflavin.[1]

Niacin

Niacin, B3, encompasses nicotinic acid and nicotinamide (also known as niacinamide) and is closely associated with riboflavin in cellular oxidation-reduction enzyme systems.[2,3,7] After absorption in the intestines, niacin is rapidly converted into nicotinamide, the metabolically active form of the vitamin.[2] Nicotinamide is then incorporated into two different coenzymes, nicotinamide adenine dinucleotide (NAD) and nicotinamide adenine dinucleotide phosphate (NADP).[2,3,7] These coenzymes function as hydrogen-transfer agents in several enzymatic pathways involved in using fat, carbohydrate and protein.[2,7] Most animals can also synthesize niacin as an end product of the metabolism of the essential amino acid tryptophan.[1,2]

Niacin is a reasonably stable vitamin, and processing conditions may release some bound niacin, increasing availability.[1] Niacin deficiency may occur when foods low in niacin and tryptophan are eaten, such as corn and other grains. This deficiency results in a condition called pellagra, or black tongue. Signs seen are dermatitis, diarrhea, dementia and death. Clinical deficiencies in dogs are not common, as most commercial foods are adequately supplemented. However, cats can develop deficiencies when fed high cereal diets because they cannot synthesize substantial niacin from tryptophan and require preformed niacin.[1]

Niacin can be found in many foods, the most significant levels being found in yeast, animal and fish by-products, cereals, legumes and oilseeds. Unfortunately, a large portion of the niacin found in many plant sources is in a bound form and unavailable for absorption. The niacin found in animal sources is primarily in the unbound, available form.[1,2] Niacin is less vulnerable to destruction during food processing and storage than the other water-soluble vitamins.[3]

Pyridoxine

Vitamin B6 comprises three different compounds: pyridoxine, pyridoxal and pyridoxamine. All three are convertible in the dog and cat to the coenzyme pyridoxal 5′-phosphate, which is the biologically active form of the vitamin.[1,2,7] Pyridoxine is involved in a wide range of enzyme systems, particularly associated with amino acid metabolism and to a lesser extent in the metabolism of glucose and fatty acids.[1,2,7] Pyridoxal 5′-phosphate is also required to synthesize hemoglobin and convert tryptophan to niacin.[2] The pyridoxine requirements in the diet vary based on the protein levels.[2]

All three forms of B6 are freely absorbed via passive diffusion in the small intestine.[1] The predominant form found in the blood is pyridoxal phosphate, which is tightly bound to proteins.[1] Only small amounts of vitamin B6 are stored in the body, with any excesses and products of metabolism being excreted in the urine.[1]

Reduced growth, muscle weakness, neurologic signs, mild microcytic anemia, irreversible kidney lesions, decreased steroid hormone activity and anorexia indicates pyridoxine deficiency.[3] Oxalate crystalluria is a notable sign of pyridoxine deficiency in cats. Naturally occurring deficiencies in dogs and cats have not been reported. Deficiencies have only been seen in specially formulated, deficient diets or owner-made deficient diets.[1]

The incidence of toxicity is very low. The earliest detectable signs include ataxia and loss of small motor control.[3]

Vitamin B6 is widely distributed in foods, occurring in the most significant concentrations in meats, whole grain products, vegetables and nuts.[1] Plant tissues contain mostly pyridoxine, whereas animal tissues contain mostly pyridoxal and pyridoxamine.[1] Pyridoxine is far more stable than either of the other two forms. Thus, processing loss is most significant in foods containing high amounts of animal tissue.[1]

Pantothenic Acid

Pantothenic acid, B5, is derived from the Greek word "pantos" meaning "found everywhere or all" because this vitamin occurs in all body tissues and all forms of living tissue.[1,2] Once absorbed, pantothenic acid is phosphorylated by adenosine triphosphate (ATP) to form coenzyme A.[1,2,7] This is one of the most critical coenzymes and is involved in the metabolism of carbohydrates, fats and some amino acids within the citric acid cycle.[1,2,7]

Coenzyme A and the acyl carrier protein are the primary forms of pantothenic acid found in foods. Both forms are degraded to pantothenic acid in the small intestine in a series of steps. Absorption occurs via a sodium-dependent energy-requiring process. At high concentrations, simple diffusion occurs throughout the small intestine. Pantothenic acid is transported in the free acid form in plasma. Red blood cells, which carry most of the vitamins, contain primarily acetyl-coenzyme A.[1]

Dogs with pantothenic acid deficiency have erratic appetites, depressed growth, fatty livers, decreased antibody response, hypocholesterolemia and can progress to coma in later stages.[1] Cats with pantothenic acid deficiencies can develop fatty livers and become emaciated. Pantothenic acid is generally regarded as nontoxic. No adverse reactions or clinical signs are seen other than gastric upset in animals consuming large quantities.[1]

Pantothenic acid is found in virtually all foodstuffs, so a naturally occurring deficiency is unlikely.[2,7] The most important sources are meats, especially liver and heart, egg yolk, dairy products and legumes.[1,2] Losses during food processing can be substantial because pantothenic acid is readily destroyed by freezing, canning and refining processes.[3]

Folic Acid

Folic acid is also known as pteroylglutamic acid.[1,7] This is a family name for a group of vitamins with related biologic activity. Other common names include folate, folates and folacin.[1] Folic acid requires enzymatic changes to form the active compound tetrahydrofolic acid. From this molecule, the folate coenzymes used in the body are made.[7]

Folic acid acts as a one-carbon methyl donor and acceptor molecule in intermediary metabolism.[1,2] An essential role of folic acid is its involvement in synthesizing thymidine, a component of deoxyribonucleic acid (DNA).[2] Vitamin B12 is also closely paired with folic acid in the production of methionine from homocysteine.[1]

Natural sources of folic acid undergo hydrolysis by intestinal enzymes and are absorbed by enterocytes. Folic acid must be reduced to participate in the one-carbon metabolic reactions (i.e., dihydro, tetrahydro).[1] It is found most commonly in the "bound" form combined with a string of amino acids (glutamate), forming a compound known as polyglutamate.[3] Intestinal enzymes hydrolyze the polyglutamate into monoglutamates and several other glutamates. These are further reduced enzymatically to the active forms.[3]

Bacteria synthesize folic acid in the intestine, which primarily meets dogs' and cats' daily requirements under normal circumstances.[7] It is required daily in the diet, as no reserves are kept in the body.[1] Naturally occurring deficiencies would be uncommon but could be seen with deficient diets and intestinal disease.[7] Clinical signs of folate deficiency are poor weight gain, anemia, anorexia, leukocytopenia (low white blood cell count), glossitis and decreased immune function. There have been no reported cases of folate toxicity as excess folate is sent to the liver, added to bile and disposed of through the intestines.[1,3]

Folic acid is found in green, leafy vegetables, organ meats and egg yolks. The vitamin is destroyed by heating, prolonged freezing and storage in water.[1,2]

Biotin

Biotin (B7) was initially known as the "bios" factor. It is a sulfur-containing vitamin that functions as a coenzyme in several carboxylation reactions.[1,2,7] It acts as a carbon dioxide carrier in reactions in which carbon chains are lengthened, specifically in specific steps of fatty acid, nonessential amino acid and purine synthesis. In its active form, it is always found covalently bound to a protein (apoprotein).[1]

After ingestion, biotin must be hydrolyzed from protein by the enzyme biotinidase to be absorbed by the intestine. After hydrolysis, free biotin is absorbed through the intestine and transported through the blood to the tissues. Bacteria in the intestines are also able to synthesize biotin for use by the body.[7]

Naturally occurring biotin deficiencies are very rare in dogs and cats. Feeding raw egg whites and oral antibiotic use are probably the two most common causes.[1] Egg white contains a compound called avidin, which binds to biotin and makes it unavailable for absorption by the body.[1,2] Cooking destroys avidin and allows the biotin in the egg to be used. Avidin can also prevent the absorption of endogenously produced biotin by intestinal bacteria.[7] Clinical signs of biotin deficiency include poor growth, dermatitis, lethargy and neurologic abnormalities.[1] Biotin toxicity has not been reported in dogs and cats.[1]

The biotin requirement is thought to be met by diet and intestinal microbes since mammalian tissue cannot synthesize it.[1] Biotin is widely found in many foods, but bioavailability varies greatly. Oilseeds, egg yolks, alfalfa meal, liver and yeast are good sources of biotin. Significant losses of biotin can occur as a result of oxidation, canning, heat and solvent extraction of foodstuffs.[1,2]

Cobalamin

Vitamin B12 is the only vitamin that contains a trace element, cobalt. Cobalamin is the largest and most complex of the B vitamins.[1] When isolated from natural sources, it is usually found in the form of cyanocobalamin. When transformed into a metabolically active coenzyme, the cyano group is replaced by another chemical group attached to the cobalt group.[7]

Cobalamin and its metabolites are essential in one-carbon metabolism during various biochemical reactions and are involved in fat and carbohydrate metabolism and myelin synthesis.[1,2] The function of vitamin B12 is closely linked to that of folate.[1,2,7]

Cobalamin absorption depends on dietary intake and adequate gastrointestinal tract function. In most animals, cobalamin absorption from the diet is facilitated by a group of glycoproteins called intrinsic factors produced by the pancreas and gastric mucosa.[1,2] The absence of these factors can lead to vitamin B12 deficiency.[1,2] Most B12 deficiencies are not due to poor intake but rather poor absorption. Inadequate absorption typically occurs either due to a lack of hydrochloric acid in the stomach or intrinsic factors.[3]

Vitamin B12 deficiency is very rare but may result in poor growth and neuropathies. A vegetarian diet may lead to deficiencies because vitamin B12 is only made by microbes and is found in animal tissues.[1] Microwave heating inactivates vitamin B12.[3] Toxicities have not been found in dogs and cats other than those given excessive amounts parenterally.[1]

Good sources of cobalamin include organ meats, fish and dairy products. This vitamin is unique in that once it is absorbed from the diet, the body can store excess amounts. The primary storage place is the liver, though muscle, bone and skin can also contain small amounts.[2] The body is efficient at storing and recycling B12 that deficiencies may take years to develop.[3]

Choline

Choline is classified as one of the B-complex vitamins, even though it does not entirely satisfy a vitamin's strict definition.[1] Choline, unlike the other B vitamins, can be synthesized in the liver from the amino acid serine. In this reaction, methionine acts as a methyl donor, with folic acid and cobalamin also being needed. It is required in much larger quantities by the body than the other B vitamins.[1,2] Because of this, even though it is an essential nutrient, not all animals require it as a dietary supplement, making it a conditionally essential nutrient.[1,3] Choline does not function as a coenzyme or cofactor as do most other vitamins but is an integral part of cellular membranes.[1]

Choline functions as an integral part of cellular membranes as the phospholipid lecithin promotes lipid transport as phosphatidylcholine, as a neurotransmitter as acetylcholine, and as a source of methyl groups for transmethylation reactions.[1–3,7]

Choline is released from lecithin in the diet by digestive enzymes in the intestinal tract and absorbed from the jejunum and ileum mainly by a carrier-mediated process. Once absorbed, choline is transported through the lymphatic system in the form of phosphatidylcholine bound to chylomicrons.[1]

Because of its synthesis in the liver, its presence in many foods, and methionine's ability to spare choline, dietary choline deficiencies have not been reported in cats and dogs.[2]

Dietary sources include egg yolks, organ meats, legumes, dairy products and whole grains.[2]

Vitamin C

Ascorbic acid can be synthesized from glucose by plants and most animals, including dogs and cats. Chemically its structure is closely related to that of the monosaccharide sugars.[1,2] Vitamin C functions in the body as an antioxidant and free radical scavenger.[1] Ascorbic acid is best known for its role in collagen synthesis though it is also involved in drug, steroid and tyrosine metabolism, as well as electron transport in cells.[1] It is required to synthesize carnitine to act as a carrier for the acyl groups across mitochondrial membranes.[1] Larger doses may play an essential role in immune function and protecting against carcinogens.[1] Ascorbic acid acts as a nitrate scavenger, thereby reducing nitrosamine-induced carcinogenesis.

Dogs and cats can synthesize adequate ascorbic acid; therefore, dietary amounts are absorbed by passive diffusion in the intestinal tract. Ascorbic acid is produced in the liver from either glucose or galactose through the glucuronate pathway.[1] Absorption efficiency in the intestines is unusually high, ~80–90%.[1] Vitamin C is transported in the plasma in association with albumin. It is widely distributed in all body tissues, with the pituitary and adrenal glands having the highest concentrations.[1] During periods of stress, the adrenal glands release vitamin C, together with hormones, into the blood.[3]

Deficiency is unlikely due to dogs and cats synthesizing most if not all of their requirements.[2] Toxicity has not been seen in dogs and cats.[1]

Sources of vitamin C include fruits, vegetables, and organ meats. Vitamin C content of most foods decreases dramatically during storage and processing as oxidative processes easily destroy it. Exposure to heat, light, alkalis, oxidative enzymes and the minerals copper and iron can all increase losses of vitamin C activity.[2]

Vitamin-Like Substances

Carnitine

L-carnitine is a natural compound found in all animal cells.[1] Its primary function is to transport long-chain fatty acids across the inner mitochondrial membrane into the mitochondrial matrix for oxidation.[1,3] It is synthesized primarily in the liver and stored in the skeletal and cardiac muscles.[1,2]

Lysine, methionine, ascorbic acid, ferrous ions, vitamin B6 and niacin are critical in L-carnitine metabolism; these nutrients are required substrates and cofactors for enzymes involved in biosynthesis.[1]

Clinical signs of L-carnitine deficiency include chronic muscle weakness, fasting hypoglycemia, cardiomyopathy, and hepatomegaly.[1] In many cases of deficiency, no clinical signs are seen.[1]

Carotenoids

This is a group of pigments that exhibit vitamin-like activities. More than 600 different compounds are classified as carotenoids. Still, fewer than 10% can be metabolized into vitamin A.[1] The carotenoids found in the most significant numbers in various foods include beta-carotene, alpha-carotene, lutein, lycopene, beta-cryptoxanthin, zeaxanthin, canthaxanthin and astaxanthin.[1]

Carotenoids are digested and absorbed into the body using bile salts. Carotenoids are incorporated into micelles, where the small intestinal lacteals absorb them by way of passive diffusion.[1] After transportation in chylomicrons in the lymphatic system, they are bound to lipoproteins and transported into the bloodstream.[1]

Carotenoids have biological activity beyond their vitamin A role. Carotenoids with nine or more double bonds function as antioxidants, and they also protect cell membranes by stabilizing the oxygen radicals produced.[1]

Carotenoids are found abundantly in orange and green vegetables, highly pigmented fruits and some fish species.[1]

Bioflavonoids

The bioflavonoids are another group of red, blue, and yellow pigments consisting of over 4,000 different compounds but are not classified as carotenoids. Like carotenoids, they also have vitamin-like activities.[1]

Flavonoids are found naturally as glycosides linked to sugars. Mammalian enzymatic systems cannot hydrolyze flavonoids, but the necessary enzymes are present in the gut microflora.[1] After hydrolysis and absorption in the small intestines, flavonoids are bound in the liver.

The flavonoids have a sparing effect on vitamin C; they also can perform similarly to vitamin C. Flavonoid reactions are involved in the antioxidant system for lipid and water environments.

Bioflavonoids are found most abundantly in the skins and peels of colored fruits and vegetables.[1]

References

1 Gross KL, Wedekind KL, Cowell CS *et al.* (2000) Nutrients. In MS Hand, CD Thatcher, RL Remillard *et al.* (eds), *Small Animal Clinical Nutrition* (4th edn), pp. 80–95, Marceline, MO: Walsworth Publishing.

2 Case LP, Carey DP, Hirakawa DA, Daristotle L (2000) Vitamins. In *Canine and Feline Nutrition* (2nd edn), pp. 29–40, St Louis, MO: Mosby.

3 Whitney E, Rolfes SR (2008) The water-soluble vitamins: B vitamins and vitamin C. In *Understanding Nutrition* (11th edn), pp. 323–57, Belmont, CA: Thomson Wadsworth.

4 Delaney SJ, Fascetti AJ (2012) Basic nutrition overview. In AJ Fascetti, SJ Delaney (eds), *Applied Veterinary Clinical Nutrition*, pp. 13–4, Chichester, West Sussex, UK: Wiley-Blackwell.

5 Hynd P (2019) Introduction to animal nutrition. In *Animal Nutrition from Theory to Practice*, p. 39, Boston, MA: CABI Publication.

6 Whitney E, Rolfes SR (2008) The fat-soluble vitamins: A, D, E, and K. In *Understanding Nutrition* (11th edn), pp. 369–86, Belmont, CA: Thomson Wadsworth.

7 Simpson JW, Anderson RS, Markwell PJ (1993) Nutrients and the requirements of dog and cats. In CJ Price, B PCG, JB Sutton (eds), *Clinical Nutrition of the Dog and Cat*, pp. 30–7, Cambridge, MA: Blackwell.

7

Minerals

Introduction

Minerals are the inorganic portion of the diet. Some are required in large quantities because they form a significant part of the body's structural components. In contrast, others are only required in small quantities for the chemical processes of metabolism.[1]

As with most other nutrients, problems with minerals in the diet are usually related more to excesses or imbalances with other nutrients than actual deficiencies in the diet.[2] Because of this, in a diet known to be nutritionally complete in its mineral content, further supplementation is at best wasteful and at worst dangerous to the animal's health.[1]

More than 18 minerals are believed to be essential for mammals. By definition, macrominerals are required by the animal in the diet in percentage amounts, whereas microminerals are required at a part per million (ppm) level.[3] Unlike vitamins, minerals are inorganic compounds that always retain their original chemical structure. Once they enter the body, they will remain there until excreted. Minerals can also not be destroyed by heat, air, acid or mixing.[4]

Minerals are used by the body for structural components as seen with calcium, phosphorus and magnesium in bones and teeth, as portions of body fluids and tissues as with the electrolytes sodium, potassium, phosphorus, chloride, calcium and magnesium, and as catalysts/cofactors in enzyme and hormone systems as seen with iodine and selenium and

in the oxygen delivery system as seen with iron in hemoglobin.[3]

The mineral content of a plant is determined primarily by the soil type, plant species, stage of plant growth and the climate in which it is grown.[5] The minerals available to a plant while growing are found exclusively in the soil, either through the minerals found there or those provided through supplementation in fertilizers. Generally, those required at higher doses by plants than by animals are unlikely to cause deficiencies. The most likely mineral deficiencies in animals are seen with potassium, copper, iodine, selenium and cobalt.[5]

Many things can affect the availability of minerals from the diet and how effectively the individual animal can use the mineral. These include the chemical form of the mineral, which affects solubility, the amounts and proportions of other dietary components that the mineral interacts with metabolically, the age, gender and species of the animal, the intake of the mineral, the body's need (the amount found in the body's stores) and environmental factors.[3]

Meat-derived foods are considered a more available source of certain minerals than plant-derived foods. The organic forms of minerals found in meats are often more available than those from inorganic mineral supplements, while those found in plants are often less available.[3] Meats, unlike plants, do not contain anti-nutritional factors, such as phytate, oxalate, goitrogens and fibers. These all have the potential to reduce mineral

Nutrition and Disease Management for Veterinary Technicians and Nurses, Third Edition. Ann Wortinger and Kara M. Burns.
© 2024 John Wiley & Sons, Inc. Published 2024 by John Wiley & Sons, Inc.
Companion Website: www.wiley.com/go/wortinger/3e

availability in the diet.[3] Different forms of minerals differ in availability based on what they are combined with. Generally, sulfur and chloride forms have the best availability, followed by carbonates, with oxides being poorly available.[3] (see Table 7.1).

Macrominerals

Calcium

Calcium has two critical functions within the body. It is necessary for the formation and maintenance of the skeleton and teeth, and it acts as an intracellular messenger that allows cells to respond to stimuli such as hormones and neurotransmitters.[3]

Calcium serves two physiologic functions in bones, as structural material and as a storage site for calcium.[3] The amount of calcium absorbed from the diet can range from 25–90%, depending on the animal's calcium status, the form of the calcium and intake in the diet.[3] The calcium found in blood, lymph and other body fluids accounts for only ~1% of the total calcium in the body. The remaining 99% is found in the bones and teeth.[3]

Calcium absorption by the body can be actively regulated by vitamin D, facilitated, or passively absorbed. Regardless of how the calcium is absorbed, vitamin D is the most important regulator of calcium absorption.[3] Vitamin D helps to make the calcium-binding protein needed for the absorption of calcium.[4] Calcium absorption is most efficient during inadequate intake and decreases as calcium needs are met. Blood calcium levels change only in response to abnormal regulatory control, not due to levels found in the diet.[4]

Deficiencies are uncommon today in well-formulated pet foods. However, calcium imbalances can occur as a result of poor feeding practices. Calcium deficiencies are most commonly seen when dogs and cats are fed "table scrap" diets or all meat diets consisting primarily of muscle and organ meats.[2,3] This diet is deficient in calcium and high in phosphorus, developing into secondary nutritional hyperparathyroidism. The low dietary levels of dietary calcium stimulate the release of parathyroid hormone (PTH). The PTH increases the resorption of calcium from the bone to increase the plasma calcium levels. Eventually, this can lead to significant bone loss with resultant pathologic fractures.[2,3] Calcium excesses are most commonly due to dietary supplementation, especially in large breed, fast-growing puppies. By over-supplementing the diet with calcium, deficiencies can be produced in other nutrients and the potential for causing an increased incidence of osteochondritis dissecans (OCD), hypertrophic osteodystrophy (HOD), and Wobbler's syndrome, to name only a few.[2,3]

A relative calcium deficiency can also be seen with eclampsia, though this is more of a problem of calcium homeostasis in the body.[2] Eclampsia is seen most often in small-breed dogs and less frequently in cats.[2] This is usually seen 2–3 weeks after parturition and is caused by a failure of the mother's calcium regulatory system to maintain plasma calcium levels when there is a loss of calcium in the milk.[2] With subnormal calcium plasma levels, seizures and tetany can be seen. The prognosis is good if treatment is started at an early stage.[2] Excess calcium supplementation to try to prevent this problem can exacerbate it. When calcium intake is high, the PTH level is low. As milk production increases, calcium is lost in the milk. Usually, PTH would be stimulated to release calcium from the bone to maintain plasma levels. The PTH cannot respond quickly enough to prevent dangerously low plasma levels from occurring in the mother.[2] The best course of preventative action is to feed a high-quality commercial diet that has been formulated for growing animals and gestation from the time of pregnancy through parturition and lactation.[2]

Calcium can be found in meat meals because of its bone content, soybean meal and flaxseed meal. Grains and meats without bones are

Table 7.1 Essential minerals and functions.

Mineral element	Symbol and electrical charge	Functions
Macrominerals		
Calcium	Ca$^+$	Component of bone Muscle contraction Nerve function Coagulation cascade
Phosphorus	P$^-$	Component of bone Component of phospholipids Component of ATP/ADP and creatine phosphate energy molecules Component of nucleic acids Component of blood buffers
Potassium	K$^+$	Nerve function with sodium Osmotic equilibrium with sodium Activatation of pyruvate kinase
Sodium	Na$^+$	/Neural function Acid-base balance Osmotic homeostasis Absorption of glucose and amino acids
Sulfur	S$^-$	Component of sulfur amino acids (cysteine and methionine) Component of insulin, thiamine, biotin and coenzyme A Major component of hair (as cysteine)
Chlorine	Cl$^-$	Acid-base balance Component of HCl- in gastric secretions
Magnesium	Mg$^+$	Neuromuscular function Numerous enzyme systems
Trace elements		
Iron	Fe$^+$	Heme synthesis
Zinc	Zn$^+$	Component of carbonic anhydrase for acid-base homeostasis Component of thymidine kinase for DNA synthesis
Copper	Cu$^+$	Iron transport and heme synthesis Component of tyrosinase Component of enzyme linking disulfide bridges
Molybdenum	Mo$^+$	Component of xanthine oxidase, aldehyde oxidase and sulfite oxidase
Selenium	Se$^-$	Component of glutathione peroxidase Antioxidant
Iodine	I$^-$	Component of the thyroid hormones T3 (tri-iodothyronine) and T4 (tetra-iodothyronine)
Manganese	Mn$^+$	Enzyme activator
Cobalt	Co$^+$	Component of cobalamin (vitamin B12)

Source: Hynd, Philip et al.[5]/Csiro Publishing.

poor sources of calcium. The most common supplements used in pet foods include calcium carbonate (limestone), calcium sulfate, calcium chloride, calcium phosphate and bone meal.[3]

Phosphorus

After calcium, phosphorus is the largest constituent found in bones and teeth. Phosphorus is a structural component of RNA and DNA and energy-generating compounds such as ATP (adenosine triphosphate), as part of the phospholipids found in cell membranes, and combined with structural proteins as with phosphoproteins.[3,4]

Phosphorus salts in the form of phosphates are found in the bones and teeth and all the cells in the body and as part of the major buffer system regulating the acid-base balance in the body.[4] These functions make it essential for cell growth and differentiation, energy use, transfer and metabolism, fatty acid transport and amino acid and protein formation.[3,4] Generally, phosphorus is more available from animal-based ingredients than from plant-based ingredients.[3] Phosphorus found in meats is primarily in the organic form, while that found in plants is in the form of phytic acid, which is only about 30% available to monogastric animals.[3] Phytic acid is a phosphorus-containing compound that can bind other minerals, including calcium, and make them unavailable for absorption.[2]

Regulation of phosphorus within the body involves the coordinated efforts of both the intestines and the kidneys. When dietary intake is low, intestinal absorption is highly efficient, and the kidneys decrease urinary losses. When dietary intake is high, intestinal absorption decreases, and urinary losses increase.[3]

High levels of phosphorus can be found in meats, eggs and milk products. The primary supplements used in pet foods include calcium phosphate, sodium phosphate and phosphoric acid.[3]

Magnesium

Magnesium is the third largest mineral constituent found in the body after calcium and phosphorus.[3] It is involved in the metabolism of carbohydrates and lipids and acts as a catalyst for a wide variety of enzymes. As a cation (a positively charged particle) in the intracellular fluid, magnesium is essential for the cellular metabolism of both carbohydrates and proteins. Protein synthesis also requires the presence of ionized magnesium.[2] Magnesium can be found in soft tissue and bone as well as intracellular and extracellular fluids.[2] Over half of the magnesium found in the body is located in the bones.[4] Several dietary and physiologic factors can negatively impact magnesium absorption, including high levels of phosphorus, calcium, potassium, fat and protein, in the diet.[3]

Magnesium homeostasis within the body is controlled primarily through the kidneys; because of this, certain drugs can cause increased renal excretion of magnesium. These would include diuretics, aminoglycosides, cisplatin, cyclosporine, amphotericin and methotrexate.[3]

A magnesium deficiency in the diet results in signs of weakness, and ataxia with eventual progression to seizures. Naturally occurring magnesium deficiency is usually not seen in healthy dogs and cats.[2] Avoiding excess magnesium is recommended to prevent the formation of struvite crystals and stones in the urine.[3] In sick animals, magnesium deficiencies can be seen with gastrointestinal and kidney diseases.[3]

Sources of magnesium in the diet include ingredients containing bone (bone meals), oilseeds (flaxseed and soybean meal) and unrefined grains and fiber sources (wheat bran, oat bran, beet pulp). Common supplements found in pet foods are magnesium oxide and magnesium sulfate.[3]

Sodium and Chloride

Sodium and chloride are the major electrolytes of extracellular fluids and are essential for maintaining osmotic pressure, regulating acid-base balance and transmitting nerve impulses and muscle contractions.[2,3] Sodium ions must also be present in the intestinal lumen to absorb sugars and amino acids.[3] Calcium absorption and mobilization are affected by sodium, and the absorption of several vitamins such as riboflavin, thiamin and ascorbic acid is sodium-dependent.[3]

Sodium and chloride are readily absorbed from the small intestine, with excretion primarily in the urine though small amounts can be in the feces and perspiration.[3] In very low sodium diets, the body has a remarkable ability to conserve sodium by excreting very low amounts in the urine.[3]

Various hormones regulate the body's sodium concentration to maintain a constant sodium/potassium ratio in the extracellular fluid.[3] Sodium requirements are influenced by reproductive status, lactation, rapid growth and heat stress.

When consuming a diet with high sodium levels, a secondary increase in water intake is seen and an increase in urination with high salt excretion by the kidneys.[2] Studies have indicated that dogs and cats are resistant to salt retention and hypertension when fed diets high in sodium compared to humans.[2]

Fish, eggs, dried whey (milk protein), poultry by-product meal and soy isolate are high in sodium and chloride.[3] Typical dietary supplements added to pet foods include salt, sodium phosphates, calcium chloride, choline chloride, potassium chloride and sodium acetate.[3]

Sulfur

Sulfur is an essential component in the sulfur-containing amino acids methionine and cysteine. Sulfate is the oxidized form of sulfur, which is commonly found in food and water.[4,5]

As a structural component of proteins, sulfur helps stabilize protein structures by using disulfide bridges. Many of the more rigid protein structures in the body have high sulfur content, including fur, nails and skin.[4] Sulfur in the amino acids functions in tissue respiration and is a component of the B-vitamins thiamine and biotin.[6]

Because sulfur requirements are met with normal protein intake, there are no recommended dietary levels. Deficiencies are only seen when severe protein deficiencies in the diet.[4]

Microminerals

Iron

Iron is present in several enzymes and other proteins responsible for oxygen activation, electron transport and oxygen transport. Iron found in food exists primarily as heme iron present in hemoglobin and myoglobin and as nonheme iron found in grains and other plants.[3] The amount of iron absorbed from food depends on the body's iron status, the availability of dietary iron, and the amounts of heme and nonheme iron found in the food.[3]

Ferrous iron has lost 2 electrons and has a net positive charge of +2. When the iron has been oxidized, it loses another electron for a net loss of 3 electrons, giving it a positive charge of +3, resulting in ferric iron.[4] Ferrous iron can be oxidized to ferric iron. Ferric iron can be reduced to ferrous iron.[4] These different forms of iron allow it to participate in the electron transport chain that transfers hydrogen and electrons to oxygen, forming water and making ATP for energy use.[4]

Iron is transported by plasma to the bone marrow, where it is used for hemoglobin synthesis in red blood cells.[3] It is stored primarily as ferritin and hemosiderin in the liver, bone marrow and spleen.[3] Excretion of iron is limited, with only small amounts being found in the urine. The iron appearing in the feces is primarily unabsorbed, though it is continually lost in sweat, hair and nails.[3]

Excess iron in the diet should be avoided because of potential antagonism with other minerals, primarily copper and zinc.[3] Chronic blood loss will eventually deplete iron stores and cause microcytic, hypochromic anemia. This is seen most commonly with parasitic infections, both intestinal in hookworms and externally with fleas and ticks.[3] Young animals are especially at risk due to their low iron stores and the low iron content in milk.[3]

Some dietary factors in foods can bind with nonheme iron, inhibiting absorption from the gastrointestinal tract. These include phytate (phytic acid) found in legumes, whole grains, and rice; vegetable proteins in soybeans, other legumes, and nuts; calcium found in milk and polyphenols in grain products.[4]

High iron levels are found in most meats, especially organ meats. Other sources include beet pulp, soy mill run and peanut hulls.[3] Typical iron additives in pet foods include ferrous sulfate, ferric chloride, ferrous fumarate, ferrous carbonate and iron oxide.[3] Iron oxide is not biologically available to dogs and cats but is added to foods to give them a "meaty red" color.[3]

Zinc

Second, only to iron, zinc is the most abundant micromineral found in the body. It is crucial for carbohydrate, lipid, protein and nucleic acid metabolism. It is necessary for the maintenance of normal skin integrity, taste and immunologic functioning.[2,3] Zinc also helps with growth and development, synthesis, storage and release of the hormone insulin from the pancreas.[4]

Homeostasis is controlled through absorption and excretion. Absorption occurs primarily in the small intestine. This absorption is markedly affected by other dietary components.[3] Phytate, found in many plants, decreases zinc absorption while certain materials such as citrate, picolinate, EDTA and amino acids such as histidine and glutamate increase zinc absorption.[3] The liver is the primary organ involved with zinc metabolism. Storage of

zinc is limited except in the bone. Stores only increase slightly when dietary levels increase.[3]

Zinc can be recycled from the pancreas to the intestines and back to the pancreas in the enteropancreatic circulation of zinc.[4] Once outside the intestines, zinc is transported in the plasma bound to albumin and transferrin.[4]

Signs of zinc deficiency can be seen in animals being fed high cereal diets due to their phytate content. This, in combination with calcium, combines to form an insoluble complex of phytate, calcium and zinc.[3] Deficiency can be seen even when zinc levels in the diet are lower than recommended levels.[3] The only reported cases of toxicity have been due to dietary indiscretion, as seen with the eating of pennies, die-cast nuts from animal carriers and baby lotions containing zinc.[3] Excesses in the diet can interfere with the absorption of other minerals, primarily iron and copper.[3]

Zinc can be found in most meats, fiber sources and dicalcium phosphate. Zinc supplements used most often include zinc oxide, zinc sulfate, zinc chloride and zinc carbonate.[3]

Copper

The body uses copper for iron absorption and transport, and hemoglobin formation. Most of the copper found in the body is bound to the plasma protein ceruloplasmin. This protein functions as a carrier of copper and in the oxidation of plasma iron. Copper is also required to convert the amino acid tyrosine to the pigment melanin, synthesize connective tissues collagen and elastin, and produce ATP.[2] Copper is needed for normal osteoblast activity during skeletal growth.[2] Like iron, copper is needed in many metabolic reactions related to the release of energy.[4]

Absorption of copper occurs throughout the intestinal tract, with a significant portion being in the small intestine.[3] The liver is the primary site of copper metabolism, with hepatic concentrations reflecting an animals' intake and copper status.[3] Excess copper is excreted in the bile.[2]

Copper deficiency results in hypochromic, microcytic anemia similar to that seen with iron deficiency. Other signs of deficiency can include depigmentation of colored hair coats and impaired skeletal development in young animals.[2] Excessive copper can result in interference with zinc and iron metabolism.[3]

The richest sources of copper include legumes, whole grains, nuts, shellfish and seeds. Most organ meats are also rich in copper.[4] Typical dietary supplements include cupric sulfate, cupric carbonate and cupric chloride.[3]

Selenium

Selenium shares some of the chemical characteristics of the mineral sulfur, allowing it to substitute for sulfur in the amino acids methionine, cysteine and cysteine.[4] Selenium is an essential component of the enzyme glutathione peroxidase, which helps to protect cellular and subcellular membranes from oxidative damage.[2,3] Glutathione peroxidase deactivates lipid peroxides that are formed during the oxidation of cell membrane lipids.[2] Vitamin E protects the polyunsaturated fatty acids (PUFAs) in cell membranes from oxidative damage, preventing the release of lipid peroxides. By reducing the number of peroxides that are formed, vitamin E spares the cellular use of selenium.[2] Selenium also helps to spare vitamin E by preserving the pancreas, allowing for normal fat digestion and thus normal vitamin E absorption, and reducing the amount of vitamin E required to maintain lipid membrane integrity through the availability of glutathione peroxidase.[3]

Selenium deficiencies or toxicities have not been reported in dogs and cats.[3] Selenium availability in food is highly influenced by whether the selenium is from foods or found as a supplement[3] Selenium availability averages ~30% in ingredients of animal origin and ~50% in ingredients of plant origin.[3]

Sources of selenium include fish, eggs and liver. Common supplements found in pet foods include sodium selenite and sodium selenate.[3]

Iodine

The body requires iodine for the synthesis of the hormones thyroxine and triiodothyronine by the thyroid gland.[7] Thyroxine stimulates cellular oxidative processes and regulates the basal metabolic rate.[2] This affects thermoregulation, reproduction, growth and development, circulation and muscle function.[3]

The thyroid gland effectively traps iodine daily to ensure adequate supplies for the production of thyroid hormones.[3] This trapping mechanism regulates a more or less constant iodine supply to the thyroid glands over a wide range of plasma levels.[3] Iodine requirements are influenced by physiologic state and diet.[3] Lactating animals require more dietary iodine because of loss through the milk.[3] The hypothalamus regulates thyroid hormone production by controlling the release of the pituitary's thyroid-stimulating hormone (TSH).[4]

The principal sign of iodine deficiency is goiter, an enlargement of the thyroid gland.[2] Naturally occurring dietary deficiency does not usually occur, but diets containing "goitrogenic compounds" can lead to this. Certain compounds found in peas, peanuts, soybeans and flaxseed can bind iodine, making it unavailable for use.[3]

Fish, eggs, iodized salt and poultry by-product meal are good sources of iodine. Common supplements found in pet foods include calcium iodate, potassium iodide and cuprous iodide.[3]

Chromium

Chromium participates in carbohydrate and lipid metabolism. Like iron, it also has different charges, with the Cr+++ ion being the most stable.[4] Chromium helps to maintain glucose homeostasis by enhancing the activity of the hormone insulin. Research has not shown that chromium supplements effectively improve glucose or insulin response in diabetics, though.[4]

Chromium can be found in various foods such as liver, brewer's yeast and whole grains.[4]

References

1 Simpson JW, Anderson RS, Markwell PJ (1993) Nutrients and the requirements of dog and cats. In CJ Price, B PCG, JB Sutton (eds), *Clinical Nutrition of the Dog and Cat*, pp. 27–30, Cambridge, MA: Blackwell.

2 Case LP, Carey DP, Hirakawa DA, Daristotle L (2000) Vitamins and minerals. In *Canine and Feline Nutrition* (2nd edn), pp. 123–8, St Louis, MO: Mosby.

3 Gross KL, Wedekind KL, Cowell CS *et al.* (2000) Nutrients. In MS Hand, CD Thatcher, RL Remillard *et al.* (eds), *Small Animal Clinical Nutrition* (4th edn), pp. 66–80, Marceline, MO: Walsworth Publishing.

4 Whitney E, Rolfes SR (2008) Water, and the major minerals. In *Understanding Nutrition* (11th edn), pp. 408–24, Belmont, CA: Thomson Wadsworth.

5 Hynd P (2019) Introduction to animal nutrition. In *Animal Nutrition from Theory to Practice*, pp. 23–31, Boston, MA: CABI Publication.

6 Jurgens M, Bregendahl K (2007) Nutrients and digestive systems. In *Animal Feeding and Nutrition* (10th edn), vol. **54**, Dubuque, IO: Kendall/Hunt Publishing.

8

Digestion and Absorption

Introduction

The role of digestion is to break up the large complex molecules found in many nutrients into their simplest, most soluble forms so that absorption and use by the body can occur.[1] The two basic types of action involved in this process are mechanical digestion as seen with chewing and the peristaltic action in the stomach and intestines, and chemical or enzymatic digestion as seen with the splitting of chemical bonds of the complex nutrients.[1]

The three major types of foods requiring digestion are fats, carbohydrates and proteins. Before fats can be absorbed, they need to be hydrolyzed to glycerol, free fatty acids and some mono- and diglycerides. Complex carbohydrates are broken down into the simple sugars of glucose, fructose and galactose. Proteins are hydrolyzed to their simple amino acids units and some dipeptides.[1,2] The digestion process begins when food first enters the mouth and continues until the excretion of waste products and the undigested portion of the foods in the feces.[1]

Digestive Tract

The digestive tract can be described as a hollow tube that starts at the mouth and continues to the anus.[3] Within this tube, various changes occur to allow ingested nutrients to be processed and utilized.[3]

Mouth

In all species, the mouth brings food into the body and starts the initial breaking down by chewing and mixing the food with saliva.[1] Saliva is produced in response to the sight and smell of food. It acts as a lubricant to make chewing and swallowing easier and liquefy the parts of the food that stimulate the taste buds and impart flavor to the food.[1,2] Saliva is composed of water, salts, mucus, and in dogs, amyline hormone.[4] Cats lack salivary amylase, which in other animals starts carbohydrate digestion in the mouth.[5]

The tongue serves to help move the food bolus around the mouth, and when the food bolus begins to liquefy, it allows the animal to taste the food it has consumed.[4] Unlike many herbivores that thoroughly chew their food, dogs, and cats often swallow large bites of food with little or no chewing.[1-3] The teeth of dogs and cats have few flat chewing surfaces, as would be seen with an herbivore. An additional distinction can be seen with cats, which have fewer premolars and molars than do dogs. The additional teeth provide dogs with an increased capacity to chew and crush their food.[1,2] The dental pattern seen with dogs suggests a more omnivorous diet, while cats are typical of the pattern seen with most other obligate carnivores.[1]

From the mouth, the food passes into the esophagus. When empty, the esophagus is a collapsed tube with longitudinal folds.[3] The esophagus lining contains many goblet

Nutrition and Disease Management for Veterinary Technicians and Nurses, Third Edition. Ann Wortinger and Kara M. Burns.
© 2024 John Wiley & Sons, Inc. Published 2024 by John Wiley & Sons, Inc.
Companion Website: www.wiley.com/go/wortinger/3e

cells that secrete a large amount of mucus to further assist in the lubrication of food during swallowing.[1,3] At the end of the esophagus is the cardia or cardiac sphincter. This muscular ring allows food to pass into the stomach but constricts back down to prevent the reflux of the stomach contents into the lower esophagus.[1-3]

Swallowing involves three steps; the first is under voluntary control, the remaining two are involuntary.[3] Swallowing is initiated by forming a bolus of food within the mouth; this is then pushed against the hard palate by the tongue and projected back into the pharynx.[3] Sensory receptors in the pharynx start the second step of swallowing by detecting the food bolus and closing the nasopharynx by upward movement of the soft palate. The pharyngeal muscles contract forcing the bolus of food into the esophagus, the last phase of swallowing involves detecting the food bolus within the cranial esophagus. This detection produces a peristaltic wave moving the food bolus down the esophagus into the stomach. A second peristaltic wave will often follow, ensuring that the food has been completely emptied into the stomach.[3]

Stomach

The stomach acts as a reservoir for ingested food and initiates the digestion process.[3] By acting as a reservoir, the stomach allows ingestion of a few large meals throughout the day rather than multiple smaller meals.[1] The stomach in cats is smaller than that found in dogs. Cats consume several smaller meals throughout the day (usually 10–20 meals); therefore, they do not need a large capacity stomach.[2,5]

The stomach is divided into four regions, the cardia, fundus, body, and pylorus. Food enters through the cardiac sphincter, which is located between the lower esophagus and the stomach. This is a strong muscular ring that helps to prevent the reentry of ingesta into the esophagus.[6] The fundic wall is thin and easily

expandable, while the body region is folded with longitudinal pleats called rugae. The rugae flatten as the stomach expands during ingestion of a meal. The pyloric region empties into the duodenum through the pyloric sphincter. This area has thick muscular walls, which contract to forcefully mix the ingesta and help to empty the contents into the duodenum.[6]

Chemical digestion of protein starts in the stomach and mixing the food with the gastric secretions.[1] The gastric secretions are composed of mucus to protect the stomach lining and further lubricate the food, hydrochloric acid to provide the proper pH for the necessary enzymatic reactions to occur, and pepsinogen, a proteolytic enzyme.[1] Hydrochloric acid converts the pepsinogen into the active enzyme pepsin. This initiates the hydrolysis of protein molecules into smaller polypeptide units.[1] Intrinsic factor, a glycoprotein necessary for cobalamin absorption in the small intestine, is also produced in the stomach.[6] Gastrin, a hormone produced by the pyloric cells, stimulates the production and release of histamine, which helps regulate acid production in the stomach.[6]

The stomach's acidic environment protects the animal from bacterial growth and kills most bacteria entering the body through the mouth.[4] The sight, smell and taste of food, together with the presence of food in the stomach, stimulate the secretion of hydrochloric acid and pepsinogen.

The stomach has a built-in pacemaker that produces five slow waves per minute, which initiate muscular contractions.[3] These peristaltic movements slowly mix the ingested food with the gastric secretions, preparing it for entry into the small intestine.[1] Thorough mixing of the ingested food produces a semifluid mass of food called chyme. Chyme must pass through the pyloric sphincter of the stomach to enter the small intestine for further digestion. The pyloric sphincter acts to control the rate of passage of chyme into the small intestine. The emptying rate can also be affected by osmotic pressure, particle size and viscosity of the chyme.[1] Generally, larger meals have a slower rate of emptying than smaller meals, liquids leave the stomach faster than solids, and very high-fat meals may cause a decrease in stomach emptying rate.

Diets containing soluble fiber, such as pectin, guar gum or fructooligosaccharides (FOS), can cause a slower emptying rate than diets containing insoluble dietary fibers such as cellulose, peanut hulls, and hemicelluloses.[1] At this stage of digestion, even though the food is now semisolid chyme, the carbohydrates and fats are almost unchanged in composition. Still, the proteins have been partially hydrolyzed into smaller polypeptide units.[2] The majority of digestion up to this point has been primarily mechanical, which is all about to change.[1]

Small Intestine

The small intestine starts at the pylorus and ends at the ileocecocolic junction. It is divided into three parts, the duodenum, jejunum and ileum. The duodenum is the first and shortest portion of the small intestine and is where the pancreatic and bile ducts enter the intestine.[3] The jejunum and ileum form the main portion of the small intestine. There are no clear divisions between the different parts of the small intestine.[3]

The small intestinal lining is composed of numerous villi with crypts in between. The cells lining the villi and the crypts are called enterocytes. Enterocytes are usually simple columnar cells, and those involved with absorption have numerous microvilli. The villi increase the absorptive surface of the small intestines, and the microvilli increase the surface area further. The surface of the microvilli is called the brush border, and the enzymes produced here are the brush border enzymes.[6]

Goblet cells are scattered throughout the epithelium and are responsible for the production of mucin. The mucin limits the number of bacteria reaching the epithelium and controls the bacterial interactions with the host immune system.[7]

Further mechanical digestion can also occur in the small intestine through the contraction of the muscle layers.[1] These contractions continue to mix the food with intestinal secretions, increasing the exposure of digested food particles to the surface of the intestine and slowly propelling the food mass through the intestinal tract.[1]

The pancreas and glands in the duodenal mucosa secrete enzymes into the intestinal lumen that begin the chemical digestion of fat, carbohydrate and protein. These enzymes include intestinal lipase, aminopeptidase, dipeptidase, nucleotidase, nucleosidase and enterokinase.[1] Intestinal lipase converts fat to monoglycerides, diglycerides, glycerol and free fatty acids.

Aminopeptidase breaks the peptide bond located at the terminal end of the protein molecule, slowly releasing single amino acid units from the protein chain.[1] Dipeptidase breaks the peptide bond of dipeptides to release two single amino acid units. Both nucleotidase and nucleosidase hydrolyze nucleoproteins to their constituent bases and pentose sugars.[1] Nucleoproteins are compound proteins consisting of a protein linked to a nucleic acid, either DNA or RNA.

Enterokinase converts inactive trypsinogen secreted by the pancreas into its active form of trypsin. Once activated, trypsin can activate more of itself as well as the other protease enzymes.[3] The brush border cells that line the intestines complete the final digestion of carbohydrates through the secretion of the enzymes maltase, lactase and sucrase—the brush border enzymes. These convert the disaccharides maltose, lactose and sucrose into glucose, fructose and galactose base monosaccharides.[1]

The pancreas is responsible for secreting the enzymes trypsin, chymotrypsin, carboxypeptidase and nuclease.[1] Most of these are secreted inactive and activated by other components in the small intestine after release.[1] The pancreas also produces lipase and amylase, which are responsible for the hydrolysis of fats and starches into smaller units. The acidic chyme produced in the stomach is neutralized by bicarbonate salts produced in the pancreas. This helps to adjust the intestinal pH to provide an optimal environment for the digestive enzymes to work.[1,4]

In dogs and cats, the chemical digestion of food is completed in the small intestine. Absorption involves the transfer by the body of digested nutrients from the intestinal lumen into the blood or lymphatic system for delivery to tissues throughout the body.[1] Like digestion, the primary site of absorption also occurs in the small intestine.[1]

Bile Salts

Bile salts are essential for producing a lipid/water interface to permit lipase digestion of triglycerides.[3] They are produced in the liver from cholesterol and concentrated and stored in the gall bladder. Bile's primary function in the small intestine is the emulsification of dietary fat and the activation of specific lipases.[1,4] The intestinal contractions ensure thorough mixing of the fat, lipase and bile salts. This produces an emulsion of small fat droplets called micelles.[3]

Hormones in Digestion

The endocrine cells located in the upper half of the villi comprise the largest endocrine gland in the body. These cells produce hormones such as secretin, cholecystokinin, ghrelin, peptide tyrosine–tyrosine (PYY) and glucagon-like peptide-1 (GLP-1).[6]

Hormonal control of digestion in the small intestine involves several parts. The duodenal mucosa produces secretin in response to the entry of chyme from the stomach.[1] Secretin stimulates the release of bicarbonate from the pancreas and controls the rate of bile release from the gall bladder. Cholecystokinin is also released from this portion of the duodenal mucosa in response to the presence of fat in the chyme. This hormone stimulates gall bladder contraction, causing the release of bile into the intestinal lumen.[1] Cholecystokinin is also called pancreozymin and stimulates the release of pancreatic enzymes.[1]

Ghrelin is often called the hunger hormone because it increases food intake by regulating energy homeostasis. Ghrelin activates the anterior pituitary gland and hypothalamus. It has been linked to creating hunger and feeding behaviors. Ghrelin does not increase meal size but does affect meal frequency.[6]

Digestion After the Intestines

Amino acids units are absorbed into the enterocytes lining the small intestine by specific carriers using an energy-dependent active process. Different carriers are used for different classes of amino acids.[3] Once absorbed, the amino acids are sent to the liver via the portal vein.[3] Peptides longer than four amino acids are not absorbed by the small intestine. However, the transporter system readily absorbs di- and tri-peptides and rapidly breaks these down into amino acids using cytoplasmic proteases.[6]

After the brush border enzymes have broken down the carbohydrates into their smallest particles, they are absorbed by the enterocytes using specific carriers in an active energy-requiring process. When the monosaccharides are in the enterocytes, they are rapidly released into the capillaries and transported to the liver.[3]

The majority of fat digestion occurs in the duodenum by pancreatic lipase and bile acids. The monoglycerides, long-chain fatty acids, phospholipids, cholesterol and fat-soluble vitamins form micelles with the emulsifying bile acids.[6] These micelles are absorbed passively into the enterocytes.[3] Within the enterocyte, the fatty acids reform into triglycerides and attach to lipoproteins to form chylomicrons. These chylomicrons are released into the lacteal, the part of the intestinal lymphatics that absorb fats for transportation to the thoracic duct at the heart to enter systemic circulation.[3,6] The bile remains within the intestinal lumen and eventually travels down to the jejunum to be reabsorbed and circulated back to the liver for reuse.[1] Medium-chain fatty acids can directly enter the enterocytes without being hydrolyzed and cross into the portal vein directly, bypassing the lacteals and the lymphatics.[6]

Water and electrolytes both flow across the intestinal mucosa in response to osmotic pressure.[1] Most minerals are absorbed by the body in the ionized form, meaning they carry an electrical charge. The water-soluble vitamins are absorbed by passive diffusion, though some may be absorbed by active processes when dietary levels are especially low.[1]

The liver further processes the absorbed monosaccharides and amino acids that arrive through the portal vein.[1] Some monosaccharides are converted to glycogen for storage, and some are secreted directly into the circulation. Some amino acids are released directly into the bloodstream, where they are available to the tissues for absorption into the cells. Excess amino acids are either converted to nonessential amino acids or metabolized by the liver and converted to fat for storage.[1] Once these amino acids are converted to fats, they can no longer be used for protein production.

Large Intestine

The large intestine begins at the ileocecal valve and continues as the cecum, ascending, transverse, and descending colon, rectum and anus.[3] These divisions are demarcated based on their location within the abdomen.[3]

The contents of the small intestine enter the colon through the ileocecocolic valve.[1,3] The cecum is small in dogs and cats and consists of an intestinal pocket next to the colon and small intestine junction, and serves no known function in these animals.[3] In nonruminant herbivores such as rabbits and horses, the cecum is quite large and has highly enhanced digestive capacities.[1]

The colon has three primary functions: the absorption of water and electrolytes, the fermentation of food residues by the resident bacterial population and the storage of feces in the rectum.[3]

Unlike the small intestine, the large intestine has no villi or brush border enzymes, and therefore has limited capacity for absorption of nutrients. It can absorb water and electrolytes quite well, though it has no mechanisms for active transport.[1,6] The absorption of water by the large intestine is very important in ensuring the passage of formed feces and preventing dehydration.[3] Normally, water is passively absorbed from the colon following the active energy-dependent absorption of sodium chloride. Goblet cells in the colon are responsible for producing large volumes of mucus, which helps to lubricate the digesta as it passes through.[6]

The bacterial colonies of the large intestine can digest some of the insoluble fiber and other nutrients in the diet that has escaped digestion in the small intestine. These dietary fibers are digested by extracellular enzymes, such as cellulases, hemicellulases and pectinases, produced by the bacteria. These enzymes produce short-chain fatty acids (SCFAs), biotin, vitamin K, carbon dioxide and methane.[8] The most important SCFA is butyrate (butyric acid), which the colonocytes use for energy in the form of ketone bodies rather than glucose or amino acids.[1,6] Acetate (acetic acid) is used directly by the peripheral tissues for energy, while propionate (propionic acid) is converted to glucose in the liver.[6]

There is no absorption of amino acids in the large intestine. When amino acids reach the colon undigested, the bacteria produce the amines indole and skatole. In addition, hydrogen sulfide gas is produced from sulfur-containing amino acids.[1,6] Hydrogen sulfide gas, indole and skatole impart strong odors to the feces and are responsible for flatulence.[1] Certain carbohydrates found in legumes such as soybeans are resistant to digestion by the small intestinal enzymes. When these carbohydrates reach the colon and the resident bacteria, intestinal gas (flatulence) is produced from the bacteria's fermentation of these resistant fibers. The degree to which flatulence and strong fecal odors occur in dogs and cats that are fed poorly digestible materials varies with the amounts and types of materials fed as well as the resident bacteria that are present in the individual animals.[1,2]

Any material that survives the digestive process in the stomach, small and large intestines is considered nondigestible waste material.[4] By the time feces have been excreted, the body has extracted all the usable energy, vitamins, minerals and fiber found in the food.

More information on the gastrointestinal microbiome is provided in Chapter 10.

References

1 Case LP, Carey DP, Hirakawa DA, Daristotle L (2000) Digestion and absorption. In *Canine and Feline Nutrition* (2nd edn), pp. 53–60, St Louis, MO: Mosby.

2 Case LP (2003) The cat as an obligate carnivore. In *The Cat: Its Behavior, Nutrition, and Health*, pp. 303–8, Ames, IA: Iowa State Press.

3 Simpson JW, Anderson RS, Markwell PJ (1993) Anatomy and physiology of the digestive tract. In CJ Price, B PCG, JB Sutton (eds), *Clinical Nutrition of the Dog and Cat*, pp. 1–18, Cambridge, MA: Blackwell.

4 Whitney E, Rolfes SR (2008) Digestion, absorption, and transport. In *Understanding Nutrition* (11th edn), pp. 71–89, Belmont, CA: Thomson Wadsworth.

5 Kirk CA, Jacques D, Jane AP (2000) Normal cats. In MS Hand, CD Thatcher, RL Remillard *et al.* (eds), *Small Animal Clinical Nutrition* (4th edn), pp. 291–337, Marceline, MO: Walsworth Publishing.

6 Hynd P (2019) Digestion in the mono-gastric animal. In *Animal Nutrition from Theory to Practice*, pp. 42–62, Boston, MA: CABI Publication.

7 Pelaseyed T, Bergstrom JH *et al.* (2014) The mucus and mucins of the goblet cells and enterocytes provide the first defense line of the gastrointestinal tract and interact with the immune system. *Immunol Rev.* **260**(1): 8–20. https://www.ncbi.nlm.nih.gov/pmc/articles/PMC4281373/ Accessed 10/26/21.

8 Gross KL, Jewell DE, Yamka RM *et al.* (2010) Macronutrients. In MS Hand, CD Thatcher, RI Remillard *et al.* (eds), *Small Animal Clinical Nutrition* (5th edn), pp. 74–5, Marceline, MO, Walsworth Publishing.

9

Energy Balance

Introduction

Energy in food is different from nutrients in that intake must be kept close to requirements. Energy balance is when an animal's intake is sufficient to meet its needs, and minimal changes in the energy stored by the body occur.[1,2] Positive energy balance happens when caloric intake exceeds energy expenditure, and weight gain occurs.[2] In growing and pregnant animals, excess energy is converted primarily into lean body tissue. In adult animals, excess energy is stored primarily as fat, with only some increase in lean body tissue.[1,2] A negative energy balance occurs when caloric intake is insufficient to meet energy expenditures. When this is the case, weight loss and decreases in fat and lean body stores can occur.[1,2] A particular amount of energy is required by animals to maintain a given body weight. Slight variations in this requirement can result in increases and decreases in body weight.[3]

Units of Measure

Energy is the capacity of the body to do work. To measure the energy used, the calorie is typically used. A calorie is defined as the amount of heat required to raise the temperature of 1 ml of water from 14.5 to 15.5 °C (1 °C).[3]) Because this amount of energy is very small, what is used in nutrition to express energy content is actually a kilocalorie or 1000 cal. You may see this expressed as "kcal," "kilocal" "big calorie" or "Calorie" (note the uppercase "C"). In large animal nutrition, a megacalorie (Mcal) may be used, which is equivalent to 1,000,000 calories or 1000 kcal.

While a calorie is considered a metric expression, the actual metric unit used to designate energy measurement is the joule.[3] To convert from calories to joules, multiply calories by 4.184 to obtain joules. As with calories, joules are a very small unit of measure and are more commonly expressed as kilojoules (1000 J) and megajoules (1,000,000 J).[3]

The energy content of food is expressed as the amount of energy (kcal) per unit of weight or volume. The weight of a given volume of food will vary based on the density of food, which can vary greatly.[3]

Daily Energy Requirements

The daily energy requirement (DER) for dogs and cats depends on the amount of energy that the body uses daily.[2] Energy balance, though, is achieved by matching input and output over a long period of time.[1] Even a small imbalance maintained over a long period of time can cause weight gain or weight loss depending on the direction of the imbalance.[1]

The principal mechanism for control of energy balance is thought to be through intake regulation, though some variation in output can be important.[1] The energy requirement of the animal and the energy density of the

Nutrition and Disease Management for Veterinary Technicians and Nurses, Third Edition. Ann Wortinger and Kara M. Burns.
© 2024 John Wiley & Sons, Inc. Published 2024 by John Wiley & Sons, Inc.
Companion Website: www.wiley.com/go/wortinger/3e

food will determine the quantity of food eaten daily.[1] But a highly palatable food can lead to excess intake over energy expenditure, and food with poor palatability can lead to an insufficient intake to meet energy requirements. Regulation of intake is considered a negative feedback system, meaning that as weight increases, intake will decrease, and when weight decreases, intake will increase.

Energy expenditure can be divided into four major areas, resting energy requirement (RER), voluntary muscular activity expenditure, body heat production and meal-induced thermogenesis.[2]

Resting Energy Requirements

RER, also called resting metabolic rate (RMR), accounts for the largest portion of an animal's energy expenditure representing ~60–75% of daily intake.[2] RER is the amount of energy used while resting quietly in a thermoneutral environment in a non-fasted animal.[1,2,4] This represents the energy required to maintain homeostasis in all of the body's integrated systems during rest.[2] Factors influencing RER include sex and reproductive status, thyroid and autonomic nervous system function, body composition, body surface area and nutritional status.[2] As an animal's lean body mass or body surface area increases, RER also increases.[2]

Common Measurements of Energy

Basal Energy Requirement (BER)

The energy requirement for a normal animal in a thermoneutral environment, awake but resting in a fasting state. Also, known as basal metabolic rate (BMR) or basal energy expenditure (BEE). It is difficult to have an animal cooperate with the activity restrictions required to measure BER. Resting energy expenditure (REE) is more commonly used in veterinary medicine.[3]

Resting Energy Requirement (RER)

The energy requirement for a normal animal at rest in a thermoneutral environment, awake but not fasted. RER accounts for energy used for digestion, absorption and metabolism of nutrients and recovery from physical activity. Also known as RMR or REE.

Maintenance Energy Requirement (MER)

The energy requirement for a moderately active adult animal in a thermoneutral environment. MER accounts for energy used for obtaining, digesting and absorbing nutrients in an amount to maintain body weight, as well as the energy used for spontaneous activity. MER is the amount of energy required to maintain an animal at its current weight and body composition. It is also known as metabolic energy expenditure (MEE).

Daily Energy Requirement (DER)

The energy required for the average daily activity of any animal, dependent on lifestyle and activity. DER includes energy necessary for work, gestation, lactation, growth and the energy needed to maintain normal body temperature.

Gross Energy (GE)

The total amount of heat produced by burning a specific amount of food in a bomb calorimeter. Neither water nor minerals in the form of ash are combustible. Therefore, they contribute no calories or energy to the GE of a diet.

Digestible Energy (DE)

The energy in food left over after digestion. The energy remaining in feces is subtracted from GE to obtain this amount.[5]

Metabolizable Energy (ME)

The energy in food available to the animal after losses from feces, urine and combustible gasses are subtracted from GE.[5]

Kilocalorie (kcal)

The energy needed to raise the temperature of 1 gram of water from 14.5 to 15.5 °C. 1 kcal = 1000 cal

3500 kcal

The amount of energy change required to lose or gain 1 pound. To lose or gain 1 kilogram, multiply 3500 by 2.2 to obtain 7700 kcals.[3,4,6]

Energy Expenditure

Voluntary muscular activity, or exercise, is the most variable area of energy expenditure. Muscular activity accounts for ~30% of total energy expenditures.[2] The amount of energy expended is directly affected by the duration and intensity of the activity, though the amount of energy used can also increase as weight increases.[2]

RER can be affected by body composition, age, caloric intake and hormonal status.[2] RER also naturally decreases as animals age and lose lean body tissue.[2] Changes in RER can also occur secondary to energy restriction. When caloric intake decreases, hormones will cause an initial decrease in energy requirements to conserve body tissue.[2,6] If caloric restriction continues, RER will be readjusted and would not be corrected until levels of lean body tissue return to normal.[2] Persistent overeating, or positive energy balance, can lead to an increase in energy expenditure in part due to the increase in lean body mass with weight gain, but also due to increased meal-induced thermogenesis. Accumulating fat in adipose tissue does not increase the energy requirements for the animal, except through increased energy used to move.[2,6]

Reproductive status affects energy requirements, with neutered animals having significantly lower estimated RER than intact animals. The decrease in energy requirements occurring immediately after neutering is estimated to be ~25%. This is due to a change in body composition (less lean body tissue), decreased activity levels and hormones.[2] Intact animals tend to be more active during the breeding season and in territorial disputes that are usually not as much of a concern for a neutered animal. The loss of the androgenic hormones decreases the lean body mass of the neutered animal.

Body Heat Production

Body heat is also known as heat increment. This is the energy associated with the ingestion, digestion, absorption and metabolism of food. Heat increment accounts for ~10–15% of dogs' and cats' total daily energy expenditure.[3] The degree of heat produced during digestion can vary based on meal size and the nutrient composition of the meal. A high-protein diet will produce the greatest heat, while a high-fat diet will produce the least heat.[3]

The ingestion of nutrients causes heat production through the process of digestion and absorption.[2] The use of digestive enzymes by the body allows these chemical reactions to occur at the relatively low temperatures found within the body. Achieving the same results in an industrial process would require much more extreme conditions of temperature, pH or highly reactive ingredients.[6] The final amount of calories used is ultimately dependent on the diet composition and the animal's nutritional status.[2]

Facultative Thermogenesis

Facultative thermogenesis refers to the energy required to maintain body temperature when an animal is outside its thermoneutral zone. For adult dogs, the thermoneutral zone is considered to be between 20–25°C and 30–35°C (68–77°F and 86–95°F). For cats, the thermoneutral zone is not entirely known but is estimated to be between 30 and 38°C (68–100°F).[3]

Adaptive thermogenesis is the change in the RER secondary to environmental stresses. These stresses include changes in ambient temperature, both heat and cold, alterations in food intake and emotional stress.[2] This process allows the body to maintain the energy balance despite changes in caloric intake by being less efficient in energy use.[2]

For animals living outdoors, facultative thermogenesis can be a significant source of energy expenditure if they experience temperatures well outside of their thermoneutral zones.[3]

Voluntary Oral Intake

Voluntary food intake is regulated by both internal physiologic controls and external cues.[2] The animal receives cues from the body in the form of physical signs such as stomach contractions when empty stimulating eating or stomach distention when fully inhibiting eating.[6] Numerous neural and hormonal mechanisms provide direct stimulation or inhibition of eating. Glucagon and insulin would be examples of two such hormones.[6] Glucagon is a peptide produced in the intestines that causes a decrease in food intake. On the other hand, insulin is produced by the pancreas and stimulates hunger and increased food intake.[2] The administration of exogenous steroids can affect insulin on hunger and food intake. Exogenous steroids do not increase the energy required for the body but do increase appetite. This can commonly be seen with the administration of corticosteroids.

External controls of food intake include stimuli such as diet palatability, food composition, food texture, and meals' timing and environment.[2] Feeding a highly palatable diet is considered a primary environmental factor contributing to the overconsumption of food, leading to obesity.[2] This can be seen with high-fat diets, calorically dense diets and foods that offer a variety of palatable flavors.[2]

Both dogs and cats have definite taste and texture preferences. Most dogs prefer canned and semimoist foods over dry food, with beef being the preferred flavor and cooked meat preferred over raw.[2] Dogs also have a strong preference for sucrose, while cats have been shown to lack the taste receptors in their tongues even to detect sugars.[2,7,8] Dogs and cats can detect several specific amino acids that are only weakly bitter to people. These amino acids and peptides help to give foods their meaty and savory aromas and tastes. They also respond to selected nucleotides and fatty acids that appear to increase the meaty taste perception in foods. A nucleotide that accumulates in decomposing meat is distasteful to cats, but not to dogs. This may help explain the dog's fascination with dead animals.[8] Both dogs and cats prefer warm food over cold food, with increasing palatability seen with increased fat levels in the diet.[2]

The timing of meals and the environment that they are offered in can affect eating behavior.[2] Dogs and cats rapidly become conditioned to receive their meals at a specific time of day; this can be seen with behavioral and physical signs.[2] Activity will generally increase at anticipated mealtimes, and gastric secretions and motility increase in anticipation of eating.[2]

The number of animals being fed can also increase the amount of food consumed with each meal. In dogs, this is a phenomenon called social facilitation. This causes a moderate increase in interest in food and an increased rate of eating. The degree that this affects individual dogs can vary greatly.[2] Social hierarchies between dogs can also affect the amount of food eaten, with subordinate dogs eating less in the presence of dominant dogs during mealtimes.[2]

For cats, the smell of food is the primary determinant of food acceptance. When they are unable to smell, they will continue to refuse all attempts to feed them.[9] Cats do not appear to participate in social facilitation in eating or by the presence of another cat during mealtimes.[9]

The frequency of meals can affect both food intake and metabolic efficiency. With increased meal frequency, there is an increase in energy loss through increased thermogenesis. With smaller, more frequent meals, the body uses more energy to digest, absorb and metabolize the food than when one or two larger meals are fed.[2]

Nutrient Composition

The food's nutrient composition can affect both the nutrient metabolism and the amount of food voluntarily eaten by the animal.[2] Most animals will decrease their intake of a high-fat diet to compensate for energy needs. However, the greater caloric density of the diet with increased palatability can still cause increased energy intake in some animals.[2] The body is also metabolically more efficient at converting dietary fat to body fat for storage than converting dietary carbohydrates or protein to body fat. Because of this, if an animal is eating calories above its requirements of a high-fat diet, it will gain more weight than if they were consuming the same number of calories in a high protein or high carbohydrate diet.[2]

The addition of treats and table scraps to the diet can also override the body's satiety cues. These treats tend to be highly desirable and appealing, and even if not hungry, the animals will not turn them down.[2] This leads to increased energy intake and obesity because owners seldom decrease the amount of "regular food" offered to the pet when also giving treats. Feeding a variety of new food types can also cause the same effect by introducing novelty.[2]

Estimated Energy Requirements

Many formulas have been used to calculate the estimated energy requirements for animals.

Table 9.1 Formula(s) for calculating RER in adult maintenance in kcals/day, using body weight (BW) in kilograms.

Canine	Feline
$70 \times (\text{body wt in kg})^{0.75}$	$70 \times (\text{body wt in kg})^{0.75}$
$(30 \times \text{body wt in kg}) + 70$	$(40 \times \text{body wt in kg})$

Source: Adapted from Pet Nutrition Alliance [11]

Dogs represent a unique challenge in that their sizes have one of the widest ranges in the animal kingdom, from the 4# Chihuahua to the 200# Great Dane.[10] Cats tend to have a smaller range of sizes, usually between 4 and 20#. Some use algometric formulas, some linear equations, and some use body surface area (BSA). All of these formulas are helpful, but all still are only estimates of actual caloric needs. Numerous charts have also been devised that allow quick access to estimate energy needs. (see Table 9.1).

If using a calculator that does not have an exponential key, one of the linear formulas will need to be used. When using a smartphone for calculation, turning the phone sideways will produce a square root key. All of these formulas have been compared, and when calculated, the results are within a reasonable value of each other. Charts that have the MER calculated out can be used to determine the kcals requirements. Ultimately all energy estimates will need to be adjusted based on the desired response from the animal; weight gain, weight maintenance or weight loss. Variability between individual animals, sexual status and environmental living conditions can result in a difference up or down of up to 25% of the calculated energy need.[2]

Using these equations and the energy density of the food, the amount of food to be fed to the individual animal can be calculated.[2] (see Figure 9.1).

Certain life stages can cause increased energy needs. These would include growth, gestation, lactation, periods of strenuous physical work and exposure to extreme

Table 9.2 Life stage factors.

Life stage – Canine	Energy requirement
Growth	2–3 × RER
Late gestation	1.6–2.0 × adult RER
Intact adult	1.8 × RER
Neutered adult	1.6 × RER
Critical care/hospitalized	1.0 × RER
Weight loss/obese	0.8–1.0 × RER
Overweight/inactive	1.0–1.2 × RER
Lactation	2–6 × RER
Prolonged physical work	2–4 × adult RER

Life stage – Feline	Energy requirement
Growth	2–3 × RER
Late gestation	2–3 × adult RER
Intact adult	1.4 × RER
Neutered adult	1.2 × RER
Critical care/hospitalized	1.0 × RER
Weight loss/obese	0.8–1.0 × RER
Overweight/inactive	1.0 × RER
Lactation	2–6 × RER

Source: Adapted from Pet Nutrition Alliance.[11]

environmental conditions.[2] Life Stage Factors or LSF is used to calculate the extra calories above RER.[2,11,12] Conversely, LSFs are also helpful when calculating energy needs during weight loss. An LSF can range from 0.8 (80%) of RER to 4.0, or 400% of RER. As with all calorie calculations, these are best guesses as to what the animal requires. If weight loss is seen when it was not planned for, increased calories need calories need to be provided.

Example:
Using the linear formula

10# dog = 4.5 kg
$RER = (wt \ in \ kg) \times 30) + 70$
$DER = RER \times 1.3$
$DER = [(30 \times 4.5 \ kg) + 70] \times 1.3$
$DER = 205 \times 1.3$
$DER = 266.5 \ kcal/day$

Using the logarithmic formula

10# dog
$RER = 70 \times (body \ wt \ in \ kg)^{0.75}$
$DER = RER \times 1.3$
$DER = [(4.5 \times 4.5 \times 4.5)\sqrt{}\sqrt{} \times 70] \times 1.3$
$DER = 216 \times 1.3$
$DER = 281 \ kcal/day$
Diet A = 326 kcal/cup
Feeding amount = 266–281 kcal/day/326 kcal/cup
Feeding amount = 0.8–0.86 cup/day
This is based on a standard 8 oz measuring cup.

Figure 9.1 Calculation of Resting Energy Requirements (RER) and Daily Energy Requirements (DER).

If weight gain is seen, when not planned for, fewer calories need to be fed. (see Table 9.2). Water requirements can be expressed in one of two ways, either 2–3 × the dry matter (DM) intake of the food, expressed in grams, or using the MER kcal/day estimates to calculate water requirements.[2] The best recommendation is to have plenty of clean, fresh water available at all times, regardless of the animal's physiologic state, caloric intake, or DM intake.[2]

References

1 Will JM (1996) Basic principles of nutrition and feeding. In N Kelly, J Wills (eds), *Manual of Companion Animal Nutrition and Feeding*, pp. 19–21, Ames, IA: Iowa State Press.

2 Case LP, Carey DP, Hirakawa DA, Daristotle L (2000) Energy balance. In *Canine and Feline Nutrition* (2nd edn), pp. 75–88, St Louis, MO: Mosby.

3 Delaney SJ, Fascetti AJ (2012) Determining Energy Requirements. In AJ Fascetti, SJ Delaney (eds), *Applied Veterinary Clinical Nutrition*, pp. 23–42, Ames, IO: Wiley-Blackwell.

4 Gross KL, Wedekind KL, Cowell CS *et al.* (2000) Nutrients. In MS Hand, CD Thatcher, RL Remillard *et al.* (eds), *Small Animal Clinical Nutrition* (4th edn), pp. 31–3, Marceline, MO: Walsworth Publishing.

5 Gross KL, Jewell DE, Yamka RM *et al.* (2010) Macronutrients. In MS Hand, CD Thatcher, RI Remillard *et al.* (eds), *Small Animal Clinical Nutrition* (5th edn), p. 55, Marceline, MO: Walsworth Publishing.

6 Burger IH (1993) A basic guide to nutrient requirements. In JM Wills, W Simpson Kenneth (eds), *The Waltham Book of Companion Animal Nutrition*, pp. 6–10, Tarrytown, NY: Pergamon.

7 Xia L, Weihua L, Hong W, et al. Pseudogenization of a sweet-receptor gene accounts for cats indifference toward sugar a www .plosgenetics.org, July 2005. **1**(1):27–35

8 Crane SW, Griffin RW, Messent PR (2000) Introduction to commercial pet foods. In MS Hand, CD Thatcher, RI Remillard, P Roudebush (eds), *Small Animal Clinical Nutrition* (4th edn), p. 123, Marceline, MO: Walsworth Publishing.

9 Horwitz D, Soulard Y, Junien-Castagna A (2008) The feeding behavior of the cat. In P Pibot, V Biourge, D Elliott (eds), *Encyclopedia of Feline Clinical Nutrition*, p. 445, Aniwa SAS: Aimargues, France.

10 Case LP (1999) Nutrient requirements. In *The Dog: Its Behavior, Nutrition, and Health*, p. 279, Ames IO: Iowa State Press.

11 Pet Nutrition Alliance. Calculating Calories Based on Pet Needs. http:// petnutritionalliance.org/site/wp-content/ uploads/2017/05/MER.RER_.PNA_.pdf. Accessed 10/28/21

12 Donoghue S (1996) The underweight patient. In N Kelly, J Wills (eds), *Manual of Companion Animal Nutrition and Feeding*, p. 103, Ames, IA: Iowa State Press.

10

Gastrointestinal Microbiome

Introduction

When mammals are born, their intestinal tract is sterile. Within the first 24 h, microbes begin to populate the GI tract. Evolution has led to a mutualistic relationship between the host and these microbes. The microbial population is called the microbiota. This relationship benefits both the host and the microbes found within it, providing a stable environment for both organisms.[1] This relationship is complex, and science is just beginning to understand the microbiota and how it influences health and disease.

Microbiome

The microbiome comprises living microorganisms, including bacteria and fungi, protozoa, viruses, parasites and archaea (single-celled organisms known as prokaryocytes).[2] The GI tract of domestic animals is home to several hundred different genera of bacteria with >1000 phylotypes. These organisms outnumber the host's cells by a factor of 100, with microbial cells numbering 10^{12}–10^{14} (10 with 12–14 zeros after it!!). Some genetic components of the microbiota exceed the hosts by 100 or more times. This is sometimes termed the "second genome."[3,4] The microbiome is seen as a functioning organ that can be affected by the nutrient composition of the diet.[5]

Commensal Microbiota

This constellation of organisms is not static but changes throughout the life of the animal.[3] The feline microbiota reaches a stable community by ~30 weeks of age.[4] Dietary changes can also affect the composition of the intestinal microbiome, with relatively small changes in certain types of dietary fiber, causing significant and detectable changes in the composition of the gut microbiome.[1]

The development of a healthy intestinal microbiome is critical to the normal development and maintenance of health in the host, and an absence of these commensal microbes is incompatible with life.[3] Typically, the host does not have a problem with this constant microbial and antigenic exposure.

If the host does not develop adequate tolerance of the accompanying massive immunological onslaught, and interact "normally" with the microbiota and prevent opportunistic pathogens from causing disease, this can contribute to a myriad of infectious and inflammatory conditions, with increasing evidence of its role in other conditions such as allergies, metabolic diseases, neoplasia and obesity.[3]

The microbiome is not confined to the intestinal tract; every part of the body that communicates with the external world will have its microbiota, the composition of which can vary between and within the various sites.

Nutrition and Disease Management for Veterinary Technicians and Nurses, Third Edition. Ann Wortinger and Kara M. Burns.
© 2024 John Wiley & Sons, Inc. Published 2024 by John Wiley & Sons, Inc.
Companion Website: www.wiley.com/go/wortinger/3e

The skin microbiota is different from the respiratory tract microbiota. The composition of the skin or respiratory microbiotas can differ between the upper and lower respiratory tracts and between the aural skin and the inguinal skin.[3]

The microbiome found in the intestines is home to one of the densest microbial populations on the planet. Alterations to this microbiota have been associated with various diseases for quite some time. The microbiota composition is viewed as a moving target, with some general aspects being understood but details remaining unclear.[3] Microbiome alterations associated with diseases are more significant than those seen in healthy animals on various diets. Dietary changes and the addition of prebiotics and probiotics can benefit the microbiota diversity and help normalize metabolite production in diseased animals.[5]

Benefits to the Host

The benefits to the host include the formation of a defensive barrier against potential pathogenic organisms, aiding in nutrient breakdown and energy release from the diet, provision of nutritional metabolites for enterocytes in the form of short-chain fatty acids (SCFAs) propionate, butyrate and acetate, regulation of the host immune system, and metabolism of drugs and xenobiotics that require metabolism by the intestinal microbes before absorption by the host.[2,3,6,7] A xenobiotic is a foreign chemical substance found within an organism that is not normally naturally produced by or expected to be present within that organism. This term can also include substances that are present in much higher concentrations than usual.[3]

The microbiome also provides competition to undesirable and pathogenic organisms by out-competing them for adhesion sites, producing toxic substances to other bacteria, secretion of antimicrobial substances called bacteriocins, assistance with GI transit time and production of vitamins and growth factors for intestinal cells.[2,3,6,7]

Production of microbe metabolites by the resident microbiome has provided a driving force behind the coevolution of the GI microbiota with the host.[2] Because of this, the type of microbiome present will depend on the composition of the diet, the environment the animal lives in, the stage of life, disease state and a myriad of other factors.[3]

Changes to the microbiome may lead to altered intestinal barrier function, damage to the brush border and enterocytes, increased competition for nutrients and vitamins and increased deconjugation of intestinal bile acids.[2]

The Immune System

The microbiome plays a significant role in the immune system, consisting of innate and adaptive mechanisms that help to protect the animal from environmental pathogens.[8] The innate immune system functions independent of previous exposure to organisms. It includes mechanical barriers such as the skin, mucous and epithelial linings and cellular components such as macrophages and neutrophils.[8]

The adaptive immune system consists primarily of B and T lymphocytes and relies on specific recognition of invading agents and generation of immunologic memory.[8] These are not two entirely different systems but act as a continuum with much overlap in response.

The adaptive immune system depends on specific recognition of invading agents and relies on "memory" produced from previous exposure to respond better and quicker when reexposed to the same antigen. This memory can be acquired either through the transfer of antibodies from colostrum, vaccination or infection.[8] Both the adaptive and innate systems are based on "immune recognition." The innate system uses germline-encoded receptors, while the adaptive system recognizes invaders based on somatically (body) generated receptors.[8]

An example of the innate systems germline-encoded receptors is the toll-like receptors (TLRs). These are transmembrane receptors for the innate immune system that recognize several types of cell components. Research has shown that saturated fatty acids in the diet can induce activation of several TLRs, while unsaturated fatty acids inhibit TLR-mediated signaling pathways and gene expression. TLRs can sense when the immune system is being exposed to pathological levels of lipids. This ability can affect eating behaviors by increasing or decreasing food intake based on lipid levels.[8]

For quite a long time, it has been known that the immune system cannot function effectively under malnutrition conditions, whether under or overnutrition. Research has demonstrated that obesity and consumption of high-fat diets, particularly those containing high levels of saturated fats, depress both innate and adaptive immune competencies. This is done by affecting the activity of immune cells, thereby enhancing the risk of severe infections and cancers.[8]

Bacteria

Historically, the assessment of the bacterial microbiota relied heavily on bacterial culture. This identification method has severe limitations because of the inability of a large percentage of the population to grow under conventional culture conditions because they are anaerobes or facilitative anaerobes, causing an underestimation of the actual bacterial numbers and diversity of species. Culture is also limited in that it is impractical to detect a population in the billions of bacteria.[3,4]

Molecular methods for bacterial identification, either quantitative PCR or reverse-transcriptase quantitative PCR, continue to evolve, allowing the assessment of complex microbial populations cost-effectively and generating massive amounts of data.[3,4] Arrays of bacterial species are possible for specific organisms, which may become economical for in-hospital analysis.[4] This method can better assess the actual bacterial populations residing in the GI tract. With that being said, the primary disadvantage of PCR panel assays is that they can miss organisms of importance, and they lack assessment of whether the bacteria found are functional.[4]

The resident intestinal microbiota plays a crucial part in the intestinal barrier system that protects the host from invading pathogens and microbial products, such as endotoxins. This happens through competition for nutrients, mucosal adhesion sites and a physiologically restrictive environment for nonresident bacteria. This restrictive environment is created through the secretion of antimicrobials, alterations in gut pH and hydrogen sulfide production.[9]

Aerobic bacteria occur in relatively higher proportions in the small intestine, while the large intestine is populated almost exclusively by anaerobic or facultative anaerobic bacteria.[9] The normal canine stomach typically contains high numbers of *Helicobacter* spp. bacteria colonizing the superficial mucosa, gastric glands and parietal cells.[9] The colonic mucosa also contains high numbers of mucosally-associated bacteria, while the small intestine has very few bacteria found within the mucosa. Except for the stomach, mucosally invasive bacteria are virtually absent in the healthy small and large intestine.[9]

The primary bacteria found in the intestinal tract of dogs and cats include *Firmicutes* spp. (~40%), *Bacteroides* spp. (~30%) and *Fusobacteria* spp. (~30%), with minor numbers, contributed by *Proteobacteria* spp. and *Actinobacteria*.[1,4,5] The specific beneficial bacterial species found in the largest amounts in dogs include *Enterococci* spp. (*Enterococcus* faecium and *Enterococcus* faecalis) and lactic acid species. For cats, the beneficial species include *Lactobacillus* spp., *Enterococcus* spp. and *Bifidobacterium* spp.[7]

A balanced microbial ecosystem is crucial for the optimal health of the host animal. Physiologically microbiota provides stimulation for the immune system, helps in the defense against invading pathogens, and provides nutritional benefits to the host through the production of SCFAs.[6] The bacterial groups most commonly depleted are important in the production of the SCFAs butyrate and acetate, which provide energy specifically to enterocytes and colonocytes and impair the capability of the host to down-regulate aberrant intestinal immune response.[2]

SCFAs provide energy directly to the intestinal cells, provide important growth factors for epithelial cells, help modulate the immune properties of the intestinal tract, inhibit pathogenic bacterial overgrowth through modulation of colon pH, and influence gastrointestinal motility.[9]

The resident intestinal microbiota is essential in the normal development of physiological gut structures. In specific-pathogen-free (germ-free) animals, altered mucosal architecture is found, involving primarily the mucosal structures. Establishing a resident microbiome early in life is crucial for developing oral tolerance to prevent the onset of an inappropriate immune response against bacterial and food antigens.[9] This can be accomplished by consuming colostrum during the early hours of life and exposure to the maternal microbiota during nursing and cleaning.

Other Components of the Microbiota

The microbiota is not composed of only bacteria, though they compromise the bulk of the organisms found. Archaea, viruses, fungi and parasites are also part of the microbiome. The archaea most likely play a minor role and may be present because they are part of the environment, and the animal is exposed to them. The viral microbiota, predominately bacteriophages, outnumber the bacterial population by a factor of 10. These only contribute 2–5% of the total DNA composition of the microbiota, though. At present, there is no easy or cost-effective way to assess the viral component of the intestinal microbiome. There have also not been any studies of the fungal component of the microbiome, even though it is recognized as present.[3,4]

Effects of Diet on the Microbiota

As mentioned above, SCFAs are used by the intestinal microbiota for energy. These SCFAs are produced primarily from dietary fibers. Dietary fibers are the edible portion of plants resistant to digestion and absorption in the small intestine. Instead, these are either entirely or partially fermented by the resident bacteria in the distal small intestine and large intestine.[10] Most of these dietary fibers are polysaccharides, meaning they are composed of long strands of carbohydrates.

Dietary fibers can be classified based on their physical or chemical characteristics and their effects on the bowel microflora. The most important characteristic for intestinal bacteria is the fermentability of these fibers.[10] Dietary fibers that can undergo bacterial fermentation include polysaccharides such as resistant starches, pectin, inulin, guar gum and oligosaccharides such as fructooligosaccharides (FOS).[10]

The degree that the microflora and fermented by-products produced utilize each fiber is influenced by the carbohydrate structure and the microflora composition within that individual animal. Complete fermentation will produce hydrogen, carbon dioxide and water; incomplete fermentation will produce methane, acetone, propionate and butyrate.[10] The end effect of providing dietary fibers in the bowel lumen is to create a selective advantage for those bacterial species adapted for its use.

When a shift in the microbiota positively affects the host animal, the fiber is defined as a prebiotic. Positive effects can be a reduction in the mucosal adherence of pathogenic bacterial species, a reduction in the numbers of pathogenic species and immune modulation of the host.[10]

The utilization of most fermentable fibers is never 100%, and most natural fiber sources contain a range of carbohydrate structures from monosaccharides and disaccharides to polysaccharides of varying fermentability. Fibers such as FOS, inulin and resistant starch can significantly increase the fermentative production of butyrate.[10] While fibers found in citrus pectin, citrus pulp, beet pulp and cellulose yield relatively low butyrate levels.[10]

In most domestic species, including dogs, butyrate is oxidized by colonocytes, and in dogs, it is also oxidized by enterocytes. Butyrate from fiber fermentation can increase colonocyte proliferation, intestinal mucosal weight, water, electrolyte absorption and brush border enzyme activity.[10] These are all seen as positive effects from fermentable fibers in the diet.

Certain fibers, such as FOS and inulin, can stimulate the growth or activity of intestinal bacteria such as *Lactobacillus* and *Bifidobacterium* spp. It has been proposed that increasing the numbers of these nonpathogenic bacterial species may positively affect the host, including outcompeting pathogenic bacteria, interfering with binding sites, and direct interaction with the mucosal immune system.[10]

Ideally, these fermentable fibers would be incorporated into the diet as functional fiber in the ingredients or actual vegetable products. Care must be taken to increase the fermentable fibers sufficiently without causing GI distress through gas production or impaired motility. Those fibers that produce a higher concentration of butyrate in the proximal colon may be more effective than less fermentable sources of fiber.[10]

Currently, insufficient information is available in feline and canine medicine to make an informed therapeutic recommendation beyond the initial introduction of mixed fermentable fiber sources and proceed with trial and error to see which is most effective with that particular animal.[10] Changes in the microbiome composition caused by dietary changes are maintained only by long-term maintenance of that specific diet.[5]

Dysbiosis

Dysbiosis refers to an imbalance in the microbiota of the animal. Maintaining a balance of the microbes is important for intestinal homeostasis, and changes in the microbiota may directly or indirectly influence metabolic host pathways.[6]

The disease can develop when the host lacks adequate immunologic tolerance to the accompanying massive immunologic onslaught from the microbiome. Inflammatory intestinal conditions may play a role in developing other conditions such as allergies, obesity, metabolic disease and cancer.[3]

Gastrointestinal disease can be caused directly by invading pathogens and by dysbiosis caused by opportunistic resident bacteria and altered communication between the innate immune system and the commensal microbes living in the intestine.[2]

Due to the complex interactions between intestinal absorption and microbial metabolism, the exact cause for changes in serum concentrations of serum metabolites is often unknown. Still, a better understanding of the physiological pathways is helpful to potentially pinpoint specific diseases.[6]

Texas A & M, Gastrointestinal Laboratory has developed a canine microbiota dysbiosis index (CDI), a PCR-based assay that qualifies the abundance of seven bacterial groups and the total bacteria typically found, and summaries them into one number.[11] This allows veterinarians to assess whether a dog has changes in the fecal microbiota composition. Using the abundance of the bacteria *Clostridium hiranonis*, the assay can predict the intestine's normal or abnormal conversion of bile acids. A lack of conversion of primary bile acids to secondary bile acids significantly contributes to abnormal microbiota.[11] The results provided by the lab will supply the DI found in the sample submitted for testing.[11] The Texas A & M site can be referenced for more in-depth information. (see Table 10.1 and Figure 10.1).

Measuring the serum concentrations of cobalamin and folate, two crucial markers for

GI health can be used to evaluate the presence or absence of disease. The uptake of cobalamin (vitamin B12) and folate (vitamin B9) from the small intestine are dependent on several factors. They can be utilized as an indirect marker for the presence of gastrointestinal disease. Disorders that may affect serum cobalamin and folate concentrations include small intestinal inflammation, exocrine pancreatic insufficiency (EPI) and small intestinal bacterial overgrowth (SIBO).

Table 10.1 Canine microbiota dysbiosis index.

Bacteria	Normal abundance*	Change observed in dysbiosis
Faecalibacterium	3.4–8.0	Decreased
Turicibacter	4.6–8.1	Decreased
Streptococcus	1.9–8.0	Increased
E. coli	0.9–8.0	Increased
Blautia	9.5–11.0	Decreased
Fusobacterium	7.0–10.3	Decreased
Clostridium hiranonis	5.1–7.1	Decreased
Dysbiosis index	<0 normal	
	0–2 equivocal	
	>2 dysbiosis	

*Numbers expressed as log DNA/gram of feces.
Source: Adapted from Canine Dysbiosis Index.[11]

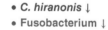

- **C. hiranonis** ↓
- **Fusobacterium** ↓
- Blautia ↓

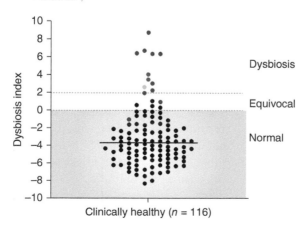

Figure 10.1 Sample dysbiosis index, compiled from 116 healthy dogs.

Cobalamin absorption is complex and requires a functioning GI tract and the presence of intrinsic factor produced in the stomach. Major disorders that interfere with cobalamin uptake are EPI, distal or diffuse small intestinal inflammatory disease, and excess bacterial utilization of cobalamin in bacterial dysbiosis. Decreased absorption ultimately leads to metabolic consequences on a cellular level.[6,11]

Dietary folate is typically present in a poorly absorbable form. In dogs, increased serum folate concentrations can be seen with proximal SIBO, as resident bacteria in the distal small intestine (i.e., ileum) and the large intestine can produce large quantities of folate.[6] Because the carriers responsible for folate uptake are located exclusively in the proximal small intestine, folate produced in distal sections of the intestine cannot be absorbed. However, if folate-producing bacteria proliferate in the proximal small intestine, the host can absorb the bacterial folate, resulting in increased serum folate concentrations. In contrast, diffuse inflammation in the proximal GI tract may damage receptors and decrease serum folate concentrations.[6]

Another critical pathway that is altered in GI disease is bile acid metabolism. Changes in intestinal bile acid metabolism have been implicated as an important factor in intestinal inflammation in human inflammatory bowel disease (IBD) patients and *Clostridium difficile* infection. The therapeutic correction of altered bile acid concentrations can lead to improvements in intestinal inflammation.[6] Unconjugated bile acids are toxic to epithelial cells, resulting in increased intestinal permeability from cellular damage. Altered bile acid profiles can lead to changes in fat absorption from the small intestine. Altered serum unconjugated bile acids have also been associated with altered small intestinal microbiota in dogs.[6,11]

A recent study has shown an increased serum D-lactate concentration in cats with various gastrointestinal diseases. The D-isomer of lactic acid is not generally found in any appreciable quantities in serum from mammals. The increase in serum D-lactate in cats with gastrointestinal disease is possibly due to disturbances in the intestinal microbiota and increased bacterial production of D-lactate. D-lactate has been shown to lead to neurological signs in some cats.[6]

Conclusion

Associations between the intestinal microbiota and health or disease must be interpreted for what they are – associations and not necessarily causation.[3] Identifying causation and associations can be difficult, particularly when there may be different influences on the disease process and microbiota, including differences in diet.[3]

As more is learned about the composition and function of the microbiome, we will also need to address ways to keep this population as healthy and happy as the host they inhabit. The microbiota plays an important role in the development, immune regulation and maintenance of health for the host animals.[3]

References

1 Middlebos, Ingmar S. Vester Boler, Brittany M. Qu, Ani, et al. Phylogenetic Characterization of Fecal Microbial Communities of Dogs Fed Diets with or without Supplemental Dietary Fiber using 454 Pyrosequencing. www.plosone.org March 2010, **5**(3), e9768. (Accessed 10/30/21).

2 Suchodolski JS (2015) The GI microbiome in domestic animals – contributions to health and disease. *ACVIM Proceedings*.

3 Weese JS (2015) The gut microbiota: can we predict and prevent gastrointestinal disease? *ACVIM Proceedings.*

4 Mansfield C (2021) Assessing when the microbiome needs to be manipulated. *ACVIM Proceedings.*

5 Pilla R, Suchodolski J (2021) The gut microbiome of dogs and cats, and the influence of diet. In D Laflamme (ed.), *Veterinary Clinics, Small Animal Practice Small Animal Nutrition*, pp. 605–15, Philadelphia, PA: Elsevier.

6 Suchodolski JS (2015) *Metabolic Consequences of Gut Dysbiosis and Inflammation*, ACVIM Proceedings.

7 Weese, J Scott. Beneficial Bacteria: Primer on Probiotics and GI Health. Nutramax Laboratories Quick Course handout.

8 Wolowcz I, Verwaerde C, Viltart O *et al.* Feeding our immune systems: impact on metabolism. *Journal of Clinical and Developmental Immunity* **2008**, Article ID 639803. doi: https://doi.org/10.1155/2008/639803.

9 Suchodolski, Jan S. Simpson, Kenneth. Canine gastrointestinal microbiome in health and disease. Veterinary Focus, Vol 23 n2/2013.

10 Cave N (2012) Nutritional management of gastrointestinal diseases. In A Fascetti, SJ Delany (eds), *Applied Veterinary Clinical Nutrition*, pp. 177–82, Ames, Iowa: Wiley-Blackwell Publishing.

11 Canine Dysbiosis Index. Texas A & M Gastrointestinal Laboratory. https://vetmed.tamu.edu/gilab/service/assays/canine-microbiota-dysbiosis-index/ (Accessed 10/30/21).

11

Prebiotics, Probiotics and Synbiotics

Introduction

Products that include probiotics, prebiotics or both (synbiotics) are readily available on the market. These can be in supplements, known as nutraceuticals, over-the-counter foods and therapeutic diets.

These products are proposed to improve the immune system and gastrointestinal (GI) function while performing many other tasks.

Definitions

According to currently adopted definitions by the Food and Agriculture Organization of the United Nations and the World Health Organization, probiotics are "living microorganisms which when administered in adequate amounts confer a health benefit on the host."[1] In contrast, prebiotics are "nondigestible food ingredients that selectively stimulate the growth and activities of specific bacteria in the gastrointestinal tract and exert beneficial effects on the host."[2] A synbiotic is a balanced combination of prebiotics and probiotics used together.[3,4] The US Food and Drug Administration defines nutraceuticals as "nondrug substances produced in a purified or extracted form and administered orally to provide agents required for normal body structure and function with the intent of improving health and wellbeing." (see Figure 11.1).[5]

As seen by these definitions, this refers to bacteria or substances that are beneficial to

Prebiotics

- Food for bacteria.
- Serve as food for intestinal bacteria and produce energy for intestinal cells.
- Plant fibers that can be easily added to pet foods or given as supplements.

Probiotics

- Live bacteria.
- Used to help adjust intestinal bacterial population.
- Difficult to add to foods.
- Available as supplements.

Synbiotics

- Combination of a probiotic and a prebiotic.
- Available as supplements.
- Not added to foods.

Figure 11.1 The difference between prebiotics, probiotics and synbiotics. *Source*: Adapted from Pan et al. [2]

bacteria in the intestinal tract. Millions of bacteria typically reside in normal, healthy animals' small and large intestines; we call this population the microflora. These bacteria help digest food, maintain intestinal mucosal integrity, participate in metabolism and stimulate systemic immune function.[6]

Because nutraceuticals are not pharmaceuticals, regulatory scrutiny over the sale of these items is minimal. Thus, it can be challenging to

Nutrition and Disease Management for Veterinary Technicians and Nurses, Third Edition. Ann Wortinger and Kara M. Burns.
© 2024 John Wiley & Sons, Inc. Published 2024 by John Wiley & Sons, Inc.
Companion Website: www.wiley.com/go/wortinger/3e

find products that do what their manufacturers say and contain viable bacteria in the types and amounts specified on the label.[7] Not all commercially available products provide the same level of usefulness, so it is crucial to understand what products, especially probiotics, have been evaluated in dogs and cats. Not all bacteria provide the same benefits with all species, nor are all products tested and evaluated to the same extent.

The Intestines

The intestines are the largest component of the immune system in the body, making up approximately 70% of the total system. The mucosal barrier in the intestines helps block the entrance of most pathogenic bacteria into the body while allowing permeable nutrients.[6] Because most pathogens enter the body through the mouth and then the intestinal tract, these intestinal defenses must be working optimally to cope with the onslaught of foreign substances and pathogens to which the intestines are constantly exposed.[6]

This defense involves the coordination of three different systems within the intestines:

● Resident intestinal microflora, which provides an environment that favors the growth and functioning of beneficial bacteria
● Intestinal mucosa, which provides a barrier against pathogenic bacteria
● Gut-associated lymphoid tissue (GALT)[6]

It would be difficult to affect the intestinal mucosa or the GALT, but the intestinal microflora can be modulated to improve the environment the bacteria are living in, which may have a positive impact on the dog or cat. Substantial research is looking at how enteral nutrition can help improve both the GALT and the intestinal mucosa barrier. Currently, prebiotics and probiotics are being used to help with this modulation of the GALT.[4]

Efforts to maintain a healthy microflora in the GI tract or rebalance the gut microbes after a disruption has focused on:

– Dietary manipulation
– Helminth therapy
– Fecal microbiota transplantation
– Prebiotic, probiotic and synbiotic use
– Antibiotics[3]

Probiotics can also help control diarrhea caused by bacterial overgrowth or parasitic infection via competitive exclusion, competition for nutrients and binding sites and increased specific and nonspecific immune responses.[6]

Antibiotics are seen as a significant destroyer of the normal GI flora and can negatively affect function. Although antibiotics are usually prescribed for a specific reason, they are not necessarily bacteria- or site-specific; instead, they destroy or kill any bacteria that fall within its spectrum, regardless of whether the bacteria are beneficial or pathogenic.[3]

Suppose an antibiotic is prescribed orally for pneumonia. In that case, it still must pass through the intestines and exert its antibacterial effect on that site and the lungs, where the actual infection is occurring. Antibiotics used as growth promoters can exert an even more significant effect on the microflora than those used intermittently.[3]

Prebiotics

Prebiotics are usually considered to be a type of carbohydrate called oligosaccharides. By definition, however, noncarbohydrates can be classified as prebiotics. The ones used most frequently are classified as soluble fibers.

These were first identified as functional food in 1995 by Marcel Roberfroid. In 2007, Roberfroid clarified that only two classes of fructooligosaccharides (FOS) fully meet the definition of a prebiotic: oligofructose (FOS) and inulin.[8]

Oligofructose is a 2–8 chain fructose-based saccharide molecule that undergoes fermentation fairly quickly in the colon, providing nourishment to the bacteria in that area.

Examples of FOS sources include soybeans, oats, beets and tomatoes.

Inulin is a longer 9–64 chain fructose-based saccharide that tends to be fermented more slowly, benefiting bacteria farther down the colon. It can also be broken down into FOS by intestinal bacteria to provide both FOS and inulin. Inulin can be found in Jerusalem artichokes, jicama and chicory root.

These two fibers are considered minimally digestible because of the β bond-based connections of the fructose molecules. Dogs and cats lack the intestinal enzyme needed to break down the β bond; instead, their enzymes break down α saccharide bonds. The resident bacteria in these animals can break the β bond, producing short-chain fatty acids (SCFAs). The most common SCFAs are acetate, propionate and butyrate.[4]

Plants do not have only one type of carbohydrate in them; some may contain both FOS and inulin in varying amounts, whereas others may contain neither. Just adding fiber to the diet may or may not provide prebiotic effects. That benefit depends on the types of fibers found in the product.[4]

The SCFAs produced by the breaking of the β bond through bacterial fermentation are an energy source for the colonocytes, lower the colonic pH and stimulate sodium and water absorption.[2] One SCFA in particular, butyrate or butyric acid, is a primary source of energy for colonocytes but may also directly enhance the cell proliferation of normal cells while suppressing the proliferation of transformed cells. Because both oligofructose and inulin are fibers, their addition to the diet can also have adverse side effects. When used at higher levels, both FOS and inulin reduce fecal protein digestibility.[2]

Studies have shown that adding FOS and fructose-based inulins to the diet generally positively affects gut microflora and host health, as evaluated through gut integrity and bacterial colonization, and animal performance, as evaluated through digestion, body weight gain and feed efficiency.[9]

Probiotics

Probiotics present an appealing approach to the treatment and prevention of many conditions because of their potential to be effective, safe and decrease the use of antibiotics in veterinary medicine.[7] Rather than encouraging the growth of beneficial bacteria and suppressing the growth of pathogenic bacteria, probiotics introduce these beneficial bacteria into the environment. Current knowledge suggests that the best use for these products is treating GI diseases, such as diarrhea and other GI abnormalities, potentially including inflammatory bowel disease.[10]

Studies in different animal species have often demonstrated bacterial strain-specific results. Thus, unless the exact product is used on the same species used in the study, at the same dose and delivery method, actual results will likely not be the same as those the researchers showed.[10]

To function as a probiotic, the bacteria must be able to:

- Survive the acidic pH and bile acids found in the GI tract.
- Adhere to the intestinal cells or transiently colonize various areas within the GI tract.
- Exclude or reduce pathogenic bacterial adherence.
- Produce acids, hydrogen peroxide, or bacteriocins that antagonize the growth of pathogens.
- Coaggregate to help achieve a normal balanced microflora population.
- Be safe, noninvasive, noncarcinogenic and nonpathogenic.[2]

The GI tract of a newborn is initially sterile but is colonized with bacteria within hours of birth. These bacteria find their niches within the intestinal tract and reach a state of equilibrium. Once this neonatal "grace period" ends, however, introducing bacteria is substantially more difficult because of gastric acidity and the introduction of bile acids to the chyme leaving the stomach.[6]

No studies have shown that supplementing pet diets with yogurt or other fermented food products, such as kimchee or sauerkraut, benefits the pets themselves. The bacteria found in these products are limited in amount and type and may not be the kind that benefits the health issue being addressed.[1,10] Research has also failed to demonstrate that routinely adding probiotics to the diet improves overall wellness in otherwise healthy animals.[10]

The primary bacterial populations in probiotics that benefit the cats and dogs are lactic acid bacteria, especially lactobacilli, bifidobacteria and enterococci. These bacteria use fermentation to transform some sugars into organic acids, mainly lactic and acetic acids. These acids lower the pH in the intestinal tract and inhibit the growth of pathogenic bacteria. (see Table 11.1).[6]

Probiotics can benefit the intestinal microflora in many ways. They can increase the fecal count of good bacteria while decreasing the number of pathogenic bacteria. Some probiotics minimize adherence to the intestinal epithelial cells and the establishment of pathogenic bacterial populations.[6]

Probiotics can produce various antimicrobial metabolites, known as bacteriocins, that can also enhance the functionality of the epithelial barrier and help modulate the mucosal immune response.[3] Compared with the large intestine, the small intestine has poor microflora colonization and limited barrier protection against pathogens. Therefore, probiotics can exert a crucial beneficial effect on the small intestines.[3,6]

The recommendation is to rely on a product for which research supports both the product and the manufacturer's claims. The most extensively researched probiotic available in veterinary medicine is Forti Flora™ (purina.com).[3]

Synbiotics

Synbiotics are a balanced combination of probiotics and prebiotics and may be advantageous for treating various GI diseases. The prebiotic portion may improve the conditions in the GI tract, enabling the probiotics to maximize survival, and may increase the proliferation and adherence of the beneficial bacteria.[4] Prebiotics may enhance or potentiate the benefits of the probiotics found in these products.

Benefits can also be obtained by using two separate products, given simultaneously, as with using a probiotic in a food that has been supplemented with prebiotic fiber.[4]

Table 11.1 Good and bad intestinal bacteria.

Beneficial	Pathogenic
Lactobacilli	*Pseudomonas aeruginosa*
Eubacteria	*Proteus* species
Bifidobacterium	Staphylococci
Enterococci	Clostridia
Streptococcus	Saccharomyces
Pediococcus	Veillonella
Leuconostoc	
Bacillus	
Escherichia coli	

Source: Adapted from Ref. [3].

Survivability and Label Claims

One of the biggest challenges for manufacturers of probiotic products is the survivability of the bacteria. Most commercially available products suffer tremendous loss of activity during storage. After 5–6 months of storage, almost no live organisms are present. Bacteria still must survive the gastric pH and duodenal bile acids before colonizing the small and large intestines. To address these concerns, some manufacturers have developed microencapsulation to protect the bacteria, while others provide a variety of bacterial species to cover more bases.[6]

A study done by Weese and Martin at the University of Guelph in Ontario, Canada, compared the actual product contents versus label statements for a variety of commercially available probiotics.[7] Of the 25 products evaluated, only 2 had acceptable correspondence between the actual production of bacteria classes and what was stated on the label. All products were evaluated before their expiration dates.[7] Prostora™ (produced at the time by the Iams Company) and Forti Flora™ were the top performers. Prostora™ was discontinued after Royal Canin acquired Iams. Forti Flora™ is still commercially available. Purina has recently introduced a synbiotic product called Forti Flora SA™ that contains both psyllium fiber and *Enterococcus faecium*.

A study looking at the multispecies symbiotic, Proviable-DC® (Nutramax Laboratories) in dogs and cats used various complementary molecular tools to evaluate the effect of a symbiotic on fecal bacterial composition.[11] The analysis suggested an increase in fecal abundance of the administered organisms during the testing period. The team was unable to verify if this increase was due to the ingestion of the probiotic stains or if they belonged to the same bacterial species but were, in fact, different strains. The results strongly suggest that the increase was due to the administered probiotic.[11] This study was conducted on healthy dogs and cats.

Conclusion

Because prebiotics is both a source of nutrition for the colonocytes and a fiber source for the animal, inclusion in the diet is relatively easy. The ingredient panel should list the fiber source but may not state whether it is a source of FOS or inulin. Ensuring familiarity with the different fiber sources used and their relative FOS and inulin contents can help evaluate a diet. When in doubt, contact the manufacturer for further information.

Unlike prebiotics, probiotics are more of a transient process based on need rather than a long-term process. Ideally, the body will supply the bacterial population to support the best intestinal health. But when this does not occur or challenges that could affect intestinal health are expected, probiotics can be easily added to the diet to help support the bacterial populations there. Unlike with the use of long-term antibiotics, no detrimental effects have been seen with long-term prebiotic or probiotic use in animals.[4]

When evaluating prebiotic or probiotic products, ensure that research supports the claims given, that the products contain the stated levels of additives, and that the products promote normal intestinal microflora.

Weese and Arroyo's review of probiotics in commercial dog and cat foods demonstrated that few products meet these guidelines.[1] Alternately, evaluation in a controlled clinical setting can provide firsthand knowledge of the effectiveness of the products used. By applying this strategy, it can be assured that the best product to support a happy, healthy intestinal tract with a hard-working population of beneficial bacteria is provided.

References

1 Weese JS, Arroyo L (2003) Bacteriological evaluation of dog and cat diets that claim to contain probiotics. *The Canadian Veterinary Journal* **44**(3): 212–6.

2 Pan XD, Chen FQ, Wu TX *et al.* (2009) Prebiotic oligosaccharides change the concentrations of short-chain fatty acids and the microbial population of mouse bowel. *Journal of Zhejiang University. Science. B* **10**(4): 258–63.

3 Marks S. Probiotics—not just for people anymore. Proceedings of the 2017

Western Veterinary Conference, Las Vegas, Nevada.

4 Steiner JM. Understanding the benefits of prebiotics. *dvm 360*. July 1, 2009. veterinarycalendar.dvm 360.com/veterinary-team-understanding-benefits-prebiotics-sponsored-iams. Accessed 10/31/21.

5 Lerman A, Lockwood B (2007) Nutraceuticals in veterinary medicine. *The Pharmaceutical Journal* **278**: 51.

6 Kelly M. The role of probiotics in GI tract health. Nestle Purina PetCare Company. purinaproplanvets.com/media/1181/role_of_probiotics.pdf 2006.

7 Weese JS, Martin H (2011) Assessment of commercial probiotic bacterial contents and label accuracy. *The Canadian Veterinary Journal* **521**: 43–6.

8 Roberfroid M (2007) Prebiotics: the concept revisited. *The Journal of Nutrition* **137**(3 Suppl 2): 830S.

9 Verdonk JM, Shim SB, Van Leeuwen P, Verstegan MW (2005) Application of inulin-type fructans in animal feed and pet food. *The British Journal of Nutrition* **93**(Suppl 1): s125–38.

10 Heinz CR Good bugs/bad bugs: the confusing world of probiotic supplements. *Pet Foodology* vetnutrition.tufts.edu/2017/06/probiotics. Accessed 10/31/21.

11 Garcia-Mascorro JF, Lanerie DJ, Dowd SE *et al.* (2011) The effect of multi-species symbiotic formulation on fecal bacterial microbiota of healthy cats and dogs as evaluated by pyrosequencing. *FEMS Microbiology Ecology* **78**(3): 542–4 https://academic.oup.com/femsec/article/78/3/542/601835. Accessed 10/31/21.

12

Nutrition Calculations

Introduction

Math is a part of our everyday world; we find it everywhere, from balancing your checkbook to calculating calories for Mrs. Smith's overweight Bassett. The more comfortable we are with doing these calculations, the more accurate our results will be. While not as potentially devastating as a drug dosage error, miscalculating calories, energy or food intake can have equally poor outcomes for our patients.

Ideally, the veterinarian will tell you what diet requirements they want, and you can take everything from there. You can determine caloric requirements, figure feeding volumes and even the percent of weight loss desired. The better your skills, the more challenged and less bored you will be in your work every day, and the more you can help your patients.

Units of Measure

In the United States, we commonly use the US customary units—the pounds, ounces, inches and feet that we are all familiar with.[1] As we all know, there is no consistency between weight, volume and length, and you have to memorize the conversions. Weight is measured in ounces, pounds and tons, length is measured in inches, feet, yards and miles, and volume in ounces, cups, pints, quarts and gallons. Conversions between the various units are tedious and often confusing. We learn early on that:

1 cup (c) = 8 ounces (oz)
16 ounces (oz) = 1 pound (lb or #)
2 pints (pt) = 1 quart (qt)
4 quarts (qt) = 1 gallon (gal)
12 inches (in or ") = 1 foot (ft or ')
3 feet (ft) = 1 yard (yd)
5,280 feet (ft) = 1 mile (m)
2,000 pounds (lb or #) = 1 ton (t)

There is no rhyme or reason for the units; we need to know them. ☺

The metric system was developed after the French Revolution in 1795 to make measuring more consistent and remove regional differences. The most significant advantage of this unit of measure is that it is divided into equal parts throughout the entire system. By simply moving decimal points, you can go from one unit of measure to another. Also, conversions between weight, length and volume are easier to figure out than US Customary units.

For metric units, weight is measured in grams, volume is measured in liters and length is measured in meters. By moving your decimal point to the right or the left, you can divide or multiply the unit being measured and easily convert from, for example, milligrams to kilograms. Everything is determined by units of 10, maintaining consistency throughout the entire system. We know that:

1 millimeter (mL) = 1 centimeter (cc)
1000 mL = 1 liter (L)
1000 grams (g) = 1 kilogram (kg)
1 kilogram (kg) = 1 liter (L)

Nutrition and Disease Management for Veterinary Technicians and Nurses, Third Edition. Ann Wortinger and Kara M. Burns.
© 2024 John Wiley & Sons, Inc. Published 2024 by John Wiley & Sons, Inc.
Companion Website: www.wiley.com/go/wortinger/3e

10 centimeters (cm) = 1 decimeter (dm) = 0.10 meter (m)

Each space to the left of the decimal point increases the value by a power of 10. Conversely, each space to the right of the decimal point decreases the value by a power of 10. The most common units seen in medicine include:

Deci- 10^{-1} (d)
Centi- 10^{-2} (c)
Milli- 10^{-3} (m)
Micro 10^{-6} (μ)
Deca- 10^{1} (d)
Hecto- 10^{2} (h)
Kilo- 10^{3} (k)

You determine the number of spaces to move your decimal point right or left to convert from one unit to another. This provides much more consistency and straightforward math than the US Customary units.

Converting Units

The biggest problem we have with the two most common units of measure, the US Customary units, and the metric units, is that they have very little in common. If you are like most technicians, you weigh your patients in pounds on the scale and then have to convert this to kilograms to calculate drug dosages or fluid rates. We have given ourselves an extra step by not using metrics in our everyday lives. 🙂 If we send medications or foods home with clients, we have to reconvert these amounts back to a value that they can utilize and recognize, resulting in even more conversions for us!

Like the US Customary units, we have to know the conversions to do these calculations accurately.

\# - 2.2 kg
1 kg = 0.45 #
1 teaspoon (tsp) = 5 mL
1 tablespoon (Tbl) = 15 mL
1 oz = 30 mL

1 cup = 240 mL
1 centimeter = 2.54 inches

The hardest part is remembering what needs to be done where and using what conversion. The most common nutrition calculation we deal with is converting between pounds and kilograms.

Example:

1 # = 2.2 kg
1 kg = 0.45 #
A 10# cat would weigh 4.5 kg

$$10\#/2.2 = 4.5$$

A 25# dog would weigh 11.4 kg

$$25\#/2.2 = 11.4$$

To convert from kilograms to pounds, you would multiply rather than divide by 2.2

Example:

A 5 kg cat would weigh 11#

$$5 \text{ kg} \times 2.2 = 11\#$$

A 25 kg dog would weigh 55 #

$$25 \text{ kg} \times 2.2 = 55\#$$

If these conversions are done incorrectly, the result would be an over twofold increase or decrease in the desired value. This is a pretty significant amount. When converting from pounds to kilograms, your final number should be smaller. When converting from kilograms to pounds, your final number should be bigger.

Calculating Resting Energy Requirements (RER)

This is our base calculation when figuring out daily calorie requirements. You can use either a linear formula such as:

$$\left(\text{wt in kg} \times 30 \right) + 70 = RER$$

Or a logarithmic formula such as

$$70 \times \text{kg body weight}^{0.75}$$

Using the linear formula is easier mathematically but is not as accurate over a wide range of body weights (<2 kg and >30 kg) as the logarithmic formula.

Example:

Body weight 28#
Convert to kg = 28/2.2 = 12.7 kg
RER = (BW kg × 30) + 70 = (12.7 × 30) + 70 = 451 kcal/day

The logarithmic formula is more complex, especially when using a four-function calculator, but it can be done.

Example:

Body weight 28#
Convert to kg = 28/2.2 = 12.7 kg
RER = 70 × (BW in kg$^{0.75}$) = (kg × kg × kg, $\sqrt{}, \sqrt{}$) × 70
(12.7 × 12.7 × 12.7 $\sqrt{}, \sqrt{}$) = 6.7 × 70 = 471 kcal/day

As both of these formulas are estimates of the animal's actual energy requirements, the animal should determine any intake adjustments. If they are hungry or losing weight, then increase the volume being fed. If they are gaining weight or are vomiting, then decrease the volume being fed.

Calculating Daily Energy Requirements (DER)

Daily energy requirements (DER) are calculated from the RER but utilize the animal's activity level to supply any extra calories required for daily maintenance.[2]

$$\text{DER} = \text{RER} \times 1.0 - 1.6 \text{ (dependent on}$$
$$\text{energy expenditure)}$$

Refer to Chapter 9 for more information on Life Stage factors.

Example:

Body weight 28# or 12.7 kg
RER = 451 – 471 kcal/day
DER = 451 – 471 × 1.0–1.6

Our dog is moderately active and goes on (2) 60-min walks/day. We will select 1.4 as our DER Life Stage factor.

$$\text{DER} = 451 - 471 \times 1.4 = 633 - 659 \text{ kcal/day}$$

As with RER, cut back if the animal is gaining weight on the amount of food fed. If they are hungry or losing weight, increase the amount fed.

Calculating Feeding Amounts

The feeding amounts are determined by the caloric density of the food selected and the kcal requirements for that animal. If you choose to follow the package direction on feeding volume, the animal will most likely not lose weight and may very well gain weight as calories are not a "one size fits all" equation.

Take the kcals required and divide that by the caloric density of the food selected.

Example:

Calories needed/day = 633–659 kcal
Calorie density of the food:
259 kcal/cup (standard 8 oz measuring cup)
417 kcal/can
633–659/259 kcal/cup = 2.44–2.54 cups.
633–659/417 kcal/can = 1.5–1.58 cans.

As we want to make this as user-friendly as possible for the owner, we need to select a unit of measure they can achieve. It is unlikely that a client will know how to get 0.44 parts of a cup but could easily do 0.5. The same is true for the canned volume. We can tell the client to feed 0.58 parts of a can. What is the likelihood that they will be able to comply with this request? They can quickly figure out 0.5 parts of a can, though.

I would recommend either 2.5 cups of dry food/day or 1.5 cans of canned food/day for this animal. Many clients like to feed a combination of canned and dry foods. How will that affect your feeding volumes?

Take the kcals/day, determine how much canned you want to feed/day or how much dry you want to feed/day, and then determine the remaining amount.

Example:

BW 28#/ 12.7 kg
DER = 633–659 kcal/day
259 kcal/cup (standard 8 oz measuring cup)
417 kcal/can

The owner wants to feed one can of food divided into two feedings, with the remaining calories supplied by the dry food.

$$DER = 633 - 659 - 417 \ (1 \ can \ of \ food)$$
$$= 216 - 242 \ calories \ remaining$$
$$that \ can \ be \ supplied \ by \ dry \ food$$

$$216 - 242/259 \ kcal/cup$$
$$= 0.83 - 0.93 \ cups/day.$$

I would likely recommend a "scant" 1 cup of dry food. This is taking the measuring cup and not quite filling it up. Make sure that clients understand what is meant by 1 cup. A level cup, not a heaping cup. ☺ A standard 8 oz measuring cup is used in the kitchen, not a 7/11 Big Gulp cup!!

Tube Feeding Calculations

When feeding through a feeding tube, whether it's a nasoesophageal, esophagostomy, gastrostomy or jejunostomy, you are going to be feeding in mls instead of cups or cans.

Diets that go through feeding tubes are either a liquid diet or a gruel. The consistency will vary based on the tube diameter. Typically, a liquid diet is needed for tubes smaller than 12 fr (external diameter in millimeters multiplied by 3 = the French size). A 12 fr tube would be 4 mm outside diameter. A gruel diet can usually be used in a tube >12 fr but may

still need to be thinned with water to ease the passage. Remember, when adding water to any diet, this dilutes the calories in that diet.

The RER and DER calculations are exactly the same. When you get down to how much to feed/day, the final amount will be in mls, and each meal fed will also be in mls.

Using our 28# dog from above, an 18 fr esophagostomy tube was placed due to facial trauma. We want to feed him Hills a/d™ diet three times daily.

Example:

Bodyweight 28# or 12.7 kg
RER = 451–471 kcal/day
DER = 451–471 × 1.4 = 631–659 kcal/day
Hill's a/d™ diet has 1.1 kcal/mL, 180 kcals/ 5.5 oz can.
631 kcal/day ÷ 1.1 kcal/mL = 574 mL/day
659 kcal/day ÷ 1.1 kcal/mL = 599 mL/day
If giving 3 equal feedings/day
574–599 mL/3 = 191–200 mL/meal
Each can = 180 kcal
191–200/180 kcals = 1–1.1 can/meal

Converting Guaranteed Analysis to Energy Density

Energy density is the percent in the diet of a nutrient x the modified Atwater factor for that nutrient = kcal/100 gm of food. Energy density differs from metabolizable energy (ME) in that nondigestible energy lost through feces and urine is not accounted for. The energy lost through "dietary thermogenesis" is also not accounted for. This is the energy required for the digestion and assimilation of nutrients in the body. Also, remember that when working with the Guaranteed Analysis, the numbers are represented as minimums (protein and fat) and maximums (crude fiber and moisture) and not the actual values found in that food. As long as the food meets these numbers, the actual values can vary significantly.

Modified Atwater factors for protein and carbohydrates are 3.5 kcal/g. For fats, they are

8.5 kcal/g. This is the number of calories for that nutrient found in 1 g of food.

Example Dog Kibble Guaranteed Analysis

P 6.0% × 3.5 = 21 kcal/g protein
F 2.8% × 8.5 = 23.8 kcal/g fat
CHO 14.7% × 3.5 = 51.45 kcal/g CHO
    96.25 kcal/g/100 kcal

Note: Carbohydrates are not usually listed on the Guaranteed Analysis. They must be extrapolated from the nitrogen-free extract, or the manufacturer can be contacted for the actual digestible carbohydrate content.

Energy Density Equals

Energy density is useful to determine the actual percentage a particular nutrient contributes to the caloric content. Take the calculated kcal/g and divide that by the total kcals/g for all nutrients. Multiply by 100 to find the percent.

Example:

P 21/96.25 × 100 = 22%
F 23.8/96.25 × 100 = 25%
CHO 51.45/96.25 × 100 = 53%

The Guaranteed Analysis would assume that only 2.8% of the calories come from fat. By calculating the energy density, you can see that, in fact, 25% of the calories come from fat.

Calculating Nutrients as a Percent Metabolizable Energy (ME) Total Calories in 100 g of Food

Protein = 3.5 kcal/g X grams in food
Fat = 8.5 kcal/g X grams in food
Carbohydrate = 3.5 kcal/g X grams in food
Total calories/100 g = protein calorie + fat calorie + carbohydrate calorie

Percentage of ME Contributed by Each Nutrient (Caloric Distribution)

Protein = (protein calories/100 g divided by total calories/100 g) X 100 = % ME

Fat = (fat calories/100 g divided by total calories/100 g) X 100 = % ME

Carbohydrate = (carbohydrate calories/100 g divided by total calories) X 100 = % ME

Example Dry Dog food (as Fed)

Moisture 8%
P 21.4% × 3.5 = 74.9 kcal/100 g of food
F 10.1% × 8.5 = 85.85 kcal/100 g of food
CHO 52.3% × 3.5 = 183.05 kcal/100 g of food
Total calories per 100 g = 344 kcal
    ME Estimate

P = (74.9/344) × 100 = 22%
F = (85.85/344) × 100 = 25%
CHO = (183.05/344) × 100 = 53%

Calculating Meals per Can/Cup/Bag

When we send food home, the client wants to know how long the food will last. This is a more straightforward calculation with canned food but can be more of a mental math challenge to come up with dry foods. The main reason for this challenge is that we are feeding the food in cups, but the manufacturer is selling it in pounds. ☺

We can determine how many ounces are in each cup of food by weighing it on the baby or small animal scale and then seeing how many "meals" are in the bag.

Example:

We want to feed 2.5 cups of dry food/day to our patient. We sell the client a 20# bag of food. How long will this bag be expected to last the client?

1 cup of food = 5.5 oz (if this was water 1 cup = 8 oz, but food is usually less dense)

20# bag of food = _____ ounces (oz)

Remember 1# = 16 oz

20# × 16 = 320 oz

Take the 320 oz/5.5 oz/cup = 58 cups of food

Each meal is 2.5 cups

58 cups/2.5 cups/day = 23 days' worth of food

Cost of Feeding

Many clients assume that the better the food brand, the more expensive it will be to feed. By calculating the cost/meal, we can demonstrate that the actual cost is not that much higher or maybe even lower between different brands of foods.

We just covered how to figure out the number of meals in a bag of food. By taking that amount and dividing the food's actual cost, you can determine the cost/meal. Again, this is easier to do with canned food, but make sure that when comparing, you compare dry food to dry food and canned food to canned food. With the substantial differences in moisture content, canned food is inherently higher in price than dry food.

When using a therapeutic diet, it is often helpful to equate feeding the food to allow less medication to be administered, thus decreasing the overall cost of medication and ease of administration. Therapeutic diets are more expensive than over-the-counter (OTC) foods, but they provide benefits that cannot be achieved with OTC foods. Often, there is no equivalent food available OTC because you need to have a veterinarian managing the disease processes, not the client.

Example:

Canned food-
Your patient requires 1.25 cans of food twice daily. The cost/can is $0.89/can.

$$(1.25 \times 2) \times 0.89 = \$2.23/\text{day} \times 30$$
$$= \$66.75/\text{month}$$

Dry food-
Therapeutic dog diet
20# bag = $43.00

20# × 16 = 320 oz
Take the 320 oz/5.5 oz/cup = 58 cups of food
Each meal is 2.5 cups
58 cups/2.5 cups/day = 23 days' worth of food
On a per meal basis $43.00/23 days = $1.87/day to feed

If we look at a "less expensive" brand of OTC food that is cheaper, lacks the therapeutic value of the veterinary diet, but is also less digestible, we will see that the OTC food may actually be more expensive or similar cost to feed.

Low-Cost Dog Food

20# = $32.00
1 cup of food = 5.5 oz (if this was water 1 cup = 8 oz, but food is usually less dense)
20# bag of food = _____ ounces (oz)

Remember 1# = 16 oz

20# × 16 = 320 oz
Take the 320 oz/5.5 oz/cup = 58 cups of food
Each meal is 3.5 cups (less caloric density than therapeutic diet)
58 cups/3.5 cups/day = 16 days' worth of food
On a per meal basis $32.00/16 days = $2.00/day to feed

This calculation shows that because you have to feed more of the less expensive food, you get fewer feeding days/bag, and the overall cost/meal is more expensive.

Conclusion

By knowing how to do these standard calculations, we can offer our patients and clients better nutrition. Go forth and use your calculator with confidence and astound those around you.

References

1 Bill R (2000) *Medical Mathematics and Dosage Calculations for Veterinary Professionals*, Ames, IO: Blackwell Publishing.

2 Ramsey JJ (2012) Determining energy requirements. In S Delaney, A Fascetti (eds), *Applied Veterinary Clinical Nutrition*, pp. 23–45, Ames, IA: Wiley-Blackwell.

Section II

Nutritional Requirements of Dogs and Cats

13

History and Regulation of Pet Foods

Introduction

Until the mid-1800s, dogs and cats were fed primarily table scraps with supplemental scavenging.[1] Some owners may have fed homemade formulas made from human foods, but no commercial pet foods were available until 1860.[1,2]

The first commercially prepared dog food was produced by James Spratt, an American living in London, in 1860.[1,2] On his trip across the Atlantic to England, he was not impressed with the dry biscuits fed to his dog aboard the ship. Once in London, he developed a dry kibble or "dog cake" that he sold to the English huntsman for their dogs.[1] These biscuits were oven-baked and made from vegetables, beef blood, wheat and beetroot.[3] Following his success with this food in England, he expanded his sales to include the United States, where production was continued until the late 1950s when General Mills purchased it.[1,2]

In the early 1900s, several other people saw the success that Mr. Spratt was having with his dry "dog cakes" and began to develop and sell their own formulas. In 1907 F.H. Bennett, an Englishman developed and produced Milk-Bone dog biscuits in New York City.[1,2] At that time, Milk-Bones was marketed as complete dog food.[1]

Until the early 1920s, Mr. Spratt and Mr. Bennett were the two primary producers of commercial pet food. In the early 1920s, the Chappel brothers of Rockford, Illinois, produced the first batches of canned commercial food. They began by canning horse meat for dogs under the Ken-L-Ration brand name, followed by dry food in the 1930s. [1,2] By the mid-1920s, Samuel and Clarence Gaines of the Gaines Food Company from Sherburne, New York began selling a new type of dog food called meal in 100-pound bags; this was the beginning of "Gaines Dog Meal." The food differed from previous food in that several dried, ground ingredients were mixed together to form the food.[2] The advantage of this to pet owners was they could buy the food in reasonably large quantities, and very little food preparation was necessary before feeding.[2]

In the 1930s, many new brands, including Cadet and Snappy, helped make canned pet foods more popular than dry foods.[1] This continued until World War II, as pet foods were classified as "non-essential," the tin used to produce the cans was diverted to the war effort. By 1946, dry foods were about 85% of the total pet food market in the United States.[1]

Marketing of Pet Foods

In the early years of commercial pet foods, direct marketing was through feed stores. The National Biscuit Company (Nabisco) purchased Milk-Bones in 1931 and began the first attempt to market its product in grocery stores.[2] At this time, selling pet foods in human markets met with much resistance. Because most pet foods were made from by-products of human foods, customers and store owners

Nutrition and Disease Management for Veterinary Technicians and Nurses, Third Edition. Ann Wortinger and Kara M. Burns.
© 2024 John Wiley & Sons, Inc. Published 2024 by John Wiley & Sons, Inc.
Companion Website: www.wiley.com/go/wortinger/3e

considered it unsanitary to sell them next to foods meant for human consumption.[2] The convenience and economy of buying pet foods at the grocery store rapidly overcame consumer concerns.[2] Improved distribution and availability resulted in increased sales and popularity of commercial pet foods.

Today foods are heavily marketed both in commercials and advertising but also through social media sites. Many clients will do a quick Google search when looking for information.[3] Unfortunately, many people do not understand that misinformation is prevalent and seem more intent on evoking fear than providing helpful information.[3]

Production of Pet Foods

The development of the extrusion process of food production was introduced by researchers at the Purina Laboratories in the 1950s. Extrusion involves mixing all the food ingredients together, rapidly cooking the mixture, and forcing it through an extruder. The extruder is a specialized pressure cooker that allows the food to be rapidly cooked and shaped into bite-sized pieces. This process also increased the digestibility and palatability of the food produced.[2] After extrusion and drying, a coating of fat or some other palatability enhancer was usually sprayed onto the outside of the food pieces.[2] In 1957, Purina Dog Chow™ was first introduced to the commercial market. Within a year, it became the best-selling dog food in the United States and maintains a number 2 position in total dog food sales today.[1,2]

During this same time, General Foods created Gaines Burger, which combined dry food's convenience with canned food's palatability. This was the first semimoist dog food product. Ralston-Purina followed this in the 1970s with the introduction of Tender Vittles, the first semimoist cat food.[1]

Science Diet™, produced by Hill's Pet Nutrition, was initially produced as a consistently high-quality food for research kennels. In 1968, this became the first specialty product line designed for different life stages.[1] Hill's Pet Nutrition had been producing pet foods in cooperation with Dr. Mark Morris Sr. since 1948: this was the Prescription Diet™ foods that we are all familiar with. The first food produced was Hill's Science Diet K/D™ diet canned. Initially produced in Dr. Morris' office for dogs with kidney disease in his practice, this was the first food designed to aid in the dietary management of a disease.[1]

During this time, little was known about the nutrient requirements for dogs and cats. This lack of nutrition knowledge leads many manufacturers to produce the same product for both species, with only different labeling.[2] As more knowledge was acquired about different nutrient needs for dogs and cats, separate foods were formulated for each.[2] As knowledge continues to grow, more companies are developing diets that are specifically designed for specific life stages, physiologic states (low activity, moderate activity and performance diets), breed differences (small breed, large breed and long-haired) and health problems.[2]

Regulatory Agencies

Association of American Feed Control Officials

Several agencies and organizations regulate the production, marketing and sales of commercial pet foods in the United States.[2] The American Association of Feed Control Officials (AAFCO) was formed in 1909 and is composed of feed control officials from states and territories within the United States and Canada.[4] AAFCO provides a forum for local, state and federal regulatory officials to discuss and develop uniform and equitable laws, regulations and policies regarding pet foods. AAFCO formed a permanent Pet Food Committee to address the need for information about pet nutrition and pet food regulations.[4] The AAFCO remains the recognized information source for pet food labeling, ingredient definition, official terms and standardized feed testing methodology.[4]

Because the AAFCO is an association and not an official regulatory body, its policies must be voluntarily accepted by state feed control officials for actual implementation.[2] Pet food regulations can vary from state to state, and using the AAFCO's policy statements, regulations promote uniformity in feed regulations throughout the United States.[2] Today, AAFCO ensures that nationally marketed pet foods are uniformly labeled and nutritionally adequate.[2]

During the 1990s, AAFCO developed the practical nutrient profiles to be used as standards for the formulation of dog and cat foods. The profiles are based on ingredients commonly included in commercial foods, and nutrient levels are expressed for processed foods at feeding.[2] Before this, nutrient minimums were based on the recommendations of the National Research Council (NRC).[4] The NRC recommendations are based on data obtained from purified foods, assuming 100% nutrient availability for only one life stage and only giving minimum levels without any safety margins.[4] The AAFCO's nutrient profiles provide suggested levels of nutrients to be included in pet foods rather than minimum levels, as does the NRC recommendation, as well as maximum levels of selected nutrients.[2] AAFCO also publishes minimum feeding protocols for dog and cat foods. Pet food manufacturers use these minimum feeding protocols for substantiating the nutritional adequacy of pet foods using feeding trials and determining the metabolizable energy found in dog and cat food.[4] The NRC provides different requirements for growth and reproduction in dogs and cats[5] (see Table 13.1)

FDA

The Food and Drug Administration (FDA) requires that all pet food manufacturers correctly identify pet foods, provide a net quantity statement on the label, provide the proper listing of ingredients and the manufacturer's

Table 13.1 Regulatory agency that covers this area of Pet Food, and what their role is.

Agency	Role
AAFCO	Information source for pet food labeling, ingredient definition. Official terms and standardized feed testing
FDA	Government agency tasked with ensuring pet food manufacturers correctly identify pet foods, provide ingredient list, net quantity statement and address
FSMA	A congressional act that increased FDA authority to oversee and enforce supply chains
CVM	Department within FDA that regulates the use of any health claims on pet food labels
USDA	Government dept that inspects animal ingredients used in pet foods. Also inspects animal research facilities
NRC	A nonprofit organization that evaluates and compiles research conducted by others
PFI	Represent commercially prepared dog and cat food manufacturers in the USA

Source: Adapted from Case et al. and Roudebush et al.[2,4]

name and address are available and use acceptable manufacturing procedures.[2,4] Feed control officials within each state inspect facilities and enforce these regulations, although the FDA is authorized to take direct action if necessary to address any violations.[2,4]

In 2011, Congress passed the FDA Food Safety Modernization Act (FSMA). This act updated regulations regarding food production, both for human and animal foods, and it gave the FDA more authority to oversee and enforce food supply chains. The focus was also shifted from the FDA responding to contamination complaints to helping to prevent contamination from occurring.[3]

Under the FSMA regulation, animal food production facilities must register with the FDA and create and implement a food safety plan that includes hazard analysis and steps to reduce or eliminate any potential food safety hazards.[3]

Facilities registered with the FDA comply with good manufacturing practices, including baseline standards for manufacturing, processing, packing and holding commercial pet food to ensure it is safe for the animal to eat.[3]

The Center for Veterinary Medicine (CVM), a department of the FDA, regulates the use of any health claims on pet food labels. One type of health claim, a drug claim, is the assertion or implication that consuming food may help treat, prevent or reduce a particular disease.[2] If a health claim is considered a drug claim, the CVM will not allow its use on the label.[2] An example of a health claim would be "Feeding this food will prevent the development of hypertension in adult dogs" as opposed to a non-health claim of "this food may be beneficial in the prevention of blood pressure-related issues in adult dogs."

USDA

The United States Department of Agriculture (USDA) ensures that pet foods are clearly labeled to prevent human consumers from mistaking these products for human foods and eating them.[2,4] The USDA inspects animal ingredients used in pet foods to ensure proper handling and to guarantee that such ingredients are not used in human foods.[2,4] The USDA is also responsible for the inspection and regulation of animal research facilities. All kennels and catteries operated by pet food companies, private groups, or universities must fulfill USDA requirements for the physical structure, record keeping, housing and care of animals and sanitation.[2,4] Once these facilities have passed their initial certification, they are subject to unannounced inspections by the USDA at least once yearly.[2,4]

Some pet food manufacturers maintain their own kennels, while others contract their feeding trials out to private research kennels or universities. Long-term feeding trials make up a large portion of the testing conducted on quality commercial pet foods. The USDA ensures that these facilities maintain proper care of their animals and conform to recommended sanitation practices.[2]

NRC

The NRC is a private, nonprofit organization that evaluates and compiles research conducted by others. The NRC functions as the working portion of the National Academy of Sciences, the National Academy of Engineers and The Institute of Medicine.[4] The NRC was created in 1916 in response to the increased need for scientific and technical services during World War I.[4] The NRC is not part of the United States government, is not an enforcement agency and is not a primary research organization with laboratories of its own.[4] The NRC does not regulate the pet food industry and has requested that its recommendations not be used to substantiate the nutritional adequacy of pet foods.[4]

PFI

In 1958, the Pet Food Institute (PFI) was organized to represent commercially prepared dog and cat food manufacturers in the United States.[2,4] The PFI works closely with the Pet Food Committee of the AAFCO to evaluate current regulations and make recommendations for changes.[2,4] The PFI also works closely with veterinarians, humane groups and local animal control officers to sponsor public and owner education programs that encourage responsible dog and cat ownership.[4] They do not have any direct regulatory powers over the production of pet foods, pet food testing or statements included on labels. However, they represent the pet food industry before legislative and regulatory bodies at the federal and state levels.[4]

States

Individual states are responsible for adopting and enforcing pet food regulations. Many, but not all, have adopted regulations that follow those established by AAFCO. The State Department of Agriculture administers pet food regulation and enforcement in most states, regulatory and protection division or state chemist[4]

Most of the control over the nutrient content of pet foods, ingredient nomenclature and label claims is regulated by AAFCO. The Model Feed Bill that the AAFCO developed and implemented is a template for state legislation.[2] Each year, the AAFCO publishes an official document that includes a section containing the current regulations for pet foods. These regulations govern the definition and terms, label format, brand and product names, nutrient guarantee claims, types of ingredients, drug and food additives, statements of caloric content and descriptive terms that are to be used with or included in commercial pet foods.[2] The AAFCO-sanctioned feeding protocols for proving nutritional adequacy and metabolizable energy are also included in this document.[4]

Food Recalls

The FDA reports recalls and withdrawals of both pet food and treats issued by manufacturers.[3] Most recalls are not associated with illnesses, though this can occasionally happen. Though recalls garner much attention, the overall incidence of pet food and treat recalls is substantially lower than those issued for human foods.[3]

While commercial food contaminated with various bacteria is classified as unfit for sale, it is not illegal to sell contaminated raw foods, commonly used for home-cooked and raw food diets.[3]

Regulations

The definition and terms section of the AAFCO's pet food regulations identifies the principal display panel (PDP) as part of the container's label and is intended to be displayed to the consumer for retail sales.[2] Statements that are allowed on labels are described and strictly regulated; these are called "statements of nutritional adequacy" or "purpose of the product." If a product states that it is "complete and balanced nutrition for all stages of life," the claim must be substantiated through one of two ways.[2] The first way involves using a series of feeding trials to demonstrate that the food satisfactorily supports their health in a group of dogs or cats throughout all life stages of gestation, lactation and growth.[2] The second way requires that the manufacturer formulate the food to contain ingredients in quantities that are sufficient to provide the estimated nutrient requirements for all life stages in the dog or cat.[2] This can be shown through a simple calculation of ingredients using standard ingredient tables or through laboratory analysis of nutrients.[2] The AAFCO nutrient profiles for dog and cat foods are used as the standard against which nutrient content is measured.[2] The AAFCO also requires that all products labeled "complete and balanced" include specific feeding directions on the product label.[2] The pet food company does not need to include how these numbers were reached. The amount to be fed usually does not specify any information other than animal size, age, activity level or sexual status but does have a bearing on the amount to be fed. This is typically measured in standard household measurements, such as "cup."

The brand name refers to the name by which a pet food manufacturer's products are identified and distinguished from other pet foods.[2] The AAFCO regulates both brand and product names.[2] Any product claims of "new and improved" are only allowed to be stated on the PDP and can be used for a maximum of 6 months.[2]

The AAFCO identifies acceptable terms for designating the guaranteed analysis for specific nutrients. Comparisons between nutrient levels in the pet food and the AAFCO nutrient profiles must be listed in the same units as those used in the published profile.[2] AAFCO also requires that no pet food, except for those labeled as sauces, gravies, juices or milk replacers, contain a moisture level greater than 78%.[2]

Artificial food colors can only be added to pet foods if they are harmless to pets or "generally recognized as safe" or GRAS.[2] Such additives are approved and listed by the FDA.[2]

In 1994, AAFCO accepted the inclusion of an optional caloric content statement on pet food labels.[2] This statement must be presented separately from the guaranteed analysis table, and the energy must be expressed as units of kcals/kg. The caloric content may also be expressed as kcal/lb, cup or another commonly used household measuring unit.[2] This claim must be substantiated by calculation using modified Atwater factors or feeding trials following AAFCO protocols.[2] The method used must be stated on the label.[2]

In 1998, the AAFCO regulations specified the acceptable use of the terms "light/lite," "less or reduced calories," "lean," "low fat" and "less or reduced fat."[2] Specific maximum energy contents are designated for all pet foods marketed using the term "light/lite." A food designated as "less or reduced calories" must include the percentage of reduction from the comparison product and a caloric content statement.[2] The terms "lean" and "less fat" must provide the maximum percentages of fat within different categories of dog and cat food and include the percentage of reduction from the product of comparison.[2]

Conclusion

Anyone can make and sell commercial pet food, but not all companies or products are of equal quality. This can make it challenging for owners to know what is best for their pets.

The World Small Animal Veterinary Association (WSAVA) is a global community of more than 200,000 veterinarians from around the world, whose goal is "to advance the health and welfare of companion animals worldwide through an educated, committed and collaborative global community of veterinary peers"[3] WSAVA established the WSAVA Global Nutrition Committee, which has created guidelines comprising eight criteria for selecting diets made by reputable companies. Recommending diets made by companies that meet the WSAVA Guidelines is one way to distinguish reputable and high-quality pet food companies from the rest.[3] The Guidelines can be accessed here: https://wsava.org/global-guidelines/global-nutrition-guidelines/.

References

1 Cowell CS, Stout NP, Brinkerman MF *et al.* (2000) Making commercial pet foods. In MS Hand, CD Thatcher, RI Remillard, P Roudebush (eds), *Small Animal Clinical Nutrition*, 4th edn, p. 129, Marceline, MO: Walsworth Publishing.

2 Case LP, Carey DP, Hirakawa DA, Daristotle L (2000) History and regulation of pet foods. In *Canine and Feline Nutrition*, 2nd edn, pp. 143–51, St Louis, MO: Mosby.

3 Sanderson SL (2021) Pros and cons of commercial pet foods. In D Laflamme (ed.), *Veterinary Clinics, Small Animal Practice Small Animal Nutrition*, vol. **51**, Number 3, pp. 529–46, Philadelphia, PA: Elsevier.

4 Roudebush P, Dzanis DA, Debraekeleer J, Brown RG (2000) Pet food labels. In MS Hand, CD Thatcher, RI Remillard, P Roudebush (eds), *Small Animal Clinical Nutrition*, 4th edn, pp. 147–50, Marceline, MO: Walsworth Publishing.

5 Delaney SJ, Fascetti AJ (2012) Basic nutrition overview. In AJ Fascetti, SJ Delaney (eds), *Applied Veterinary Clinical Nutrition*, pp. 20–1, Ames, IO: Wiley-Blackwell.

14

Pet Food Labels

Introduction

Pet food labels are legal documents regulated primarily at the state level, with state feed control officials making sure that the labels found on pet foods comply with guidelines published in the most current *Official Publication* of the Association of American Feed Control Officials (AAFCO).[1,2] State feed control officials operate under the Food and Drug Administration (FDA) in the jurisdiction of the United States. Regulations that apply to pet food labeling and testing of foods for nutritional adequacy are published in the AAFCO Manual.[1] This manual is updated yearly and provides definitions for the various terms used in pet food labeling.[1,3]

Definition of Terms

Complete

A nutritionally adequate feed for animals other than man; by a specific formula, it is compounded to be fed as a sole ration and can maintain life and promote production without any additional substance being consumed except water.[1]

Balanced

A term that may be applied to a diet, ration or feed that has all the required nutrients in proper amount and proportion based upon

Table 14.1 Percentage of content in food (using chicken as an example).

Chicken	Chicken must be at least 70% of the total product
Chicken dinner, Chicken platter, Chicken entree	Chicken must be at least 10% of the total product
with Chicken	Chicken must be at least 3% of the total product
Chicken flavor	Chicken must be recognizable by the pet, usually less than 3% of the total product
Canned foods	Moisture not greater than 78%
Gravy, stew, broth, sauce, juice or milk replacer	Moisture can be greater than 78%

Source: Roudebush et al.[4]/Mark Morris Institute.

recommendations of recognized authorities in the field of animal nutrition, such as the NRC, for a given set of physiological requirements. The species for which it is intended and the functions such as maintenance or maintenance plus reproduction shall be specified.[1] See Table 14.1

Regulations

Current regulations require that all labels for pet foods manufactured and sold in the United States contain the following items: product

Nutrition and Disease Management for Veterinary Technicians and Nurses, Third Edition. Ann Wortinger and Kara M. Burns.
© 2024 John Wiley & Sons, Inc. Published 2024 by John Wiley & Sons, Inc.
Companion Website: www.wiley.com/go/wortinger/3e

name; net weight; name and address of the manufacturer; guaranteed analysis for crude protein, crude fat, crude fiber and moisture; list of ingredients in descending order of pre-dominance by weight; the terms "dog food" or "cat food" and a statement of nutritional adequacy or purpose of the product.[1,3,5] A statement must also indicate the method used to substantiate the nutritional adequacy claim. This can either be through the AAFCO feeding trials or by formulating the feed to meet AAFCO *Nutrient Profiles.* An expiration date indicating the time span from the date of pro-duction to the date of expiration of the product is optional, as is a "best if used by" date.[1,5]

Principal Display Panel

The required information can be found on either the principal display panel (PDP) or the information panel. The FDA defines the PDP as "the part of the label that is most likely to be displayed, presented, shown or examined under customary conditions of display for retail sale."[4] This is the primary means of

attracting the consumer's attention to a prod-uct and should immediately communicate the product's identity. AAFCO requires that the PDP contain only three things: the product name, the intended species to be fed to and the net quantity of the product contained within the package.[2] The information panel is defined as "that part of the label immediately contigu-ous and to the right of the PDP" and usually contains information about the product.[4] Any information contained on the label must be both truthful and substantiated or proven.[2] See Figure 14.1 and Table 14.2.

The product identity is the primary means of identification of pet foods by consumers.[4] In the United States, the product identity must legally include a product name but may also include a manufacturer's name, a brand name or both.[4] The brand name is the name by which the pet food products of a given company are identified.[4] The product name provides infor-mation about the individual identity of a particular product within that brand.[4]

The PDP must identify the species for which the food is intended, such as "dog food" or "cat food." This statement is intended to help guide

Sample Label

**Dr D's
Natural Food**

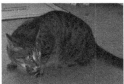

Field mouse
for cats

Complete and balance as nature designed for adult maintenance

Ingredients: Water sufficient for processing, Michigan grown whole ground wild field mouse

Guaranteed analysis: Crude protein min. 20%, crude fat min. 10%, crude fiber max. 1%, moisture max. 65%, ash max. 4%

AAFCO feeding studies substantiate complete and balanced for adult maintenance

Manufactured by MICE, Belleville MI USA (269) 543-6789

Feeding recommendations:

Size	1−5#	6−10#	11−15#	16−20#
Amt fed	0.5−0.6 can	0.6−1 can	1−1.5 can	1.5−2 can

Figure 14.1 This is an example of a pet food label with the information that is required provided. *Source*: Ann Wortinger(Book Author).

Table 14.2 Important elements found on pet food labels in the United States and Canada.

Principal display panel	Information panel
Product identity (required)	Ingredient statement (required)
Manufacturer's name	
Brand name	
Product name	
Designator or statement of intent (required)	Guaranteed analysis (required)
Net weight (required)	Nutritional adequacy statement (required)
Product vignette or picture (optional)	Feeding guidelines (required)
Nutritional claim (optional)	Manufacturer or distributor (required)
Bursts or flags (optional)	Universal product code (optional)
	Batch information (optional)
	Freshness date (optional)
	Caloric content (optional)

Source: Roudebush et al. [4]/Mark Morris Institute.

consumer purchases.[1] This does not mean that the food cannot be fed to an alternate species but has only been tested and formulated for the indicated species. This is called the "designator" or "statement of intent."[4]

The net weight indicates the amount of food in the specific container, often given in pounds/ounces or kilograms/grams, or both.[1] This is found on the PDP and must be placed within the bottom 30% of the panel.[4]

A product vignette refers to any graphic or pictorial representation of a product on a pet food label.[4] The product vignette should not misrepresent the contents of the package by looking better than the actual product or ingredients.[4]

Nutrition statements on the PDP include the terms "complete and nutritious," "100% nutritious," "100% complete nutrition" or similar

designations. Nutritional adequacy statements indicate which species the food is formulated for and the life stage the food is appropriate to feed.[2] The term "all life stages" indicates that it can be fed to gestating or lactating females, growing animals and adults. These claims must be substantiated by a nutritional adequacy statement on the information panel.[4]

Product Naming

Product names are typically used to convey information to the owner and often emphasize a particular ingredient or aspect of the food.[3] As seen in the following table, there are complicated and precise methods for naming pet foods. What the consumer reads or sees and what the actual ingredients are can be vastly different. See Table 14.3.

Nutritional Adequacy

Nutritional adequacy can be established using three methods; the first is to conduct a feeding trial or protocol using the food fed to the designated species in a controlled setting using a defined protocol.[2] Alternately, adequacy can be established using a computer formulation to a specific nutritional profile established by AAFCO. Finally, adequacy can be established following the "family product rule," which allows foods that are similar in ingredients and that have been tested to match or exceed key nutrient levels of another food that has passed a feeding trial or protocol to claim that the unfed "family member" food has passed a feeding trial or protocol for the same life stage.[2] There is no way to tell from the label if the "family product rule" has been used.

Bursts and flags are areas of the PDP designated to highlight information or provide specific information with visual impact.[4] New products, formula or ingredient changes and improvements in taste are most often highlighted.[4] "New" or "new and improved"

Table 14.3 Common pet food ingredients.

Description	Example	Contribution to diet
Meat (muscle)	Skeletal muscle, tongue, diaphragm and heart	Animal fat, protein and energy
Meat by-products	Lung, spleen, kidney, brain, blood, bone and intestine	Animal fat, protein and energy
Meat meal, meat and bone meal, fish meal and blood meal	Dry rendered product from animal tissue	Animal fat, protein and energy
Cereals	Corn, wheat, oats, barley and corn gluten meal	Carbohydrate, protein, fiber and energy
Soy flour, soy meal	Vegetable protein sources including Textured Vegetable Protein (TVP)	Protein, texture/chunks (usually the meaty chunks in foods)
Animal fat, vegetable oil	Tallow, chicken fat, corn oil and soy oil	Fats, fatty acids, essential fatty acids and energy
Egg	Egg powder	A protein of high biologic value
Milk	Skim milk powder, whey	Milk protein
Grain hulls, root crops	Bran, beet pulp, chicory root	Dietary fiber
Humectants	Sugars, salt and glycerol	Reduction in water availability, energy
Digest	Hydrolyzed liver or intestine	Flavor and palatability enhancer, some protein and fat
Preservatives	Sodium benzoate, sodium and potassium sorbate	Retard spoilage from molds and bacteria
Flavors	Natural and artificial and "nature identical" flavors, process reacted flavors, key character compounds	Improvement in taste, smell and mouthfeel
Coloring agents	Natural and artificial colorings	Improvement in owner appeal
Aromas	Natural and artificial aromas and tones	Improvement in owner and animal appeal
Vitamins, minerals	Vitamin and mineral premixes	Nutrients and dietary balance
Antioxidants	BHT, BHA, ascorbic acid and mixed tocopherols (vit E)	Prevents fat rancidity

Source: Roudebush et al. [6]/Iowa State University Press.

can only appear on the label for 6 months, while comparisons such as "preferred 5 to 1 over the leading national brand" can appear on the label for one year unless it is resubstantiated.[4]

Information Panel

The information panel is usually the second place where consumers look for information about the food.[5] The list of ingredients must be arranged in decreasing order by predominance by weight. The terms used to describe the products must be those assigned by the AAFCO, or names commonly accepted as a standard in the feed industry.[5] No single ingredient can be given undue emphasis, nor can designators of quality be included.[5]

Most grocery stores and generic brands are formulated as "variable formula diets."[5] This means that the ingredients used in the food will vary from batch to batch, depending on market availability and pricing. In contrast, most premium foods sold in feed stores, pet stores and through veterinarians (i.e., therapeutic diets) are produced using fixed formulas.[5] Although the cost for a fixed formula food may be more than a variable formula diet, the consistency between batches of food is a distinct advantage to the dog or cat consuming the food.[5] This will help eliminate the GI distress that can often accompany a diet change, even if the brand of the food itself has not changed.

The ingredient list must be listed on the packaging in decreasing order of inclusion based on weight before cooking, drying or other processing.[2,3] It also does not indicate the quality of the ingredients used in the food. These ingredients can vary in digestibility, amino acid content and bioavailability, mineral availability and the number of indigestible materials they contain.[5] Unfortunately, there is no way to determine the quality of the ingredients from the ingredient list.

Some premium foods with high-quality ingredients may have an ingredient list almost identical to generic food containing poor ingredients with low digestibility and poor nutrient availability.[5] This can be seen in products that claim to be "the same as" another higher-priced product. As with most anything else, consumers get what they pay for. Ingredients must be listed using their AAFCO or FDA-defined names using generic names only. Brand or trade names cannot be used.

References to the "quality, nature, form, or other attributes of an ingredient shall be allowed when the designation is not false or misleading; [and] the ingredient imparts a distinctive characteristic to the pet food because it possesses that attribute and the reference to quality or grade of the ingredients do not appear in the ingredients statement." It is common to see references on the ingredient panel stating that chicken is a natural source of glucosamine. However, references stating that the ingredient is "USDA choice beef" are not allowed.[2]

Another misleading practice is the splitting of ingredients to place them lower on the ingredient list. This occurs when several different forms of the same product are listed separately (e.g., wheat germ meal, wheat middlings, wheat bran and wheat flour). Because the requirement is to list by weight, by splitting the ingredients, they each weigh less and can be placed further down the ingredient list when they compromise a significant portion of the product. Dry ingredients also appear lower on the list than those that are naturally higher in moisture. This allows most "meat" products to appear higher on the ingredient list than the dry grains and starches, which may be found in a higher percentage in the diet.[4] By their very nature, meats, which contain a higher portion of water than other ingredients, will appear higher on the ingredient label. Consumers are continually told that meat-based products are more desirable ingredients than plant-based products. Hence, the manufacturer has a lot of incentive to manipulate the label to appeal to consumers.

Pet food additives such as vitamins, minerals, antioxidant preservatives, antimicrobial preservatives, humectants, coloring agents, flavors, palatability enhancers and emulsifying agents that the manufacturer lists must also be included on the ingredient list. See Table 14.4.[4]

In the United States, pet food manufacturers must include minimum percentages for crude protein and crude fat and maximum percentages for crude fiber and moisture.[4] These percentages generally indicate the "worst case" levels for these nutrients in the food and may not accurately reflect the exact or typical amounts included.[4] Also, notice that these indicate only minimums or maximums found in the foods. Actual values may differ dramatically.

Crude protein estimates the total protein in food obtained by multiplying analyzed nitrogen levels by a constant numerical value.[4,5] Crude protein is an index of protein quantity but does not indicate amino acid content, protein quality or digestibility.[4,5]

Table 14.4 This table provides a list of common pet food ingredients, and what they contribute to the diet.

Ingredient rule	Contents	Example
95%	Simple names indicating ingredient	Beef for dogs
	Must be at minimum 95% of named product	Tuna for cats
	If in water, the named ingredient must be at minimum 70% of the product	
25% or dinner/entrée/nuggets	Descriptive term	Beef dinner for dogs
	Must be at minimum 25% of the named product.	Salmon entrée for cats
	If in water, the named ingredient must be at minimum 10% of the product	
3% or with	Intended to highlight ingredients on PDP.	Dog food with beef
	Allows the presence of minor ingredients to be noted, but not in a sufficient quantity to qualify as dinner or entree	Cat food with cheese
Flavor	A percentage is not required but must be contained in sufficient quantity to be detectable.	Beef dog food with milk
	Seldom used except for bacon or smoke flavors	Chicken-flavored cat food

Source: FDA [3].

Crude fat is an estimate of the lipid content of food obtained through the extraction of the food with ether.[4,5] This procedure also isolates certain organic acids, oils, pigments, alcohols and fat-soluble vitamins. But it may not be able to isolate some complex lipids such as phospholipids.[4,5]

Crude fiber represents the organic residue that remains after the plant material has been treated with dilute acid and alkali solvents and after extracted mineral components.[4,5] Although crude fiber is used to report the fiber content of commercial foods, it usually underestimates the actual level of fiber found in the food.[4] The values also do not indicate the intestinal bacteria's solubility or fermentability of that fiber, which releases additional energy from the food.

The amount of water found in an individual product can significantly affect the values of the other nutrients listed in the guaranteed analysis. Most pet foods display nutrients on an "as-fed" basis rather than a "dry-matter" basis.[4,5] "As-fed" means that the percentages of nutrients were calculated directly, without accounting for the proportion of water in a product.[4,5] It is important to convert these guarantees to a dry-matter basis when comparing foods of differing moisture contents, such as canned versus dry foods, to represent the actual nutrients accurately.[4,5] Most dry foods contain 6-10% water, while canned foods contain up to 78% water.[4,5] It is also possible to use metabolizable energy when comparing different foods; this will give the percentage of each nutrient in the food on an as-fed basis, taking into account the different caloric amounts of each nutrient in the food. Metabolizable energy provides the percent of protein, fat and carbohydrates found in the food, as these are the only energy-containing nutrients.

Maximum ash guarantees are not required in the United States but are often included on pet food labels.[4] Ash consists of the noncombustible materials in food, usually composed of salt and other minerals. This is determined by burning the food in a bomb calorimeter and incinerating all non-mineral-based components. High ash content in dry and semi-moist foods generally indicates high mineral content, specifically magnesium.[4] The ash content of canned cat foods usually correlates poorly with the magnesium content of that food.[4]

Except for treats or snacks, all pet foods in interstate commerce must contain a statement and validation of nutritional adequacy.[4,5] Current AAFCO regulations allow four primary types of nutritional adequacy statements:

Complete and Balanced for All Life Stages

The food has been formulated to provide complete and balanced nutrition for gestation, lactation, growth and maintenance.

Limited Claim

The food provides complete and balanced nutrition for a particular life stage such as adult maintenance or growth.

Intermittent or Supplemental

The food has been formulated for only intermittent or supplemental use and is not intended for full-time feeding.

Therapeutic

The food is intended for therapeutic use under the supervision of a veterinarian.[4,5]

The foods must also indicate what method was used to establish the nutritional adequacy claims. The use of feeding trials is the most thorough and reliable method of evaluation. The terms "feeding tests," "AAFCO feeding test protocols" or "AAFCO feeding studies" all validate that the product has undergone feeding tests with dogs or cats. If the substantiation claim states only that the food has met the AAFCO's *Nutrient Profiles*, feeding trials were not done on the food.[4,5] The nutrient levels can be calculated in a laboratory after production, or the diet can merely be formulated using a standard table of ingredients.[5] Neither of these methods considers digestibility or availability of individual nutrients or loss of nutrients through processing or excesses found in the ingredients.

Feeding guidelines are required on all foods labeled as completed and balanced for any life stage.[4] These directions must be given in standard terms and must appear prominently on the label. At a minimum, these should state "feed (weight/unit of product) per (weight unit) of dog or cat" with a stated frequency. The guidelines are general at best and do not consider the individual pet's sexual status, activity level or environmental factors like exposure to heat and cold. Because of individual variations, specific animals may require more or less food than recommended on the label to maintain optimal body condition and health.[4] An exception to this rule is therapeutic diets, which can state "use only as directed by your veterinarian"[2]

A statement of caloric content must be expressed on a kcals/kg basis. It must be separate from the guaranteed analysis and appear under the "caloric content" heading. The statement is usually based on kilocalories of metabolizable energy (ME) on an as-fed. Manufacturers are also required to express the kcals in familiar household units, given as kilocalories per familiar household measures such as kcal/cup or kcal/can.[3,4]

In the United States, the name and address of the manufacturer, distributor or dealer of the pet food must be found on the label, usually on the information panel.[3,4] This information is not required to be complete and may only include the distributor and city of origin. Most premium foods include their name, mailing address, phone number with hours of operations and a website address. This makes it much easier for the consumer to contact the manufacturer with any problems or questions.

Although not a legal requirement, most manufacturers include the Universal Product Code (UPC) or bar code on the label. Other information, such as batch numbers and date of manufacture, can also frequently be found on the labels. There may also be a freshness date included on the label.[4]

Other Label Claims

Many terms are applied to pet foods, but do they provide any information to the consumer above marketing claims? The terms "premium," "super-premium" or even "ultra-premium" convey that a product is unique and potentially contains higher quality ingredients.[3] Unfortunately, these are just labels, and the products are not required to contain any different or higher-quality ingredients. They are also not held to any higher standards than being required to be complete and balanced.

Another term seen commonly is "natural." This term is construed as lacking in artificial flavors, colors or preservatives.[3] Artificial flavorings are seldom used in commercial pet foods, and color additives are typically for the owner's benefit. If these are used in pet food, they are required to be from approved sources.[3] The use of preservatives, especially with higher-fat foods, is necessary to prevent rancidity. Rancidity renders that nutrient, usually a fat, or no value to the animal, adversely affecting the taste and texture of the product (think soured milk!). Natural preservatives, such as mixed tocopherols, can be used but tend to be less effective and require large volumes to achieve the same effect of preventing rancidity.[3]

Natural is not the same as "organic." Organic refers to the condition in which the plants or animals are grown or raised. No official rules govern the labeling of organic foods for pets in the US currently.[3]

References

1 Buffington CA, Holloway C, Abood SK (2004) Diet and feeding factors. In *The Manual of Veterinary Dietetics*, pp. 43–8, St Louis, MO: Elsevier.

2 Delaney S, Fascetti A (2012) Using pet food labels and product guides. In S Delaney, A Fascetti (eds), *Applied Veterinary Clinical Nutrition*, pp. 69–74, Ames, IA: Wiley-Blackwell.

3 FDA Pet food labels-general. https://www .fda.gov/animal-veterinary/animal-health-literacy/pet-food-labels-general. Accessed 11/5/21.

4 Roudebush P, Dzanis DA, Debraekeleer J, Glenn BR (2000) Pet food labels. In MS Hand, CD Thatcher, RI Remillard, P Roudebush (eds), *Small Animal Clinical Nutrition* (4th edn), pp. 151–7, Marceline, MO: Walsworth Publishing.

5 Case LP, Carey DP, Hirakawa DA, Daristotle L (2000) Pet food labels. In *Canine and Feline Nutrition* (2nd edn), pp. 153–63, St Louis, MO: Mosby.

6 Kelly NC (1996) Food types and evaluation. In N Kelly, J Wills (eds), *Manual of Companion Animal Nutrition and Feeding*, p. 34, Ames, IA: Iowa State University Press.

15

Nutrient Content of Pet Foods

Introduction

Nutrient content refers to the levels of various nutrients in the food and the digestibility and availability of all essential nutrients.[1] Since we are feeding a specific food to provide nutrients, knowledge of the levels of these nutrients is important to know. There are four different ways that the nutrient content of a product can be determined.[2]

1. Laboratory analysis of the final product can be done.
2. The target values can be obtained from the manufacturer.
3. Nutrient content can be calculated based on published values for the ingredients.
4. The information found on the label guaranteed analysis and typical analysis can be used.[2]

Laboratory Analysis

Laboratory or proximate analysis provides information on a specific nutrient group and will not usually contain all the nutrients found in food. The nutrients typically looked at are expressed as percentages: Moisture, crude protein, crude fat ash (minerals) and fiber.[3] The guaranteed analysis found on the product label is generated from the proximate analysis. If a company wants to provide additional material to the consumer or veterinary professional above what is allowed on the label, product information can be found online, through product brochures and in product reference guides.[3]

If the contact information is provided for the product, contacting the manufacturer can also be a source of additional information. Of course, this is dependent on the level of customer support provided by the manufacturer. Using the label-guaranteed analysis to determine actual nutrient levels in the food is the least accurate method due to how these values are given. Moisture, fiber and ash as reported as maximum levels, which may or may not be close to what is found in the product, and protein and fat are reported as minimum levels.

If food is formulated to meet the nutrient profile of a specific life stage, nutrient levels should be equal to or greater than the nutrient profile minimums and equal to or less than the nutrient profile's maximums.[4] This method of evaluating nutrient content is not recommended due to severe limitations and discrepancies in the calculated values.[2]

Calculation

Calculating nutrient content based on published values of ingredients also has limitations; there is a lack of complete and accurate data for the nutrient content of many ingredients used in commercial pet foods. Because of this, manufacturers rely on lists containing approximations of the types of ingredients

Nutrition and Disease Management for Veterinary Technicians and Nurses, Third Edition. Ann Wortinger and Kara M. Burns.
© 2024 John Wiley & Sons, Inc. Published 2024 by John Wiley & Sons, Inc.
Companion Website: www.wiley.com/go/wortinger/3e

used.[1] These lists may also contain outdated or misleading information, resulting in inaccurate values being used.[1] The National Research Council (NRC) published values are often used to evaluate the level of nutrients in pet foods.[3]

The quality of the ingredients is not taken into account when using the calculation method; this can affect the level and availability of nutrients in the finished product.[1] The standardized tables represent average nutrient content for individual ingredients, and therefore may not represent ingredient quality among various raw ingredients.[3] Processing methods can further affect ingredient quality, with nutrient losses occurring during processing and storage.[1] Studies have shown that digestibility and nutrient availability of animal-based and plant-based ingredients are significantly affected by processing methods.[1] This method would likely be used for determining the nutrient content of homemade diets, though adequate time and knowledge to perform the calculations would be a significant limitation.[2]

Most pet food manufacturers will supply target values for the nutrient content of their foods upon request.[2] Though these values often reflect actual average nutrient levels, occasionally, they will vary significantly from the actual values found in the food.[2] Since no laws govern the accuracy of target nutrient levels, the manufacturer does not have to have the food within these levels.[2] Remember, the manufacturer only has to ensure the food is within the stated maximum and minimum levels. Overall, these values should be a reasonable approximation of nutrient levels and adequate for most instances.

Final Product Analysis

Of the methods listed above, the most accurate way to determine the nutrient content is through laboratory analysis of the final product; this provides the proximate analysis.[1] A proximate analysis tests for a limited number of parameters, including moisture content, crude protein, crude fat, ash (minerals) and fiber contents.[1] Nitrogen-free extract (NFE) represents a rough estimation of the soluble carbohydrate content of the food and can be calculated by simple subtraction. Starting at 100%, subtract the moisture, protein, fat, ash and fiber percentages. What is left is the NFE.[2] The guaranteed analysis panel is generated from the proximate analysis results and reports only the maximum or minimum levels.[1]

Digestibility

Digestibility provides a measure of the final diet's quality because it directly determines the proportion of nutrients in the food available for absorption into the body.[1] Currently, the AAFCO regulations do not require companies to determine or provide digestibility levels for their foods.[3]

Digestibility should always be considered when evaluating various pet foods. Digestibility is a measure of the actual level of nutrients that are available for the body for use.[3] Feeding trials are the most accurate method used to determine the digestibility of nutrients and measure the disappearance of nutrients as they pass through the animal's digestive system and are absorbed by the body for use.[3] Information about the nutrient content of a diet has little meaning if the digestibility is unknown.[1]

For example, two diets that each contains 28% protein if the digestibility of one diet is 70%, and the digestibility of the second diet is 85% the actual protein available to the animal is less than 20% in the first diet and over 24% in the second diet.[1] While this difference may not seem significant, the amount of protein provided to the animal can become significant over time. Even though laboratory analysis would show that they have similar protein contents, digestibility shows that the second diet provides significantly more digestible protein than the first diet.[1]

Digestibility also affects fecal volume, form and frequency. As a diet's digestibility increases, fecal volume decreases significantly. Additionally, a highly digestible diet produces firm and well-formed feces.[1]

Manufacturers are not required to conduct feeding trials to determine the digestibility of their foods. Reputable companies that produce quality products always conduct these trials to ensure that their foods contain levels of nutrients that will meet an animal's daily requirements for absorption into the body.[1] A food can pass a feeding trial without meeting a nutrient profile's values. Because of this, no assumptions can be made on nutrient levels of food based solely on the absence or presence of feeding trials. Examples of this can be seen in many therapeutic diets that do not meet AAFCO nutrient profiles but have undergone feeding trials. This also explains why these foods are prescription diets, which should only be fed when the animal is under the supervision of a veterinarian monitoring for any nutrient deficiency caused by restricted diets.[4] This is also why OTC foods for specific disease management do not exist, as the animals would not be monitored to determine if nutrient deficiency or excesses exist.

Feeding Trials

In the United States, the AAFCO testing procedure for adult maintenance diets is done over six months, requires only eight animals per group, and monitors only a limited number of parameters.[2] The food being evaluated is fed to a group of animals, and feces and urine are collected throughout the testing period. The energy found in the feces and urine is subtracted from the total energy found in the food before feeding to evaluate actual digestibility. (6) This data provide digestible energy (DE) or metabolizable energy (ME) of that specific food. Passing such tests does not ensure that long-term nutrition or health-related problems will not occur or that problems with an occurrence rate of less than 15% would not be seen.[2] The protocols are also not designed to ensure optimal growth or maximize physical activity.[2]

DE measures the amount of energy found in food absorbed across the intestinal wall. ME accounts for any energy lost in the urine and feces, as well as what is absorbed across the intestinal wall.[3] ME provides a more accurate assessment of the energy available to the animal for use, rather than measuring the total amount of energy found in the food (gross energy). Digestion is not 100% efficient, and ME reflects the degree of inefficiency in a specific species. Remember that each individual animal may be more or less efficient at digestion than their species' average, especially when disease processes are factored in.

If these factors are of concern due to disease, additional long-term feeding trials need to be evaluated. Numerous premium pet food manufacturers conduct long-term studies to optimize the response to various nutrients and therapeutic treatment protocols.

Food Comparisons

When trying to compare various foods or different types, what method is best to use? If foods are compared on a dry-matter basis (DMB), differences seen with different food types can be eliminated, but differences in energy content are not addressed. The energy content for protein and carbohydrates is calculated at ~3.5 kcal/g, while fat is calculated at ~8.5 kcal/g. The nutrient density should be evaluated as a proportion of ME to evaluate different diets accurately.[1] Nutrient density accounts for differences in water content and energy content. It expresses nutrient levels in pet foods based on the energy available for the animal to use as ME.[1]

Nutrient density is expressed as grams/100 kcal of ME for each nutrient.[1] Since all animals are fed to meet their energy requirements, the amount of food consumed and the number of nutrients received depend on the energy density of the food.[1] When an animal is fed calorically dense food, the percentage of nutrients by weight in these foods must be higher to meet the essential nutrients' needs since the animal will consume less food.[1] The inverse is also true. When feeding a calorically dilute food, the number of nutrients provided in that food must be available at a level that the animal can meet when consuming the volume of food that meets its energy requirements.

Metabolizable Energy

The easiest way to express nutrients is as a percentage of ME or as units per 1000 kcal of ME instead of a weight percentage. Nutrient densities of foods with different moisture contents can be compared because water does not contribute any calories to the distribution.[1] Unfortunately, this method does not consider the calories in the foods or the amount the animal must consume to meet energy requirements.[1]

Caloric distribution is helpful when finding a higher or lower diet than another diet in particular nutrients. The three primary nutrients that are evaluated are protein, fat and carbohydrates. These are usually expressed as a percentage and given as pie charts or line charts in the product reference guides available from the manufacturers. (see Figure 15.1).

These two last diets are the same brand; notice the different caloric distribution between the canned and dry foods. (see Table 15.1).

If the grams of nutrient/100 g of food is not given, then using the guaranteed analysis and kilocalories/100 g, the following formula

can be used. Because metabolic or fecal/urine losses are not accounted for, these values are not as accurate as the ME values. (see Table 15.2).

By converting the nutrients into a percentage of ME, dry foods can be compared to canned foods produced by any manufacturer. This is the most accurate way to compare foods. It will also allow us the best way to find a food that meets a specific nutrient profile (i.e., low fat or high protein).

Diet A-dry food (renal diet)

Nutrient density (gm/100 kcal ME)
Crude protein - 3.44
Crude fat - 3.59
Crude fiber - 0.23
Carbohydrate - 14.07

Guaranteed analysis DM
Crude protein 15.4%
Crude fat 16.04%
Crude fiber 1.03%
Moisture 10%

Metabolizable energy calories ME
Protein 13.1%
Fat 33.2%
Carbohydrate 53.7%

Caloric distribution

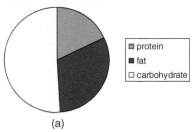

(a)

Figure 15.1 Examples of nutrient density and caloric distribution (Purina ProPlan Veterinary Diets Product Reference Guide).[5]

Diet B-canned food (recovery diet)

Nutrient density (gm/100 kcal ME)

Crude protein - 7.95
Crude fat - 7.36
Crude fiber - 0.15
Carbohydrate - 2.46

Guaranteed analysis DM

Crude protein 40.58%
Crude fat 37.54%
Crude fiber 0.74%
Carbohydrate 12.53%

Metabolizable energy calories ME

Protein 28.1%
Fat 63.2%
Carbohydrate 8.7%

Caloric distribution

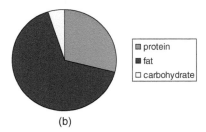

(b)

Figure 15.1 (*Continued*)

Diet C-dry food (intestinal diet)

Nutrient density (gm/100 kcal ME)

Crude protein - 6.67
Crude fat - 3.09
Crude fiber - 0.26
Carbohydrate - 12.09

Guaranteed analysis DM

Crude protein 27.7%
Crude fat 12.86%
Crude fiber 10.9%
Moisture 10%

Metabolizable energy calories ME

Protein 25.4%
Fat 28.6%
Carbohydrate 46%

Caloric distribution

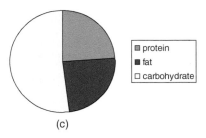

(c)

Figure 15.1 (*Continued*)

Diet D-canned food (intestinal diet)

Nutrient density (gm/100 kcal ME)

Crude protein - 9.33
Crude fat - 4.67
Crude fiber - 0.21
Carbohydrate - 8.23

Guaranteed analysis DM

Crude protein 38.35%
Crude fat 19.18%
Crude fiber 0.85%

Metabolizable energy calories ME

Protein 32.3%
Fat 39.2%
Carbohydrate 38.5%

Caloric distribution

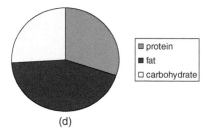

(d)

Figure 15.1 (*Continued*)

Table 15.1 Nutrients as a percentage of metabolizable energy.

Total calories in 100 g of the food

Protein = 3.5 kcal/g × g in food

Fat = 8.5 kcal/g × grams in food

Carbohydrate = 3.5 kcal/g × grams in food

Total calories/100 g = protein calorie + fat calorie + carbohydrate calorie

Percentage of ME contributed by each nutrient (caloric distribution)

Protein = (protein calories/100 g divided by total calories/100 g) × 100 = % ME

Fat = (fat calories/100 g divided by total calories/100 g) × 100 = % ME

Carbohydrate = (carbohydrate calories/100 g divided by total calories) × 100 = % ME

Source: Case et al.[1]

Table 15.2 Energy density from guaranteed analysis.

% in the diet of nutrient × mod. Atwater factor = kcal/100 g of food

Divided % nutrient by total calories to get nutrient distribution

Work Sheet Examples

No Name Dog Food Guaranteed Analysis

Protein 21%

Fat 5%

Moisture 12%

Insoluble fiber 12%

Ash 3%

Protein 21% x 3.5 = calories from protein per 100 g of food

73.5 protein Calories

Fat 5% x 8.5 = calories from fat per 100 g of food

42.5 fat calories

Carbohydrates need to be calculated from given values, usually not provided

((100 −(protein + fat + insoluble fiber + moisture + ash))

Carbohydrate = ((100 −(21 + 5 + 12 + 12 + 3)) = 47% × 3.5 = calories from carbohydrate per 100 g of food

164.5 carb calories

Total calories = 73.5 + 42.5 + 164.5 = 280.5 kcal/100 g

Metabolizable Calories equals

Protein 73.5/280.5 × 100 = 26.2%

Fat 42.5/280.5 × 100 = 15%

Carbohydrate 164.5/280.5 × 100 = 58.6%

Source: Hand and Purina ProPlan.[2,5]

References

1 Case LP, Carey D, Hirakawa DA, Daristotle L (2000) Nutrient content of pet foods. In *Canine and Feline Nutrition* (2nd edn), pp. 165–86, Mosby: St Louis, MO.

2 Hand MS, Thatcher CD, Remillard RI (2000) Small animal clinical nutrition: an iterative process. In MS Hand, CD Thatcher, RI Remillard, P Roudebush (eds), *Small Animal Clinical Nutrition* (4th edn), pp. 7–11, Marceline, MO: Walsworth Publishing.

3 Case LP, Daristotle L, Hayek MG, Raasch MF (2011) Nutrient content in pet foods. In *Canine and Feline Nutrition* (3rd edn), pp. 141–60, St Louis, MO: Mosby.

4 Delaney S, Fascetti A (2012) Using pet food labels and product guides. In S Delaney, A Fascetti (eds), *Applied Veterinary Clinical Nutrition*, pp. 69–74, Ames, IA: Wiley-Blackwell.

5 Purina ProPlan 202 Product Guide pgs.

16

Types of Pet Foods

Introduction

Until the early 1900s, there were few options on what to feed dogs and cats; they ate what we ate. After the start of commercial pet food production, the available options have continued to expand at an alarming rate to encompass the amazing variety of foods, flavors and treats found today.

While clients typically decide what food to feed their pets themselves, many clients wish their veterinary team would recommend a specific diet.[1] American Animal Health Association (AAHA) and the World Small Animal Veterinary Association (WSAVA) have made the recommendations and developed guidelines to make nutritional assessments and recommendations for the fifth vital assessment, along with temperature, pulse, respiration and pain on routine physical exams.[2,3] While every veterinary professional cannot hope to know about the estimated 175 pet food manufacturers in the United States, developing a working knowledge of the most popular or your favorite foods is essential.[1]

Pet Food Library

With the easy availability of information on the internet, it would be thought that accessing the information on various pet foods and treats would be more accessible when in fact, it has become more challenging. This difficulty is due primarily to the overwhelming variety of foods out there.

The Pet Nutrition Alliance (PNA) has produced a chart with most of the information in one site on their website that provides information on the Nutrition Guidelines offered by WSAVA. This area is called The Pet Food Manufacturer Evaluation Report and provides an easy-to-consult chart organized by the brand name of the food where the WSAVA information is collected and foods can be compared. This report can also be used to see which company produces which foods and which companies were unwilling to provide information on their diets.

https://petnutritionalliance.org/chart/index
.php/manufacturer-report[4]

Commercial Diets

It has been reported that over 90% of dogs and cats in the US consume more than half of their daily calories in the form of commercial pet foods.[1] These commercial diets are available in several forms that vary according to their processing methods, the ingredients used and the method of preservation.[5] The foods can be further classified based on their nutrient content, the purpose of use, the quality of the ingredients and the water content of the diet.[5,6]

Commercial pet foods are available in four primary forms: dry, canned, semi-moist and raw diets.[1,5] Knowing the potential advantages

Nutrition and Disease Management for Veterinary Technicians and Nurses, Third Edition. Ann Wortinger and Kara M. Burns.
© 2024 John Wiley & Sons, Inc. Published 2024 by John Wiley & Sons, Inc.
Companion Website: www.wiley.com/go/wortinger/3e

and disadvantages each of these types of diets offers is helpful for client communication and when making diet recommendations.[1]

Dry Pet Foods

Dry or kibble foods are the most common type of pet food fed to dogs.[1] Dry pet foods contain between 3% and 11% moisture and 90% or more dry matter (DM).[1,5] They are generally sold in the form of kibbles, biscuits, meals and expanded extruded pellets.[5–7] These may be "complete and balanced" for all life stages or designed for a specific life stage. They may also be formulated only to be a treat or snack.[5–7] This is the food choice when the owners feed ad lib.[1] This type of food also tends to be the most economical to feed.[1]

A certain level of starch content must be included in expanded products to allow for proper processing of the product. This generally is met through the inclusion of cereals, cereal by-products and soy meals.[5] The loss of nutrients, particularly vitamins, through processing is limited because the baking or extrusion processes do not require excessive temperatures or time, and sufficient supplements are added to counterbalance processing and storage losses.[6] Because of the low moisture content of the food, they usually do not contain enough water for bacterial or fungal growth and have a long shelf-life if kept in cool, dry storage conditions.[6]

Kibbles and biscuits are prepared in much the same way, though the final shapes are different.[5] In both cases, the ingredients are mixed to form a dough similar to cookie dough, then baked. When biscuits are made, the dough is formed or cut into desired shapes, and the individual biscuits are baked like cookies.[5] With kibbled foods, the dough is spread onto large sheets and baked. After cooling, the large sheets are broken into bite-sized pieces and packaged.[5] Most dog and cat treats are baked biscuits, though some companies still produce complete and balanced kibble.[5] Dry meal foods are prepared by mixing several dried, flaked and granular ingredients to form a dog and cat version of "trail mix."[5,7]

The development of the extrusion process by Purina in the 1950s resulted in the almost complete replacement of meals and kibbles with extrusion in commercial foods.[5] The extrusion process produces expanded pet foods and involves mixing all the ingredients together to form a dough. This dough is then cooked under conditions of high pressure and temperature in an extruder. When the cooked dough reaches the end of the extruder (within 20-60 seconds), it exits through a small die. This die forces the soft product into the desired shape(s), and a rotating knife cuts the pieces into the desired kibble size.[5] The extrusion process causes rapid cooking of the starches within the product, resulting in increased digestibility and palatability. After cooling, a coating of fat or digest (a type of flavor enhancer produced by chemical or enzymatic breakdown of proteins) is usually applied to the outside of the food in a process called enrobing. The enrobing further enhances the palatability of the food. Hot air drying reduces the total moisture content to 10% or less.[5]

Dry foods contain a greater concentration of nutrients and energy per unit weight than foods with higher moisture content. Because of this, relatively small amounts are needed to provide a particular quantity of nutrients.[6,7] Unless they contain a large amount of nondigestible fiber such as cellulose or hemicellulose, the overall digestibility of dry foods is good but often lower than that of meats or canned foods.[6] Dry foods are better digested by dogs than by cats due to the higher carbohydrate content found in the diets.[6] Since most cat foods have higher protein and lower carbohydrate levels than dog foods, this difference is negligible.

Dry foods also tend to be less expensive than canned or semi-moist diets, but this can vary based on the ingredients used and the quality of those ingredients.[7] The primary disadvantage of dry diets is that they are less palatable than meats or canned diets. Still, the process of enrobing the finished kibble can affect this by increasing palatability.[1,6] Decreased palatability can be an advantage in animals that are overweight or obese but can be problematic in finicky or underweight animals.[1] The primary advantage of dry foods would be cost and convenience.

Most popular or premium brands of dry foods may be lower in nondigestible fiber than less expensive brands and are comparable to quality canned foods in the digestibility of nutrients.[7] The stools produced will help indicate the quality of the food, with high-quality food-producing well-formed, firm stools 1-2 times/day, while a poor-quality food may result in bulky, less formed stools produced more often.[7]

The availability of essential fatty acids (EFAs), especially linoleic acid for the dog and arachidonic acid for the cat, can be affected by prolonged storage in less than optimal conditions for some completely dry foods. This would include those foods stored in warm, damp environments (kitchens) or exposed to sunlight. This is a particular problem if beef tallow (fat) is used as the fat source.[5,7] This can also be seen in those situations where food is bought in bulk, especially with a small dog or cat, and stored in an open container in the kitchen for prolonged periods (6 months or more).[5,7]

Moist Pet Foods

Moist diets are no longer just found in "cans" but also in plastic trays, foil containers, plastic cans and pouches. These products have a moisture range of 60-87% on an "as-fed" basis.[1,7] Moist diets can either be "complete and balanced" or designed to be used for supplemental feeding, as with a treat.[5] Cats, unlike dogs, are more likely to receive most of their calories from moist diets.[1]

Moist diets are prepared by first blending the meat and fat ingredients with measured amounts of water. Measured amounts of dry ingredients are then added, and the entire mixture is heated.[5] Canning occurs on a conveyor line. After filling, the cans are sealed, washed and labeled. Pressure sterilization of canned products is called retorting.[5] Temperatures and times can vary with the product and size, but typically at 250 °C/480 °F for 60 minutes.[5] After exiting the retort, the cans are cooled under controlled conditions to ensure the sterility of the food and the integrity of the sealed product. After cooling, paper labels are then applied.[5]

For processing methods, there are three main types of moist foods-loaf, chunks or chunks in gravy and chunk-in-loaf combinations.[5] See Table 16.1.

Depending on the ingredients used, these products can vary greatly in nutrient content, digestibility, and nutrient availability.[5] These diets are often higher in fat, sodium and phosphorus when compared to dry foods.[1] Many owners assume that the "meaty chunks" found in the food are meat. More commonly, these chunks are textured soy products (TSP) similar to tofu. These chunks provide the owners with the visual appeal they are looking for while keeping the cost down for the manufacturer.[5]

Table 16.1 AAFCO recognizes these various 3 main types of moist pet food products.

Loaf	Ground cereal and chopped meat, fish and poultry. Has a solid meatloaf-like appearance
Chunks, chunks in gravy	Ground cereal and chopped or pre-formed meat. It may be meat-based, fish-based, or meat and cereal-based. May appear as balls, shapes or chunks together with gelling agents and mineral/vitamin supplements in gravy or jelly
Chunk-in-loaf	A combination of the chopped loaf appearance and the chunks in gravy foods

Source: Burger.[6]

Moist diets tend to be more palatable and digestible than many dry foods, but a poor-quality moist diet would not be more digestible than a good-quality dry food.[5] The high heat and pressure used in processing a moist diet kills harmful bacteria and causes some nutrient losses.[5] Manufacturers that conduct feeding trials adjust their formulas to compensate for these losses. Companies that use the calculation method to substantiate their label claims are not required to compensate for losses because the calculation method is used before processing the ingredients.[5]

The high moisture content of these foods affects the nutrient density, meaning that these foods have fewer nutrients per 100 g of food than other food types so that more food must be eaten to satisfy energy and nutrient needs.[7] The higher moisture content and lower energy density can help provide satiety and reduce calorie intake. The higher moisture content can also be helpful when dealing with a patient where increased water intake is desirable, such as urinary tract health concerns and chronic renal failure.[1]

The most palatable diets contain little or no cereal products and are presented as meaty or fishy chunks in gravy or jelly.[6] Protein content can range from 7% to 9% in dog foods and 8-11% in cat foods on an "as-fed" basis.[6] Digestibility of moist foods for both dogs and cats is high, being 80-85% for most nutrients in quality products.[6] Energy density is the highest in moist diets on a dry-matter basis of all commercially available diets, but the water serves to dilute this. Palatability is directly related to the meat and fat content, with the foods higher in cereal being less palatable.[6]

Moist foods offer an extremely long shelf life with high acceptability by the pet. Because of their nutrient content and texture, canned foods tend to be highly palatable. If moist diets are fed free choice to an animal with low energy requirements, they can override their tendency to eat to meet energy requirements, resulting in overeating and obesity.[5]

Because the diets are sterilized using steam and heat, no other preservatives are needed. This makes them ideal for a client concerned about the use of preservatives in their pets' food.[1] Though many owners do not like the smell or mess associated with moist diets or that unused portions need to be stored in the refrigerator.[1]

Not all moist foods are complete and balanced; many are designed for supplemental feeding only. Many clients use these foods to "top dress" their pets' dry foods to improve palatability. This is what they are supposed to be used for. Still, many animals, especially cats, can easily develop "fixed food preferences" and will only eat this one food item and refuse all others regardless of nutrient balance (cats are not very good at math).[5]

Semi-Moist Foods

The third class of food products is the semi-moist or soft-moist foods. These foods generally contain between 15% and 30% water and can include fresh or frozen animal tissues, cereal grains, fats and simple sugars as their main ingredients.[5] Semi-moist foods more closely resemble dry foods in nutrient content; they tend to have higher proportions of animal protein and a higher energy density on a dry-matter basis.[6] The carbohydrate portion of the diet is mainly disaccharides (sucrose).[6] Digestibly can be as high as 80-85%.

Preservation is achieved through the use of humectants and certain preservatives.[5,6] Humectants such as sugars, salts and glycerol are included in the foods to decrease water availability for use by invading microorganisms.[5,6] This helps to retard microbial spoilage. The addition of potassium sorbate is used to inhibit the growth of yeast and molds, and small amounts of organic acids can be included to decrease the pH and further help in inhibiting bacterial growth.[5,6]

The high sugar content of many semi-moist products contributes to palatability and digestibility, especially for dogs. Cats are less likely to select a sweet food, remember that cats lack salivary amylase and sweet receptors on their tongues.[5] Semi-moist diets that contain high levels of simple carbohydrates have digestibility similar to those of moist products. However, because of their lower fat content, the energy density tends to be lower.[5] The carbohydrate content of semi-moist diets is similar to that found in dry food diets, but the carbohydrate type found is mainly in the form of simple carbohydrates, with relatively small proportions of starch, complex carbohydrates or fibers.[5] Because of the use of simple carbohydrates for preservation, these diets would not be recommended for use by diabetic animals. The use of semi-moist treats should be limited to less than 10% of the overall diet.

Semi-moist foods do not require refrigeration before use and have a relatively long shelf life. The overall cost of the foods tends to be in between dry foods and moist foods.[5] Because they are usually sold in single-serving packets, the price is usually closer to moist diets.[5] Some owners prefer semi-moist diets due to the relative lack of odor and mess associated with moist foods and because they come in shapes similar to foods they eat (e.g., burgers, vegetables, etc.). These diets can become hard and dry out if left exposed to room air for extended periods.[1]

On an "as fed" basis, semi-moist diets have the highest caloric density than dry or moist diets. They have lower moisture content than do canned foods and fewer air pockets than extruded products.[5]

Raw

Raw food diets can either be commercially prepared or homemade by the owner.[8] These may be referred to as "BARF" diets, which stand for either "bones and raw foods" or "biologically appropriate raw food" diets.[1] Some advocates for this type of diet present the theory that dogs should be fed raw meat because their wild ancestors survived and present-day relatives continue to survive on uncooked food.[8] There is no compelling scientific evidence to support statements that dogs should eat uncooked food, as did their wild ancestors.[8] Numerous studies present evidence that a raw diet tends to be unbalanced and can present significant parasite and microorganism risks to pets consuming them and their families.[8]

The two most common forms of raw food diets fed include commercially complete foods intended as sole source nutrition and combination diets where the owner purchases a supplement mix that is then combined with the raw meat they provide.[1] For the complete diets, they are available as fresh raw food, frozen raw food and freeze-dried raw diets that the owner can rehydrate before feeding.[1] With the combination diets, the owner has more flexibility in what source of meat is being fed as they purchase that to mix with the supplement.[1]

Proponents of this type of diet claim many health benefits associated with feeding raw foods. Some of these include improved coat health and dental benefits (less gingivitis and tarter). These diets' high-fat content (>50%) can account for improved coat health. Increased incidence of periodontitis and tooth fractures have been associated with the feeding of raw meats and bone. In a study conducted by Drs. Freeman and Michel, none of the homemade and commercially available raw food diets analyzed were appropriate for long-term feedings. Each diet has deficiencies or excesses in nutrient levels, some of which are significant.[8]

Significant health problems have been associated with feeding pets' raw food diets. These include the risk of nutritional imbalances, cracked or fractured teeth, gastrointestinal obstruction and perforations, bacterial contamination of the pet's GI tract and the environment in which the food is prepared and fed, and the potential for parasitic infections from contaminated meat.[1]

The overwhelming majority of raw food diets have not undergone feeding trials to detect any nutritional imbalances in their formulations. They count on the owner's ability to detect any imbalance and institute a corrective program or maintain a varied enough diet to prevent imbalances over time rather than over each meal.

Snacks and Treats

Many items can be used for treats, including some foods that people eat and others very few people would care to consume. Owners spend a considerable amount on treats, though the feeding of table scraps incurs no additional costs.[9] A 2006 study by Euromonitor showed that dog owners in the US spent more than $1.7 billion on treats for their dogs and nearly $234 million on treats for their cats in 2005.[9] The American Pets Products Association reports that consumers spent over $18 billion on food and treats in 2010 and over $36 billion in 2019.[10]

Market research showed that more than 90% of dog owners who buy specialty dog food brands treat their dogs. Biscuits comprised 65% of the money spent, 45% buy bones and 40% buy various chews.[9] A 2006 study conducted by PetPlace.com indicated that the market continues to grow significantly, with 88% of dog owners, 65% of cat owners and 73% of bird owners providing treats to their pets.[9]

Snacks and treats are usually not purchased for their nutritional value but as a way of showing love and affection for the dog or cat, as training aids, as a distraction for long times spent in a cage, and just for fun.[5,9] Though most pet owners buy treats for emotional reasons.

Nutritionists advised that not more than 10% of the total daily calories be composed of treats.[9] Remember, this is total calories, not total volume eaten. Many treats can be quite calorically dense, and what only looks like 10% volume can be significantly more calories. Excessive feeding of treats can interfere with normal appetite, unbalance a previously balanced diet, and can contribute to obesity.[9]

Inappropriate use of treats occurs when the quantity consumed is more than the manufacturer's recommendations or over 10% of the daily calories or when the treats contribute excessive volumes of cream, meat, organ tissues and processed human foods.[9]

Because of this emotional connection, palatability is of chief importance.[5] In the early years, all dog treats were in the form of baked biscuits. Since the buying of treats is usually an impulse buy on the owner's part and intended to show affection or as a training aid, the design is geared primarily to the owner.

Today's treats can be categorized into four basic types: moist, biscuits, jerky and rawhide products. Cat treats are usually in the form of either semi-moist or biscuit products, with dogs preferring rawhide and jerky treats.[5]

Although treats and snacks do not have to be nutritionally complete, a significant proportion of the products are formulated to be complete and balanced. Some may carry the same nutritional claim as dog and cat foods.[5] In general, treats and snacks are highly palatable and cost significantly more than other types of pet foods when compared on a weight basis.[5] A large portion of this cost is due to the more significant amounts of money directed toward marketing.[5] Clients should be advised that treats contribute significant calories to the pet and should not be more than 10% of the total caloric intake per day.

A class of treats that is gaining increased popularity is those composed of dried animal tissues, including items such as bovine penis (bully sticks), tendons and hoofs, pigs' ears, snouts, and feet and bovine tails and tracheas.[9] These treats forms are typically greater than 85% protein. As most of this protein is composed of collagen, the biological value is very low, and the protein is unavailable to the animal.[9]

Large volumes of treats can contribute to the obesity epidemic and unbalanced therapeutic diets for managing diabetes mellitus, urolithiasis, cardiac failure, renal failure and adverse food reactions.[9] This is an important topic to cover with clients before starting management using therapeutic diets.

A relatively new line of foods is those designed to benefit oral health. Many products are available, with claims ranging from 'flosses teeth' to 'reduces harmful bacteria.' Few studies support these claims. The Veterinary Oral Health Council (VOHC) provides a list of accepted products on its website for both dogs and cats.[11] Products that have met the VOHC guidelines can put the VOHC Seal of Approval on their products.[12]

Toxicity and Recalls

Propylene glycol is a humectant used to keep semi-moist foods and treats semi-moist.[13] While the FDA says that it is generally regarded as safe (GRAS) as a food additive, cats are particularly sensitive to it. Cats can develop Heinze body anemia from foods containing as little as 5-10% of the product. However, research has not shown the same problem with dogs. As with many other toxic chemicals, the dose makes a difference, and when consumed in small quantities, no problems have been demonstrated.[13] Propylene glycol is also commonly found in 'pet-safe' types of antifreeze.

It is not uncommon to hear of dog and cat treats that the FDA has recalled. A list of these recalls is available on their website and is included in the references. The reasons for a product to get recalled can range from excessive vitamin D levels to bacterial contamination to incorrect compliance guidelines to possible chemical contamination.[10,13,14]

The bacteria of concern include those pathogenic to animals and the humans that handle the treats and their pets. Examples include *Clostridium botulinum* and *Salmonella* spp.[10]

A secondary problem with many rawhide and dried animal tissue treats is the potential to produce a choking hazard if the animal either ingests a large piece or swallows the entire item. Vigilance is required to help prevent this from occurring.

Few things would be more devastating to an owner than to have a product bought as a treat to contribute to severe illness or death.

References

1 Delaney S, Fascetti A (2012) Food types and evaluation. In S Delaney, A Fascetti (eds), *Commercial and Home-prepared diets in Applied Veterinary Clinical Nutrition*, pp. 95–105, Ames, IA: Wiley-Blackwell.

2 https://petnutritionalliance.org/resources/ nutritional-assessment-procedure/creating-a-nutritional-plan/. Accessed 6/27/23.

3 https://www.aaha.org/globalassets/ 02-guidelines/nutritional-assessment/ nutritionalassessmentguidelines.pdf. Accessed 6/27/23.

4 Pet Nutrition Alliance Dare to Ask Manufacturer Report. https://petnutritionalliance .org/resources/pet-food-manufacturer-evaluation-report/. Accessed 6/27/23.

5 Case LP, Carey DP, Hirakawa DA, Daristotle L (2000) Types of pet foods. In *Canine and Feline Nutrition* (2nd edn), pp. 187–97, St Louis, MO: Mosby.

6 Burger I (1995) Balanced diets for dogs and cats. In JM Wills, KW Simpson (eds), *The Waltham Book of Companion Animal Nutrition*, pp. 52–5, Tarrytown, NJ: Elsevier.

7 Kelly NC (1996) Food types and evaluation. In N Kelly, J Wills (eds), *Manual of Companion Animal Nutrition and Feeding*, pp. 22–42, Ames, IA: Iowa State Press.

8 Miller EP, Ahle NW, DeBey MC (2010) Food Safety. In MS Hand, CD Thatcher, RL Remillard *et al.* (eds), *Small Animal Clinical Nutrition* (5th edn), pp. 227–9, Marceline, MO: Walsworth Publishing.

9 Crane SW, Cowell CS, Stout NP *et al.* (2010) Commercial pet foods. In MS Hand, CD Thatcher, RL Remillard *et al.* (eds), *Small Animal Clinical Nutrition* (5th edn), pp. 160–1, Marceline, MO: Walsworth Publishing.

10 Sanderson SL (2021) Small pros and cons of commercial pet foods (including grain/grain-free) for dogs and cats. In D LaFlamme (ed.), *Animal Nutrition, Veterinary Clinics of North America, Small Animal Practice*, vol. **51**, Number 3, p. 532, Philadelphia, PA: Elsevier.

11 Veterinary Oral Health Council. http://www.vohc.org/accepted_products_dogs.html. Accessed 6/27/23.

12 Logan EI, Wiggs RB, Scherl D, Cleland P (2010) Periodontal disease. In MS Hand, CD Thatcher, RL Remillard *et al.* (eds), *Small Animal Clinical Nutrition* (5th edn), p. 994, Marceline, MO: Walsworth Publishing.

13 Scheidegger, J. Propylene glycol: Educate yourself and your veterinary clients. https://www.dvm360.com/view/propylene-glycol-educate-yourself-and-your-veterinary-clients. Accessed 6/27/23.

14 https://www.fda.gov/animal-veterinary/safety-health/recalls-withdrawals. Accessed 6/27/23.

17

Raw Food Diets

Introduction

It is generally accepted that dogs, *Canis familiaris*, were domesticated from an unknown and extinct wolf; the period of this evolution ranges from 10,000 to 135,000 years ago.[1] Accordingly, some recent DNA research shows that this occurred in stages in different areas. Not all domesticated dogs came from the same wolf species or geographic area.[1] Dogs have been shown to have originated in Europe between 32,000 and 19,000 years ago.[1] This time period is when humans were still hunter-gathers, and the agricultural revolution had not started.[1]

Ben Sacks from the University of California Davis, School of Veterinary Medicine has found genetic evidence that 6,000–9,000 years ago, ancient farmers brought dogs from Europe and the Middle East to an area of present-day China south of the Yangtze River.[2]

Early dogs in Europe and the Middle East continued to interbreed with wolves. In contrast, the dogs that had moved to China "apparently underwent a significant evolutionary transformation in southern China that enabled them to dominate and largely replace earlier western forms demographically." Dr. Sacks and his team also suggest that the ability of dogs to digest starch occurred during the domestication in China associated with the development of agriculture, specifically rice farming that had become a significant source of food for humans.[2]

The primary ancestor of the domestic cat, *Felis silvestris catus*, is believed to have been the African wild cat, *Felis silvestris libyca*. Domestication started for cats much later than for dogs, ~8000 years ago, with full domestication only 4000 years ago.[3] The time difference between these two species reflects what these animals were domesticated for: dogs were hunters and protectors, while cats were vermin killers on the farms. Our needs changed as we evolved from a hunting society to a farming society.

With this history in mind, we need to look at what food these animals have consumed since joining us in our farms and homes. Dogs did not continue to hunt and eat raw foods once domesticated; they primarily ate our leftovers and scraps. Since we have not consumed a raw food diet since fire was discovered, our dogs did not eat raw food either. Since cats were domesticated for their ability to control small vermin, they continued to eat a raw food diet for a much longer time.

Government and Professional Associations

The Centers for Disease Control's recommendation regarding raw food diets is "CDC does not recommend feeding raw food diets to pets. Germs like *Salmonella* in raw pet food can make your pets sick. Your family also can get sick by handling the raw food or by taking care of your pet"[4]

Nutrition and Disease Management for Veterinary Technicians and Nurses, Third Edition. Ann Wortinger and Kara M. Burns.
© 2024 John Wiley & Sons, Inc. Published 2024 by John Wiley & Sons, Inc.
Companion Website: www.wiley.com/go/wortinger/3e

The American Veterinary Medical Association (AVMA) position statement "discourages the feeding to cats and dogs of any animal-source protein that has not first been subjected to a process to eliminate pathogens because of the risk of illness to cats and dogs, as well as humans."[5]

The American Animal Hospital Association (AAHA) position statement is that "… homemade raw food diets are unsafe because retail meats for human consumption can be contaminated with pathogens…Many of the pathogens found in raw protein diets can be transmitted to the human population by contact with the food itself, pet or environmental surfaces… Feeding a raw protein diet no longer concerns only each individual pet but has become a larger community health issue; for this reason, AAHA can no longer support or advocate the feeding of raw protein diets to pets."[6] This position statement was further endorsed by the American Association of Feline Practioners (AAFP) and the National Association of State Public Health Veterinarians.

Nutritional Content

There is no scientific evidence showing that raw food diets are nutritionally superior to processed foods. All processed foods must conform to American Association of Feed Control Officials (AAFCO) standards for sale in the United States. These standards can be met in one of two ways. The food can be "formulated" to meet AAFCO standards or feeding trials. Feeding trials are the preferred method of substantiating AAFCO certification.[7] This considers nutrient content and nutrient loss due to processing and digestibility.

Raw food diets overall are not marketed as "complete and balanced" and therefore do not need to meet AAFCO standards. However, some frozen diets are marketed as "complete and balanced" and have AAFCO statements on the labels, but most have not undergone feeding trials. The claim is that these diets are "complete and balanced" over a period of time but not for each meal.

There are three main types of raw food diets.

- Commercially available complete raw food diets.
  - o These diets are intended to be complete and balanced without additional supplements. They are typically sold in frozen form.
- Homemade complete raw food diets (many recipes for homemade raw food diets are available in books, articles and the internet).
  - o These diets expect the owner to balance the diets out in the long term as each meal is not in itself balanced.
- Combination diets.
  - o These consist of commercially available mixes of grains and supplements. This mix is, in turn, combined with raw meat.[8]

Granted, raw food diets may be nutritionally superior to some commercially processed foods. Those would be the poor quality foods that have not gone through feeding trials, use lower grade ingredients and have high cereal contents. Feeding any premium quality food would improve the animal's hair coat, activity and overall health due to the increased quality of the ingredients used.

Since the majority of raw food diets have not gone through feeding trials, it is not easy to know if they are nutritionally balanced or not. Drs. Freeman and Michel conducted a study that looked at the nutrient content of various raw food diets, both home-prepared and commercially available. None of the diets studied were balanced, and all had nutrient deficiencies or excesses. The authors note that these deficiencies and excesses may have been balanced out in the long term, but this is not guaranteed.[8]

Pet food manufacturers know what changes occur with their foods with the various processing methods and supplement them to maintain optimum nutrient levels. As with any science, we continue to discover new ways to use diets to modulate various diseases or conditions every day. Pet food manufacturers continue to change and improve their foods.

Bacterial Contamination in Food

Pet food manufacturing facilities inspected by the FDA must establish and implement a food safety system. A preventative control measure must be implemented when a hazard has been identified.[9] This is designed to help prevent contaminated products from entering the food stream. This is especially important in regard to bacterial contamination and parasites. As few raw food diets come under the review of the FDA, these measures do not need to be implemented unless the diet is labeled as complete and balanced.

Numerous studies have found bacterial contamination in the food or dishes or death related to pathogenic bacteria found in raw food diets.[10–12] The bacterial contamination is directly linked to the diet being fed.[5,8,13–15] *Salmonella* spp. bacteria are normal enteric bacteria found in poultry, and consequently, contamination from undercooked or raw meat is common.[4] Human disease can occur when people ingest salmonella from undercooked meat or contaminated hands or environmental surfaces in the kitchen during preparation.[4]

The study done by Drs. Freeman and Michel looked at the nutrient content of the raw food diets and microbial analyses. One of the diets yielded growth of *Escherichia coli* 0157:H7.[5,8,15] This strain of *E. coli* has been connected to *E. coli* infections in people and is one of the more pathogenic strains.

Another study published in JAAHA reported two cats presenting for necropsy that died from septic *Salmonellosis*. One of the cases was directly traced back to the raw food diet fed. The two cases were 9 months apart in presentation but from the same household. Healthy adult cats appear to have high immunological resistance to the development of clinical *Salmonellosis*. Immunocompromised cats or those otherwise ill would be at increased risk of infection due to contaminated foodstuffs.[13]

Animals that are not sick themselves can also pose a public health concern due to the shedding of bacteria into the environment. Several bacteria can be found on raw meat and transmitted to animals and subsequently to their owners or others in contact with the animal or their stool.[15]

About 20-25% of poultry carcasses intended for human consumption test positive for *Salmonella* organisms. The raw meat used for feeding dogs is even more frequently contaminated. Most raw poultry is also contaminated with *Campylobacter* species, primarily *Campylobacter jejuni*. Foodborne infection is highly probable for dogs fed raw chicken.[14]

Shiga toxic *E. coli* strains are routinely isolated from fresh ground hamburgers. *E. coli* 0157:H7 has been identified in dog feces and would pose a hazard for environmental contamination.[14]

Yersinia enterocolitica can frequently be isolated from raw meat, especially pork. As much as 89% of the commercially available raw pork may be contaminated with this organism.[14]

Numerous food-borne parasitic infections can also affect dogs and cats. Feeding raw fish can result in infection with a variety of organisms, including *Diphyllobothrium latum,* the fish tapeworm; *Opisthorchis tenuicollis*, a trematode that infects the bile duct, pancreatic ducts and small intestines; *Dioclophyme renale*, the giant kidney worm; and *Nanophyetus salmincola,* the vector for *Neorickettsia helminthoeca*, the agent responsible for salmon poisoning in dogs.[14]

Dogs routinely fed raw meat are commonly infected with the protozoan *Sarcocystis* spp., and infected dogs may excrete sporocysts in their feces and contaminate the environment. Dogs can become infected with *Toxocara canis* and the raccoon ascarid, *Baylisascaris proconis*, from eating raw meat. Infected dogs can develop enteritis and shed infective eggs into the environment. In humans, these two parasites cause visceral larval migrans. Dogs are also susceptible to infection with *Trichinella spiralis,* whose larvae are found encysted in meat. Undercooked or raw pork is occasionally contaminated with this parasite.[14]

Health of the Pets

The primary claim from raw food proponents is that this diet improves the health of their pets. While this is relatively nebulous and hard to prove, few medical conditions can be directly traced to nutrition other than specific nutrient excesses or deficiencies.

On average, a wolf in the wild only survives to 8 years old. Wolves in captivity can survive up to 16 years. Most deaths in the wild are attributed to predation, disease and starvation. As Darwin showed us, life in the wild is survival of the fittest. An animal with many diseases we treat commonly in small animal medicine would not survive in the wild. That, to our pets, would be the benefit of domestication. Until recently, the medical knowledge to treat these conditions did not exist in veterinary medicine either, but as human medicine progresses, so does veterinary medicine.

It would be presumptuous to think that the conditions seen and treated in our cats and dogs do not exist in the wild and that this is solely due to the diet they consume. Furthermore, what would be the hunting ability of many of our current breeds? Could a Persian administer a cervical bite to a mouse, or is their breeding-induced malocclusion too severe to do this? What are the chances that a Frenchie would be able to catch and kill anything to eat, and considering the variety of foreign objects that a Labrador eats, would it be able to find the right food to kill and eat without developing a GI foreign body that results in its death?

Dental Health

There is significant concern among veterinarians that consumption of raw bones can lead to oral and dental trauma and esophageal and GI obstructive foreign bodies.[15] Compared to cooked bones, raw bones have a lesser potential of splintering and causing tooth fractures. However, there is still the strong possibility of sharp bone fragments being produced that can cause injury at any point along the GI tract from the mouth to the colon.[15] Grinding of bones included in the raw diets has been suggested to decrease the incidence of GI trauma, but the bioavailability of the calcium from these sources is still unknown.[15] Bones can also pose a significant risk of bacterial contamination, especially if they are allowed to remain at room temperature for extended periods.

Digestion and Digestive Enzymes

Some nutrients are destroyed by heat, but not all heat-sensitive nutrients are eliminated during cooking. This depends on the nutrient content of the food initially and how the food is processed, stored and cooked.[2]

Heat can also affect proteins. Proteins can be "denatured" by heat and pH. Once denatured, the process is irreversible. This happens with egg whites when they are cooked: the albumen becomes denatured and more accessible for the body to digest. Some proteins in meat also exist as enzymes; proponents of raw food diets contend that these enzymes become inactive when the meat is cooked.

These proteins would also become inactive in the stomach when they meet with the low pH of the gastric acids. Other enzymes are resistant to digestion (digestive enzymes) and may not be affected by stomach acid or the heat from cooking. There is little evidence for the enzymes affected by heat, suggesting that they are more beneficial to animals that eat them raw.[2]

Due to the cellulose layer found in all plant-based compounds, digestion of these nutrients is reduced until the cellulose layer breaks down, allowing the digestive enzymes to access the cell contents. This can be accomplished by chewing, grinding the food or cooking. As anyone who has watched a dog or cat eat or cleaned up vomited food knows, there is little grinding of their foodstuffs before it enters the stomach for continued digestion.

Plant-based materials are the primary source of carbohydrates for the body; these carbohydrates, in turn, are used for glucose production. If insufficient carbohydrates are available for energy, the body can also use glucogenic amino acids or glycerol from fats. If adequate dietary carbohydrates are not available, amino acids will be directed away from muscle growth, fetal growth and milk production for glucose production.[7]

As carbohydrates are heated or cooked with water, the starch contained within the cells undergoes a process called gelatinization. The greater the degree of gelatinization that occurs in the starch with cooking, the greater the digestibility for the food.

The central nervous system and the red blood cells require glucose for their energy needs, and they will not use alternate fuel sources such as ketones unless necessary. Glucose consumed over energy needs can be stored as glycogen. After glycogen stores are filled, any extra carbohydrates are converted into long-chain fatty acids and stored as fat.[7]

Options

Since feeding trials have not been done on the majority of raw food diets, their nutrient content, digestibility and supplementation levels are, for the most part, unknown. By using raw meats, clients are leaving their pets and themselves open to bacterial and parasitic infections from possibly contaminated meats. And there is also no guarantee of improved health.

What other options are available to clients in feeding their pets if they do not want to feed foods with preservatives, fillers, gluten or processing? There are numerous commercial diets available that provide similar nutrient profiles to those with raw food diets or do not contain grain, preservatives or offer natural ingredients.[15]

If the owner is determined to feed a homemade diet, a cooked formula designed by a trained veterinary nutritionist would provide an excellent option and ensure that adequate nutritional needs are being met.[15]

Conclusion

First and foremost, do not ostracize these clients; most people opting to feed a raw food diet are conscientious owners looking to do the best thing for their pets. They, unfortunately, do not have a veterinary nutritionist in their kitchens. Most importantly, getting them to cook the food being fed to their pet will address the bacterial and parasitic problems.

Find out what they do not like about commercially available diets. If they are misinformed on any issues, gently guide them in the right direction. If clients insist on feeding raw food diets or homemade cooked diets, recommend 2–4 visits/year for complete physical exams and blood screens to detect any problems before they become severe. These screenings and exams should include a complete serum biochemistry profile including T4 levels, CBC with differential and complete urinalysis.

References

1 Morell V. How wolf became dog. In Scientific America. https://www.scientificamerican.com/article/how-wolf-became-dog. Accessed 12/9/21.

2 Sacks B. Agriculture and parting from wolves shaped dog evolution in VetLearn 2/22/2013 https://www.ucdavis.edu/news/agriculture-and-parting-wolves-shaped-dog-evolution-study-finds. Accessed 12/9/21.

3 Bisno J. (1997). Cats in Ancient Egypt. Natural History Museum of Los Angeles County. https://www.academia.edu/42513082/Feline_faced_Deities_of_the_Underworld. Accessed 12/9/21.

4 Weese JS. Raw pet food and human Salmonellosis. https://www.wormsandgermsblog.com/2018/10/articles/animals/dogs/raw-pet-food-and-human-salmonellosis. Accessed 12/9/21.

5 AVMA Policy statement: raw or undercooked animal-source protein in cat and dog diets. https://www.avma.org/resources-tools/avma-policies/raw-or-undercooked-animal-source-protein-cat-and-dog-diets. Accessed 12/9/21.

6 AAHA Position statement: raw protein diet. https://www.aaha.org/about-aaha/aaha-position-statements/raw-protein-diet. Accessed 12/9/21.

7 Roudebush P, Dzanis DA, Debraekeleer J, Glenn BR (2000) Pet food labels. In MS Hand, CD Thatcher, RI Remillard, P Roudebush (eds), 4th edn *Small Animal Clinical Nutrition*, pp. 147–50, Marceline, MO: Walsworth Publishing.

8 Freeman LM, Michel KE (2001) Evaluation of raw food diets for dogs. *Journal of the American Veterinary Medical Association* **218**(5): 705–9.

9 FSMA Final rule on preventative controls for animal food. https://www.fda.gov/food/food-safety-modernization-act-fsma/fsma-final-rule-preventive-controls-animal-food. Accessed 12/9/21.

10 Schlesinger DP and Joffe DJ. Raw food diets in companion animals: a critical review https://www.ncbi.nlm.nih.gov/pmc/articles/PMC3003575. Accessed 12/9/21.

11 Freeman Lisa M and Chandler Marjorie L. Current knowledge about the risks and benefits of raw meat-based diets for dogs and cats. https://avmajournals.avma.org/view/journals/javma/243/11/javma.243.11.1549.xml. Accessed 12/9/21.

12 Davies RH, Lawes JR, Wales AD. Raw diets for dogs and cat: a review, with particular reference to microbiological hazards. https://onlinelibrary.wiley.com/doi/10.1111/jsap.13000. Accessed 12/9/21.

13 Stiver Shane L, Frazier KS, Manuel MJ (2003) Septicemic Salmonellosis in two cats fed a raw meat diet. *Journal of the American Animal Hospital Association* **39**(6): 538–42.

14 LeJeune JT, Hancock DD (2001) Public health concerns associated with feeding raw meat diets to dogs. *Journal of the American Veterinary Medical Association* **219**(9): 1222–4.

15 Delaney S, Fascetti A (2012) Commercial and home-prepared diets. In S Delaney, A Fascetti (eds), *Applied Veterinary Clinical Nutrition*, pp. 104–5, Ames, IA: Wiley-Blackwell.

18

Grain-Free and Boutique Diets

Introduction

Grains have been standard in commercial pet foods until approximately 10-15 years ago.[1] The exclusion of grains from pet foods was driven primarily by marketing and not scientific evidence. Marketing claims were made that grains were used as fillers in pet food or that the grains used in pet foods had been rejected for human consumption and were therefore inferior in quality. Claims were also made that associated grains with allergies and other more nebulous problems.[1]

Marketing Versus Science

Marketing of pet foods that excluded grains was used to vilify certain ingredients while promoting others. Certain grains (specifically corn, wheat and rice) were the primary ingredients of concern and animal by-products.

This exclusion effort was occurring in pet foods while human doctors were trying to encourage the consumption of whole grains as having proven healthful benefits to people.[1]

Approximately $1.7 billion was spent on grain-free pet foods from September 2012 to September 2013 in US pet specialty stores. This accounts for a 28% increase in sales, making this one of the fastest-growing segments of the pet food market.[2,3] Food sales only account for a portion of the total pet food sales through these outlets.

Grain-free is marketed as a healthy alternative to conventional grain-inclusive pet foods. However, there is no scientific evidence comparing nutrient levels or ingredients in these foods versus conventional pet foods.[1]

No long-term safety studies have been done on these grain-free diets, except for those markets by companies that meet WSAVA guidelines. As this is such a fast-growing segment of the pet-food market, and consumer demand was high, even premium pet food manufacturers jumped on the bandwagon.[1]

Grains

Botanically speaking, grains are the reproductive parts of many types of grass that have been cultivated from wild plants over the millennium by human farmers. Grains provide a rich source of nutrients, including essential amino acids, essential fatty acids, antioxidants, vitamins and minerals, energy through starches and fats and fiber.[1]

Grains also contain protein in the form of glutens. In particular, one gluten protein, gliadin, has raised many concerns through marketing.[1] Gliadin is a type of gluten protein found in wheat, barley and rye. Non-gliadin gluten proteins are found in corn and rice.[1] In humans, gliadin has been associated with celiac disease. This sensitivity in veterinary medicine is exceedingly rare, confined to 1 inbred strain of Irish setters in Europe.[3]

Nutrition and Disease Management for Veterinary Technicians and Nurses, Third Edition. Ann Wortinger and Kara M. Burns.
© 2024 John Wiley & Sons, Inc. Published 2024 by John Wiley & Sons, Inc.
Companion Website: www.wiley.com/go/wortinger/3e

Science has demonstrated that with proper processing, plant proteins are nearly as digestible as animal-based proteins. An additional benefit to grains is that contrary to current marketing claims, allergies to grains are very rare.[3] Most allergies are to proteins, not carbohydrates, the primary nutrient in most grains.[3]

Carbohydrate Digestion

By mapping the dog and wolf genomes, scientists have identified novel genome adaptations that allowed ancestors of modern dogs (and modern dogs themselves) to thrive on a starch-rich diet compared to wolves.[2]

While cats are obligate carnivores and require certain nutrients that can only be provided from animal sources, they can digest carbohydrates well. They produce amylase to break down dietary starches and have a glucose transport system in the intestines, to move these mono-and di-saccharides into the enterohepatic circulation for use by the rest of the body.[2] No studies have shown that grain-inclusive foods are harmful to cats and dogs or cannot provide the nutrients they need to live and thrive.[2]

Grain Substitutes

When grains are removed from a diet, alternative carbohydrate sources are still required, especially for dry foods, which need carbohydrates in their processing methods to help hold the product together. These alternative ingredients include legumes or pulses, potatoes, sweet potatoes and tapioca/cassava.[2] Legumes refer to the individual plants, while pulses are the plants' seeds.

A study looked at feline grain-free foods specifically and identified peas, cranberries, potatoes and carrots as the most common grain substitutes.[4] While cranberries have been suggested as helping with urinary tract health in humans, this has not been studied in cats. Furthermore, the number of cranberries included in the food is negligible, contributing nothing to the overall composition of the food.[4]

Nutrient Profiles

While grain-free therapeutic diets have been available for nearly 20 years, these diets meet or exceed WSAVA guidelines and are complete and balanced, as demonstrated through feeding trials.[1]

Very few commercially available grain-free diets have undergone feeding trials, and their nutrient profiles may be higher or lower in carbohydrates than similar grain-inclusive foods. Just substituting carbohydrate sources does not improve the quality of the food.[3]

Additionally, while the use of grains in pet foods has a long history with a lot of research behind it, no long-term safety studies have been done on these ingredients.[1] We do not know what the long-term implications of inclusion in pet foods can cause.[1]

Dilated Cardiomyopathy

One specific area of concern has been the recent development of diet-associated dilated cardiomyopathy (DCM) in dogs. Beginning in 2018, the cases of DCM reported to the Food and Drug Administration (FDA) went up significantly, from 3 cases reported in 2017, 320 cases reported in 2018, 619 cases in 2019 and 170 cases in 2020.[5] The majority of these dogs were fed dry food (88%), with 90% of the foods fed being marked as grain-free and 93% of the diets having peas and/or lentils in them in a significant proportion[5] See Figure 18.1.

Cases were reported in breeds typically associated with DCM and breeds (including mixed breeds and mutts) not associated.[6] For cases being fed grain-free diets, an improvement in symptoms was seen with a change to a

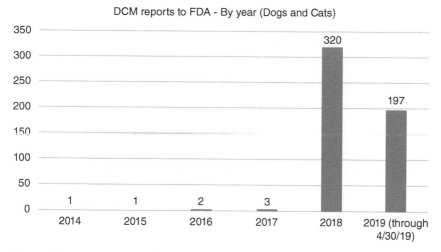

Figure 18.1 Reports of Dilated Cardiomyopathy in dogs and cats received by the FDA by year. *Source*: FDA[5]/U.S Food & Drug Department https://www.fda.gov/animal-veterinary/outbreaks-and-advisories/fda-investigation-potential-link-between-certain-diets-and-canine-dilated-cardiomyopathy.

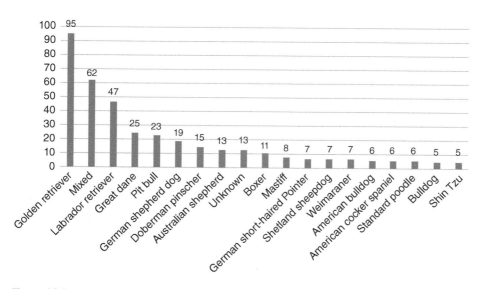

Figure 18.2 DCM cases: Breeds most frequently reported to the FDA. *Source*: FDA[5]/U.S Food & Drug Department https://www.fda.gov/animal-veterinary/outbreaks-and-advisories/fda-investigation-potential-link-between-certain-diets-and-canine-dilated-cardiomyopathy.

grain-inclusive diet, and medications, though significant numbers of these dogs are dying from this disease. See Figure 18.2.

Unlike dogs with genetic DCM, the diet-associated cases have tended to live longer with appropriate treatment. Interestingly, two studies have shown occult disease in asymptomatic dogs, with larger heart size and weaker contractions found on echocardiograms, reflecting damage to the heart.[6] Research is ongoing to determine the source of the problem with these foods. More information on diet-associated DCM can be found in Chapter 45. See Figure 18.3.

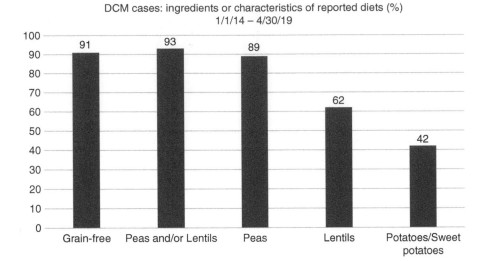

Figure 18.3 Primary ingredients or characteristics of diets reported to the FDA. *Source*: FDA[5]/U.S Food & Drug Department https://www.fda.gov/animal-veterinary/outbreaks-and-advisories/fda-investigation-potential-link-between-certain-diets-and-canine-dilated-cardiomyopathy.

Boutique Foods

The term "boutique" is defined by Merriam-Webster as "a small company that offers highly specialized services or products."[7] Regarding pet foods, this term refers to foods manufactured by small companies, that may not perform research or use ingredients and recipes approved by veterinary nutritionists, and backed by years of research on their digestibility and nutrient profiles.[6]

The gold standard of pet food testing is feeding trials following the AAFCO guidelines. Few of these boutique pet food manufacturers spend the money required to perform these tests and instead attain their AAFCO certification through chemical analysis or recipe analysis of their ingredients. This method provides no information on digestibility, nutrient interactions or palatability.

These foods tend to be heavily marketed and may use exotic ingredients that veterinary nutritionists have not used or researched extensively. We have years of research on chicken, beef and lamb as protein sources in pet foods and rice, wheat and corn as carbohydrate sources.

No evidence demonstrates that kangaroo, bison or pheasant are better protein sources for pet foods or that spelt (an ancient wheat grain), peas or sweet potatoes are better carbohydrate sources.[4]

Boutique foods are much more expensive than comparable foods that have met WSAVA guidelines and have undergone feeding trials using commonly found ingredients. Presumably, this extra cost is associated with exotic ingredients and marketing.[3]

References

1 Sanderson SL (2021) Small pros and cons of commercial pet foods (including grain/grain-free) for dogs and cats. In D LaFlamme (ed.), *Animal Nutrition* *Veterinary Clinics of North America, Small Animal Practice* Vol 51, Number 3, pp. 529–50, Philadelphia, PA: Elsevier.

2 Phillips-Donaldson D. Grain-free pet foods are all the rage, but are they really better for dogs-and are they sustainable? https://www.petfoodindustry.com/articles/ 4107-riding-the-grain-free-petfood-wave Riding the grain-free petfood wave. Accessed 12/10/21.

3 Freeman LM, Linder DE, Heinze CR. Grain-free diets-Big on marketing, small on truth. https://vetnutrition.tufts.edu/2016/ 06/grain-free-diets-big-on-marketing-small- on-truth. Accessed 12/10/21.

4 Heinze CR. New insight into grain-free cat diets. https://vetnutrition.tufts.edu/2017/07/ research-update-new-insight-into-grain-free- cat-diets. Accessed 12/10/21.

5 FDA investigation into potential link between certain diets and canine dilatated cardiomyopathy. https://www.fda.gov/ animal-veterinary/outbreaks-and- advisories/fda-investigation-potential-link- between-certain-diets-and-canine-dilated- cardiomyopathy. Accessed 12/11/21.

6 Freeman LM. Risk of heart disease in boutique or grain-free diets and exotic ingredients. https://vetnutrition.tufts.edu/ 2018/06/a-broken-heart-risk-of-heart-disease- in-boutique-or-grain-free-diets-and-exotic- ingredients. Accessed 12/11/21.

7 Boutique. Merriam-Webster. https://www .merriam-webster.com/dictionary/boutique Accessed. 12/11/21.

19

Additives and Pet Food Preservatives

Introduction

Preservatives are added to foods to help prevent microbial growth and oxidative damage to a food or food product. They also function to retard spoilage or help maintain certain desired qualities in foods, such as softness or crunchiness.[1–4] On the other hand, additives can make the food more appealing to the consumer. By using various colors, flavor enhancers, either artificial or natural, can make the food more palatable to the animal, and texture enhancers and nutrient additives are used to fortify or maintain the nutritional quality of foods.[4] In general, additives other than vitamins and minerals are found in the smallest amounts in moist foods and the largest quantities in dry foods, semi-moist foods, treats and snacks.[3]

Antimicrobial agents are designed to prevent microbial growth in or on pet foods.[4] Colors are used to increase the eye appeal to the consumer and offer little to the pet as they cannot differentiate the colors used.

Food manufacturers are responsible for ensuring that their foods remain free from bacterial contamination and harmful toxins and are protected from nutrient loss during storage.[1] The Food and Drug Administration (FDA) is concerned with additives and their food safety. A manufacturer must ensure that the additives are effective, detectable and measurable in the final product, and safe.[4]

Safety is defined as not causing cancer, birth defects or other injuries when consumed in

Table 19.1 Methods of preservation.

Dry foods	Low moisture content helps to inhibit the growth of most organisms
Moist foods	Heat sterilization and an anaerobic environment kill all microbes
Semi-moist foods	Low pH and humectants bind water in the food, making it unavailable to bacteria and fungi
Frozen foods	Protected by storage conditions and low temperatures
Irradiated foods	Sterilized by radiation

Source: Linda et al.[1] 2011/with permission of Elsevier.

large quantities by animals under controlled conditions. Many substances are exempted from FDA compliance because they are Generally Recognized as Safe (GRAS). This designation is based on their extensive, long-term use in foods or current scientific evidence.[4] Several hundred substances are on the GRAS list, including sugar, salt, caffeine and many spices[4] See Table 19.1.

Antioxidants

An antioxidant is any substance that significantly delays or prevents oxidation of that food product when added to food.[5] Foods that have no added antioxidant preservatives at the time of processing may contain ingredients such as animal fat, fish meal and fat-soluble vitamins preserved with antioxidants.[6]

Nutrition and Disease Management for Veterinary Technicians and Nurses, Third Edition. Ann Wortinger and Kara M. Burns.
© 2024 John Wiley & Sons, Inc. Published 2024 by John Wiley & Sons, Inc.
Companion Website: www.wiley.com/go/wortinger/3e

The primary nutrients that require protection during storage are fats in the form of vegetable oils or animal fats and the fat-soluble vitamins A, D, E and K.[1] It takes as little as 0.05% of the fat to react with oxygen to produce rancidity.[6] This oxidation of fats is called lipid peroxidation. The first stage is when a free radical, usually oxygen, attacks a poly-unsaturated fatty acid (PUFA) forming a fatty acid radical. This fatty acid radicals continue to react to oxygen, forming peroxides. These newly formed peroxides react with other fatty acids to form more fatty acid radicals and hydroperoxides.[1] This process is called propagation because the reaction continues on its own without the use of a catalyst. The reaction only ends when all the available fatty acids and fat-soluble vitamins have been oxidized.[1] Decomposition of the hydroperoxides contributes to the offensive odors, tastes and changes in texture found in rancid foods. One only has to think about rancid milk to understand the changes that have occurred to change a sweet liquid substance into a bitter, solid.

Oxidation of fats results in loss of calorie content and the formation of toxic peroxides that can be harmful to health.[1] A study done on growing Coonhounds found that dogs that ate diets containing oxidized fats had reduced serum vitamin E levels and compromised antioxidant status.[1] Antioxidant do not reverse the effect of oxidation once it has started. Still, they retard the oxidative process and prevent further destruction of fats. Therefore, they must be included in the diet when initially mixed and processed to be fully effective.[6] Ingestion of inadequately preserved rancid fats may be more harmful to the pet's health than any adverse effects of the preservatives.[6]

Naturally Derived Antioxidants

Naturally-derived antioxidants are commonly found in certain grains, vegetable oils, herbs and spices.[1] These antioxidants have been processed to make them more available for use.[1] No naturally-derived antioxidants do not undergo extensive processing to make them usable.

Mixed tocopherols, incorrectly called vitamin E, are obtained primarily from distilling soybean oil residue. Further processing separates α (alpha), λ (delta) and δ (gamma) fractions. Alpha-tocopherol, accurately called vitamin E, is the most biologically active form but provides little protection against oxidation in foods. Delta and gamma tocopherols have lower biological activity than alpha-tocopherol but are more effective as antioxidants.[1] Mixed tocopherols using both alpha and delta-tocopherols are the most effective naturally derived antioxidants and show the greatest efficacy in protecting fats in pet foods.[1] Because tocopherols rapidly decompose as they protect fats from oxidation, the shelf-life of foods preserved with tocopherols alone is shorter than that of foods stabilized with a mix of several different antioxidants.[1]

Ascorbic acid, more commonly called vitamin C, functions as an antioxidant by scavenging oxygen; however, it is water-soluble and not easily mixed with the fat found in foods. It does work synergistically with other antioxidants such as the mixed tocopherols and butylated hydroxytoluene (BHT) when included in foods for this reason.[1]

Ascorbyl palmitate is similar to ascorbic acid but is not generally found in nature. It undergoes hydrolysis to form ascorbic acid and the fatty acid, palmitic acid, both found in nature. Citric acid is often used in combination with other naturally-derived antioxidants.[1]

Dried leaves from the shrub *Rosmarinus officinalis* (common rosemary) are used to make a refined extract (rosmarinic acid). The extract is used to avoid the herb's influence on the taste and odor of the food.[1,2] This extract is effective in high-fat diets and has been shown to enhance antioxidant efficiency when combined with mixed tocopherols, ascorbic acid and citric acid.[1]

Effective antioxidants must have good carry-through. This is the retention of antioxidant functions after being subjected to the high heat, pressure and moisture of pet food processing.[1] Because most naturally derived antioxidants have poor carry-through, excessive amounts must be included to compensate for the high losses during processing.[1] Since naturally derived preservatives tend to be significantly more expensive than synthetic ones, it is not easy to achieve necessary levels of protection using only naturally derived products without production becoming cost-prohibitive.[1]

Marigold extract, obtained from common marigold flowers, is a source of lutein, a naturally occurring carotenoid antioxidant that may also positively affect immune and eye function.[1] This can also impart an attractive golden color to foods.

Lecithin, modified starches, monoglycerides and diglycerides are naturally derived compounds that act as emulsifying agents. This prevents the separation of fats from other dietary components and allows greater contact between the antioxidants and fats.[1]

Potassium sorbate is used to prevent the formation of yeast and molds in foods. Glycerol and certain other sugars are used as humectants to keep foods soft and moist.[1]

Synthetic Antioxidants

Synthetic antioxidants are made in laboratories and not from naturally derived products. The FDA has approved butylated hydroxyanisole (BHA) and BHT for use in both human and animal foods. When used together, they have a synergistic antioxidant effect, exhibit good carry-through, and increased efficiency compared with naturally derived antioxidants in protecting animal fats but have slightly lower efficacy in protecting vegetable oils.[1]

Tertiary butyl hydroquinone (TBHQ) is an effective antioxidant for most fats and is approved for human and animal use in the United States. However, TBHQ has not been approved for use in Canada, Japan or the European Union, so it is not used in foods for the international market.[1]

Ethoxyquin is approved for use in human and animal foods and has been used since 1959.[1,7] Its mechanism of action is similar to those of BHA and BHT in that it reduces oxidative damage of polyunsaturated fatty acids, vitamins A and E, and other fat-soluble substances by stopping free radical formation.[7] Ethoxyquin is more efficient than either BHA or BHT in protecting oils with high levels of polyunsaturated fatty acids such as linoleic, alpha-linolenic and arachidonic acids. This allows for lower levels of antioxidants to be added to the final product.[1]

Ethoxyquin has a toxicity rating of 3 and is considered moderately toxic. This rating is slightly higher than for tetracycline or penicillin and lower than for aspirin or caffeine.[6] Ethoxyquin is readily absorbed, metabolized and excreted in the urine and feces. Residual levels are found in the liver, gastrointestinal tract and adipose tissue.[6]

Before ethoxyquin gained FDA approval, the manufacturer (Monsanto, St Louis MO) conducted an l-year chronic toxicity study in dogs in which "no observable effect level" was determined to be 150 ppm (150 mg/kg) of food.[1] Mild changes were seen histopathologically in the liver and kidneys at much higher doses of 360 ppm (360 mg/kg) of food, with more pronounced signs of toxicity observed at 500 and 1000 mg/kg.[7] The Center for Veterinary Medicine (CVM) requested, as of July 31, 1997, that manufacturers voluntarily lower the maximum level of ethoxyquin in complete dog food to 75 ppm (75 mg/kg) of food, from the allowed 150 ppm to increase further the margin of safety for lactating females and puppies.[1,8]

Ethoxyquin and other synthetic preservatives have been blamed for widespread infertility, neonatal illness, death, skin and coat problems, immune disorders, thyroid dysfunction, liver and pancreas dysfunction and behavioral problems.[2,3,7] Reports of adverse reactions have been almost exclusively in dogs, the majority of these being purebred or

Table 19.2 Characteristics of some antioxidants.

Antioxidant	Carry-through	Effectiveness
Naturally derived		
Mixed tocopherols	Poor	Low
Ascorbic acid	Poor	Low
Ascorbyl palmitate	Poor	Low
Synthetic		
Butylated hydroxyanisole	Good	High
Butylated hydroxytoluene	Good	High
Tertiary butyl hydroquinone	Good	High
Ethoxyquin	Excellent	High

Source: Linda et al.[1] 2011/with permission of Elsevier.

inbred ones.[3,7] To date, the FDA has found no scientific or medical evidence that ethoxyquin used at approved levels is harmful to human or animal health.[2] After gaining FDA approval for ethoxyquin, Monsanto conducted an additional study of a multigenerational group of dogs over 5 years using foods with two times the approved level of ethoxyquin at that time (i.e., 360 ppm).[7] No adverse effects, especially those noted by breeders, were found in these dogs. See Table 19.2.

Antimicrobials

Bacteria can affect foods in two ways; one is relatively harmless—causing the food to lose flavor and attractiveness. The other way bacteria can affect food is by causing food-borne illnesses such as food poisoning.[4]

The most widely used antimicrobials found are ordinary salt and sugar. Salt has been used throughout history to preserve meat and fish. Sugar serves the same purpose in semi-moist foods.[4] Both of these products work by capturing water and making it unavailable to the bacteria.

Nitrites are also added to foods to preserve color, enhance the flavor by inhibiting the rancidity of fats and protect against bacterial growth.[4] Because of the concerns over nitrosamine formation when nitrites are heated, minimal amounts are used in food products to achieve the desired results.[4]

Food-borne infections can be caused by microorganisms such as *Escherichia coli* and species of *Salmonella, Neorickettsia, Vibrio, Yersinia* and *Campylobacter*. Illness can also be caused by ingestion of the toxins produced by such microorganisms as *Clostridium botulinum, Bacillus cereus, Staphylococcus aureus* and various mycotoxins.[2] Properly preserved foods kill most microorganisms by cooking/sterilization and prevent the proper conditions for growth in the final product. While cooking and sterilization can effectively kill bacteria contaminating food, they do not affect the toxins potentially produced by these bacteria.

Functional Ingredients

Functional ingredients are those added to food to provide a specific type of health benefit. In human foods, this is governed by the Dietary Supplemental Health and Education Act(DSHEA) passed in 1994.[1] The CVM, a division of the FDA, argues that this does not apply to pet foods but does allow the inclusion of functional ingredients made from AAFCO-approved ingredients or nutrients for which specific veterinary health claims are not made.[1] With this caveat in mind, if the CVM determines that a food is making a drug claim, instead of being used as a feed-ingredient, it can intervene and require that the ingredient in question be classified as a drug and undergo required testing and approval.[1] This can make the label claims on pet foods tricky. Using glucosamine as an example, a claim that it "supports joint health" is acceptable, but claims of reduces joint inflammation or decreases lameness are not acceptable.[1]

Chondroprotective ingredients for joint health in humans and pet foods include glucosamine and chondroitin sulfate. Others include green-lipped mussel powder, a source of glycosaminoglycans, omega-3 fatty acids and other nutrients.[1]

Coat shine and skin health are associated with overall health, and adding modified levels of omega-3 and omega-6 fatty acids, conjugated linoleic acid and formulations that combine various oils and B vitamins can be done.[1]

The gastrointestinal function can be supported by including moderately fermentable fibers and a combination of fibers in pet foods. These are typically the fructooligosaccharide (FOS) and mannanoligosaccharide (MOS) fibers. Fiber can also be added to foods to help manage furball formation in cats.[1]

Functional ingredients that support lower urinary tract health in cats include agents that may control inflammation and reduce the risk of crystal or stone formation. These formulations that are available OTC cannot make the same claims that veterinary therapeutic urinary diets can make.[1]

Colors

Only a few artificial colors remain on the FDA's approved list of additives for pet foods. Colors derived from natural sources must also meet the same purity and safety standards as synthetic colors.[4] Food color additives are common in pet foods and are used primarily for the consumer's benefit.[9]

Artificial Flavors and Flavor Enhancers

Natural and artificial flavors and flavor enhancers are the largest single group of food additives.[4] In people, the taste is confined to four primary groups: sweet, salty, bitter and acidic. Dogs and cats can also taste several amino acids that taste only weakly bitter or acidic to people.[5] These amino acids contribute to the meaty and savory aromas of pet foods.

Dogs can taste and demonstrate a preference for simple sugars, while cats show little interest in sweet flavors.[5] Foods acidified with a phosphoric or citric acid appeal to cats, though this is decreased in moist cat foods. Dogs do not seem to appreciate any significant changes in the pH of their foods.[5]

Texture and Mouth Feel

The mouthfeel of a particular food has a tremendous effect on food preferences for both dogs and cats.[5] The size and shape of expanded kibbles can be important in food acceptance. Dogs prefer larger kibbles over smaller kibbles of the same formula. Cats prefer one specific shape to others in identical formulas and may develop strong preferences for mouthfeel and can be found with a pile of sorted-out shapes sitting next to their food dishes.[5]

In moist diets, gums can be added to thicken sauces and help form gels that may appeal to certain animals.[4] Neither cats nor dogs like sticky foods.[5]

Smell

We know that dogs and cats have highly developed senses of smell compared to people. Despite this, foods must also provide a taste for animals to maintain a sustained interest in a particular diet.[5] The smell of moist foods can be intensified by heating to slightly below body temperature. This can be used to interest an animal in a particular food but obviously cannot be relied on to maintain interest. See Table 19.3.

Need for Additives

The need for antioxidants in pet foods is obvious. Therefore, questions about the safety of preservatives need to be balanced against the pets' needs. Canned or frozen foods have

Table 19.3 Common food additives.

Antioxidant— natural derived	Mixed tocopherols (vitamin E)
	Ascorbic acid (vitamin C)
	Ascorbyl palmitate
	Citric acid
	Rosemary extract
	Marigold extract
Antioxidant— synthetic	BHA
	BHT
	TBHQ
	Ethoxyquin
Antimicrobial	Sugar
	Salt
	Nitrite
	Potassium sorbate
	Glycerol
	Sterilization
Functional ingredients	Chondroitin sulfate
	Glucosamine
	FOS
	MOS
	Linoleic acid
	Omega-3 and omega-6 fatty acids
Texture enhancer	Guar gum
	Lecithin
Artificial color	GRAS colors
	Sodium nitrite
Flavor enhancer	Phosphoric acid
	Citric acid

Source: Adapted from.[1,4,5]

the lowest levels of antioxidants because either heat or cold-not antioxidants preserve them. Some pet food manufacturers produce dry foods preserved with naturally derived antioxidants, although they may contain small amounts of synthetic antioxidants in the vitamin premix. When buying a food preserved with only naturally derived antioxidants, look for a "best if used by" date, and use the food within this time frame. If no date is included on the package label, contact the manufacturer for information on when the product was manufactured and its shelf-life.

The FDA requires that preservatives in quantities high enough to affect the final product be listed on food labels. If the preservative is present in trivial amounts or no longer serves a technical or functional effect, it may be exempt from inclusion on the label.[10] This applies to premixes or vitamin additives in foods. Ethoxyquin is an exception to this regulation; the FDA CVM has stated that ethoxyquin should be declared on labeling regardless of the source or final level in the food.[10]

Manufacturers of premium pet foods conduct feeding trials on their products to detect deficiencies or other problems before foods are released for sale. Check the labels on the foods to see whether feeding trials have been done. Manufacturers must state how they have met AAFCO standards. The label should also list all the ingredients from largest amount to smallest.

Color, taste and texture will help maintain an interest in a specific food. Preservatives can help to maintain these factors, ensuring that the animal will continue to consume a particular food and not become ill in the process.

References

1 Case L, Daristotle L, Hayek MG, Raasch F (2011) Melody. Nutrient content of pet foods. In *Canine and Feline Nutrition* (3rd edn), pp. 155–60, St. Louis, MO: Mosby.

2 Zicker SC, Wedekind KJ (2010) Antioxidants. In M Hand, C Thatcher, R Remillard *et al.* (eds), *Small Animal Clinical Nutrition* (5th edn), pp. 149–55, Marceline, MO: Walsworth Publishing.

3 Roudebush P (1993) Food additives. *Journal of American Medical Association* **203**: 1667–70.

4 Whitney E, Rolfes SR (2008) Consumer concerns about food and water. In *Understanding Nutrition* (11th edn), pp. 682–5, Belmont, CA: Thomson Wadsworth.

5 Zicker SC, Wedekind KJ (2010) Antioxidants. In MS Hand, CD Thatcher, RI Remillard *et al.* (eds), *Small Animal Clinical Nutrition* (5th edn), pp. 149–55, Marceline, MO: Walsworth Publishing.

6 Dodds WJ, Donoghue S (1994) Interactions of clinical nutrition with genetics. In JM Will, KW Simpson (eds), *Waltham Book of Clinical Nutrition in the Dog and Cat*, pp. 114–5, Tarrytown, NY: Pergamon.

7 Dzanis D (1991) Safety of ethoxyquin in dog foods. *Journal of Nutrition* **121**: S163–4.

8 FDA Center for Veterinary Medicine: Labeling and use of ethoxyquin in animal feed. https://www.fda.gov/animal-veterinary/ingredients-additives/labeling-and-use-ethoxyquin-animal-feed. Accessed 12/12/21.

9 Crane SC, Cowell CS, Stout NP *et al.* (2010) Commercial pet foods. In MS Hand, CD Thatcher, RI Remillard *et al.* (eds), *Small Animal Clinical Nutrition* (5th edn), p. 169, Marceline, MO: Walsworth Publishing.

10 Dzanis D. (2009). US Pet Food Regulation Hot Topics in Focus on Nutrition CompendiumVet.com October 2009. http://vetfolio-vetstreet.s3.amazonaws.com/mmah/73/d04185a6234b8cb5ca482a5ed2b40a/filePV_31_10_462.pdf. Accessed 6/27/23.

20

Homemade Diets

Introduction

Counseling clients on feeding is one of the most critical client education services the veterinary team can offer.[1] Even though most pet owners in the United States enjoy the convenience, economy and reliability of commercially produced diets, some owners still prefer to prepare homemade diets for their pets.[2] The vast majority of dogs and cats in the United States are fed table food at some point in their lives.[3] Many pets learn of the availability of table scraps after a family meal and are very determined to share in the leftovers. As long as the supplementation of scraps does not exceed 10% of the caloric intake, this is not usually a problem as long as the food is not toxic (i.e., onions, chocolate and grapes)[3]

The reasons that clients choose to feed a home-prepared diet vary greatly. Some of the more common reasons are:

- They adopt a traditional approach among a minority of owners not using commercially prepared food.
- Induced food preference in pets by exposure to home-cooked food from kitten or puppy-hood.
- Anthropomorphism: giving human food preferences to pets.
- Picky eaters will "hold out" for tasty home-cooked treats
- Veterinarian-recommended home-prepared "elimination diets" may work better in some food-related diseases, such as skin problems.

- Poor owner perception of commercially prepared foods as "unwholesome" or unappetizing.
- Wanting to feed "what nature intended."
- Veterinary therapeutic diets may lack palatability or acceptability, particularly in advanced illnesses.
- Wanting to be involved in the care of their pet especially older or ill animals.
- Wish to use ingredients that are fresh, wild-grown, organic or natural
- Concerned that the ingredient list is an indecipherable list of chemicals.
- They hope to construct a nutritional profile for the dietary management of a disease for which no commercial food is available.
- They wish to provide food variety as a defense against malnutrition or because of the popular idea that animals need variety.
- They wish to lower feeding costs through the use of significant quantities of table foods and leftovers
- They wish to feed a pet according to human nutritional guidelines such as low fat or low cholesterol.
- They want to feed their pet according to their diet preferences, such as vegetarian/vegan diets.[4,5]

While many pet owners consulted their veterinary team for nutrition information regarding their pets, as many as 17% of owners cited the internet as their primary source of information.[6] The concerning part of this number is the vast amount of misinformation

Nutrition and Disease Management for Veterinary Technicians and Nurses, Third Edition. Ann Wortinger and Kara M. Burns.
© 2024 John Wiley & Sons, Inc. Published 2024 by John Wiley & Sons, Inc.
Companion Website: www.wiley.com/go/wortinger/3e

regarding dog and cat nutrition found on the internet. Feeding unbalanced, homemade diets can lead to many medical complications such as osteodystrophy, osteopenia, secondary nutritional hyperparathyroidism and pansteatitis.[6]

Even when recommended by the veterinarian, as many as 90% of the homemade diets were not balanced and were not nutritionally adequate to support the requirements for adult maintenance.[6] The primary problem with many homemade diet recipes is they contain too much protein instead of too little. This high protein level leads to one of the most common inverses, that of Ca:P ratio imbalances. This inverse ratio can lead to calcium deficiencies, vitamins A and E, and potassium, copper and zinc levels. For homemade cat diets, insufficient fat content or fat source is common.[1,6] Remember that cats require the essential fatty acid, arachidonic acid, which is only found in animal-sourced fats.

Compared to AAFCO requirements for specific life-stage nutrition, 55% of the veterinary recommended diets found in commonly used books had inadequate protein. All diets were deficient in the amino acid taurine, 64% had inadequate vitamin levels and 86% were deficient in minerals.[7]

Why Home Made?

When clients elect to feed homemade diets, it is essential to understand their reasons and motivations. It is possible to address their concerns and recommend an appropriate commercial diet that will meet everyone's needs in many cases.[5] In those instances where a client is insistent about cooking for their pet, it is always better to provide them with a well-designed homemade recipe, rather than allowing them to prepare food according to their own or a breeder's well-intentioned formulation that may have significant nutrient excesses and deficiencies.[5]

Any ingredient used in homemade diets should be safe for human consumption and preferably cooked. The quality of the nutrients depends on the source and digestibility of the ingredients.[4] One of the problems with preparing homemade diets is that many of the available recipes have not been adequately tested for nutrient content and availability.[2] Poor feeding management rather than faulty diets are responsible for many nutritional problems.[1] Even if a balanced diet is offered, clients will usually "adjust" the ingredients to their likes, very likely upsetting any balance that the diet did have, or will supplement with treats or snacks above 10% of the caloric requirements. This practice is commonly referred to as "diet drift."[3,7]

It should be noted that the most prevalent form of malnutrition that is seen in dogs and cats today is obesity. This would be even more likely to occur when an animal is fed a homemade, highly palatable diet with unknown nutrient density (i.e., caloric concentration).

Food Preparation

Any food fed to a pet needs to be properly cooked before feeding. Cooking improves digestibility and kills bacteria and parasites that might cause disease.[8] However, cooking does not eliminate the problem caused by endotoxins released from dead bacteria such as *E. coli* and *Clostridium botulinum*.[8] These endotoxins can be found in meats previously contaminated by bacteria.[8] Nothing can be done to decontaminate a food containing endotoxins.[8] Antibiotics are also ineffective in treating a pet who has ingested these endotoxins as they are not bacteria themselves. However, there are antitoxins available for some of these endotoxins, but not all are commonly found in most veterinary practices.

When foods are prepared at home, safe food handling and preparation methods determine whether or not the final diet will be safe for consumption.[8] Safe handling of food by owners begins at the store and continues in the home. Safe handling prevents or minimizes hazards associated with biological (bacteria), chemical (cleaning agents) and physical (equipment) causes.[8]

According to the Centers for Disease Control (CDC), handwashing is the single most important means of preventing the spread of infection from bacteria, pathogens and viruses, causing disease and food-borne illnesses.[8] Most importantly, food preparation includes hand washing done before and after handling each ingredient in the diet.[8] In addition to handwashing, counters, equipment, utensils and cutting boards should be sanitized with a dilute bleach solution.[8] Frozen foods should never be thawed at room temperature. Thawing should be done in the refrigerator, the microwave or a cold water bath.[8]

All ingredients used in the diet should always be cooked thoroughly. Freezing or rinsing with cold water is not an acceptable method for destroying bacteria.[8] Once a diet is cooked, it may be stored in the refrigerator and reheated later before serving.[8]

All diets should be prepared according to the specific recipe recommended, with no substitutions, additions, or omissions done by the client or veterinarian.

Ingredient Choices

Many owners choose their pet's diet ingredients based on their preferences, product availability or affordability.[5] Other pets are fed a variety of leftovers such as fat trimmings, vegetable skins, crusts and condiments. These diets rarely represent the owner's diet and are not "complete and balanced" for the pet.[5] Diet drift is commonly encountered when a client starts to substitute ingredients based on cost or perception of change needed by the pet. Each ingredient in a diet is important and provides specific nutrients to the diet. Inappropriate substitutions can contribute to the advancement of a disease process or change

the palatability of the overall diet.[6,7] Feline foods designed by clients are often deficient in fat and energy density or may contain an unpalatable fat source such as vegetable oil.[3]

Owners may also choose the ingredients based on current human nutrition trends. These include grain-free, gluten-free or vegetarian/vegan diets.[7] As we know, there are several differences between canine, feline and human nutrition and nutrient digestion and needs. Clients who feed their pets vegetarian/vegan diets are at the greatest risk of feeding an unbalanced, inadequate diet. Several commercially prepared canine vegetarian diets are complete and balanced.[5] Clients should be strongly discouraged from feeding cats vegetarian/vegan diets. Cats are obligate carnivores and have specific nutrient requirements that are only found in meat-based food sources, such as the amino acid taurine and the essential fatty acid arachidonic acid. Without adequate supplementation (usually available from only meat-based products), cats fed vegetarian or vegan diets are at high risk for taurine, arginine, tryptophan, lysine, arachidonic acid and vitamin A deficiency. These deficiencies are life-threatening and can lead to the death of the cat.[5]

Due to inconvenience, expense or failure to understand its importance, many clients eliminate the vitamin and mineral supplements in homemade diets. This would cause a recipe that was crudely balanced to become grossly imbalanced.[5] While vitamins and minerals do not contribute calories to the diet, they are the sole source of essential nutrients required for the normal, daily function of the animal.

Assess the Recipe

If possible, offer the client a nutritionally adequate recipe rather than making their own or using one from a non-veterinary source. There are several sources for clients to have nutritional balanced homemade diets formulated to meet their pet's needs. See Table 20.1.

Table 20.1 Sources of homemade diet recipes from veterinary nutritionists.

• Pet diet evaluations
www.PetDiets.com
www.Balanceit.com
https://acvn.org/nutrition-consults/ accessed 9/2/23
ACVN Diplomate Directory
https://acvn.org/directory/

The homemade formulation can be checked for nutritional adequacy and adjusted using the "quick check" guidelines below:[5]

- Do all five food groups appear in the recipe?
  - Carbohydrate/fiber source
  - Protein source, preferable animal origin
  - Fat source
  - Mineral sources, primarily calcium
  - Multivitamin and trace mineral source
- Carbohydrate source cooked and presented in higher or equal quantity than the protein source?
  - Feline carbohydrate: protein 1 : 1 to 2 : 1
  - Canine carbohydrate: protein 2 : 1 to 3 : 1
- What is the type and quantity of the primary protein source?
  - Final food should contain 25–30% cooked meat for dogs and 35–50% cooked meat for cats. Skeletal muscle meat is preferred. Liver can be used once weekly. If feeding lacto-ovo vegetarian diets, eggs are the best protein source. If feeding a vegan diet, soybeans provide the next best protein source but have an incomplete amino acid profile.[5] For cats, organ meats have higher taurine concentrations than muscle meats. Taurine levels can also be affected by cooking, specifically boiling leaches out available taurine rendering it unavailable to the animal.[7] Raw food diets have also been shown to have decreased taurine availability compared to commercial and cooked diets.[7]
- Is the primary protein source lean or fatty?
  - If using "lean" meat, an additional fat should be added either of animal, vegetable or fish source
  - 2% of the total formula weight for dogs
  - 5% of the total formula weight for cats
- Is a source of calcium and other minerals provided?
  - Absolute calcium deficiency is most common in homemade diets
  - Milk products usually contribute inadequate amounts of calcium to the diet
- Is a source of vitamins and other nutrients provided?
  - An adult over-the-counter supplement that contains no more than 200% of the recommended daily allowances for humans usually works well for dogs and cats
  - Give ½-1 tablet per day, based on pet size.
  - Cats should receive additional taurine supplementation, between 200 and 500 mg/day, depending on the diets' calculated taurine content
  - Iodized salt should be used to meet the iodine requirement[5]

Selecting a Diet

Software programs are available to help formulate a balanced diet from scratch. Contacting a member of the American College of Veterinary Nutrition (ACVN) for food recommendations is also recommended. Many veterinary schools offer help with homemade recipes. In addition, there are many published recipes available. Critically evaluate the source and see if any testing has been done on the recipe. References 1 and 4 contain a variety of recipes and acceptable substitutions. The sources listed in Table 20.2 can provide appropriate, balanced homemade recipes. There is usually a fee for this service. See Table 20.2.

Table 20.2 Veterinary schools/hospitals offering nutritional support services accessed 12/14/21.

- The University of Missouri, College of Veterinary Medicine, Veterinary Medical Teaching Hospital Nutrition Consultations

https://vhc.missouri.edu/small-animal-hospital/nutrition/

- The Ohio State University

https://vet.osu.edu/vmc/companion/our-services/nutrition-support-service

- Tufts Cummings School of Veterinary Medicine

https://vetnutrition.tufts.edu/

- University of California, Davis, School of Veterinary Medicine

https://www.vetmed.ucdavis.edu/hospital/small-animal/nutrition

- University of Florida, Small Animal Hospital, College of Veterinary Medicine

https://smallanimal.vethospital.ufl.edu/clinical-services/integrative-medicine-services/nutrition/nutrition-services-offered/

- University of Tennessee

https://vetmed.tennessee.edu/vmc/smallanimalhospital/small-animal-nutrition/nutrition-services/

- Virginia Tech Veterinary Teaching Hospital

https://vth.vetmed.vt.edu/inpatient-outpatient-services/nutrition.html .

Additional Instructions

Be sure to provide specific instructions for preparing, storing and feeding homemade foods to the pet owners. These diets do not contain preservatives and are high in moisture. They are more susceptible to bacterial and fungal contamination when left at room temperature for prolonged periods.[6] Food that is not immediately fed to the pet should be stored in an airtight container in the refrigerator for no more than a few days.[6] When the food has been stored in the refrigerator, it should be warmed to body temperature before feeding to increase palatability. If using a microwave,

make sure the food is mixed well before feeding to prevent the development of hot spots in the food.[6] If desired, a small amount of water can be added to the food to either increase the water intake or improve the consistency of the food. Any food not consumed at that meal should be discarded and not saved for the next meal.[6]

Explain the importance of each ingredient and the proper proportions to be used. Foods should be checked daily for any changes in color or odor that may indicate spoilage or deterioration.[5]

Patient Assessment and Monitoring

Dogs and cats fed homemade diets should be brought to the clinic for veterinary evaluations 2-3 times per year. The physical examination should include an assessment of body condition, body weight, and if indicated, CBC chemistry and urinalysis testing.[7] This will help identify any diet problems before they become too big to fix.[5]

The purpose of these exams is to evaluate the effectiveness of a diet by noting the patient's body weight, body condition and activity level. Laboratory levels such as albumin, red blood cell number and size and hemoglobin concentration are gross estimations of the animal's nutritional status. More specifically, the skin and hair should be examined closely, and an ophthalmic evaluation should be performed, looking specifically at the lens and retina. Stool quality needs to be also assessed.[5]

The diet history should be updated at every visit to determine if any changes to the diet have been done by the owner or need to be done by the veterinarian.[7] Often, what appear to be simple substitutions on the client's part can result in significant changes in the nutrition distribution in the diet.[7] A list of board-certified veterinary nutritionists can be located through the ACVN at www.acvn.org.

References

1 Strombeck DA (1999) Introduction. In *Home-Prepared Dog and Cat Diets, A Healthful Alternative*, pp. 3–19, Ames, IA: Iowa State Press.

2 Case L, Daristotle L, Hayek MG, Raasch F (2011) Melody. Types of pet foods. In *Canine and Feline Nutrition* (3rd edn), pp. 173–4, St. Louis, MO: Mosby.

3 Remillard RL, Crane SW Making pet foods at home. In MS Hand, CD Thatcher, RI Remillard *et al.* (eds), *Small Animal Clinical Nutrition* (5th edn), pp. 207–19, Marceline, MO: Walsworth Publishing.

4 Kelly NC (1996) Food types and evaluation. In N Kelly, J Wills (eds), *Manual of Companion Animal Nutrition and Feeding*, pp. 38–41, Ames, IA: Iowa State Press.

5 Remillard RL, Crane SW (2010) Making pet foods at home. In M Hand, C Thatcher, R Remillard *et al.* (eds), *Small Animal Clinical Nutrition* (5th edn), pp. 207–20, Marceline, MO: Walsworth Publishing.

6 Schenck P (2010) Homemade diets. In *Home-prepared Dog and Cat Diets* (2nd edn), pp. 5–13, Ames, IA: Wiley-Blackwell.

7 Delaney S, Fascetti A (2012) Commercial and home-prepared diets. In S Delaney, A Fascetti (eds), *Applied Veterinary Clinical Nutrition*, pp. 98–105, Ames, IA: Wiley-Blackwell.

8 Strombeck DA (1999) Food safety and preparation. In *Home-Prepared Dog and Cat Diets, A Healthful Alternative*, pp. 43–61, Ames, IA: Iowa State Press.

21

Resources for Alternative Diets

Introduction

When presented with clients who, for various reasons, do not want to feed a commercially prepared diet that follows World Small Animal Veterinary Association (WSAVA) guidelines, how do we ensure that their diet choices are the best for their pets? Marketing has introduced several nebulous terms with a significant emotional impact but may not provide the benefits that owners believe they will.

Descriptors

Terms like all-natural, corn-free, grain-free, gluten-free, raw, BARF, freeze-dried, fresh and ancestral sound good, but what do they provide or remove from an animal's diet?

Natural

The American Association of Feed Control Officials (AAFCO) defines natural as a feed or ingredient derived solely from plant, animal or mined sources, either in its unprocessed state or having been subject to physical processing, heat processing, rendering, purification, extraction, hydrolysis, enzymolysis or fermentation, but not having been produced by or subject to a chemically synthetic process and not containing any additive or processing aids that are chemically synthetic except in amounts as might occur unavoidably in good manufacturing processes.[1,2]

Is this the definition that consumers are using when looking for all-natural products? Also, this definition only applies to products sold commercially that have AAFCO certification on their labels. This would exclude some boutique, locally produced foods or those that are not complete and balanced.

This definition **does not** exclude the use of genetically modified organisms (GMOs), plants grown with chemical fertilizers and herbicides or foods containing synthetic preservatives.[1] The term natural is not defined for human foods.

Free in Foods

As discussed in Chapter 18 on grain-free and boutique foods, the simple act of pointing out that what a product does not have something in it raises concerns that the presence of this ingredient is bad.

Corn-free foods are marketed under the assumption that corn is a filler, it is not well-digested by dogs and cats, and is linked to allergies.[2] None of these are true. Corn is an excellent source of complex carbohydrates, linoleic acid (an essential fatty acid), fiber and some carotenoids that impart its golden color.[2]

Marketing has portrayed grains as associated with food allergies, increasing the risk of diabetes mellitus and obesity.[2] Grains, including corn, do not significantly contribute to food

Nutrition and Disease Management for Veterinary Technicians and Nurses, Third Edition. Ann Wortinger and Kara M. Burns.
© 2024 John Wiley & Sons, Inc. Published 2024 by John Wiley & Sons, Inc.
Companion Website: www.wiley.com/go/wortinger/3e

allergies. The ingredients most associated with allergies include beef, dairy products and wheat in dogs, to a lesser degree, lamb, chicken, eggs and soy products.[2] In cats, food-related allergies are most often associated with beef, dairy products and fish.[2]

In dogs and cats allergies most often present as skin disease. With <1% of all skin allergies related to a food ingredient. Seldom does food allergies present as gastrointestinal signs.[2]

When grains are removed from foods, they are often replaced with ingredients such as potato, tapioca or sweet potatoes, which can be lower in protein, and higher in simple carbohydrates when compared to oats and corn.[2]

The extremely low incidence of gluten intolerance in dogs and cats was covered in Chapter 18. This is not seen as a problem in dogs and cats, and by removing gluten from a product, an important source of protein is also removed.[2]

Organic

Organic refers to the handling and processing of ingredients but does not describe the quality of a product. If this term is applied to pet food, the company must comply with the United States Department of Agriculture's (USDA) Natural and Organic Program regulations.[3] This program regulates the sourcing, ingredient handling, manufacturing, labeling and certification of products.[3]

Raw Foods

As covered in Chapter 17, raw food diets or BARF diets can be incomplete and expose the pets and humans to harmful bacterial contamination and parasites.[2] A 2013 study showed that dogs have more genes than wolves for digesting starches, as they've evolved to live with humans.[2] As most of these diets are not complete and balanced and have not undergone AAFCO feeding trials, the chances of being nutritionally unbalanced are significant.[2]

Client Communications

The WSAVA recommends that veterinary teams discuss foods, and feeding programs and make nutritional recommendations for every pet at every visit.[4] This can be done as a simple checkoff form or through the use of open-ended questions. These questions are designed to clarify and ensure a complete picture of what the dog or cat consumes. Ideally, this information can be used to determine if the caloric intake is sufficient to support the animal at its current life stage, or more likely, point to why the animal is overweight or obese.[2,4]

If clients are feeding an atypical food or type of food, this is an excellent time to identify the reasons for this choice and correct any misconceptions regarding commercially available pet foods. With this information, clients can be directed to a better OTC or therapeutic food to address their concerns or offer options for more balanced and complete homemade diets.[2]

Guidelines

The American Animal Hospital Associations' (AAHA) guidelines for dogs and cats, published in 2010, provide a list of nutritional assessments to enhance the pets' quality of life and provide optimal animal care.[5]

These guidelines involve asking questions of the owners and assessing the dog or cat's health. Body condition scoring (BCS) and muscle condition scoring (MCS) can provide information on the quantity and quality of the diet being fed.[5] An ideal BCS is 2.5–3 out of 5. MCS is graded as normal, mild loss, moderate loss or severe loss.[6] These scores are independent of each other. This means that a very athletic dog may have a low BCS but a normal

MCS. Conversely, an obese animal could have a high BCS and a low MCS.[5,6]

WSAVA also provides guidelines for selecting pet foods directed specifically at the food. Does the company employ a nutritionist, who formulates the diets, what method is used to meet AAFCO certification requirements, is contact information provided to reach the manufacturer, and who makes the food (the distributor or a third-party manufacturer)?[7]

Trying to obtain this information can be a tedious prospect, but the Pet Food Alliance (PNA) has already compiled a list accessed through its website.[8] Their Pet Food Manufacturer Evaluation Report page provides the answers or lack of answers for many commercially available foods. As an overall guideline, the less information available, the lower this should be as a food recommendation.

Options

If, after an in-depth discussion with the owners, a complete physical and BCS and MCS assessment, the owner is unwilling to feed a commercially available complete and balanced diet. What options are available to ensure that the pets' nutritional needs and the owner's needs are met?

As covered in Chapter 20, homemade diets formulated by a board-certified veterinary nutritionist is the preferred option.

Names and links to several ACVIM (Nutrition) specialists who provide nutritional consults and diet formulations are available in Chapter 20. If a client is feeding raw, encourage them to cook the food before feeding. This will help to kill any pathogenic bacterial contamination.

As with all recommendations to clients, be sure to record any nutritional recommendations provided to the client for future reference.

Our goal is to provide the soundest nutritional recommendations based on the available science, follow current regulations and address client concerns. Review the clients' concerns, address those that can be addressed and make sound recommendations for the animal's long-term health. There are many resources listed to assist in this endeavor.

References

1 Pet Food Institute Debunking Pet food myths and misconceptions, Ryan Yamka https://www.petfoodindustry.com/blogs/10-debunking-pet-food-myths-and-misconceptions/post/6807-navigating-pet-food-product-claims-part-3-natural. Accessed 12/20/21.

2 Alternative pet diets, Ed Carlson https://todaysveterinarynurse.com/articles/alternative-pet-diets-grain-free-raw-and-other-trends/. Accessed 12/18/21.

3 USDA National Organic Program regulation. https://www.ams.usda.gov/rules-regulations/organic. Accessed 12/20/21.

4 WSAVA Global nutrition guidelines. https://wsava.org/global-guidelines/global-nutrition-guidelines/. Accessed 12/19/21.

5 AAHA Nutritional assessment guidelines for dogs and cats. https://www.aaha.org/globalassets/02-guidelines/nutritional-assessment/nutritionalassessmentguidelines.pdf. Accessed 12/19/21.

6 WSAVA Muscle condition score. https://wsava.org/wp-content/uploads/2020/01/Muscle-Condition-Score-Chart-for-Dogs.pdf. Accessed 12/20/21.

7 WSAVA Guideline on selecting pet foods. https://wsava.org/wp-content/uploads/2021/04/Selecting-a-pet-food-for-your-pet-updated-2021_WSAVA-Global-Nutrition-Toolkit.pdf. Accessed 12/20/21.

8 Pet Food Manufacturer Evaluation. https://petnutritionalliance.org/resources/pet-food-manufacturer-evaluation-report/

Section III

Feeding Management for Dogs and Cats

22

Feeding Regimens for Dogs and Cats

Introduction

To understand normal feeding behaviors in domestic dogs and cats, you first need to understand where these behaviors developed and how they differ from those still found in their wild counterparts.

Feeding behaviors include searching, hunting and caching of prey, as well as postprandial grooming and sleeping.[1] An obvious difference between domestic dogs and cats and their wild ancestors is the amount of energy expended in obtaining a meal and the time required.[2] Wild ancestors of domestic dogs and cats expended considerable amounts of energy locating and time capturing a meal, and their success was not guaranteed.

Wild canids, such as wolves, foxes and coyotes, can spend up to 60% of their day searching for food.[6] No animal evolved to acquire food from walking up to a filled bowl.[6] Wild animals do not have a reliable and consistent food source for the most part.[2] To maintain access to food, additional energy was expended on territorial behaviors.[1] Our domestic pets are usually provided with a consistent source of nutritious and palatable foods and expend only the effort required for begging to obtain this.[2]

Dogs

Wolves, our modern-day dogs' wild ancestors, hunt in packs, using cooperative behavior to prey on large animals that otherwise would be unavailable to an animal hunting on its own.[2] This cooperative behavior allows for more significant amounts of food to be obtained and dictates the type of feeding behavior seen, that of gorging themselves immediately after a kill and then not eating for extended periods.[2] Food is consumed rapidly and in a predetermined order within the pack. Any food that is left over is hoarded or cached for consumption later when food is not so readily available[2].

These gorging and hoarding behaviors can be seen in some of our domestic dogs today. This can lead to choking and swallowing large amounts of air during eating (aerophagia)[2]. Dogs may also eat more rapidly and consume more food if fed in a group situation rather than alone.[3] Changing the feeding situation can help curb the gorging behavior if this occurs in a pack situation. Removing the dog from the pack and feeding them by themselves may decrease the desire to gorge and overeat.

If the dog is consuming the food too quickly, sometimes changing the type of food being fed can help and change how that food is offered. Eating large amounts of canned food out of a bowl is easier than eating large amounts of dry food fed off a flat tray.[2] There are also unique bowls with a raised center that make the dog work harder to obtain individual kibbles from around the side. This decreases the ability to consume large amounts of food in a short time (see Figure 22.1).

Conversely, the presence of another dog may stimulate the appetite of a poor eater, so they consume more food than if fed alone.[2]

Nutrition and Disease Management for Veterinary Technicians and Nurses, Third Edition. Ann Wortinger and Kara M. Burns.
© 2024 John Wiley & Sons, Inc. Published 2024 by John Wiley & Sons, Inc.
Companion Website: www.wiley.com/go/wortinger/3e

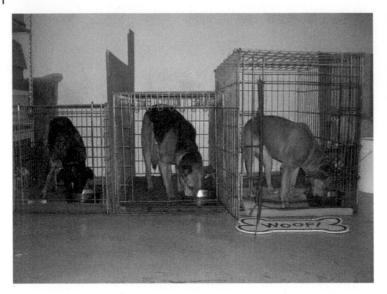

Figure 22.1 Dogs being group fed using the portion-controlled method. *Source*: Courtesy Heidi Reuss-Lamky LVT, VTS (Anesthesia and Analgesia) (Surgery).

Dominance may also play a part in the amount of food consumed within a group, with the dominant dog eating more than its share. Separating the dogs at mealtime may help, as well as designating feeding locations or bowls for each dog.[2]

Domestic dogs still hoard choice food items, as can be seen with buried bones in the yard and treats hidden in furniture and under beds.[2] Unlike their wild ancestors, domestic dogs often forget about these hidden items, leading to quite a collection in various places within the house and yard.[3]

If we look to the wolf for our domestic dog's feeding schedule, large meals fed infrequently would seem to be the natural way to feed.[2] However, when domestic dogs are given free-choice access to food, they tend to eat small meals frequently throughout the day.[1,2] This pattern is similar to that seen with cats, except that dogs tend to only eat during the day.[2] Our domestic dogs can readily adapt to several feeding regimes, the primary ones being portion-controlled feeding, time-controlled feeding and free-choice or ad libitum feeding.[2]

It has been shown that dogs can learn food preferences for novel flavors from other dogs in the house.[4] They also learn to follow human pointing gestures during feeding and have been known to select a smaller portion of food over another larger portion in the pointing direction of the owner.[4] Given that the vast majority of dogs live in multi-dog households, the presence of another dog during feeding and directions from the owner can significantly influence individual eating behaviors.

Cats

Domestic cats look like their wild cousins, tiger and lion, but they are descendants of the much smaller African wildcat, *Felis sylvestris libyca*. This distinction is important because the larger cats eat larger meals less frequently, while the smaller African wildcat consumes multiple small meals throughout the day. The primary prey for *F. libyca* is small rodents similar to our common field mouse.[4] This leads to a more ad libitum feeding schedule for the smaller cats.[1] There is no convincing evidence that the smaller cats engage in cooperative hunting behaviors, even when living in large groups[1] (see Figure 22.2).

Because these cats hunt alone and consume small meals frequently, they tend to consume their meals slowly and are uninhibited by the

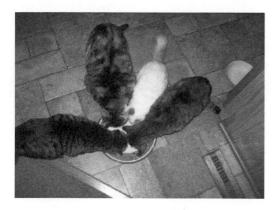

Figure 22.2 Cats being group fed using ad libitum feeding.

presence of other animals.[2,3] This same type of behavior can readily be seen with our domestic cats. If fed free choice, they will nibble at their food throughout the day and night. It is not unusual for a cat to eat between 9 and 16 meals per day, with each meal having a calorie content of about 23 kcal. The average caloric value of a typical field mouse is ~30 kcal/animal.[4] If a 10# cat needs ~235 kcal/day, this would be ~8 mice/day to meet their caloric requirements. That assumes that the mice are all adults and in good nutritional status before being caught and eaten.

Like the dog, the cat can adapt to several different feeding regimes, though time-controlled feeding with cats does not work as well as dogs due to their nibbling behavior and desire for small meals frequently.[2] The feeding method used often depends on the owner's preference rather than the ingrained preference of an individual species.[3]

What to Feed

As listed in Chapters 16, 17, and 18, the food choices for owners include dry, semi-moist, moist, raw and homemade diets. Most owners prefer the convenience, cost-effectiveness and reliability of feeding commercial foods. If the choice is made to feed a homemade diet, care

must be exercised to ensure that the diet is complete and balanced and that all ingredients and the final product are safe to consume, provide all the essential nutrients, and are stored properly.[2] Surveys have shown that more than 90% of owners feed commercial foods to their pets.[2]

One of the most important considerations when deciding what food is fed is the pet's life stage.[2] Nutrient and energy needs will differ according to an animal's age, activity level, reproductive status and health.[2] Specific diets have been developed by commercial pet food manufacturers to address pets' needs during different ages, physiologic states and disease conditions.[2,4]

When evaluating a diet to be fed, some other important considerations for all life stages are:

- Does the food provide all the essential nutrients in adequate amounts and proper balance to meet the lifestyle and life-stage needs?
- Does the food supply sufficient energy to maintain ideal body condition and weight and support optimal tissue growth?
- Is the food palatable enough to ensure that the animal willingly consumes it when fed as the primary diet over an extended period?
- Does extended use support proper gastrointestinal function and consistently produce regular, firm and well-formed stools?
- Is the animal subjectively healthy with good coat quality, healthy skin condition, proper body physique and muscle tone and sufficient energy to function as desired with extended use?[2]

While many of these qualities are subjective and can only be assessed over an extended period, some can be found in the product reference guides supplied by pet food manufacturers. Have feeding trials been done on this food? What are the life-stage rating, the metabolizable energy of the diet and the diet's nutrient density? Many clients do not connect the quality of the diet being fed to their pet to the skin and coat condition, the stool quality or the lack of endurance when exercising.

If pet owners are reluctant to follow the dietary recommendations, use the list above to compare the diet they are currently feeding with recommended ones. Point out the significance of each point and how the current food compares to the desired food. Referencing the Pet Food Manufacturer Evaluation Report site from the Pet Nutrition Alliance can provide information on individual foods. https://petnutritionalliance.org/resources/pet-food-manufacturer-evaluation-report/.

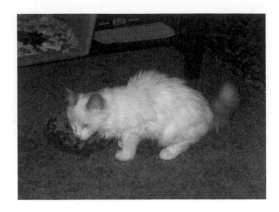

Figure 22.3 Adlib feeding a special needs kitten in a multi-cat household to ensure adequate food intake.

Feeding Regimens

The three primary feeding choices available for dogs and cats are free-choice or ad libitum, time-controlled feeding and portion-controlled or measured feeding.[2]

The method used will be determined by the owner's daily schedule, the number of animals being fed, the type of food being fed and the acceptability of the method to the pet or pets.[2]

Free-Choice Feeding

Free-choice feeding is having a surplus of food available at all times. This enables the pet or pets to consume as much food as desired at any time of the day.[2] This feeding method relies on the animal's ability to self-regulate food intake so that only the actual energy and nutrient needs are met and no excess energy is consumed.[2] Dry food is the best choice for this method as it will not spoil or dry out as quickly as other products. This does not mean that by feeding dry food, the dishes do not need to be cleaned or the food refreshed daily, though.[2]

Compared to the other methods, free-choice feeding requires the least amount of work and knowledge by the owner.[2] The food and water supply are only replenished once daily (or less often), and the owner does not need

to determine the pet's exact daily energy requirements (DERs).[2] When dogs are fed free choice, they tend to consume frequent small meals throughout the day. This feeding pattern has the advantage of more significant meal-induced energy loss through digestion when compared to dogs eating larger meals less frequently.[2] However, this increased energy loss is usually more than compensated for by increased energy intake by most dogs (see Figure 22.3).

Free-choice feeding can be a helpful way to feed those animals that are "poor doers" or have higher energy expenditure and do not or cannot eat sufficient calories to support themselves when fed time-controlled meals.[3] This allows them to eat multiple small meals throughout the day, increasing their overall energy intake. This method can also be helpful for animals that work at a very high energy level, such as hunting dogs, service dogs and search and rescue dogs, by allowing them to replenish their energy reserves throughout the day.[2]

Free-choice feeding can be a disadvantage if animals have problems with anorexia or overconsumption. These problems may go undetected for an extended time as the owners are not feeding and monitoring the intake daily.[2] If these problems are related to a medical condition, valuable treatment time may be lost until the animal is sick enough for the owner to notice a change in the condition. If the animal were meal or portion fed, the problem with increased or decreased intake would be evident to the owner within a short period.[2]

Obesity is a common problem with animals that are fed free-choice food. The usual regulatory mechanisms used to control food intake are easily overridden by a highly palatable diet and a sedentary lifestyle.[2] In young growing animals, this overconsumption of energy has been shown to cause an accelerated growth rate and increased fat deposition within the body, further contributing to obesity later in life.[2] This increased growth rate has also been linked to the development of degenerative joint diseases as the animal matures and decreased overall life expectancy.[3,5]

Time-Controlled Feeding

Time-controlled feeding involves controlling the amount of time that the animal is given access to the food, but they can eat as much as they want or can within this time.[2] Time-controlled may also pertain to portion-controlled feeding where the food is only given at a specific volume for a controlled time. If this volume of food is not consumed within this time, it is removed until the next feeding.[4] This method also relies on the animal's ability to regulate its energy intake. A surplus amount of food is supplied at mealtime, and the animal is allowed to eat for a predetermined period.

For most dogs and cats that are not physiologically stressed, 15–20 minutes is sufficient to meet their energy requirements.[2] This is usually done in either one or two meals daily. While most animals can eat a sufficient amount of food when fed once daily, twice daily is healthier and more satisfying for the animal.[2] Twice daily feeding will also help reduce hunger between meals and decrease food-associated behaviors such as begging and stealing food.[2]

Some animals do not adapt well to time-controlled feedings. Some may not consume a sufficient quantity within the time allotted, while others will gorge themselves throughout the entire time, leading to overeating and obesity. Time-controlled feedings may encourage gluttonous behavior because animals quickly learn that they have to "beat-the-clock.[2]"

Picky eaters or those who are intimidated by the presence of other animals during mealtime may not be able to consume enough calories to meet their energy requirements. Some will only pick at their food but hold out for table food and scraps from the owner's more frequent meals, thus defeating the purpose of time-controlled meals.[4]

Portion-Controlled Feedings

Portion-controlled feedings are the preferred method in most situations.[2] By feeding a predetermined amount of food once, twice or more daily, the owner is given the most significant amount of control over the pet's diet. Portion-controlled feedings also allow the owners to monitor the food intake more closely and quickly notice any changes in intake or behavior.[2] This method provides the most control over growth rate and weight and can be adjusted as needed to maintain the desired effect.[2] By doing this, conditions related to overweight, underweight or inappropriate growth can be corrected early[2] (see Figure 22.4).

Portion-controlled feeding also demands the most amount of knowledge and effort by the owner. Guidelines for feeding amounts are provided on the bags or containers of food. These can be used as a starting point to determine the amount of food to be fed to the animal.[2] The DER can also be calculated using the pets' weight, activity level and the food's energy density. The energy density of the food is found on the product label, usually under the feeding guidelines. Internet sites maintained by the manufacturer will often contain

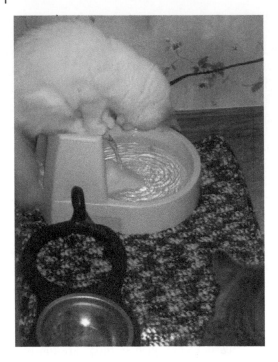

Figure 22.4 Portion control of the same special needs cat as an adult. He often got distracted by the waterer.

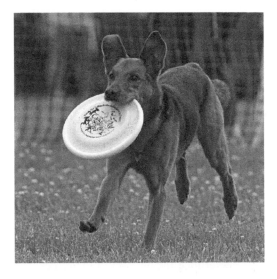

Figure 22.5 Active dog competing in Frisbee tournament. *Source*: Courtesy Heidi Reuss-Lamky LVT, VTS (Anesthesia and Analgesia) (Surgery).

the energy density of the food and the nutrient distribution. When in doubt, always contact the manufacturer for the correct information (see Figure 22.5).

Guidelines for expectations need to be provided to owners as to desired outcomes for using portion-controlled feedings. We need to ensure that adequate food is being fed to meet the animal's energy requirements and provide the necessary nutrients in the correct portions. This is an excellent time to introduce the concept of Body Condition Scoring (BCS) and give clients a lesson on how to conduct these at home and the desired number to achieve. It is also important to ensure that you and the clients discuss the same measure unit when determining feeding volumes. A standard 8 oz measuring cup does not provide the same volume of food as the standard 7/11 Big Gulp cup, but both constitute a "cup."

The time commitment for portion-controlled feeding is usually not a problem for most owners unless many animals are being fed at any one time. The easiest method is to coordinate the pets' meal time with the owners, decreasing begging at the table because they are eating their own food.[2]

The amount of food being fed can be adjusted based on the individual animal's activity level, growth rate, body condition and lifestyle changes. Any treats being fed will need to be figured into the total caloric allotment for each animal. There are no free calories, and portion-controlled feeding does not work if treats and snacks are not controlled. This also allows the owner to monitor food intake more closely and make any adjustments as needed before significant changes have occurred in the animal's body condition (see Figure 22.6).

Many timed feeders on the market are designed to help with portion-controlled feeding that requires less effort by the owner. They usually provide a specific amount of food delivered using a timer set by the owner. This

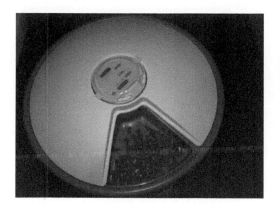

Figure 22.6 Automated timed feeder.

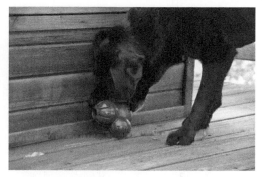

Figure 22.7 A dog using a Kong™ puzzle feeder. *Source*: Courtesy Judy Conley LVT.

method can also help animals with extreme begging behavior by removing the owner from the feeding process. These timed feeders can be set for multiple feedings per day and are also helpful for those owners who have unreliable schedules and are not always at home at the designated mealtime.

Puzzle Feeders

Introducing feeding puzzles can move food into an interactive activity and away from only a source of nutrition. There is a wide variety of feeding puzzles ranging from just scattering the food so that it has to be "hunted" to complex, expensive ones available at pet stores and online. It is also reasonably accessible to DIY many of these toys, keeping the pet engaged.[7]

A feeding puzzle can be any toy or object containing food and requires the pet to find a way to get to that food.[5,7] Most people are familiar with Kong™ toys, hollow rubber toys stuffed with food or treats. The goal for this type of feeder is to slowly release the food, with some effort on the animal's part.[7] If the animal gets at the food too quickly, freezing the filled toy can slow them down and prolong the

activity. When using toys that involve canned foods or soft treats, it is usually a good idea to offer them inside a crate or on a harder, easy-to-clean surface. A mess will be produced (see Figure 22.7).

For many animals feeding puzzles can provide all of their food, not just treats. A popular type of feeding puzzle is the food balls. These tend to be knocked under furniture and into corners, making locating them for the next feeding challenging.

Behavioral Problems

A study done by Beth Strickler looked at owner engagement and six specific behavioral issues.[8] She demonstrated that the more involved the owners were in engaging their cats daily, the fewer behavioral-related issues were present. This engagement was primarily through playing. Owners, who played with their cat for 5 minutes daily, reported fewer behavioral problems than those who did not.[8] The two most frequently reported behavior problems were aggression toward the owners (36%) and periuria (24%).[6] Feeding puzzles offer another way for owners to provide enrichment for their cats, encourage mental stimulation and decrease overeating.

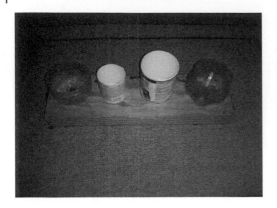

Figure 22.8 A DIY puzzle feeder made out of bottles.

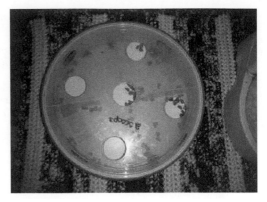

Figure 22.9 The amount to be placed into the feeder is written on the top. The difficulty of this feeding method is easily increased by taping over the holes or placing balls inside.

Introducing Puzzles

How are feeding puzzles introduced to animals? It is easier to introduce these if the pet is hungry and begins with the simpler toys first, and for those overachieving pets, some are quite difficult and can challenge even a herding dog's brain.[5,6]

Start by placing some fragrant treats inside the toy to attract initial attention. They may need assistance to understand that food is inside. For some animals using peanut butter or baby food can help attract their attention.[6] As they perfect the technique involved in getting the treats out, slowly switch out, placing food in the puzzle instead of the bowl (see Figure 22.8).

For this method to work, portion control is essential. Determine the desired volume of food per day, and divide this into two to three smaller feedings dispensed in one or multiple puzzles. Increasingly more difficult puzzles for some animals may be required, or the puzzle's difficulty can be increased by closing off or narrowing the openings.

To increase their mental stimulation, have a selection of puzzles that can be rotated daily. To further increase the stimulation, hide them around the house, so more hunting is involved. This is a wonderful way to increase environmental enrichment, control feeding amounts and provide mental stimulation (see Figure 22.9).

References

1 Voith VL (1994) Feeding behaviors. In JM Wills, KW Simpson (eds), *The Waltham Book of Clinical Nutrition of the Dog and Cat*, pp. 119–27, Tarry Town, NY: Elsevier.

2 Case L, Daristotle L, Hayek MG, Raasch F (2011) Melody. Feeding regimens for dogs and cats. In *Canine and Feline Nutrition*, 3rd edn, pp. 191–7, St. Louis, MO: Mosby.

3 Case L (1999) Feeding management throughout the life cycle. In *The Dog, Its Behavior,* *Nutrition and Health*, pp. 311–28, Ames, IA: Iowa State Press.

4 Case L (2003) Feeding management throughout the life cycle. In *The Cat, Its Behavior, Nutrition and Health*, pp. 329–40, Ames, IA: Iowa State Press.

5 14-year life span study in dogs. https://www.purinainstitute.com/science-of-nutrition/extending-healthy-life/life-span-study-in-dogs. Accessed 12/21/21.

6 Tony Buffington. Trouble with Food Puzzles? Here are Six Tips. VetStreet March 7, 2017. https://www.vetstreet.com/our-pet-experts/trouble-with-food-puzzles-here-are-six-tips. Accessed 6/27/23.

7 Tripp R. Food puzzles. http://www.animal-behavior.net/LIBRARY/AllPets/PPM/PetFood-Puzzles.htm. Accessed 12/21/21.

8 Strickler BL (2014) An owner survey of toys, activities and behavior problems in indoor cats. *Journal Veterinary Behavior* **9**(5): 207–14 www.journalvetbehavior.com/artilces/S1558-7878(14)00088-4/pdf. Accessed 12/21/21.

23

Nutritional Assessment

Introduction

A nutritional assessment should be done in the same systemic way as a physical examination. Using a check-off form is an easy and convenient way to ensure important questions are not missed or that the conversation drifts away from nutrition.

A nutritional assessment is a 2-step process.[1] A screening evaluation is performed on every pet at every visit. If the animal is healthy without any risk factors, no additional assessment is needed. An extended evaluation is needed when one or more nutrition-related risk factors are present or suspected based on the screening evaluation.[1]

Screening Evaluation

A nutritional screening evaluation is easily included in the routine history taking and physical examination taken for every animal. Information collected should include the current diet (brand name and manufacturer), the type of food (canned, kibble, semi-moist), the volume consumed, the method of feeding (ad lib, timed, feeding puzzles), treats fed and any dietary concerns of the owners.[1] Diet changes may be recommended based on this evaluation. However, if the animal is doing well and the owner is happy, no further action may be needed.

Extended Evaluation

An extended evaluation is warranted for patients at risk for nutrition-related problems found during the screening evaluation.[1]

If nutrition is likely to play an important role in managing or development of an underlying disease, an extended evaluation is recommended. This is done to obtain additional information, including historically relevant factors affecting the pet's condition.[1]

An extended evaluation looks at animal factors, such as changes in food intake or behavior, skin condition, results of a diagnostic workup and current medical conditions and medications.[1] Diet factors, such as the caloric density of the current diet, evaluation of other sources of nutrients, including treats, supplements, foods used to administer medications and chew toys.[1] Evaluations of the diet, including the presence of Association of American Feed Control Officials (AAFCO) certification, whether the diet is marketed as complete and balanced or for supplemental use only, which life stage it is formulated for, and whether feeding trials have been done.[1] Checking the Pet Nutrition Alliance Pet Food Manufacturer Evaluation Report page can provide information on the food manufacturer.[1,12]

If the clients are feeding a homemade diet, specific questions about the recipe, preparation, storage, recipe rotation or ingredient substitution should be asked. A board-certified veterinary nutritionist can evaluate the current diet or formulate a new homemade diet if the current diet is deficient or excessive in ingredients.[1]

The feeding method and environmental factors include determining the primary feeder for the pet, how and when they are fed and the presence or issues with other pets in the house. Enrichment for the pet can include toys, housing and the presence of other pets or food delivery devices.[1]

The activity level and type can help assess the energy level and amount of activity the animal engages in daily and determine the life-stage factor used to calculate the daily energy requirement (DER).[1]

Environment stressors such as recent changes to the household, such as people moving in or out, or babies being present, uncontrollable outdoor stimuli, resource conflicts over food or access to the owner or conflict between animals.[1] Remember that what the pet finds stressful may differ from what the owner perceives as stressful to the pet.

The final step of the extended evaluation is the interpretation, analysis and action steps. Determine if the current food type and volume are appropriate for that animal. Calculate resting energy requirement (RER) and DER based on activity level and life stage using the life-stage factors.[1]

If the pet is hospitalized at the time of the evaluations, create monitoring and feeding plans and a transition plan for after discharge from the hospital. Unlike a plan for an animal at home, a hospitalized pet's plan needs to include information on the feeding route, including the use of appetite stimulants, coax feeding or feeding tubes, to ensure adequate nutrient intake.[1]

For nonhospitalized pets, a monitoring and feeding plan is developed incorporating the preferred diet, route and amount of feeding and any changes in the frequency of meals.[1] Providing clear, written directions is best, with reference to appropriate websites if needed.[1]

The recheck frequency for monitoring response to the feeding plan can vary based on the disease process being addressed and the pet's response to the nutritional recommendations. Teaching clients how to perform a Body Condition Score(BCS) is a helpful, at-home monitoring tool.[1] At every blood work or physical exam recheck, a nutritional evaluation should be done to determine if any changes are necessary based on the response to the current plan.

For hospitalized patients, daily monitoring should be done. The feeding orders and response need to be evaluated daily, with changes done to ensure adequate nutrition is being provided. Is the current route of intake working? If not, what changes are needed?[1] Remember that an animal needs to be consuming, at minimum 85% of their RER, to continue using the oral feeding route.

As most animals are discharged from the hospital, before complete resolution of their disease, a transition plan needs to be provided to the owner with the specific diet being recommended, the meal route and frequency, and any medications or supplements needed. Ensure that the plan provides clear instructions on the current feeding plan and what needs to be done if the nutrient goals are not met.[1]

Body Condition Scoring

Body condition and percent of body fat can be assessed with humans using body mass indexing (BMI). For most humans, this method is a helpful way of determining body condition and if the person is underweight, ideal or overweight/obese. Unfortunately, our patients' sizes are too broad and their body types too diverse to make this system usable for veterinary medicine.

In an attempt to determine the ideal weight for our patients, several systems have been developed. The use of weight/height charts is impractical, especially for dogs, because of their different body types and the difficulty in obtaining information on a moving, happy animal.[2,3] Zoometric methods, similar to anthropometric methods used in humans, have been developed but are more useful in a research setting as they are challenging to use daily on pets. Morphometric methods have also been developed but require acquiring several measurements and plugging these into a complex formula to determine percent body fat. Due to the difficulty in obtaining these measurements and the complexity of the formula, errors are common, making this method impractical.[3] In animals, the subcutaneous fat adheres more to muscle than to skin, making skin-fold thickness a questionable means for determining body fat in cats and dogs[4] (see Table 23.1).

BCS is a subjective (not objective) assessment of an animal's body fat and, to a lesser extent, protein stores.[6] The scoring system considers the animal's frame size independent of its weight. BCS involves visual and physical assessment through palpation to assess body fat over the rib, abdomen, lumbar area and tail base[3] (see Figures 23.1 and 23.2).

The primary scoring system uses a 9-point scale. This system uses defined criteria to help make the subjective process of body evaluation more objective, but all subjectivity cannot be removed when assigning a score to an animal. For this reason, the same person must try to assign the score each time the animal is evaluated.[6]

Studies have shown that body fat increases 5–7% for each whole increment increase using

Table 23.1 9-point body condition score.

BCS	What you see	What you feel
1/9 Emaciated	Obvious ribs, pelvic bones, and spine, no body fat or muscle mass	Bones with little covering of muscle
2/9	Obvious ribs, pelvic bones, and spine, minimal body fat, minimal loss of muscle mass	Bones with some covering of muscle
3/9 Thin	Ribs and pelvic bones, but less prominent; tips of spine, an "hourglass" waist (looking from above), a tucked up abdomen (looking from side)	Ribs and other bones with no palpable fat, but more muscle is present
4/9 Ideal	Minimal fat covering, waist is easily seen from above, abdominal tuck evident	Ribs easily palpated, muscle mass present
5/9	Less prominent hourglass and abdominal tuck	Ribs without excess fat covering
6/9 Heavy	Slight fat covering, waist evident when viewed from above, but not prominent, abdominal tuck apparent	Ribs palpable with slight excess fat covering
7/9	General fleshy appearance, hourglass, and abdominal tuck hard to see	Ribs, with difficulty, noticeable fat deposits over the lumbar area and at the base of the tail
8/9	Heavy fat deposits over lumbar area and at base of the tail, waist absent, no abdominal tuck evident, obvious abdominal distension	Ribs not palpable under heavy fat cover, obvious fat deposits over lumbar and at base of the tail, abdominal palpation difficult
9/9 Obese	Sagging abdomen, large deposits of fat over chest, abdomen, and pelvis	Nothing, except general flesh

Source: Buffington et al.[5]/Saunders, St. Louis.

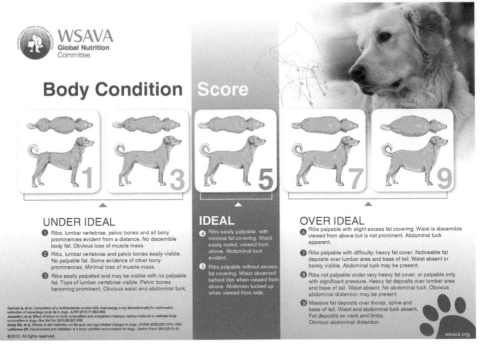

Figure 23.1 Canine body condition scorecard. *Source*: WSAVA[7], Courtesy of World Small Animal Veterinary Association (WSAVA).

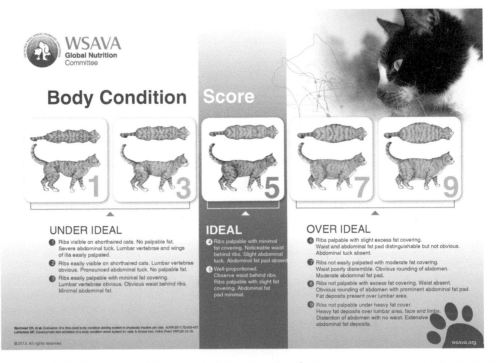

Figure 23.2 Feline body condition scorecard. *Source*: WSAVA[8], Courtesy of World Small Animal Veterinary Association (WSAVA).

a 9-point scale with mid-range scoring dogs (4/9–5/9) having 15–20% of their body mass as fat.[4] For cats, a mid-range score would be consistent with a body fat percentage of 25-30%.[3] When trying to detect small changes in body fat, the use of BCS scores would probably not be the best monitoring choice. For monitoring and routine care, however, it is quick, easy and painless. BCS are ideally used with body-weight measurement, not in place of weighing the animal at every visit.

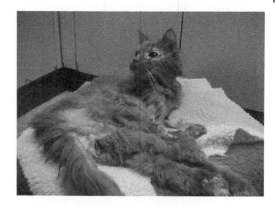

Figure 23.3 A cat with a BCS of 1/9 had undergone 3 months of starvation.

Body Condition Score Uses

A BCS should be recorded with the weight each time an animal is examined. Bodyweight alone does not indicate how appropriate the weight is for that individual animal. The BCS puts in perspective what an individual animal should weigh[1] (see Figures 23.1 and 23.2).

In general, dogs and cats with an optimal body conditions have:

- Normal body contours and silhouettes.
- Boney prominences are easily palpated but not seen or felt above the skin surface.
- Intra-abdominal fat that is insufficient to obscure or interfere with abdominal palpation.

Normal BCSs are 4/9–5/9. When scores are below 3/9 or above 7/9, action should be taken to bring the animal into a more normal BCS[6] (see Figures 23.3 and 23.4).

Studies have shown that people are more likely to underestimate their own pet's BCS. This may be due to daily exposures, making the clients more accepting of any increases that may have occurred or accepting a heavier body condition as normal.[3] As a veterinary health care team, we are often willing to ignore and not bring the owner's attention to increases in body condition. Whether this is due to a failure to appreciate the problems that being over-weight or obese can pose to the animal or an unwillingness to engage the owner in a discussion on obesity management is undetermined.

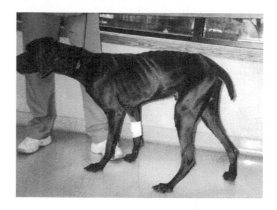

Figure 23.4 A dog with a BCS of 1/9. The ribs and vertebral spines are clearly evident, as are the wings of the ilium.

In an extensive survey of veterinary practices in the United States, ~28% of the dogs and cats were scored as overweight or obese. Still, only 2% had this problem recorded as an issue on the medical record[3] (see Figure 23.5).

Best practice would dictate that the weight be recorded at every visit to the clinic, a BCS be done at every physical exam, and a discussion with the client regarding any abnormalities at every visit.[3] Sometimes, this can seem like we are talking to a brick wall when discussing overweight and obesity issues with clients, but our job is to advocate for the pet. Our knowledge of obesity-related issues continues to grow at least as fast as the obesity problem in our patients. We also need to remember to

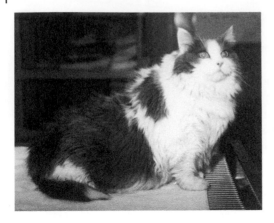

Figure 23.5 A cat with a 9/9+ BCS. This cat would be at a high risk of malnutrition in the hospital despite its extra fat stores.

encourage those owners with pets within a normal range to continue with the excellent work.

Just because an animal score a 9/9 does not mean that this is the maximum size or weight that this animal can attain. Animals can be scored as a 9/9+ if morbid obesity is present. There is no "maximum" amount of body fat compatible with life.[6]

Using BCS is an effective means of monitoring an animal's condition and weight and can be quickly learned by most pet owners and done at home. By teaching clients how to do this, our assessment should come as less of a surprise and involve them in maintaining a healthy weight in their dogs and cats. This should be instituted early in the client/patient/veterinary team relationship to prevent obesity and associated problems.

Muscle Condition Scoring

Muscle condition scoring (MCS)is a visual and palpation assessment, similar to BCS. Muscle loss is typically seen first over the abdominal area's epaxial muscles along the spine. Other sites used for assessment include over the temporal muscles along the sides of the head, scapulae, crest of the skull and over the wings of the ilium[9,10] (see Table 23.2).

The muscle condition is scored as normal (0), mild loss (1), moderate loss (2) or severe loss (3). It is important to remember that overweight animals can still have significant muscle loss, while athletic animals with a low body condition can have minimal muscle loss.[10] Using both BCS and MCS scoring should be done together to get a complete picture of each patient's condition.[10-12] (see Figure 23.6).

Muscle loss tends to be greater in animals with many acute and chronic diseases than in healthy animals with weight loss primarily involving fat stores.[9] Catabolism of muscle mass through cachexia and sarcopenia causes muscle loss and can adversely affect strength, immune function, wound healing and reduces the ability to recover from illness, surgery or injury[9,13] (see Figure 23.7).

Table 23.2 Muscle condition scoring.

MCS	What you see	What you feel
Normal (0)	Normal musculature	No loss of muscle mass
Mild loss (1)	Mild loss of musculature	Some loss of muscle mass over boney prominences
Moderate loss (2)	Moderate loss of musculature with increased muscle weakness	Significant loss of muscle mass over boney prominences
Severe loss (3)	Significant loss of musculature with extreme muscle weakness	Extreme loss of muscle mass all boney prominences

Source: Michel.[9,11]

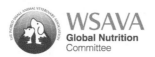

Muscle Condition Score

Muscle condition score is assessed by visualization and palpation of the spine, scapulae, skull, and wings of the ilia. Muscle loss is typically first noted in the epaxial muscles on each side of the spine; muscle loss at other sites can be more variable. Muscle condition score is graded as normal, mild loss, moderate loss, or severe loss. Note that animals can have significant muscle loss even if they are overweight (body condition score > 5/9). Conversely, animals can have a low body condition score (< 4/9) but have minimal muscle loss. Therefore, assessing both body condition score and muscle condition score on every animal at every visit is important. Palpation is especially important with mild muscle loss and in animals that are overweight. An example of each score is shown below.

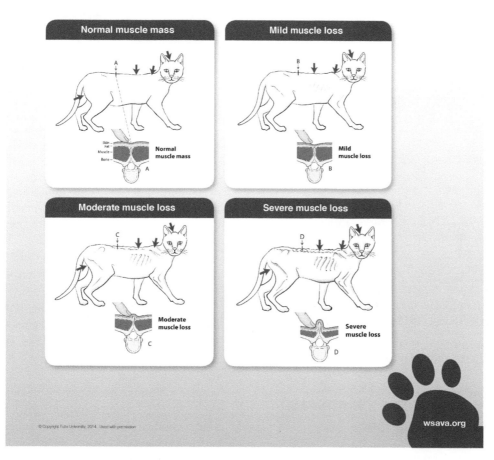

Figure 23.6 Muscle condition Scoring, demonstrating the differences in muscle mass with various stages of muscle loss.[10] new content. *Source*: Courtesy of Tufts University.

With a normal MCS, there is no muscle wasting noted on palpation over the boney prominences. With mild muscle wasting, muscle loss is felt over the boney prominences. With moderate and marked muscle wasting, increasing loss of muscle mass is noted on palpation[9,11,13] (see Figure 23.8).

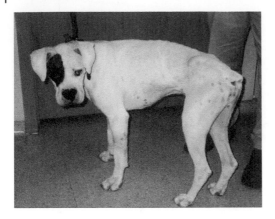

Figure 23.7 A dog with an MCS of 3-extreme loss. The wings of the ilium are clearly visible, as are the vertebral body indicating loss of the epaxial muscles along the spine.

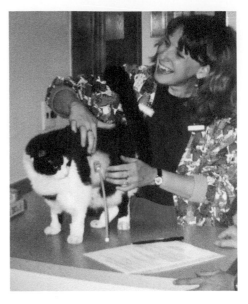

Figure 23.9 A hospital discharge for a cat with hepatic lipidosis. The technician explains how to implement the feeding plan, monitor the response, and when the next recheck appointment is. The written directions can be seen on the table.

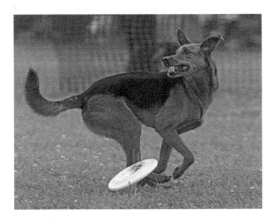

Figure 23.8 A frisbee dog with a MCS of 0-normal. Even though the ribs are evident in this image, this dog is very athletic and has a BCS of 4/9. *Source*: Courtesy of Heidi Reuss-Lamky LVT, VTS (Anesthesia/analgesia)(Surgery).

Communicating a Nutritional Recommendation

Client communication and a good rapport will help the team achieve their nutritional support goals. Technicians can be integral in this process through their nutritional knowledge and communication skills. When developing a feeding and monitoring plan, include the client in the decision-making process and clearly communicate expectations (see Figure 23.9).

Demonstrating how to perform BCS, MCS, and routine weight checks can ensure the client is involved in the pet's progress.

Written directions and website links can increase client compliance and understanding. Expectations and goals should be specific, achievable and follow-up directions to monitor progress and compliance.[1] Scheduling regular weigh-ins or happy visits can allow the veterinary team to monitor the progress and encourage the owner to reach their pet's nutrition goals (see Figure 23.10).

WSAVA provides a Nutritional Assessment Checklist at https://wsava.org/wp-content/uploads/2020/01/Nutritional-Assessment-Checklist.pdf. This template can be used as-is or adapted to your individual setting.

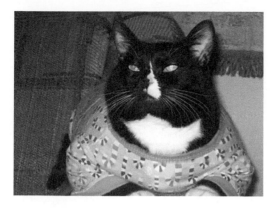

Figure 23.10 This cat developed diabetes mellitus after years of obesity.

References

1 WSAVA. Nutritional Assessment Guidelines. https://wsava.org/wp-content/uploads/2020/01/WSAVA-Nutrition-Assessment-Guidelines-2011-JSAP.pdf. Accessed 12/21/21.

2 Case L, Daristotle L, Hayek MG, Foess Raasch M (2011) Adult maintenance. In *Canine and Feline Nutrition* 3rd edn, pp. 239–42, St. Louis, MO: Mosby.

3 Delaney S, Fascetti A (2012) Nutritional management of body weight. In S Delaney, A Fascetti (eds), *Applied Veterinary Clinical Nutrition*, pp. 111–5, Ames, IA: Wiley-Blackwell.

4 Burkholder WJ (2000) Precision and practicality of methods assessing body composition of dogs and cats. In *Nutrition Forum Proceedings*, p. 1, 9, Ralston Purina Co: St Louis MO.

5 Buffington CA, Holloway C, Abood SK (2004) Nutritional assessment. In *Manual of Veterinary Dietetics*, pp. 4–5, St. Louis, MO: Saunders.

6 Toll PW, Yamka RM, Schoenherr WD, Hand MS (2010) Obesity. In MS Hand, CD Thatcher, RI Remillard *et al.* (eds), *Small Animal Clinical Nutrition* (5th edn), pp. 501–35, Marceline, MO: Walsworth Publishing.

7 WSAVA. 2013 Canine BCS. https://wsava.org/wp-content/uploads/2020/01/Body-Condition-Score-Dog.pdf.

8 WSAVA. 2013 Feline BCS. https://wsava.org/wp-content/uploads/2020/01/Cat-Body-Condition-Scoring-2017.pdf.

9 Gruen, ME, Duncan LB, Colleran E, Johnson J, Marcellin-Little D. https://www.aaha.org/aaha-guidelines/nutritional-assessment-configuration/bcs-and-mcs/ Accessed 1/2/22.

10 https://wsava.org/wp-content/uploads/2020/01/Muscle-Condition-Score-Chart-for-Dogs.pdf Accessed 1/2/22.

11 Michel K (2015) Nutritional assessment in small animals. In D Chan (ed.), *Nutritional Management of Hospitalized Small Animals*, pp. 3–4, Ames IA: Wiley-Blackwell.

12 https://petnutritionalliance.org/resources/pet-food-manufacturer-evaluation-report/#report-about Accessed 6/27/23.

13 Freeman L. What's your Pet's Score? Assessing Muscle Condition in https://vetnutrition.tufts.edu/2017/11/mcs/ Accessed 11/16/17.

24

Pregnancy and Lactation in Dogs

Introduction

Nutrition for the bitch during gestation and lactation should take place long before being bred or the litter is whelped. Before breeding, both the sire and the dam should be in excellent physical condition, moderate body condition (BCS 4-5/9) and well-exercised. They should both have complete physical exams done by a veterinarian, be current on all preventative health programs, such as vaccinations, heartworm medications and intestinal dewormers, and be tested for the presence of brucellosis and herpes virus.[1,2] If this is a purebred litter, both parents should also be screened for any congenital problems, such as hip dysplasia, elbow dysplasia or retinal problems, as well as shown to adhere to established breed standards.[1]

If the bitch is underweight, she may not be able to consume enough food during the pregnancy to provide for both her physical needs and the needs of her developing puppies. Lack of proper nutrition in the bitch can decrease conception rates, decrease birth weight, increase neonatal mortality and perform poorly during lactation.[1,3] Puppies born to underweight bitches have been shown to have decreased birth weights, have increased incidence of experiencing hypoglycemia, and show lower survival rates.[3]

A bitch that is overweight at the time of breeding may experience lower ovulation rates, have smaller litters and perform poorly during lactation.[3] They are predisposed to the development of very large puppies and resultant dystocia due to fetal-maternal disproportion, which puts the life of both the bitch and puppies at risk. It is recommended that overweight bitches lose weight before breeding to optimize fertility and decrease the risk of developing dystocia.[4]

Pregnancy

In general, gestation for dog's averages 63 days (+/- 2 days) and can be divided into 21-day trimesters.[1] Gestation is a unique situation where nutritional requirements increase markedly over a relatively short time.[4] The bitch's energy requirements do not increase substantially until the last third of gestation (~days 42-63).[3]

During gestation, the average bitch will gain approximately 15-25% of their prepregnancy weight.[3] Actual energy requirements for gestation peak anywhere between 30% and 60% of the pre-breeding requirements. This variation is dependent on the size of the litter and the activity level of the bitch.[3] These increased energy requirements continue to rise after whelping and into lactation, reaching their highest levels approximately 3-5 weeks after whelping.[3]

It is suggested to increase the amount of food fed to the bitch by 15% each week from the fifth week of gestation until parturition. Following this regimen would mean that the bitch should be eating 60% more food than

Nutrition and Disease Management for Veterinary Technicians and Nurses, Third Edition. Ann Wortinger and Kara M. Burns.
© 2024 John Wiley & Sons, Inc. Published 2024 by John Wiley & Sons, Inc.
Companion Website: www.wiley.com/go/wortinger/3e

when she was mated by the time she whelps.[5] As the pregnancy advances, it is reasonable to decrease the size of the meals and offer them more frequently. This allows a bitch with a large litter and little free abdominal space to still meet her energy requirements.[5]

Lactation

Lactation presents the biggest test of nutritional adequacy of any feeding regimen.[5] The bitch must eat, digest, absorb and use large amounts of nutrients to produce sufficient milk of adequate quality to support the growth and development of several puppies.[5] Not only does she need to meet the entire energy requirements for the rapidly growing puppies, but she must also be able to meet all of her energy and nutrient requirements. The amount of energy needed to meet these multiple requirements is dependent on the average energy intake of the bitch, and the size and age of the litter.[5] A 5# Maltese with 2 puppies would require must less energy per pound than a 15# Beagle with 6 puppies.[5] The bitch does not require additional vitamin or mineral supplements if a balanced diet suitable for gestation and lactation is being fed[5] (see Table 24.1).

After whelping, the bitch's energy requirement steadily increases and peaks between 3- and 5-weeks post-partum to a level 2-4 times higher than Daily Energy Requirements (DERs) for non-lactating adults.[4] The energy requirements return to normal levels about 8 weeks post-partum.[4] If the energy density of the food is too low, the bitch may not be able to physically consume enough food to meet both her and the puppies' energy requirements. If this happens, her milk production will decrease, she will lose weight, and she may display signs of severe exhaustion.[4] This is most pronounced in giant-breed dogs with large litters.[4]

During lactation, most dogs can be fed ad-lib or small meals frequently to allow them to

Table 24.1 Recommended nutrient levels during canine pregnancy and lactation.

Nutrient	Recommended Levels in Food
Protein	25-35% ME
Fat	20% ME (higher if needed)
Carbohydrates (soluble)	23% ME
Calcium	1-1.7% ME
Phosphorus	0.7-1.3% ME
Calcum:Phosphorus ration	1.1 : 1-2 : 1

Source: Debraekeleer et al.[6]

meet their energy requirements while producing adequate milk for the puppies.[3] The exception to this would be a bitch that experiences fetal loss and is only left with 1-2 puppies to care for. This dog will not experience increased energy requirements at the same level as a bitch with a larger litter.[3]

A common misconception is that other mammal milk can replace or supplement the bitch's milk. The milk produced by a dog has twice the protein and fat of cow's milk and more protein than goat's milk[6] (see Table 24.2).

The Puppies

Although the puppies are developing rapidly, they are very small until the last third of the 63-day gestation.[1] They have little impact on the bitch's weight and nutritional needs until after the fifth week of pregnancy. After the fifth week, fetal size and weight increase rapidly for the remaining 3-4 weeks of gestation. In the dog, greater than 75% of the weight and at least half of the fetal length are attained between the 40th and 55th day of gestation.[1]

What to Feed

If the breeding pair is in good physical and nutritional condition, no special foods need to

Table 24.2 Composition of mammals' milk as related to the growth rate.

Species	Days required to double birth weight	Protein (%)	Fat (%)	Calcium (%)	Phosphorus (%)
Man	180	1.6	3.75	0.03	0.014
Cow	47	3.3	3.7	0.12	0.10
Goat	22	2.9	3.8	na	na
Dog	9	7.5	9.5	0.24	0.18
Cat	9.5	7.5	8.6	0.18	0.16
Rabbit	6	11.5	15.0	0.61	0.38

Source: Debraekeleer et al.[6].

be fed before or during the breeding. Feeding a complete and balanced, highly digestible diet that has undergone feeding trials for pregnancy and lactation would be recommended.[1,2,4] It is not unusual for the bitch to have a slightly depressed appetite during estrus; this can be due to hormonal changes and nervousness.[1,4] The diet should be changed if needed early in her reproductive cycle to fully adjust to the new food before breeding and help prevent any abrupt change in diets during gestation or lactation.[1]

As lactation progresses, the bitch will gradually start weaning the puppies. The number of calories offered can be reduced correspondingly. Not only does this help prevent the development of obesity in the bitch, but it will also help reduce the amount of milk that she is producing. Once weaning has been completed, usually by 6-8 weeks, the bitch should be back to the number of calories she consumed before breeding.[3]

Nutrients

There are no special nutrient requirements during estrus in the dog. Breeding sires also do not have any unique nutrient requirements, though both intact males and females may require more energy than neutered males and females.[6]

Water

Water is of utmost importance during lactation. Inadequate water intake leads to a significant decrease in the quantity of milk produced. Water is needed to produce the milk as well as for thermoregulation.[6] Water requirements are roughly equivalent to the energy requirements in kcals.[6] Fresh, cool water should always be readily available to the lactating bitch, allowing her to determine optimal water intake.[1]

Protein

Protein requirements for mating are the same as for maintenance for young adult dogs and do not increase substantially for the first 2 trimesters of pregnancy. When entering the third trimester, protein requirements increase from 40% to 70% above maintenance as the puppies do their most growth.[6] At this point, the food should contain ~4 g of digestible protein/100 kcal of metabolizable energy. The recommended crude protein allowance for foods fed during gestation and lactation ranges from 20% DM (NRC)[7] to 22.5% DM (AAFCO).[8] Because very few proteins are 100% digestible, the recommended dietary amounts of proteins found in diets fed during gestation and lactation would be between 25% and 35% DM.[6]

Protein deficiency during pregnancy may decrease birth weight, increase mortality during the first 48 hours of life and decrease the immunocompetence of the puppies.[6] The protein requirement increases faster during lactation than the energy requirement.[6]

Fats

Fats provide increased energy compared to proteins or carbohydrates, provide essential fatty acids and absorb fat-soluble vitamins.[6] Increased fat intake has also been shown to improve food efficiency during lactation.[6] Increased fat intake by the bitch may increase the fat content of the milk. As puppies have very low energy reserves, this can increase the energy available through the milk.[6] The minimum recommended level of fat found in food for late gestation on into lactation is 8.5% DM (AAFCO)[8] and 8.5% DM (NRC).[7] Remember that the National Research Council (NRC) and Association of American Feed Control Officials (AAFCO) recommendations are minimums. The aim is for optimal performance. The recommended levels for bitches with fewer than 4 puppies would be at least 20% DM crude fat. For giant breeds dogs, the recommendation would also be 20% DM crude fat, and higher levels may be needed to meet energy requirements for those dogs with larger litters.[6]

Increased fat intake for both the bitch and the puppies' results in better food efficiency during lactation. Puppies are born with very low energy reserves. Sufficient energy needs to be provided through milk, which serves as their only source of nutrition for the first 4-6 weeks of life. Increasing the caloric density of the food the bitch eats has the effect of increasing the fat content in the milk that she produces.[6]

The omega 3 ($n-3$) and omega 6 ($n-6$) fatty acids have received much attention lately related to pregnancy and lactation. The diet should ideally be supplemented with both fatty acids in a ratio of 5 parts $n-3$: 1 part $n-6$

up to 10 parts $n-3$: 1 part $n-6$.[9] The $n-3$ docosahexaenoic acid (DHA) is essential for puppies' normal neurologic and retinal development. Adult animals have a limited ability to synthesize DHA from alpha-linolenic acid; the best way to ensure that the developing fetuses have enough DHA for optimal development is by supplementing the bitch's diet.[9]

Carbohydrates

While the body does not have a "requirement" for carbohydrates, feeding carbohydrate-free diets to pregnant bitches may result in weight loss, decreased food intake, reduced birth weight in the puppies and decreased neonatal survival with a possible increased risk of stillbirth.[6]

With more than 50% of the energy required for fetal development being supplied by glucose, bitches have an increased requirement for glucose during the last trimester of pregnancy. While gluconeogenic amino acids can supply glucose, this is an expensive way to supply glucose. When using fats for energy production, the risk of ketosis increases during late pregnancy.[6] A diet providing approximately 20% of the energy from soluble carbohydrates (i.e., starches and glycogen) is sufficient to prevent the harmful effects of a carbohydrate-free diet.[6] Foods fed during lactation should contain at least 23% DM from digestible carbohydrates.[6]

Calcium and Phosphorus

For most breeds of dogs, calcium and phosphorus requirements are the same for the first 2 trimesters of pregnancy as they are for adult maintenance (Ca:P ratio 1 : 1 to 1.5 : 1).[6] Due to rapid fetal skeletal growth during the final weeks of pregnancy, the requirements for calcium and phosphorus increase by 60%.[6] The NRC recommends a minimum recommended allowance for calcium in foods intended for

Table 24.3 Sample calculation of bitch and puppy feeding requirements.

Example
60# Labrador (prepregnancy weight) with 7 puppies
60# = 27.3 kg
RER = (30 × wt kg) + 70
RER = (30 × 27.3 kg) + 70 = 889 kcals
Lactation = RER × 1.9 = 1689 kcal/day
25% for each puppy 0.25 × 7 = 1.75 DER
7 puppies = RER × 1.75 = 889 × 1.75 = 1555.75 kcal/day
Bitch + puppies = 1689 + 1555.75 = 4644.75
Commercial dry Puppy food = 375 kcal/cup
3244.75 kcals/375 kcal/cup = 8.6 cups/day
Feed 8 2/3 cups/day or 2 rounded cups (2.15 cups) QID
If the energy content of the food is increased to 454 kcal/cup, 3244.75 kcal/454 kcal/cup = 7.14 cups/day
Feed 7 cups/day or 2 1/3 cups TID
The feeding amount could be decreased to 7 cups and still meet energy requirements

late gestation and peak pregnancy is 0.8% DM. AAFCOs recommendations are 1.2% DM.[6] Excessive calcium intake during late pregnancy may decrease parathyroid gland activity and predispose the bitch to develop eclampsia during lactation.[6] Because of this, a balance needs to be found between meeting minimum calcium levels without over-supplementing. The recommended calcium level is 1-1.7% DM, phosphorus levels of 0.7-1.3% DM with a calcium-phosphorus ratio of 1.1 : 1 to 2 : 1.[6] These levels also apply to large and giant breed dogs. If fed an appropriately balanced commercial diet, calcium supplementation is not recommended during gestation or lactation.[6] (see Table 24.3).

Digestibility

During late gestation, the actual caloric requirements for the bitch and fetuses may exceed what she can consume. This occurs most often if the food is poorly digestible. Digestibility is determined through feeding trials to measure the energy found in the food and the amount of energy available to the animal through digestion. The higher the digestibility, the more energy is available to the bitch. While there is no digestibility requirement, a food with an energy density of 4 kcal ME/gram or higher will have more fat and less fiber, increasing overall digestibility.[6]

DERs for a lactating bitch would be 1.9 × RER as a rough estimate. Each puppy would account for an additional 25% (0.25) of DER for each puppy.[6]

References

1 Case LP, Carey DP, Hirakawa DA, Daristotle L (2010) Pregnancy and lactation. In *Canine and Feline Nutrition* (3rd edn), pp. 199–206, St Louis MO: Mosby.

2 Buffington CA, Holloway C, Abood SK (2004) Normal dogs. In *Manual of Veterinary Dietetics*, pp. 9–11, St Louis MO: Saunders.

3 Delaney S, Fascetti A (2012) Feeding the healthy dog and cat. In S Delaney, A Fascetti (eds), *Applied Veterinary Clinical Nutrition*, pp. 82–3, Ames IA: Wiley-Blackwell.

4 Debraekeleer J, Gross KL, Zicker SC (2010) Introduction to feeding normal dogs. In MS Hand, CD Thatcher, RI Remillard, P Roudebush (eds), *Small Animal Clinical Nutrition* (5th edn), pp. 251–5, Marceline MO: Walsworth Publishing.

5 LeGrand-Defretin V, Munday HS (1995) Feeding dogs, and cats for life. In I Burger

(ed.), *The Waltham Book of Companion Animal Nutrition*, pp. 57–9, Tarrytown NY: Elsevier.

6 Debraekeleer J, Gross KL, Zicker SC (2010) Feeding reproducing dogs. In MS Hand, CD Thatcher, RI Remillard *et al.* (eds), *Small Animal Clinical Nutrition* (5th edn), pp. 281–90, Marceline MO: Walsworth Publishing.

7 National Research Council (2006: Beitz Donald C; Bauer, John E; Behnke, Keith C, Dzanis, David A, et al.) *Nutrient Requirements of Dogs and Cats. 2006*, Washington DC: The National Academies Press https:// nap.nationalacademies.org/read/10668/ chapter/1#vii. Accessed 6/27/23.

8 Association of American Feed Control Officials Ingredient Standards 2006. Champaign, IL https://www.aafco.org/consumers/ understanding-pet-food/ingredient-standards/. Accessed 6/27/23

9 Case LP, Daristotle L, Hayek MG, Raasch MF (2011) Pregnancy and lactation. In *Canine and Feline Nutrition* (3rd edn), pp. 199–206, St Louis MO: Mosby.

25

Pregnancy and Lactation in Cats

Introduction

As with dogs, any cat being considered for breeding should be in excellent physical condition, moderate body condition, normal muscle condition and well-exercised. Both the queen and tom should have complete physical exams by a veterinarian, be current on all preventative health programs, such as vaccinations, heartworm medications and intestinal dewormers, and be tested for the presence of feline leukemia virus and feline immunodeficiency virus.[1,2] If this is a purebred litter, both parents should also be screened for any congenital problems as well as shown to adhere to established breed standards.[1] If the queen is significantly underweight (BCS 3/9) or overweight (BCS >6/9), she should not be bred until she is closer to her ideal body weight and condition.[3]

Queens that are underweight or in poor body condition may fail to conceive, abort or bear small underweight kittens. They may also have markedly reduced lactation. Obesity in cats can lead to large kittens resulting in an increased incidence of dystocia.[3,4]

First Heat Cycle

Domestic cats generally have their first heat cycles between 6 and 9 months of age. This does not mean that they are physically ready to have a litter of kittens. Before 10-12 months of age, queens are still growing, and if they

become pregnant, they must support their continued growth and that of their kittens.[4] The best age for breeding is between 1.5 years and 7 years of age. Queens older than 7 years should not be bred due to reproductive complications, irregular estrous cycles and reduced litter size.[4]

Cats are seasonally polyestrous and with repeated estrous cycles throughout the breeding season.[5] In cooler regions, 2 heat cycles per year are typical, while a third heat cycle can often occur in warmer regions.

The cat is an induced ovulator and requires mating to end a heat cycle. The spines on the male's penis provide the stimulation required to induce ovulation. Multiple males can contribute to the fertilization of a single litter.[5]

Pregnancy

The gestational length for cats is 63 days (+/- 2 days). The fetal sacs can be palpated as early as 14-25 days gestation. Ultrasound can detect a pregnancy as early as 11 days.[5] Radiographs require skeletal ossification and are unreliable until 45 days gestation.

Unlike most species, weight gain in a queen increases linearly from conception to parturition. This weight gain in early pregnancy is not associated with significant growth of reproductive tissues or fetal growth. It appears to be stored in energy deposits (presumably as fat) to support lactation.[1,4]

Nutrition and Disease Management for Veterinary Technicians and Nurses, Third Edition. Ann Wortinger and Kara M. Burns.
© 2024 John Wiley & Sons, Inc. Published 2024 by John Wiley & Sons, Inc.
Companion Website: www.wiley.com/go/wortinger/3e

Energy intake parallels the linear pattern of weight gain. The weight gain is also independent of the number of fetuses being carried.[3] This stored energy can account for up to 60% of the weight gained during the pregnancy and is gradually lost during lactation.[1] Energy requirements increase to 90-100 kcal/kg of body weight/day.[3] The average weight gain should be about 40% of the pre-mating weight.[4] Energy needs can be met by providing RER × 1.6 at the time of breeding, with a gradual increase to RER × 2 at birth.[5]

Lactation

Lactation presents the biggest test of nutritional adequacy of any feeding regimen.[6] The queen must eat, digest, absorb and use large amounts of nutrients to produce sufficient milk of adequate quality to support the growth and development of several kittens.[6] Not only does she need to meet the entire energy requirements for the rapidly growing kittens, but she must also be able to meet all of her energy and nutrient requirements. The amount of energy needed to meet these multiple requirements depends on the queen's regular energy intake and the size and age of the litter.[6]

Lactation is considered the most physically demanding life stage regarding energy and nutrient requirements.[3] When lactating, energy needs for the queen increase with a peak at 7 weeks post parturition, though peak lactation amounts are reached at 3 weeks post parturition.[3] This discrepancy can be explained by looking at the calories consumed by the queen for maintenance and lactation and including the calories consumed by the kittens from both lactation and oral intake of the queen's food.[3]

The queen should be eating 2-3 times her maintenance energy requirements during lactation, depending on litter size.[1] A general guideline is to feed 1.5 times DER during the first week of lactation, 2 times DER during the second week, and 2.5-3 times DER during

the fourth week of lactation.[1] If the energy density of the food is too low, the queen may not be able to physically consume enough food to meet both her and the kittens' energy requirements. If this happens, her milk production will decrease, she will lose weight, and she may display signs of severe exhaustion.[4]

Lactation begins at birth. Colostrum is produced for the first 24-72 hours. Milk production depends on litter size and stage of lactation.[5] Peak lactation occurs between 3-4 weeks post-partum.[4] The kitten's continuous weight gain is the best indicator of adequate milk production by the queen.[5]

A common misconception is that other mammal milk can replace or supplement the queen's milk. The milk produced by a cat has more than twice the protein and fat of cow's milk and more protein and nearly 3 times the fat found in goat's milk[5] (see Table 25.1).

The Kittens

Kittens should exhibit steady weight gain, have good muscle tone and suckle vigorously. Young kittens are quiet between feedings.[4] Kittens that are restless and cry excessively may not be receiving enough milk due to poor lactation. Gastric distension is not a good indicator of adequate nursing. Excessive swallowing of air during nursing can give the appearance of gastric fullness, despite inadequate milk intake.[4] Kitten mortality reportedly varies from 9% to 63% depending on the source of the cats and the cattery.[4] Several genetic, husbandry and nutritional factors contribute to high mortality. If kitten death or cannibalism by the queen is high, all three areas should be investigated.[4]

What to Feed

The queen should be fed a diet intended for reproduction throughout gestation and lactation.[1,4] The amount of food should be gradually increased, beginning at the second

Table 25.1 Composition of mammals milk as related to the growth rate.

Species	Days required to double birth weight	Protein (%)	Fat (%)	Calcium (%)	Phosphorus (%)
Man	180	1.6	3.75	0.03	0.014
Cow	47	3.3	3.7	0.12	0.10
Goat	22	2.9	3.8	na	na
Dog	9	7.5	9.5	0.21	0.18
Cat	9.5	7.5	8.6	0.18	0.16
Rabbit	6	11.5	15.0	0.61	0.38

Source: Case et al.[1]/with permission of Elsevier.

week of gestation and continuing until parturition. At the end of gestation, the queen should be consuming about 25–50% more food than during her normal maintenance needs.[1] Due to the high energy demands during pregnancy and lactation, free choice or ad-lib feeding is recommended to allow the queen to meet her increased energy demands.[3]

After parturition, approximately 40% of the weight gained during pregnancy is lost. By the time the kittens are weaned (7-8 weeks post-parturition), the queen should be back to her pre-breeding weight.[3]

Once the kittens are weaned, the queen can be returned to her regular maintenance diet to maintain optimal body condition score (BCS) and muscle condition score (MCS)[3] (see Table 25.2).

Nutrients

Few studies have established the nutritional requirements for queens or toms used for breeding. Most recommendations have been extrapolated from growth studies, results from other species and clinical experience.[5]

Ideally, a pregnant queen will be fed a complete and balanced diet designed to support gestation and lactation.[5] The nutritional requirements for toms and queens during mating do not appear to be significantly different from the requirements for young adults.[5]

Table 25.2 Recommended nutrient levels during feline pregnancy and lactation.

Nutrient	Recommended levels in food
Protein	35-50% DM
Fat	10-30% DM
Omega 3: Omega 6 FA ratio	5 : 1-10 : 1
Digestible carbohydrate	>10% DM
Calcium	1.1-1.6% DM
Phosphorus	0.8-1.4% DM
Calcium:Phosphorus	1 : 1–1.5 : 1% DM

Source: Armstrong et al.[5]/Mark Morris Institute.

Water

Water is important for normal reproduction. Expansion of extracellular fluid compartments and maternal and fetal tissue development during pregnancy increases the daily water requirement.[5]

Water is the most crucial nutrient the queen consumes during lactation. Because milk has an estimated 78% water content, inadequate water intake leads to a significant decrease in the quantity of milk produced.[1] As lactation increases post-parturition, the queen's water requirements will increase significantly.[1] Fresh, cool water should always be readily available to the lactating queen.[1]

If the queen is fed dry kitten food during pregnancy and lactation, the volume of water required will be higher than if she is fed canned food. This is due to the inherently higher water content found in canned diets. If water intake is insufficient, switching from dry to canned food can help, as can adding additional water to a canned diet.[5]

Protein

Protein synthesis in the queen is significantly increased during gestation.[5] Providing a high-quality protein in a sufficient quantity is required to provide the essential amino acids needed during this time.[5] Feeding a diet that meets the minimum AAFCO requirement of 30% dry matter is essential for optimal production and growth during gestation and into lactation. (AAFCO 2013) Due to the carnivorous nature of cats, attention also needs to be paid to the type of protein that the queen is consuming. Animal-based proteins are preferred as the primary dietary source of protein, as they tend to be more digestible and have the essential amino acids (EAA), taurine. Taurine, an essential amino acid for cats, can only be found in animal-based protein sources. When insufficient taurine is in the diet, the conception rate and neonate birth weights decrease.[1] Additionally, when queens are fed a protein-restricted diet during late gestation and lactation, their kittens can have delayed home orientation. This means they have a delayed ability to orient to and return to the nest. Aberrant locomotor development and decreased emotional responsiveness can also be seen in the kittens.[5]

During peak lactation, milk protein output for a 4 kg queen, nursing a large litter, can reach as high as 19 g crude protein/day.[5] Due to variations in food digestibility and ingredient quality, the recommended crude protein allowance for lactation is at least 35% DM, with a range of 35-50% DM.[5]

Fat

Due to its increased caloric density, the easiest way to increase caloric content is to increase the fat quantity. AAFCO recommends a minimum crude fat content of 9.0% DM for late gestation and lactation. (AAFCO 2013) For optimal reproductive performance, foods given to queens should have at least 18% DM, with a range of 18-35% DM.[5]

Litter size can be positively influenced by the fat level found in the queen's diet. This fat should include essential fatty acids (EFAs) and arachidonic acid. Arachidonic acid is an EFA for cats and can only be found in fats obtained from animal sources.[1]

The omega 3 ($n − 3$) and omega 6 ($n − 6$) fatty acids have received much attention lately related to pregnancy and lactation. The diet should ideally be supplemented with both fatty acids in a ratio of 5 parts $n − 3$: 1 part $n − 6$ up to 10 parts $n − 3$: 1 part $n − 6$.[1] The $n − 3$ docosahexaenoic acid (DHA) is essential for kittens' normal neurologic and retinal development. Adult animals have a limited ability to synthesize DHA from alpha-linolenic acid; the best way to ensure that the developing fetuses have enough DHA for optimal development is to supplement the queen's diet.[1] Common ingredients such as fish and poultry meals represent a good source of DHA for queens.[5]

For queens in late gestation and peak lactation, the minimum recommended allowance of DHA plus eicosapentaenoic acid (EPA) is at least 0.01% DM. The DHA part needs to be at least 40% of the total DHA/EPA amount or 0.004% DM.[5]

Long-term deficiency of the EFA, arachidonic acid, causes reproductive failure in cats. AAFCO recommends 0.02% DM for Foods that meet AAFCO label statements for growth or reproduction and should provide sufficient amounts of arachidonic acid.[5,7]

Digestible Carbohydrates

Although cats do not have a digestible carbohydrate requirement, digestible carbohydrates can protect against weight loss in queens during lactation.[5] Digestible carbohydrates also spare protein required to maintain blood glucose and provide a substrate for lactose during milk production. Until further studies are done to define the optimal level of digestible carbohydrates during lactation, at least 10% DM should be included in the queen's food.[5]

Calcium and Phosphorus

Calcium and phosphorus are required at greater levels during gestation and lactation to support fetal skeletal development and milk content. The AAFCO minimum recommended levels are 1.0% DM for calcium and 0.8% DM for phosphorus. Levels at or greater than these are found in commercial cat foods meeting AAFCO certification requirements.[5] Unlike dogs, eclampsia is uncommon in cats; it can occur.[5]

References

1 Case LP, Carey DP, Hirakawa DA, Daristotle L (2011) Pregnancy and lactation. In *Canine and Feline Nutrition* (3rd edn), pp. 199–206, St Louis MO: Mosby.

2 Buffington CA, Holloway C, Abood SK (2004) Normal dogs. In *Manual of Veterinary Dietetics*, pp. 9–11, St Louis MO: Saunders.

3 Delaney S, Fascetti A (2012) Feeding the healthy dog and cat. In S Delaney, A Fascetti (eds), *Applied Veterinary Clinical Nutrition*, pp. 81–2, Ames IA: Wiley-Blackwell.

4 Armstrong PJ, Gross KL, Becvarova I, Debraekeleer J (2010) Normal cats. In MS Hand, CD Thatcher, RI Remillard, P Roudebush (eds), *Small Animal Clinical Nutrition* (5th edn), pp. 361–71, Marceline MO: Walsworth Publishing.

5 Armstrong PJ, Gross KL, Becvarova I, Debraekeleer J (2010) Feeding reproducing cats. In MS Hand, CD Thatcher, RI Remillard, P Roudebush (eds), *Small Animal Clinical Nutrition* (5th edn), pp. 401–11, Marceline MO: Walsworth Publishing.

6 LeGrand-Defretin V, Munday HS (1995) Feeding dogs and cats for life. In I Burger (ed.), *The Waltham book of Companion Animal Nutrition*, pp. 57–9, Tarrytown NY: Elsevier.

7 AAFCO Procedures Manual. https://www.aafco.org/Portals/0/SiteContent/Regulatory/AAFCO_Procedures_Manual.pdf. Accessed 7/16/22.

26

Neonatal Puppies and Kittens

Introduction

The neonatal period of a dog or cat's life is considered the first 2 weeks of their life.[1] The first week of this period is critical for its survival. Newborn puppies and kittens are physiologically immature, with low percentages of body fat, 1–2% compared to 12–35% in adults. This immaturity is termed altricial, which means that they are born immature and are therefore wholly dependent on their mother for survival.[1] If they are orphaned, that care will depend on their foster parents until they mature enough to start caring for themselves.

Nutrition

Surveys indicate that many deaths before weaning are due to a relatively small number of causes: infectious diseases, congenital defects and malnutrition.[2] Infectious diseases are more of a concern with neonates who did not receive adequate colostrum from their mothers and are therefore deficient in passive immunity. Milk is assumed to be a complete food for neonates until weaning, with the composition changing as the puppies and kittens needs change as they grow.[3] The cause of malnutrition is usually from the mother's death or neglect, lactation failure or a litter that is too large for the milk supply.[2]

Water

Water is one of the most essential nutrients for neonates, as the proportion of their total body weight composed of water is much higher than it is for adults. A typical kitten contains 78.8% body water at one week of age. An adult cat is composed of only 61.7% water.[4] A typical puppy requires 132–220 mL/kg body weight daily, while a typical kitten requires 155–230 mL/kg body weight/day.

Protein

The minimum protein requirement for neonates has not been established. It is assumed to be comparable to that for weanling, with approximately 30% DM for kittens and 22.5% DM for puppies.[5]

Bitch milk contains high levels of arginine, lysine and branched-chain amino acids. These inclusions are vital when formulating commercial milk replacers.[3] For kittens, arginine and histidine are the amino acids of primary concern in milk replacers.[4]

In kittens, taurine is vital for normal growth and development. Queens fed a taurine-deficient diet have significantly lower taurine levels in their milk. Cows being strict herbivores, have very low taurine levels in their milk. For milk replacers based on cow's milk, additional taurine must be supplemented to provide the levels that kittens require.[4]

Fat

Fat serves as a source of energy and essential fatty acids for neonates. The fat content of the milk produced will gradually increase during the lactation period.[4] The milk's fat content and composition often reflect the mother's dietary intake.[3] Bitch milk contains high levels of unsaturated fatty acids and is rich in linoleic acid. Queen milk contains the essential fatty acids linoleic and arachidonic acids. Both bitch and queen milk have much higher linoleic acid levels than cow's milk.[3] The *n*−3 fatty acid, docosahexaenoic acid (DHA), is essential for normal retinal and brain development, while linoleic acid is required for normal growth.[3,4]

Carbohydrate

The disaccharide lactose is the primary carbohydrate in milk. It is broken down into its constituent monosaccharides (galactose and glucose) during digestion. Lactose is unique among the disaccharides in that it is linked with ß-bonds instead of α-bonds. This bonding makes lactose a less suitable substrate for bacteria that may infect the mammary gland or the neonate's GI tract.[3] While the lactose concentration varies during the lactation cycle, the average concentration in bitch milk is 14.5% DM, and queen milk varies from 14–26% DM.[3,4]

Calcium and Phosphorous

Calcium concentration in colostrum is low, increasing throughout the lactation cycle. However, the Ca:P ratio remains consistent at around 1.3:1.[3,4] This increasing calcium content is needed for bone mineralization and growth.

Colostrum

The first nutritional concern for newborns is receiving colostrum immediately after birth. All of the components of colostrum are critical to the survival of the newborn. Colostrum is milk produced by the mother during the first 24–72 h after parturition. Colostrum provides nutrients, water, growth factors, digestive enzymes and maternal immunoglobulins (antibodies).[6] Most of the immunoglobulins and other factors transmitted through the colostrum are in the form of large proteins. Once absorbed across the intestinal barrier, they confer passive immunity to the neonate.[1] The ability of the neonate to absorb these large proteins across the intestinal barrier is lost after the first 24–72 h. Continuation of colostrum after this period provides no additional immunity to the neonate. It is important to remember the neonate can only receive protection from diseases the mother has either been vaccinated for or has contracted and developed natural immunity to. This passive immunity will help to protect the neonate until into the weaning period and is considered gone by ~16 weeks of age.[1]

Milk

The main difference between colostrum and milk is the water content and nutrient composition.[6] The water content of colostrum is lower than that of milk, which accounts for its sticky, concentrated appearance compared with regular milk. The water content found in the milk will gradually increase from day 1 to day 3.[6]

Lactose concentrations found in colostrum are also lower than those found in milk with higher protein and fat levels. The energy content found in milk also increases throughout lactation.[6] Due to their immaturity, neonates do not develop adequate glycogen reserves until after the first few days of nursing.[2] This lack of glycogen reserves means that they need to nurse or be fed frequently, sometimes as often as every 2 h for the first week or so of life.

The ratio of casein: whey in the milk is also different for each species. Casein is the solid protein found in milk, while whey is the liquid protein found in milk. The amount of casein found in milk can affect protein digestion, mineral utilization, and the milk's amino acid composition. The ratio for cats is 60:40, while for dogs is 70:30.[1] Queen's milk would also be inadequate for puppies because of inadequate lactose and calcium levels. Bitch's milk contains almost twice as much protein as cow's milk. It also provides branched-chain amino acids and high levels of arginine and lysine.[3] (see Table 26.1).

If the puppy or kitten is raised by its mother, it should be allowed free access to her. They should be monitored to ensure adequate nutrition and have received colostrum during the first 24 h of life.[3] During the first few weeks of life, they should nurse at least 4–6 times per day. In healthy puppies and kittens, the mother's milk supports normal growth until approximately 4 weeks of age.[7] Supplemental feedings should only be necessary with unusually large litters or maternal rejection.[7] After 4 weeks of age, milk alone does not provide adequate calories or nutrients for continued normal development.[7]

Thermoregulation

Maintenance of body temperature is the second most crucial concern for newborns. Neonatal puppies and kittens are unable to thermoregulate and must be kept in an environment of 85–90 °F/29–32 °C during the first week of life, and 80–85 °F/26–29 °C during the second week.[2] If the neonates are not kept warm enough and develop hypothermia, they will be unable to nurse, and if tube-fed, they will be unable to digest the food. This failure to eat may result in rejection by the bitch or queen.[2] The best source of warmth is the mother. After 6 days, the neonates can shiver but are still very susceptible to chilling. Keeping the environment warm and free of drafts is of utmost importance during the first few weeks of life.[7] (see Table 26.2).

Orphans

Neonates are considered orphaned if they lack adequate maternal care for continued survival from birth to weaning.[3] Orphaned neonates have the same requirements as neonates with a mother; they still need adequate nutrition and warmth. The best course for the young puppy or kitten would be to have a foster mother; if this is not available, they can be hand-raised. If they are hand-raised, not only do they need

Table 26.1 Nutrient composition of various milks.

Nutrient	Queen's milk	Bitch's milk	Cow's milk	Goat's milk
Moisture (g/100 g)	79	77.3	87.7	87.0
Crude Protein (g/100 g)	7.5	7.5	3.3	3.6
Crude Fat (g/100g)	8.5	9.5	3.6	4.1
Lactose (g/100 g)	4.0	3.3	4.7	4.0
Calcium (mg/100 g)	180	240	119	133
ME (kcal/100 g)	121	146	64	69

Source: Armstrong et al. [6]/Mark Morris Institute.

Table 26.2 Optimal environmental temperatures for orphans.

Age	Celcius	Fahrenheit
Week 1	29–32	84–90
Week 2	26–29	79–84
Week 3	23–26	73–79
Week 4	23	73

Source: Debraekeleer et al. [3]/Mark Morris Institute.

to be fed, but they also have to have their urination and defecation stimulated. The mother would do this by licking the anogenital area. Since the foster parent is unlikely to consider this option, a dry dish rag or cotton ball can provide the same stimulation. If using a damp cloth, make sure that the area is thoroughly dry after defecation/urination, or chapping can occur in this very delicate area. This will need to be continued until the puppy or kittens are between 16 and 21 days old.[3]

Milk Replacers

Milk from other species is an inadequate substitute for mothers' milk. The protein, fat and calcium levels found in goat and cow milk are too low for puppies or kittens.[3]

Commercially available milk replacers can supply or supplement the nutritional needs of neonates. Most milk replacers are based on cow or goat's milk and modified to resemble the nutrient profile for bitch and queen's milk.[8]

While there are "homemade" recipes for milk replacers for puppies and kittens, most of these recipes were developed through trial and error, and their actual nutrient content is unknown.[7] If fed straight cow's milk, neonate puppies develop severe diarrhea. Cow's milk contains nearly three times the lactose in bitch's milk.[7] Cow's milk also contains an excessive proportion of casein for neonatal puppies and kittens and supplies insufficient calories for both.[7]

Commercial milk replacers are the preferred source of nutrition for orphans or as supplemental feeding to those neonates who are not receiving enough nutrition from their mothers.[7] A product that has been tested for the specific purpose of raising neonatal puppies or kittens should be selected. Even though the nutrient content and bioavailability are guaranteed, commercial formulas vary in their ability to provide adequate nutrition and calories.[7] Most commercial replacement formulas have a nutrient density of ~1 kcal/mL, though dilution with water will reduce that.[9] Feeding recommendations vary from 13–18 mL/100 g of body weight, using a formula with ~1 kcal/mL.[9] This amount will gradually increase as the neonate gains weight. Frequent reassessment of the feeding plan should be done, looking at the overall health, appearance, activity level, hydration status and weight gain of the orphans.

For kittens, the expected weight gain would be ~18–20 g/day. Due to the greater variation in size, puppies are ~1 g of weight gain for every 2–5 g of milk consumed during the first 5 weeks of life.[9] Chronic whimpering or vocalization may indicate discomfort or hunger and warrant a reassessment of the feeding plan.[9]

The American Association of Feed Control Officials (AAFCO) does not provide detailed guidelines for testing milk replacers. Obtaining the manufacturers' information related to nutrient composition, nutritional integrity and feeding efficacy is helpful in selecting the best replacement.[7] It is important to remember, even the best milk replacer cannot provide the neonate with the antibodies found in colostrum. Therefore, extra care must be taken to maintain a clean environment and prevent disease transmission.[7] Feeding materials such as bottles, nipples and tubes should be cleaned and disinfected between feedings. The milk replacer itself should be made fresh or refrigerated between feedings to decrease the incidence of bacterial contamination. Only the volume of milk replacer consumed within 24 h should be made up. Any milk replacer that is not used at that feeding should be stored in the refrigerator.[4]

Weaning

Weaning is a gradual process with two phases. The first phase begins when the neonate begins to eat solid food between 3 and 4 weeks of age.[6,7] This can be encouraged by mixing a commercial food specifically made and tested for all life stages, or puppies and kittens, or a thick gruel made by mixing a small amount of warm water with the mother's food which has also been made and tested for all life stages, including lactation.[1,9]

Cow's milk should not be used to make the gruel as the lactose level is too high and may contribute to diarrhea.[1] This semisolid food should be provided in a shallow dish, with the puppies or kittens allowed free access to the fresh food several times per day.[6,7] The food should be removed after 20–30 min to discourage bacterial growth. A homemade weaning formula should not be fed, as the nutrient content would be unknown, leading to nutrient, vitamin and mineral imbalances, and the caloric density is unknown.[1]

Initially, the food intake will be minimal, but by 5–6 weeks of age, the deciduous teeth will have begun to erupt, enabling the puppies and kittens to chew and eat dry food.[6,7] As the food intake increases in the neonates, the mother's milk production will decrease. By 6 weeks of age, the second weaning stage can begin with the puppies and kittens obtaining their complete nutrition from their food and not from their mother (nutritional weaning).[6,7] Even though some mothers will continue to nurse their young past this time, very little milk is being produced with little nutrition being obtained. It is believed that the psychological and emotional benefits of suckling may be as significant as the nutritional benefits in animals that are older than 5 weeks of age.[7] For this reason, complete weaning (behavioral weaning) should not be done until puppies and kittens are at least 7–8 weeks of age.[7]

References

1 Case LP, Daristotle L, Hayek MG, Raasch MF (2010) Nutritional care of neonatal puppies and kittens. In *Canine and Feline Nutrition* (3rd edn), pp. 209–17, St Louis, MO: Mosby.

2 Buffington CA, Holloway C, Abood SK (2004) Normal dogs. In *Manual of Veterinary Dietetics*, pp. 11–2, St. Louis, MO: Saunders.

3 Debraekeleer J, Gross KL, Zicker SC (2010) Feeding nursing and orphaned puppies from birth to weaning. In MS Hand, CD Thatcher, RI Remillard, P Roudebush (eds), *Small Animal Clinical Nutrition* (5th edn), pp. 295–309, Marceline, MO: Walsworth Publishing.

4 Gross KL, Iveta B, Debraekeleer J (2010) Feeding nursing and orphaned kittens from birth to weaning. In MS Hand, CD Thatcher, RI Remillard *et al.* (eds), *Small Animal Clinical Nutrition* (5th edn), pp. 415–27, Marceline, MO: Walsworth Publishing.

5 AAFCO Procedures Manual https://www. aafco.org/Portals/0/SiteContent/Regulatory/ AAFCO_Procedures_Manual.pdf (Accessed 7/16/22).

6 Armstrong PJ, Gross KL, Becvarova I, Debraekeleer J (2010) Normal cats. In M Hand, CD Thatcher, RI Remillard, P Roudebush (eds), *Small Animal Clinical Nutrition* (5th edn), pp. 361–71, Marceline, MO: Walsworth Publishing.

7 Case LP, Carey DP, Hirakawa DA, Daristotle L (2000) Nutritional care of neonatal puppies and kittens. In *Canine and Feline Nutrition* (2nd edn), pp. 233–43, St Louis, MO: Mosby.

8 LeGrand-Defretin V, Munday HS (1995) Feeding dogs and cats for life. In I Burger (ed.), *The Waltham Book of Companion Animal Nutrition*, pp. 61–5, Tarrytown, NY: Elsevier.

9 Delaney S, Fascetti A (2012) Feeding the healthy dog and cat. In S Delaney, A Fascetti (eds), *Applied Veterinary Clinical Nutrition*, p. 83, Ames, IA: Wiley-Blackwell.

27

Growth in Dogs

Introduction

The dog is unique among other mammals in that it has the broadest range of normal adult body weight within any single species, ranging in size from adult Yorkshire Terriers and Chihuahuas weighing only 3# (1.4 kg) to adult Great Danes and Mastiffs that can top 200# (90 kg).[1] Because of this wide range in sizes, growth in the early stages of life is very rapid, and in general, most breeds of dogs will reach 50% of their adult weight between 5 and 6 months old.[1] Different breeds will continue to mature at different rates, with some of the larger breeds not reaching their full mature size until almost 2 years of age. Initial weight gain should be between 2 and 4 g/day/kg of anticipated adult weight for the first 5 months of life.[2] While this can be helpful in purebred dogs, where anticipated adult weight can at least be guessed, for mixed-breed dogs where the adult size of both parents may not even be known—this does not provide much helpful information.

After nursing, postweaning growth is the most nutritionally demanding period in a dog's life. With large and giant breed dogs, the length and speed of their growth pose an even higher nutritional demand. First, average growth will be addressed, and then how this differs between large and giant breeds. What works nutritionally for a Chihuahua would not necessarily work for an Irish Wolfhound.

Normal Growth

Growth is a complex process involving interactions between genetics, nutrition and other environmental factors.[3] Nutrition can affect the growth and development of growing dogs. It directly affects the immune system, body composition, growth rate and skeletal development.[3]

The most rapid period of growth is seen during the first 6 months of life. With this comes an increased requirement for all nutrients, with energy and calcium being of particular concern.[3] Most small breed dogs will have reached their adult size by 8–12 months, medium breed dogs by 12–18 months and large and giant breed dogs not reaching their mature size until 18–24 months of age.[4] By maturity, most dogs will have increased their birth weight by 40–50 times.[4]

The growth rates for young dogs are affected by the nutrient density (kcal/can or cup) and the amount of food fed.[3] Young dogs should be fed to grow at an optimal rate for bone development and body condition instead of maximal growth rate.[3] Feeding for a maximal growth rate increases the incidence of skeletal deformities, and 1 study has shown a decrease in overall longevity.[3]

Diet restriction, and thus energy restriction, has been shown to affect the life span of dogs, with the primary research being done on Labrador Retrievers over the span of 15 years.

Nutrition and Disease Management for Veterinary Technicians and Nurses, Third Edition. Ann Wortinger and Kara M. Burns.
© 2024 John Wiley & Sons, Inc. Published 2024 by John Wiley & Sons, Inc.
Companion Website: www.wiley.com/go/wortinger/3e

All dogs were housed in the same conditions, received the same level of care and were fed the same food; the only difference between the two groups was the amount of food consumed. One group of 24 dogs was designated the control group and was fed 62.1 kcal of ME/kg of estimated ideal body weight. The remaining 24 dogs were fed 25% less than their pair-mate. The group fed the larger amount had a BCS of 6-7/9, while the restricted-feeding group had a BCS of 4-5/9. On average, the group that received the larger amount of food died 2 years younger than their pair-mates, developed osteoarthritis 1.1 years sooner, and developed chronic health conditions 6 months sooner.[5] The only difference between these two groups was the amount of food fed. Following body condition scoring, none of the group fed the larger amounts were obese, and none of the restricted-fed dogs were emaciated; these were all "average" sized Labradors.

This group of Labradors was fed controlled amounts from the time they entered the study at 6 weeks of age until they either died or were euthanized.[5] Because of the rapid growth seen in dogs during the first 12–18 months, this restriction can become very important when looking at the development of orthopedic problems later in life. While these problems occur later in life, they do not develop later in life but while the dog is going through this rapid growth phase.

The most helpful indicator of a healthy growth rate in puppies is its body condition score (BCS). A BCS should be evaluated and reassessed at a minimum at every vaccination appointment, ideally every 2 weeks. This allows for adjustments in the volume fed before the puppy gets overweight.[3]

Everyone loves the image of the roly-poly puppy. This ideal needs to be adjusted to prevent skeletal deformities from occurring and prevent the formation of excess adipocytes early in life. Once an adipocyte (fat cell) has formed, it is there forever and makes active actions through hormones to maintain or gain cell contents in the form of stored fat cells.

What to Feed

Energy

Energy density is very important for growing puppies because of the quantity of food needed to meet energy requirements. If fed poor-quality food with low energy density and low digestibility, the puppies need to consume larger quantities to meet their energy requirements.[3] This intake of large volumes of food can increase the incidence of flatulence, vomiting, diarrhea, fecal volume and the development of a "pot-bellied" appearance.[3] When feeding poor-quality food, even inexpensive food can cost more to feed than higher-quality food, more expensive food, since so much of it will not be utilized by the body and will instead end up as feces.

While puppies have higher requirements for energy and other essential nutrients than adults, they also tend to have less digestive capacity, smaller mouths and smaller and fewer teeth to eat their food. This is especially true for small and toy breeds of dogs.[4] These differences limit the amount of food the puppy can consume and digest within a meal or a given amount of time.[4] It is equally important to not over-feed growing dogs; not only can this lead to an accelerated growth rate due to excess energy consumption, but it also causes a build-up of adipose tissue that can contribute to obesity later in life.[4]

Protein

The protein requirements for growing puppies are higher than those for adult dogs. This is because the puppy has normal maintenance needs, but it also needs protein to build new tissue associated with growth.[4] Since puppies eat higher amounts of energy, the total amount of protein eaten is naturally higher. Foods fed to growing puppies should contain slightly higher protein levels than those fed for adult maintenance.

Most importantly, this protein should be of high quality and highly digestible.[4] The minimum level of protein found in puppy diets should be 22.5% of the DM, with optimal levels between 22 and 32% DM. The type of protein included in the diet should be of high quality to ensure that all of the essential amino acids are being delivered to the body for growth and development.[3,4] This does not mean that only muscle meats provide adequate protein of high digestibility.

An important difference in protein requirements between growing and adult dogs is that the amino acid arginine is essential for puppies and is only conditionally essential in adult dogs.[3]

Fats and Fatty Acids

Dietary fats serve as sources of essential fatty acids (EFA), carriers for the fat-soluble vitamins A, D, E and K, and a concentrated form of energy. The EFA requirements can be provided by food containing between 5 and 10% DM of fat. Studies show that docosahexaenoic acid (DHA) is required for the normal neural, retinal and auditory development of puppies. Including fish oils as a source of DHA in puppy foods increase trainability. Unlike adults, puppies have an inefficient conversion of short-chain polyunsaturated fatty acids into DHA.[3] Adding a source of DHA to puppy foods is considered essential for growth.

A 10–25% DM (dry matter) content is recommended for fat from post-weaning to adulthood to meet energy requirements. The minimum recommended level of DHA plus eicosapentaenoic acid (EPA) is 0.05% DM, with no more than 60% of this amount composed of EPA and at least 40% composed of DHA.[3]

Calcium and Phosphorus

Even though calcium is essential for bone growth, the actual requirements in puppies are quite low. The American Association of Feed Control Officials (AAFCO) *Nutrient Profiles* 2014 recommends that dog foods formulated for growth contain a minimum of 1.2% DM calcium.[4] In general, calcium absorption from food is dependent on requirements and calcium intake.[3] In puppies under 6 months of age, intestinal calcium absorption never falls below 40%, even if increased calcium levels are in the food. Supplementation of calcium in this age group of puppies causes an artificially high calcium level, increasing retention.[3]

Foods for large and giant breed puppies should contain between 0.7 and 1.2% DM calcium and 0.6–1.1% phosphorus.[3] Acceptable calcium levels can be higher for small to medium-breed puppies, at 0.7–1.7% DM calcium and 0.6–1.3% phosphorus. Care must be taken to ensure the Ca:P ratio for small to medium-breed puppies remains between 1:1 and 1.8:1, and for large to giant-breed puppies, 1:1 and 1.5:1[3] (see Figure 27.1).

Feeding Regimens

When a new puppy is initially brought home, the diet should not be changed from what was previously fed unless the food is very poor quality. Moving to a new home and leaving the bitch and littermates is quite stressful for a young dog.[4] A new diet can be introduced 2–3 days after moving to the new home, although it is best to transition over 5–7 days. The easiest way to do this is to mix the food in quarters, so on day 1, give ¾ of the old diet mixed with ¼ of the new diet. Day 2 and 3 give ½ of the old diet mixed with ½ of the new diet, day 4 & 5 give ¼ of the old diet with ¾ of the new diet and on day 6, the transition is complete.[3] If the initial food is of poor quality, switching over all at once is acceptable, though some diarrhea may also be expected.

Free-choice and time-restricted feedings are not recommended for puppies. Free-choice feedings may increase the amount of body fat, predisposing the dog to obesity later in life and causing skeletal deformities at a young age. Studies using time-restricted feedings have shown that the puppies increase body

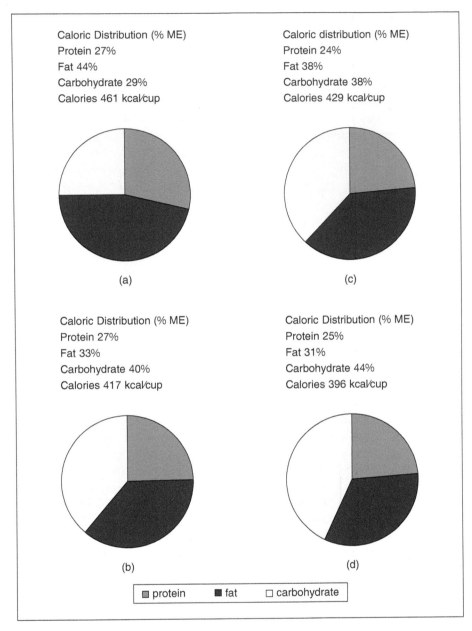

Caloric Distribution (% ME)
Protein 27%
Fat 44%
Carbohydrate 29%
Calories 461 kcal/cup

(a)

Caloric distribution (% ME)
Protein 24%
Fat 38%
Carbohydrate 38%
Calories 429 kcal/cup

(c)

Caloric Distribution (% ME)
Protein 27%
Fat 33%
Carbohydrate 40%
Calories 417 kcal/cup

(b)

Caloric Distribution (% ME)
Protein 25%
Fat 31%
Carbohydrate 44%
Calories 396 kcal/cup

(d)

■ protein   ■ fat   □ carbohydrate

Figure 27.1 Nutrient Profiles. (a) Small breed puppy food dry. (b) Large breed puppy food dry. (c) Adult Maintenance Food dry. (d) Adult maintenance large breed dry.[6]

weight, have more body fat and increase bone mineralization faster than puppies fed free-choice.[3] During periods of rapid growth, it is better to do measured feedings 2–4 times per day. The amount fed should be based on the dog's growth rate and the BCS.

The feeding guides listed on the package can be used as a starting point. Because the feeding directions on the package are designed to provide enough calories for all dogs on a specific diet, the amounts given tend to over-estimate the actual volume needed. Amounts

Table 27.1 Life-stage factors for puppies based on estimated adult size.[3]

Time frame	LSF
Weaning to 50% of adult body weight	3
50–80% of adult body weight	2.5
>80% adult body weight	1.8–2.0

should be adjusted to maintain an ideal BCS.[2] Puppies should be lean, not skinny, and not roly-poly throughout their growth phase.

The initial feeding amount can be estimated by dividing the puppy's daily energy requirements (DER) by the energy density of the food (kcal/cup or can). Remember that energy requirements are estimates, and adjustments may need to be made based on each individual puppy. Using BCS, the feeding volume should be adjusted regularly to allow for changes in the growth rate.

Ideally, owners should weigh their puppies weekly, record their body weights and food intake (including snacks and training treats) and use this information to make any adjustments in food intake needed to maintain ideal body condition[3] (see Table 27.1).

Large and Giant Breed Puppies

Nutrient excesses, rapid growth rates and excessive weight gain appear to be important factors contributing to the incidence of skeletal disorders in growing large and giant breed dogs.[7] While we continue to select increased sizes for many of our larger dogs, size itself is not detrimental to the dog. Still, management practices that allow growth rates to be maximized can cause the negative consequences seen in these dogs.[8] It has been estimated that more than 20% of orthopedic diseases in dogs are due to dietary origins, with more than 22% of these showing up in dogs under 1 year of age.[9]

It is well documented that the incidence of skeletal disease, including osteochondrosis,

hypertrophic osteodystrophy and hip dysplasia, is markedly increased in the growing large breed dog if management practices are such that this maximal genetic potential for the rate of growth is realized.[8] The primary management practice affecting growth rate and skeletal disease is nutritional support.[8]

The primary nutritional considerations implicated in skeletal disease development in growing large breed dogs are dietary concentrations of protein, energy and calcium.[8] To ensure a slower growth rate, energy intake needs to be managed through measured feedings and monitoring BCS to maintain lean body weight. A minimum of 2 meals should be fed daily, while 3–4 meals may be more appropriate for some dogs.[2] Slight underfeeding of energy during growth will slow the overall rate but has not been shown to impact the final adult size of the dog negatively.[9]

Hip Dysplasia (CHD)

Canine hip dysplasia is a common, heritable developmental orthopedic disease. Studies have shown that dysplastic dogs are born with normal hips but develop hip dysplasia due to growth disparity during their first 6 months of life.[9] Abnormal development of the hip joint results from a disparity between the strength of the soft tissues supporting the joint and the increasing biomechanical forces associated with weight gain. This causes the coxofemoral joint to not "fit" properly; this subluxation causes remodeling of the joint, including a shallowing of the acetabulum (hip socket in the pelvis), a flattening of the femoral head and eventually osteoarthritis.[7,8] Hip dysplasia can affect any breed but is more prevalent in large-breed dogs and is generally accepted as polygenic in its inheritance.[7,8] This means that the disease is not caused by one gene but by a combination of multiple genes and outside factors, and predisposition is genetic.

A controlled study conducted on Labrador Retrievers showed significantly less hip joint laxity and a lower incidence of hip dysplasia in the group of dogs receiving 25% less food than their pair-mates. The food-restricted group grew at a slower rate than those receiving 25% more food; this is believed to be the reason for the significant decrease in hip dysplasia.[5,7] In the food-restricted group, 16 of 24 dogs developed osteoarthritis with the mean age of onset of 13.3 years. For the unrestricted group, 19 of 24 dogs developed osteoarthritis, with the mean age of onset being 10.3 years.[5]

Diet will not cure hip dysplasia once it has developed. Still, it can affect the phenotypic expression if growth rates are managed in at-risk puppies by optimizing the development of the hip joints during early growth.[9]

Osteochondrosis (OCD)

Osteochondrosis (OCD) is a focal area of disruption in endochondral ossification and is characterized by impaired maturation of chondrocytes and delayed cartilage mineralization.[7,10] If this disturbance occurs in articular cartilage (the cartilage lining moving joints), OCD may develop.[9] The most commonly affected joints are the shoulder, elbow, hock and stifle. Acute pain and swelling are seen in the affected areas, with stiffness and lameness aggravated by exercise.[7]

It is believed that overnutrition caused by too much energy being taken in or a food enriched with calcium, whether from ad-lib feeding, over the calculation of a measured feeding, or addition of supplements, helps to stimulate skeletal growth, bone remodeling and weight gain in breeds already having a genetic potential for rapid growth.[9,10] This combination of rapid growth and remodeling weakens the subchondral region in supporting the cartilage surface.[10] The increasing body weight exerts excessive biomechanical forces on the cartilage and leads to secondary chondrocyte nutrition, metabolism, function and viability disturbances.[10] Acute inflammatory joint disease begins when the subchondral bone is exposed to synovial fluid. Inflammatory mediators and cartilage fragments are released into the joint and perpetuate the cycle of degenerative joint disease.[10] In a rapidly growing puppy, overnutrition can result in a mismatch between body weight and skeletal growth, leading to overloading of skeletal structures.[10]

Dietary modifications at an early stage can positively influence the spontaneous resolution of disturbed endochondral ossification. Dietary modifications will not normalize cases of OCD in which severe or complete detachment of the cartilage in the joint has already occurred.[9]

What to Feed Large and Giant Breed Puppies

Overnutrition to achieve maximal growth rate causes excessive bodyweight, which overloads the young skeleton and may contribute to the development of skeletal disorders.[7] Since fats contain over twice the caloric density of protein and carbohydrates, a diet lower in fat is recommended for large and giant breed puppies.[7]

A BCS of 4/9 should be maintained throughout puppyhood.[10] Limiting energy intake to maintain these physical parameters will not affect the dog's final adult size. It can, however, reduce food intake, fecal output, obesity and the risk of skeletal disease.[10]

Protein has not been shown to negatively affect the dog's calcium metabolism or skeletal development.[10] A minimum level of protein in the diet depends on digestibility, amino acid profile and bioavailability and should at minimum meet the AAFCO recommendations for growth.[10]

The absolute calcium level rather than a calcium/phosphorus imbalance is responsible for negatively influencing skeletal development.[10] Young, large-breed dogs fed a diet high in calcium have a significant increase in the incidence of developmental skeletal disease.[10] Large breed puppies should not be switched to an adult maintenance diet too early because of the difference in energy density between a puppy and an adult diet; the puppy would consume more calcium in an adult diet because it would need to eat more to meet its energy needs.[10] Under no circumstances should these puppies receive calcium supplements.[10]

If puppies are fed based on energy requirements, activity levels and body condition, growth diets do not increase the risk of developmental bone disease in large and giant breed dogs.[10] It is essential to feed the appropriate diet and feed the diet appropriately.[10]

References

1 LeGrand-Defretin V, Munday HS (1995) Feeding dogs and cats for life. In I Burger (ed.), *The Waltham Book of Companion Animal Nutrition*, pp. 63–4, Tarrytown, NY: Elsevier.

2 Delaney S, Fascetti A (2012) Feeding the healthy dog and cat. In S Delaney, A Fascetti (eds), *Applied Veterinary Clinical Nutrition*, p. 84, Ames, IA: Wiley-Blackwell.

3 Debraekeleer J, Gross K, L; Zicker, Steven C. (2010) Feeding growing puppies. In MS Hand, CD Thatcher, RI Remillard *et al.* (eds), *Small Animal Clinical Nutrition* (5th edn), pp. 311–7, Marceline, MO: Walsworth Publishing.

4 Case LP, Carey DP, Hirakawa DA, Daristotle L (2011) Growth. In *Canine and Feline Nutrition* (3rd edn), pp. 221–33, Mosby: St Louis, MO.

5 Kealy RD, Lawler DF, Ballam JM *et al.* (2002) Effects of diet restriction on life span and age-related changes in dogs. *JAVMA* **220**(9) : 1315–20.May 1

6 Purina ProPlan Veterinary Product Reference Guide 2020

7 Kuhlman G, Biourge V (1997) Nutrition of the large and giant breed dog with emphasis on skeletal development. *Veterinary Clinical Nutrition* **4**(3): 89–95.

8 Lepine AJ, Reinhart GA (1998) Feeding the growing large breed dog. In *Clinical Nutrition Symposium XXIII Congress of the World Small Animal Veterinary Association*. Buenos Aires Argentina, October 6, pp. 12–6.

9 Hazewinkel H, Mott J (2006) Main nutritional imbalances implicated in osteoarticular diseases. In P Pibot, V Biourge, D Elliott (eds), *Encyclopedia of Canine Clinical Nutrition*, pp. 348–79, Aniwa SAS: Aimargues, France.

10 Richardson DC (1999) Developmental orthopedics: Nutritional influences in the dog. In SJ Ettinger, EC Feldman (eds), *Textbook of Veterinary Internal Medicine, Diseases of the Dog and Cat* (4th edn), pp. 252–8, Philadelphia, PA: Saunders.

28

Growth in Cats

Introduction

Unlike dogs, cats do not have a wide variety of sizes or shapes, and they do not have as rapid of a growth phase. But like dogs, they should be fed to achieve normal growth and development.[1] Nutrient and energy needs during this phase of life exceed those for any other period, except lactation, with the most rapid growth occurring during the first 3–6 months of life.[1] The goal is to ensure that the kittens develop into healthy adults and can optimize growth and minimize risk factors for disease.[2]

Normal Growth

As young animals, kittens have a small physical capacity for food. Because of this, it is recommended to feed energy-dense foods and feed them frequently.[3] Most cats will achieve skeletal maturity at about 10 months of age even though all growth plates may not have closed by this time[2] Additional weight gain may occur after 12 months of age and represents a phase of maturation and muscle development.[2] In kittens, excessive growth rates do not cause the same orthopedic problems associated with rapid growth in dogs.[4] However, the deposition of excessive fat cells (adipocytes) during this growth phase may predispose the cat to obesity throughout its life. Once a fat cell has been formed, it will remain with the animal throughout the rest of

its life and continue to secrete hormones that encourage fat deposition.

Growing kittens have high energy requirements to meet the needs of rapid growth, thermoregulation and maintenance.[2] Feedings an energy-dense food allows for smaller volumes to be consumed to satisfy caloric needs.[2] However, growing cats with BCS of 4/5 or 6/9 should be fed foods with lower energy density to prevent obesity. The prevalence of obesity increases after 1 year of age, and overnutrition is more of a problem in most kittens than undernutrition.[2] Kittens should be fed a diet that meets the nutrient and energy requirements for growth or all life stages.[4]

There is no evidence that the age of neutering alters the growth rate. Unfortunately, energy requirements do decline with neutering, increasing the risk of obesity if energy intake is not adjusted.[2] As neutering is typically performed between 6 and 12 months of age, the caloric requirements also decrease as the animal matures. There is a corresponding decrease in caloric requirements secondary to the neutering procedure.[4]

What to Feed

Energy

Growing kittens have high energy requirements due to their rapid growth rate, thermoregulation and maintenance requirements.[2] They may grow as fast as 14–30 g/day during

Nutrition and Disease Management for Veterinary Technicians and Nurses, Third Edition. Ann Wortinger and Kara M. Burns.
© 2024 John Wiley & Sons, Inc. Published 2024 by John Wiley & Sons, Inc.
Companion Website: www.wiley.com/go/wortinger/3e

rapid growth phases. Energy requirements are highest at about 10 weeks of age, with a DER of approximately 200 kcal/kg body weight, and after this point, the energy requirements per unit of body weight gradually decrease, although they remain relatively high for at least the first 6 months of life.[2] By 10 months of age, the DER has decreased to adult levels of 80 kcal/kg body weight.[2]

Neutering reduces energy requirements by 24–33% regardless of the age of neutering.[2] The food intake or caloric requirements should be adjusted immediately after neutering and including this information on surgical discharge instructions would be helpful to the owners.

Kittens and juvenile cats that were previously fed adlib should be transitioned to measured feeding to help prevent weight gain. Also, changing the food from energy-dense, growth diets to low fat, lower-energy food can help to prevent weight gain after neutering. (6) Total energy intake can be decreased by 25% after neutering.

Obesity should be prevented in young cats as this increases the number of fat cells capable of storing fat as the cat enters adulthood.

Protein

The requirement for protein is already relatively high for the adult cat; it is even higher for growing kittens by about 10%.[3] At least 19% of the protein should be from an animal source to ensure adequate amounts of the sulfur-containing amino acids (i.e., taurine, cysteine, methionine). These are required in more significant amounts in kittens than in other species.[2] High protein diets (>56% DM) must contain the essential amino acid arginine at 1.5 times the requirement to maintain a normal urea cycle function.[2]

Taurine has a well-documented role in reproduction and growth, and all foods for growing kittens should contain adequate amounts.[2] Rapid tissue formation associated with growth accounts for much of the increased protein needs for young cats.[1] The actual percentage of protein found in the diet is not as important as the balance between protein and energy found in the food.[1]

Association of American Feed Control Officials (AAFCO) recommends a minimum protein level of 26% ME, with optimal levels as high as 29% ME.[1,2]

Fat and Fatty Acids

Dietary fats provide energy, fat-soluble vitamins and essential fatty acids to growing cats.[2] Kittens can tolerate foods with a wide variety of fat contents, but when given a choice, they will usually go with the food with the higher fat content. Optimal growth rates are achieved with a diet containing higher levels of fats.[2] Feeding diets with fat levels between 18% and 35% is preferred to enhance palatability, meet fatty acid requirements and maintain the energy density of the food.[2]

All cats require the essential omega-6 fatty acids linoleic acid and arachidonic acid, especially those still growing. Increasing evidence has shown the importance of the omega-3 fatty acids, DHA (docosahexaenoic acid) and EPA (eicosapentaenoic acid) in growth. DHA is made in the body from alpha-linolenic acid and is required for normal neural, retinal, and auditory development in kittens.[2]

Conversion of the omega-3 fatty acid alpha-linolenic acid to DHA is inefficient in cats and affected by age; therefore, supplementing omega-3 fatty acid amounts in the food with fish oil is recommended to ensure adequate intake.[1,2]

Calcium and Phosphorus

Unlike puppies, kittens are fairly insensitive to inverse calcium-phosphorus ratios in their diets.[2] Calcium excesses are not associated with developmental orthopedic diseases. However, extremely high concentrations of calcium do interfere with magnesium availability.[2] The acceptable calcium-phosphorus ratio should be 1.1:1 to 1.5:1.

Calcium deficiency and phosphorus excesses commonly occur in kittens fed unsupplemented all-meat diets. Nutritional secondary hyperparathyroidism results in osteitis fibrosa and presents as limping, pain and reluctance to move.[2] These kittens should be immediately switched to commercial kitten food without additional calcium supplementation so that rebound hypercalcemia does not develop.[2]

Potassium

The potassium requirement depends on the protein content of the food and the effect on the acid-base balance.[2] Potassium loss through the urine is increased in kittens fed high-protein, acidifying diets. To avoid hypokalemia, kittens over 8 weeks of age should not be fed acidifying diets. Some diets intended for all life stages may target urinary pH levels more appropriate for adult cats.[2]

Urinary pH

When fed similar diets, the urinary pH of kittens is lower than that of adult cats. This is caused by hydrogen ions released during bone formation, which are then excreted in the urine, lowering the pH. This continues until about 12 months old when most bone growth is completed.

Kittens fed acidifying diets have been shown to grow more slowly and plateau at lower body weights than kittens fed foods with higher pH levels. Poor bone mineralization was also found in the kittens fed acidifying diets. To avoid these effects, food fed to kittens should not produce a urine pH of less than 6.2 when fed free-choice.[2]

Deficiencies

Deficiencies in energy, protein, essential fatty acids, certain vitamins and minerals can negatively affect a growing cat's immune system, decreasing its immune response and defense.[1] Adequate levels of antioxidants included in the food help support the immune system and have the potential to enhance the immune response.[1] The most widely used nutrients that have antioxidant activity include vitamin E, beta-carotene (provitamin A), lutein (another carotenoid antioxidant), vitamin C, flavonoids, zinc and selenium.[1]

Carbohydrates

Carbohydrates are not required in the food used for growing kittens if sufficient gluconeogenic amino acids are available.[2] Cats can readily digest carbohydrates, though feeding a diet high in poorly digestible carbohydrates may result in flatulence, bloating and diarrhea.[2] This can often be seen in kittens fed cow's milk after weaning. Cow's milk has higher levels of lactose than does cat's milk, and after weaning a kitten's level of lactase, the enzyme that breaks down lactose declines.[2] This leads to incomplete digestion of the lactose, causing a digestive upset in the cat in the form of diarrhea and flatulence.

Feeding Regimens

The palatability of the food should be good enough to ensure adequate energy intake, with total digestibility of at least 80% and protein digestibility of at least 85%.[2] A high-quality commercial kitten food shown to be adequate for growth through AAFCO feeding trials is recommended.[1] Supplementation of this diet is not recommended and should not be necessary.[1] (see Figure 28.1).

It is better to change to food specifically formulated for kittens than to try balancing an inappropriate food.[2] A balanced kitten food can be fed until kittens reach adulthood at approximately 10–12 months of age, though feeding amounts should be adjusted to maintain an ideal BCS.[2] If a young adult cat shows signs of obesity, it can be switched to a balanced adult diet by 6 months of age.[3]

Caloric Distribution (% ME)

Protein 39%

Fat 41%

Carbohydrate 20%

Calories 531 kcal/cup

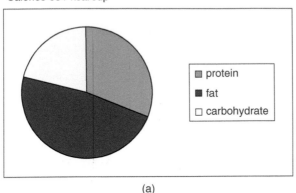

(a)

Caloric Distribution (% ME)

Protein 37%

Fat 37%

Carbohydrate 26%

Calories 509 kcal/cup

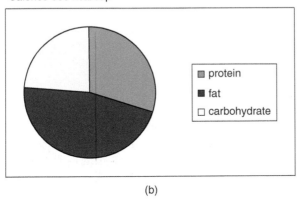

(b)

Figure 28.1 Nutrient profiles. (a) Kitten food dry. (b) Cat adult maintenance hairball dry.[5]

Free-choice feeding is often preferred with kittens because it reduces the risk of under-feeding and the marked gastric distension accompanying rapid meal feeding in kittens.[2] This feeding method may not be a good option if older cats are in the house, as they may push the kitten away from the food and eat it all themselves. Measured feedings can be used in a mixed-age household if 2–3 meals per day are offered, and everyone is fed in separate areas to allow the kitten to eat unharassed.

A good option with a kitten in a house of older cats is to either separate the kitten at mealtimes or make an area accessible to the kitten but not to the older cats and place the food there. This can be as easy as using a plastic or cardboard box, turning it upside down, and cutting an appropriate size hole in the box. Place the box where it cannot be tipped over and put the food inside out of reach of the older cats. (see Figure 28.2).

Both dry and canned foods are appropriate for weaned kittens. Dry foods are more

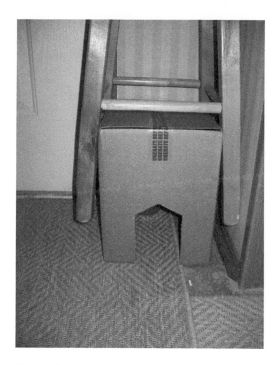

Figure 28.2 An example of an exclusion device to keep adult cats out of a kitten's food.

energy-dense per unit of food, helping kittens meet their energy requirements. Canned and moist foods tend to be more palatable, encouraging food intake.

Treats are unnecessary but can be fed if they do not compose >10% of the daily calories consumed. Fresh, clean water should be always available.[2]

Package recommendations are a good place to start determining feeding volume but fail to consider the kitten's age, body condition or activity. Using body conditions to adjust the feeding volume can ensure that the kitten continues to receive an adequate but not excessive volume of food.[2]

Body condition scores should continue to be done as the kitten grows, and food intake should be adjusted to maintain a 3/5 or 4-5/9 BCS throughout kittenhood and into adulthood. Obesity is much easier to prevent than to treat.

For very young kittens feeding out of a shallow plate or pan can facilitate access, as most bowels have sides too high for small kittens. Canned and moist foods should be fed at or slightly above room temperature but left out for prolonged periods at room temperature to prevent spoilage.[2]

Reassessment

Postweaning kittens should be weighed monthly until they are 4–5 months old. Luckily, this coincides with their vaccine booster appointments. The growth rate will vary, but a positive trend should be seen with each visit. Kittens provided with proper nutrition will be active and alert, have a good body condition, steady weight gain and have a clean glossy coat. Stools will be well-formed, firm and medium to dark brown.[2] (see Figure 28.3).

When dealing with growth in small animals, it is helpful to remember that it takes

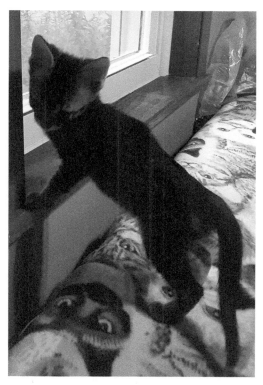

Figure 28.3 This kitten was received in foster care as part of a litter of five, was unable to compete with his litter mates for food, and was significantly underweight for his age.

3500 kcals to gain a pound. For a kitten only eating 100–200 kcal/day, having enough excess intake to gain a pound can take some time. For a very rough estimate, average kitten growth should be approximately 1#/month until 6 months of age. Debilitated and underweight kittens can take several months to reach their ideal body condition.

References

1 Case LP, Carey DP, Hirakawa DA, Daristotle L (2011) Growth. In *Canine and Feline Nutrition* (3rd edn), pp. 221–33, St Louis, MO: Mosby.

2 Gross KL, Becvarova I, Debraekeleer J (2010) Feeding Growing Kittens. In MS Hand, CD Thatcher, RI Remillard et al. (eds), *Small Animal Clinical Nutrition* (5th edn), pp. 429–34, Marceline, MO: Walsworth Publishing.

3 LeGrand-Defretin V, Munday HS (1995) Feeding dogs and cats for life. In I Burger (ed.), *The Waltham Book of Companion Animal Nutrition*, pp. 64–5, Tarrytown, NY: Elsevier.

4 Delaney S, Fascetti A (2012; pg 84) Feeding the healthy dog and cat. In S Delaney, A Fascetti (eds), *Applied Veterinary Clinical Nutrition*, Ames, IA: Wiley-Blackwell.

5 Purina ProPlan Veterinary Product Reference Guide 2020.

29

Adult Maintenance in Dogs

Introduction

Dogs that have reached mature adult size and are not pregnant, lactating or working strenuously are defined as being in a state of maintenance.[1] Depending on the breed, these are usually dogs between 1 and 7 years of age. Some breeds mature more slowly and do not reach their full mature size until 18–24 months of age, while others are fully grown by 10 months.[1,2]

Most companion dogs live indoors in a temperate environment. They are usually not pregnant or lactating, not involved in regular work or excessive exercise and are not subject to temperature extremes.[3] For an animal in maintenance, the diet must:

o Provide the correct amount, balance and availability of nutrients to sustain physical and mental health and activity.
o Promote peak condition and therefore reduce the dog's susceptibility to disease.
o Be sufficiently nutrient-dense to allow the animal to meet its nutrient requirements by eating an amount within limits set by appetite.
o Be sufficiently palatable to ensure an adequate intake.[3]

Maintenance

The ultimate goal of any maintenance diet is to minimize risk factors for disease and achieve optimal health. Maintenance of ideal body condition score (BCS) has been shown to increase dogs' quality and quantity of life.[4]

Healthy adult dogs have relatively small nutrient requirements when compared to those in the reproductive stages of life. They may be maintained for years on various diets with little apparent consequences.[5] The probability of a diet-related problem should be lower for dogs fed properly formulated commercial diets due to the Association of American Feed Control Officials (AAFCO) verification required. Dogs fed homemade diets, or those who have not undergone AAFCO certification would pose significantly higher risks for diet-related problems. An adverse consequence that has not been seen in a single animal does not mean that a diet provides superior nutrition.[5] Remember that AAFCO requirements provide the minimal levels to sustain a dog; you cannot feed minimal foods and expect optimal results.

The guidelines printed on pet food labels provide an estimate of the amount of food to feed an average adult dog living indoors and doing a moderate amount of exercise.[1] These estimates may not consider whether the animal is neutered or intact, if they engage in 2 walks a day, or are confined to the yard and go on no walks. These amounts are guidelines at best, and adjustments would need to be made based on each individual animal.

An estimate of the amount to feed can also be calculated using the dog's ideal body weight, with adjustments in intake being made based

Nutrition and Disease Management for Veterinary Technicians and Nurses, Third Edition. Ann Wortinger and Kara M. Burns.
© 2024 John Wiley & Sons, Inc. Published 2024 by John Wiley & Sons, Inc.
Companion Website: www.wiley.com/go/wortinger/3e

on changes in BCS. An animal housed outside of these conditions may require more or less food than recommended. Label guidelines are also based on the food being the only source of nutrition for the dog; this means that no treats, snacks or table food are being fed. Adding these foods can significantly change the amount of food that the dog requires. Current recommendations are that additional sources of nutrition (i.e., snacks) not compose more than 10% of the entire caloric intake.[2]

A wide variety of foods are not necessary for most dogs. The owner makes picky eaters, not the breeder. Most dogs are best managed on a balanced dog food diet with a constant fresh, clean water supply.[1] Frequent diet changes can result in the gastrointestinal tract upset with resulting diarrhea or vomiting. The cause for these GI upsets can usually be traced back to a lack of digestive enzymes to meet the diet formula. The body does not have unlimited amounts of enzymes in place at all times. It will usually take 5–7 days to adjust the enzyme production to meet the new diet's requirements.

Sometimes these changes can be seen when feeding a lower-quality commercial food brand, which utilizes a variable feed formula instead of a fixed feed formula. With a variable feed formula, the ingredient amounts and types can vary from batch to batch based on market conditions or product availability. The manufacturers can do this as long as the product conforms to the minimums and maximums listed on the guaranteed analysis. The ingredients do not change with a fixed-feed formula but remain constant from batch to batch. Unfortunately, this information is not listed on the label and can only be obtained by contacting the manufacturer.

Owners should be encouraged to weigh their dog every month or so, with adjustments in intake based on any changes seen. Dogs who are nutritionally well managed are alert and have ideal BCS (3/5, 4-5/9) with stable,

normal body weight, a healthy coat and maintain an active lifestyle. Stools should be firm, well-formed and medium to dark brown in color.[2,4]

Gender and Neuter Status

No studies have evaluated differences in nutritional requirements on intact male versus intact female dogs. Like other mammals, it is presumed that intact females require less energy intake than intact male dogs.[2]

Neutering does not appear to impact the resting energy requirements (RER) of female dogs significantly. However, neutering may significantly increase food intake, causing obesity. This is thought to be due to the loss of appetite-suppressing estrogens.[2] Monitoring BCS and decreasing food intake is recommended to prevent obesity.

Activity Level

The energy output through activity can affect the requirements of individual dogs. Energy output can range from a daily energy requirements (DER) that equals RER to 15 × RER for endurance athletes under extreme conditions (sled-dog racers).[2] Increases in lean body mass through exercise can also increase energy expenditures.

Because activity levels are often inconsistent and are challenging to define, it is best to avoid overfeeding by using a lower DER and adjusting upwards only if indicated.[2] Weekend warriors often do not require any increase in food intake, especially during days off.

Environment

The influences on energy requirements of temperature, humidity, type of housing, level of stress and degree of acclimatization need to be considered based on breed and life stage nutrient requirements. Dogs can tolerate extreme cold. However, if housed outdoors in cold weather, energy needs may increase by 90%. Energy use during periods of cold is similar to those used by endurance athletes.[2] Higher-fat foods are well suited to cold-acclimatized dogs. For long-term exposure, the amount of food fed also needs to be increased to ensure enough energy to keep the animal warm.

Compared to cold weather conditions, relatively small amounts of energy are used to dissipate heat at higher-than-normal temperatures. The metabolic rate increased by only 10% in adult dogs when the ambient temperature was 95°F/37°C.[2]

Water

Water deprivation will result in death faster than withholding any other nutrient.[2] It has been argued that this makes water the most essential nutrient. Water accounts for about 56% of an adult dog's body weight, with a limited storage capacity.

Water intake can be influenced by the environment, physiologic state, activity, disease processes and food composition.[2] A dry food diet typically contains between 8% and 12% water, while a canned or moist diet can contain upwards of 80% water.

In general, dogs self-regulate water intake based on physiologic needs. For healthy adult dogs, water requirements are roughly the same as DER in kcals. 1 kcal = 1 mL of requirement.[2] Fresh, clean water should be available during rest and before, during and after exercise. During warm weather, enough clean, fresh water must be available to compensate for evaporative loss through panting.[2]

Energy

Because DER are influenced by breed, neuter status, age, daily activity, environmental temperature and insulative characteristics of the skin and coat, it is better to calculate energy needs based on resting energy requirements (RER) and different multipliers (Life Stage Factors-LSF) to account for these differences.[2]

Most pet dogs are inactive, and their DER may approach or be the same as their RER. If fed at LSF for maintenance-1.6, these dogs will be overfed and will likely become overweight or obese.[2]

For active and working dogs, a LSF of 1.6 provides a good starting point, with adjustments being made based on their BCS and performance rate. For dogs that are not consistently active, feeding the same food as usual but increasing the amount on days of increased activity can be easily managed by most owners. For very athletic dogs, such as sled dogs participating in a race, their LSF can be as high as 15 to maintain body condition. During non-race days or shorter races, the LSF can be lower, as needed, to maintain body condition and performance.[2]

Fats and Fatty Acids

Fats are a source of energy but are also required to provide the essential fatty acids (EFAs). Fat also serves as a carrier for the fat-soluble vitamins A, D, E and K.

Linoleic acid is the base fatty acid for all omega-6 fatty acids and is considered essential in dogs. Alpha-linolenic acid is the base fatty acid for all omega-3 fatty acids and an EFA for dogs.[2]

Omega-3 FAs can modulate the proinflammatory effects of the omega-6 class of FAs, which can help manage certain inflammatory diseases. The minimum recommended level of dietary fat in foods for normal, healthy adult dogs is 8.5% DM, with at least 1% of this being linoleic acid. (2)The recommended range is 10–20% DM, though lower levels are recommended for obese-prone adult dogs of 7–10% DM.[2]

Fiber

As fiber is nondigestible by dogs, as fiber increases in a diet, the lower the energy becomes. It has been shown to increase satiety by providing bulk to the diet. As the gastrointestinal microbiome digests fiber through fermentation, it is difficult to determine the optimal fiber concentration in a diet. Up to 5% DM crude fiber appears to be adequate, though obese and overweight dogs may benefit from a level up to 10% DM.[2]

Protein

After the amino acid requirements are met for the dog, adding more protein provides no known physiologic benefits. Unlike fat stored in adipocytes and glucose, which can be stored as glycogen in the liver and muscles, the body does not store amino acids outside of each cell's small amino acid pool.

Protein consumed above the amino acids required is instead deaminated in the liver and stored as fat or glycogen. It cannot be reanimated back into a protein after this process. Instead, it becomes a costly form of stored fat or glycogen.[2]

Marketing of high-protein dog foods as necessary for carnivores misrepresents the fact that dogs are instead omnivores. The minimum crude protein content required in food is dependent on both the digestibility and quality of the protein used. The minimum recommended allowance for crude protein is 10% DM with an energy density of 4 kcal/g. The recommended range for young, healthy adult dogs is between 15% and 30% DM.[2]

Antioxidants

Oxidative stress from free radical damage has been implicated in contributing to or exacerbating cancer, diabetes mellitus, kidney/urinary tract disease, heart disease, liver disease, inflammatory bowel disease and cognitive dysfunction. Free radical damage has also been associated with the effects of aging.[2]

While the body can synthesize many antioxidant enzyme systems and compounds, it relies on the diet for others and the components. Food-sourced antioxidants are commonly supplemented, including vitamins E and C, beta-carotene and other carotenoids and selenium. Fruits and vegetables are good sources of flavonoids, polyphenols, and anthocyanidins (i.e., red, purple and blue colors in foods).[2] Remember that when a fruit or vegetable is listed toward the bottom of the ingredient list, it is unlikely to contribute any significant antioxidants to the overall diet.

Stress

Physiologic stress can affect caloric intake in several ways. It is not uncommon for working or boarding dogs to refuse to eat for no apparent reason. Conversely, a dog's appetite may improve by adding another dog to the household. If one dog is more dominant and allowed to control access to the food dish, weight loss may be seen in one dog, with weight gain seen in the other.[2]

Environmental stress can also change energy requirements. In a hot environment, increased water intake can be seen to help with cooling. In colder environments, dogs kept outdoors, even within shelters, may need increased energy intake to maintain their body temperatures.[2] If a change is seen in appetite or BCS, look at possible stressors within the dog's environment.

Obesity

Studies indicate that up to 60% of dogs within the United States seen by veterinarians were overweight or obese (BCS 4-5/5, 7-9/9).[6] By definition, obesity is the accumulation of excessive body fat.[4] Excess body weight is the

Table 29.1 Influence of age on daily energy requirements (DER) for dogs.[2]

Age in years	DER adjustment
1–2	$1.7\text{–}2.0 \times \text{RER}$
3–7	$1.4\text{–}1.9 \times \text{RER}$
>7	$1.1\text{–}1.7 \times \text{RER}$

most prominent form of malnutrition seen in companion animals.

Risk factors associated with obesity include:

o Middle age
o Neuter status
o Low activity
o High-fat, high-calorie foods

Obesity occurs twice as often in neutered dogs than in intact dogs. Neutering does not appear to have a marked impact on the resting energy expenditure of female dogs; however, it can significantly increase food intake.[2] This may be due to reducing the appetite-suppressing hormone estrogen.[2] A decrease in physical activity is also assumed to occur in many dogs after neutering and may play a more critical role in weight gain for male dogs due to decreased roaming activity.[2]

Obesity has been linked to the increased incidence of diabetes mellitus, lameness and degenerative joint disease and skin disease. By preventing the occurrence of these diseases, we can, in turn, increase the quality and quantity of life our dogs can have.[4]

It is much easier to prevent an obese animal than to treat obesity once it has occurred. Following BCS in puppyhood to get an adult in the normal to lean range is the best way to prevent obesity later in life. True obesity is the direct result of too much energy consumption without a corresponding increase in activity level (see Table 29.1).

Feeding Plan

While owners are directly responsible for selecting what food is fed to their dogs, recommendations should be made by and sought from the veterinary team. Adlib or free-choice feeding has been associated with obesity. Still, it may be of benefit for those shy animals. They may not have unlimited access to the food dish due to the presence of a more dominant animal or activity levels within the house disrupting feeding time.

Measured and timed feeding will help control the volume of food a dog consumes, but unless the appropriate amount is determined, the animal can quickly become over or underweight. Working with clients to determine the ideal food for that dog and an appropriate amount to feed and feeding method to use is part of our jobs. A good starting point when doing energy calculation is to determine RER at desired body weight. DER is calculated by taking a LSF of $0.8\text{–}1.6 \times \text{RER}$ to determine the estimated caloric intake. The caloric density of the food will need to be used to calculate the desired volume to feed. This can be found either from the product reference guide, an internet search, or by contacting the manufacturer.[2] Regular contact with clients with BCS and weight checks of dogs can help control food-related weight issues ensuring we can keep them healthy and happy for as long as possible. (see Table 29.2).

The introduction of feeding puzzles and feeding toys can prolong the feeding period, increase engagement from the dog and decrease boredom. A calculated volume is placed into the puzzle or puzzles, and the dog is allowed to figure out how to access the food. A feeding puzzle can be as easy as a muffin tin where the food is distributed into individual cups, to very complex puzzles that demonstrate just how smart some of our dogs are (see Figures 29.1 and 29.2).

Table 29.2 Calculating daily energy requirements (DER).

1. Determine ideal maintenance body weight in kilograms.
2. Determine RER using this number.
3. Determine DER by multiplying RER by the estimated adjustment factor based on age and activity.
4. Determine the caloric density of the food.
5. Take the DER divide it by the caloric density to determine volume to feed/day.
6. Divide this volume by the desired number of feedings/day.

Zeus is a 5-year-old beagle who weighs 25#, with an ideal BCS of 3/5. His owner wants to switch his food and needs help with determining the volume to feed. Zeus is a house beagle, who has access to the outdoors but does not go on many walks. The new food has a caloric density of 254 kcal/cup.

1. 25#/ 2.2 = 11.36 kg
2. RER = (wt in kg × 30) + 70 (or whichever formula you prefer) (11.36 × 30) + 70 = 411 kcal/day
3. 411 kcal/day × 1.4 (low activity level for age) = 575 kcal/day
4. 254 kcal/cup
5. 575/254 = 2.25 cups/day
6. 3 meals/day = 2.25/3 = 0.75 cup/meal

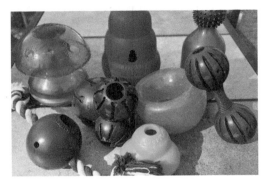

Figure 29.2 A selection of different interactive feeding toys for dogs.

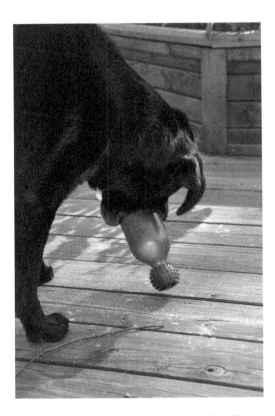

Figure 29.1 This Labrador is enjoying a Kong™ toy with some of her food. *Source*: Courtesy of Judy Conley LVT.

References

1 Case LP, Carey DP, Hirakawa DA, Daristotle L (2011) Growth. In *Canine and Feline Nutrition* (3rd edn), pp. 239–42, St Louis, MO: Mosby.

2 Debraekeleer J, Gross KL, Zicker SC (2010) Feeding young adult dogs before middle age. In MS Hand, CD Thatcher, RI Remillard *et al.* (eds), *Small Animal Clinical Nutrition* (5th edn), pp. 257–71, Marceline, MO: Walsworth Publishing.

3 Wills JM (1996) Adult maintenance. In *Manual of Companion Animal Nutrition and Feeding*, pp. 44–6, Ames, IA: Iowa State University Press.

4 Delaney S, Fascetti A (2012; pg 85) Feeding the healthy dog and cat. In S Delaney, A Fascetti (eds), *Applied Veterinary Clinical Nutrition*, Ames, IA: Wiley-Blackwell.

5 Buffington CA, Holloway C, Abood SK (2004) Normal dogs. In *Manual of Veterinary Dietetics*, pp. 15–8, St. Louis, MO: Saunders Burkholder.

6 Toll PW, Yamka RM, Schoenherr WD, Hand MS (2010) Obesity. In MS Hand, CD Thatcher, RI Remillard *et al.* (eds), *Small Animal Clinical Nutrition* (5th edn), pp. 501–40, Marceline, MO: Walsworth Publishing.

30

Adult Maintenance in Cats

Introduction

Cats that reach mature adult size and are not pregnant, lactating or working strenuously are defined as being in a state of maintenance.[1] Cats generally reach adult size between 10 and 12 months of age and reach their full mature weight by 18 months. Adult maintenance is usually the time from 12 months to 8 years.[2]

Cats as Carnivores

Cats are classified as obligate carnivores, unlike dogs, who are omnivores. This classification is based on cats' specific behavioral, anatomic, physiologic and metabolic adaptations.[3]

The predatory drive in cats is so strong that they will stop eating to make a kill.[3] From their point of view, the dead animal is going nowhere, and there's no telling when the next moving meal will appear.

Cats prefer the tastes of animal fat, protein hydrolysates (digests), meat extracts and certain free amino acids found in muscle tissue, such as alanine, proline, lysine and histidine.[3]

Unlike dogs, cats are not attracted to the taste of sugars and are repelled by flavors derived from plant products, such as glutamic acid and medium-chain triglycerides. With this being said, there is considerable variability within the cat population, with reports of cats liking cantaloupe, pumpkin, bananas and celery.[3]

Maintenance

Most companion cats live indoors in temperate environments. They are usually not pregnant or lactating, not involved in regular work or excessive exercise, and are not subject to temperature extremes.[4] For an animal in maintenance, the diet must:

- Provide the correct amount, balance and availability of nutrients to sustain physical and mental health and activity.
- Promote peak conditions and therefore reduce its susceptibility to disease.
- Be sufficiently nutrient-dense to allow the animal to meet its nutrient requirements by eating an amount within limits set by appetite.
- Be sufficiently palatable to ensure an adequate intake.[4]

Gender and Neuter Status

Differences in energy intake between the sexes appear related to gender-related differences in lean body mass. Males typically have more lean body mass than females, though this difference decreases once the animals are neutered.[3]

Neutering has been shown to decrease energy requirements, and if the amount of food fed is not adjusted after the procedure, the animals can quickly become overweight

Nutrition and Disease Management for Veterinary Technicians and Nurses, Third Edition. Ann Wortinger and Kara M. Burns.
© 2024 John Wiley & Sons, Inc. Published 2024 by John Wiley & Sons, Inc.
Companion Website: www.wiley.com/go/wortinger/3e

or obese.[3] Feeding a controlled amount of low-energy foods can reduce this risk, as can limiting the number of treats to <10% of the overall caloric intake.[3]

Environment and Activity Level

Cats prefer ambient conditions of low humidity and warm temperatures. Remember that our domestic house cats evolved from the desert cat found in northern Africa. When conditions deviate significantly from these, energy requirements can be altered.[3] In extremely high temperatures (>38 °C/100.4 °F), food intake can initially decrease by 15–40%. As the respiratory rate and grooming behaviors increase, caloric and water requirements also increase.[3]

Multi-cat environments (two or more cats) can lead to social and psychological stress, especially with overcrowding. Situations of >5 cats appear to be at increased risk for problems associated with food intake, behavioral problems and infectious disease transmission.[3] (see Figures 30.1 and 30.2).

Stress levels in multi-cat households can be reduced by modifying the environment. This can include safe outdoor areas, multi-level indoor and outdoor resting areas, visual barriers and quiet hiding spots where cats can retreat from unwanted social interactions.[3] (see Figures 30.3 and 30.4).

Water

Energy

Individual cats may have energy requirements 50% or more above or below the average for that age, sex and neuter status.[2] This can be affected by their amount of lean body mass, environmental temperatures, genetics, housing and activity level. As seen with most animals, smaller cats tend to consume more kcals/kg of body weight than larger cats. Because of

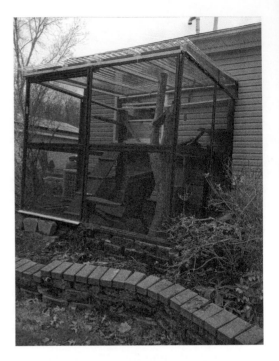

Figure 30.1 Author's catio enclosure for the cats.

this, remember that all kcal calculations are estimates only, and may need to be adjusted based on that animal's needs.[2] Alternately, controlling energy intake is important for managing and preventing obesity.

Fats and Essential Fatty Acids

While we know that cats use fats for energy and as a source of essential fatty acids (EFAs), a minimum requirement for fat has not been established. The minimum fat level, on a dry matter (DM) basis recommended by the National Research Council (NRC) is 9%.[2]

Fats enhance the palatability of food, and a preference among cats has been shown for foods with a fat level near 25%, versus those with fat contents of 10% or 50%.

Current Association of American Feed Control Officials (AAFCO) allowances for the EFAs linoleic acid and arachidonic acid are appropriate for adult cats. Because of this, if

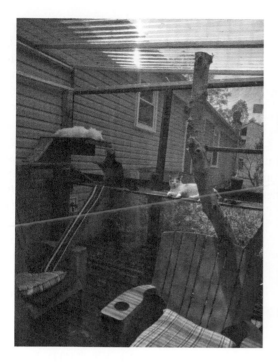

Figure 30.2 The family cats enjoy the multiple levels, the actual tree trunk and the dirt floor of their custom catio.

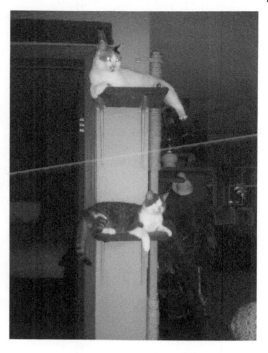

Figure 30.3 Author's multilevel indoor resting areas close to the family living area.

the AAFCO label statement provides that the food is appropriate for adult maintenance, the food should provide adequate levels of linoleic and arachidonic acids.[2]

Fiber

Cats do not have a dietary fiber requirement, though small amounts in foods can enhance stool quality and promote normal gastrointestinal function. The animals that compose the cat's natural diet contain <1% dietary fiber. This is usually from the intestinal tract of the herbivores they eat, not from plant material ingested by the cat.[2]

Fiber concentrations of <5% DM are recommended for adult maintenance. Remember that increased levels of dietary fiber can reduce the energy density of the food. Diets intended for overweight or obese cats may contain up to 15% fiber on a DM basis to help induce satiety

and decrease energy intake.[2] Fiber supplementation can also be helpful in removing excess hair that could form a hairball or trichobezoar in the stomach or intestines.

Protein

When establishing protein requirements for adult cats, this is usually done using experimental foods containing essential amino acids at or above the minimum required for growth. The NRC has used these studies to suggest a minimum protein requirement of 16%, with a minimum recommended protein requirement of 20%[2]

Commercial food prepared from natural ingredients, not purified amino acids, may have lower protein digestibility than the experimental diets used to establish these levels. AAFCO has suggested a dietary minimum of 26% DM for adult maintenance. This level is based on food containing 4.0 kcal/g.[2]

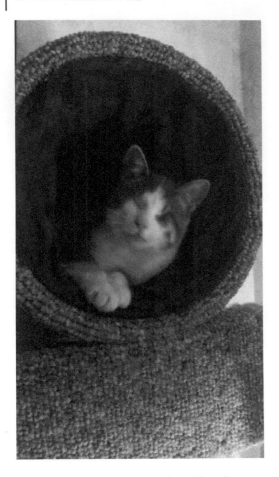

Figure 30.4 Author's cat's favorite hiding place. This is a converted 5-gallon bucket that has been padded and lined.

Protein intake in excess of the requirements for that cat will be converted to fat and stored for energy. The body has minimal capacity to store amino acids for future use.

Although cats can be fed vegetable-based foods, it is recommended that the majority of protein in the food should be provided by animal-based protein. The amino acid profile for most animal-based proteins better reflects the protein requirements for cats.[2]

Urinary pH

The urine pH of cats is based on both the food ingredients in the diet and the feeding methods being used. The normal urinary pH of cats eating mice and rats is 6.2–6.4. Dr. Buffington was able to demonstrate an increased risk of struvite precipitation was greatly reduced at urinary pH levels of <6.5.[2]

Metabolic acidosis can be seen with urinary pH < 6.0. This can contribute to increasing bone demineralization, urinary calcium and potassium loss, and an increased risk of calcium oxalate urolithiasis.[2]

Free-choice feeding helps to modulate urinary pH by dampening the normal postprandial alkaline tide that occurs 3–6 h after a larger meal. Meal feeding causes a greater alkaline tide and higher average urinary pH. Commercial foods commonly balance dietary cations and anions to allow an appropriate urinary pH.[2]

Foods that produce urinary pH values of 6.2–6.4 when fed free-choice can reduce the risk of struvite-mediated FLUTD, help avoid metabolic acidosis and reduce the risk of calcium oxalate urolithiasis in adult cats.[2]

Antioxidants

The cat's body is able to synthesize many of the antioxidants its needs for daily activity, such as superoxide dismutase. Others need to be provided in the food, such as vitamin E.[2]

Many of food-based antioxidants, such as vitamins E and C, carotenoids and thiols are also good sources of flavonoids, polyphenols and anthocyanidins.[2]

Prolonged oxidative stress, such as that caused by the production of free radicals has been shown to cause or exacerbate a wide variety of degenerative diseases. This can include various cancers, diabetes mellitus, kidney, urinary tract, heart and liver diseases. This free radical damage has also been associated with the effects of aging.[2] The body is able to defend itself against the effects of free radicals through the use of protective antioxidants. To be able to make these compounds, the base materials must be included in the diet.

Requirements

The ultimate goal of any maintenance diet is to minimize risk factors for disease and achieve optimal health and longevity of life. Healthy adult cats have relatively small nutrient requirements compared to those in the reproductive stages of life. They may be maintained for years on various diets with little apparent consequences.[5] The probability of a diet-related problem should be lower for cats fed properly formulated commercial diets due to the AAFCO testing required. Cats fed homemade diets or those fed diets that have not undergone AAFCO certification would pose significantly higher risks for diet-related problems. Just because an adverse consequence has not been seen in a single animal does not mean that a diet provides superior nutrition.[5] Remember that AAFCO requirements provide minimal levels of nutrients. You cannot feed a minimal diet and expect optimal results.

It has been shown that for dogs, maintaining a lean body condition score (BCS) throughout their lives increases the quality and quantity of their lives. We could safely surmise that these conditions would benefit cats by avoiding conditions that contribute to early mortality, such as diabetes mellitus, lameness, cardiac disease and skin diseases.[6]

The guidelines printed on pet food labels provide an estimate of the amount of food to feed an average adult cat that is living indoors and provided moderate amounts of exercise.[1] An estimate of the amount to feed can also be calculated using the cat's ideal body weight, with adjustments in intake being made based on changes in BCS. An animal housed outside of these conditions may require more or less food than recommended.

Label guidelines are also based on the food being the only source of nutrition for the cat; no treats, snacks or table food are being fed. Adding these foods can significantly change the amount of food that the cat requires. Current recommendations are that additional sources of nutrition not compose more than 10% of the entire caloric intake.[2]

A wide variety of foods is unnecessary for most cats. Picky eaters are not born but made by the owner. Most cats are best managed on a diet of balanced cat food with a constant supply of fresh, clean water.[1] Frequent diet changes can result in the gastrointestinal tract upset with resulting diarrhea or vomiting. The cause for these GI upsets can usually be traced back to a lack of digestive enzymes to meet the diet formula. The body does not have unlimited amounts of enzymes in place at all times. It will usually take 5–7 days to adjust the enzyme production to meet the new diet requirements.

Sometimes these changes can be seen when feeding a lower-quality commercial brand of food that utilizes a variable-feed formula instead of a fixed-feed formula. The contents of a variable-feed formula can vary from batch to batch based on market conditions or product availability. The manufacturers can do this as long as the product conforms to the minimums and maximums listed on the guaranteed analysis. The ingredients do not change with a fixed-feed formula but remain constant from batch to batch. Unfortunately, this information is not listed on the label and can only be obtained by contacting the manufacturer.

Neutering reduces the daily energy requirements by 24–33% compared to intact animals.[2] This decrease does not appear to be affected by the age of neutering. The reduction in energy requirements is most likely due to a reduction in basal metabolic rate since apparent changes in behavior and activity are usually not seen after neutering, especially in young cats.[2]

By nature, cats do not usually participate in heavy work or endurance-like activities. Thus, the variation in energy requirements between active and sedentary cats is small compared to dogs.[2] Even considering this, a twofold increase can be seen between sedentary and active cats' energy requirements (DER = RER × 2). According to activity level, food intake should be adjusted to maintain a BCS of 3/5, 4–5/9.

Sedentary, inactive, caged or older cats often have energy requirements very near or even below the average resting energy requirement. (DER = RER × 1 or less) Cats with unlimited activity may need 10–15% above normal energy needs.[2] Very active or "high-strung" cats may have markedly higher energy expenditures than normal cats, as much as 30% higher than average.[2]

Although different breeds of cats may have varying nutritional requirements, this variation is less pronounced than that seen with dog breeds.[2] Some of the more active breeds, such as Abyssinians and Siamese, may have higher energy requirements, while others, such as Persians or Ragdolls, tend to be very sedate and expend little energy above maintenance.[2] Disposition tends to affect energy requirements more than does breed.

Cats provided with proper nutrition are healthy and alert, have ideal body condition and stable weight, and have a clean, glossy hair coat. The owners should ideally evaluate BCS every 2 weeks, monitor daily food and water intake, and observe the cat's interest in food and its appetite. Stools should be evaluated regularly for changes in frequency or character, with normal stools being firm, well-formed and medium to dark brown in color.[2]

Canned Versus Dry Food

One of our most prevalent controversies in feeding cats currently involves discussing whether canned or dry food diets are better for the cat. We know that cats evolved to eat a meat-based diet, and in fact, due to their classification as obligate carnivores, they require meat in their diets to meet their essential nutrient requirements.[7] We also know that cats produce amylase as a pancreatic enzyme and can digest and utilize carbohydrates for energy.[6]

In the wild (which our current companions are not in), cats consumed few carbohydrates other than those already consumed by their

Table 30.1 Nutrient levels found in a rat carcass.

Nutrient	Rat carcass
Moisture %	63.6
Protein %	55
Fat %	38.1
Carbohydrate %	1.2

Source: Armstrong et al.[3]/Mark Morris Institute.

preferred prey (the digesta found in the prey's digestive tract that the cat also consumes).[7] Small rodents such as moles, voles and field mice make up 40% or more of a feral domestic cat's diet, supplemented with young wild rabbits and hares, birds, reptiles, frogs and insects, making up the remaining portion of the diet.[7] The average mouse contains approximately 30 kcal of metabolizable energy. For an active (DER = RER × 1.7–2.0), 12# cat, this would be an average caloric intake of 370–440 kcals/day. This would be approximately 12–15 mice/day.[3] Since cats eat 10–20 small meals a day, this works out well for most cats in the wild. How do we translate these behaviors and physiologic needs into a process that works for humans? (see Table 30.1).

Proponents of canned food diets cite the documented increase in water consumption when feeding a canned food diet. Canned food diets have about 80% moisture instead of 8–10% found in dry food diets. This increase in water intake may be helpful in the prevention of urinary tract problems and may decrease food intake, and help prevent obesity due to the dilution of calories with water.[6]

One other advantage cited for feeding canned food diets is the nutrient profile typically found in these diets. They tend to be higher protein, lower carbohydrate diets that more accurately reflect the nutrient profile found in their wild prey. A typical mouse only contains 3–5% carbohydrates.[3] Canned food diets can have as few carbohydrates as 0% but may also contain as much as that found in dry food diets. This would depend on the ingredients, and one cannot automatically assume that all canned food diets contain a low-carbohydrate nutrient profile.

One reason commonly given for reluctance to feed canned food diets exclusively to companion cats is the cost. With a standard 3.5 oz can contain approximately 90–100 kcals, an average 10# cat would need to be fed 2.5–3.0 cans per day. With the cost of each can ranging from $1–2/can, and most cats living in multi-cat households, this can become quite expensive very quickly.

Proponents of dry food diets cite the dental health benefits and the ability to feed a schedule more typical of their natural diet (10–20 small meals daily). Due to their processing methods, dry food diets can range from 10–50% carbohydrates based on metabolizable energy content.[3] Again, the assumption cannot be made that all dry diets have the same nutrient composition and that all dry food diets are inherently high in carbohydrate levels. The cost of feeding a dry food diet is significantly less expensive for owners and is easier to feed with our busy schedules. After all, who has time to feed their cats 10–20 small meals daily?

Cats are very sensitive to their foods' physical form, odor and taste. Mouthfeel (oral tactile sensation) is important to normal feeding behavior in cats.[3] Cats also develop fixed taste preferences early in life and may be very reluctant to eat a food that does not "feel right" to them regardless of how yummy it may taste.[3] Because of this, the recommendation to owners is to feed young cats a variety of foods to increase their exposure before these fixed taste preferences are fully developed.

In general, cats prefer solid, moist foods and do not like foods that have a powdery, sticky or greasy texture. If fed a moist diet, they prefer it to be near or at normal body temperature.[3] Even with all this information we have regarding feeding and eating preferences for cats, owners will often cite a cat who will willingly eat fruits and vegetables. After all, cats are individuals too. ☺ (see Table 30.2).

Table 30.2 Calculating daily energy requirements (DER).

(1) Determine ideal maintenance body weight in kilograms.
(2) Determine RER using this number.
(3) Determine DER by multiplying RER by the estimated adjustment factor based on age and activity.
(4) Determine the caloric density of the food.
(5) Take the DER and divide it by the caloric density to determine the volume to feed/day.
(6) Divide this volume by the desired number of feedings/day.

Stryder is a 5-year-old DSH who weighs 12#, with an ideal BCS of 3/5. His owner wants to switch his food and needs help determining the volume to feed. Stryder is a house cat who has access to a screened-in porch but does not go outdoors. The new food has a caloric density of 479 kcal/cup.

(1) $12\#/2.2 = 5.45\,kg$
(2) $RER = (wt\ in\ kg \times 40)\,(5.45 \times 40) = 218\,kcal/day$
    $RER = (wt\ in\ kg)^{0.75} \times 70\,(5.45)^{0.75} \times 70 = 247\,kcal/day$
(3) $218\,kcal/day \times 1.3$ (low activity level for age) $= 284\,kcal/day$
    $247\,kcal/day \times 1.3$ (low activity level for age) $= 321\,kcal/day$
(4) $479\,kcal/cup$
(5) $284/479 = 0.6\,cups/day$
    $321/479 = 0.67\,cups/day$
(6) 3 meals/day $= 0.6/3 = 0.2\,cup/meal$ (for both formulas)

Obesity

By definition, obesity is the accumulation of excessive body fat.[7] Excess body weight is the most prominent form of malnutrition seen in companion animals.

Studies indicate that up to 60% of cats within the United States seen by veterinarians were overweight or obese (BCS 4-5/5, 7-9/9).[3,6] The highest prevalence is seen in middle-aged cats (7–8 years old), with ~50% of this group being overweight or obese (BCS 4-5/5. 7-9/9).

Risk factors associated with obesity include:

o Middle age
o Neuter status
o Low activity
o High-fat, high-calorie foods[2]

Neutered cats have an RER of 20–25% less than intact cats of similar age. In practical terms, this means that a neutered cat would require only 75–80% of the food required by an intact cat of the same age and size, to maintain optimal body condition.[2,3]

It is much easier to prevent an obese animal than it is to treat obesity once it has occurred. Following BCS in kittenhood to get an adult in the normal to lean range is the best way to prevent obesity later in life. True obesity results from too much energy consumption with insufficient energy expenditure.

References

1 Case LP, Carey DP, Hirakawa DA, Daristotle L (2011) Adult maintenance. In *Canine and Feline Nutrition* (3rd edn), pp. 239–42, St Louis, MO: Mosby.

2 Gross KL, Becvarova I, Armstrong PJ, Debraekeleer J (2010) Feeding young adult cats: before middle age. In MS Hand, CD Thatcher, RI Remillard *et al.* (eds), *Small Animal Clinical Nutrition* (5th edn), pp. 373–87, Marceline, MO: Walsworth Publishing.

3 Armstrong PJ, Gross KL, Becvarova I, Debraekeleer J (2010) Introduction to feeding normal cats. In MS Hand, CD Thatcher, RI Remillard *et al.* (eds), *Small Animal Clinical Nutrition* (5th edn), p. 362, Walsworth Publishing: Marceline, MO.

4 Wills JM (1996) Adult maintenance. In N Kelly, J Wills (eds), *Manual of Companion Animal Nutrition and Feeding*, pp. 44–6, Ames, IA: Iowa State University Press.

5 Buffington CA, Holloway C, Abood SK (2004) Normal dogs. In *Manual of Veterinary Dietetics*, pp. 30–1, St. Louis, MO, Saunders.

6 Delaney S, Fascetti A (2012; pg 85) Feeding the healthy dog and cat. In S Delaney, A Fascetti (eds), *Applied Veterinary Clinical Nutrition*, Ames, IA: Wiley-Blackwell.

7 Pierson, Lisa. *Feeding your cat: Know the Basics of Feline Nutrition*. Catinfo.org. Accessed 4/2/22.

31

Feeding the Healthy Geriatric Dog and Cat

Introduction

Continued infection control and nutrition improvements have resulted in a gradual increase in the average lifespan of the companion cat and dog. The maximum lifespan of any given species has remained relatively fixed; genetics, health care and nutrition can affect the average lifespan within a given population.[1] It is estimated that more than 40% of the dogs and 30% of the cats in the United States are at least 6 years old, and approximately 30% of these animals are older than 11 years.[1] While we see older animals, it is important to remember that old age is not a disease, and if they are otherwise healthy, old age alone will not kill any animal.[2]

The dog's average lifespan is about 13 years, with a maximum life span of 27 years. Small breeds of dogs tend to live longer than do large and giant breeds.[1]

Aging has been defined as "a complex biologic process resulting in the progressive reduction of an individual's ability to maintain homeostasis under physiologic and external environmental stresses, thereby decreasing the individual's viability and increasing its vulnerability to disease and eventually death"[2]

While old age is difficult to define, the aging process can vary tremendously from one individual to another. Cats appear to age more slowly than dogs and do not show breed differences in aging or longevity.[1] The average life span of the domestic indoor cat is 14 years, with a maximal life span as high as 25–35 years.

Table 31.1 The onset of old age.[2-4]

Category	Body weight in pounds	Age considered senior	Age considered old
Small	Under 20#	8–9 years	11.5 years
Medium	20–50#	7 years	10 years
Large	50–90#	6 years	8.8–9 years
Giant	Greater than 90#	5 years	7.5 years
Cats		7 years	12 years

Based on the increased variety of challenges facing cats that are either indoor/outdoor or strictly outdoors, their lifespans can often be much shorter. Healthy cats are considered seniors when they are 10–12 years old.[1] (see Table 31.1).

There are breed and size differences in which dogs are considered to be geriatric. We know that larger breeds tend to age more quickly than smaller breeds, and mixed breed dogs tend to live longer than pure breeds of a similar size.[2] According to Fascetti and Delany, a survey of veterinarians revealed that clinicians believe the term "geriatric" is appropriately applied to small dogs (<20 lb) at 11.5 years of age, medium dogs (21–50 lb) at 10 years old, large breeds dogs (51–90 lb) at 9 years of age, and giant breed dogs (>90 lb) at 7.5 years old.[2] Other experts suggest that "old age" is when an animal has completed approximately 75–80% of its expected life span, or 5–7 years old.[2] (see Table 31.2).

Nutrition and Disease Management for Veterinary Technicians and Nurses, Third Edition. Ann Wortinger and Kara M. Burns.
© 2024 John Wiley & Sons, Inc. Published 2024 by John Wiley & Sons, Inc.
Companion Website: www.wiley.com/go/wortinger/3e

Table 31.2 Most common causes of mortality in cats.

Cause of death	Percentage of occurrence
Cancer	35%
Kidney disease	24.9%
Heart disease	10.7%
Diabetes mellitus	7.6%

Source: Gross et al.[5]/Mark Morris Institute.

Feeding Requirements

Though old age is not a disease, aging has biological effects on the body. These include a gradual decline in the organs' functional capacity, which begins shortly after the animal has reached maturity.[1] These changes occur in tissue structure and composition, rate of metabolism, cardiovascular and pulmonary function, renal and gastrointestinal tract excretion, special senses, skin and reproductive system and virtually all functional and structural systems of the body.[3]

Different systems age at different rates, and the degree of compromise that must occur before the onset of clinical signs also depends on many factors.[1] It is not unusual for more than one chronic disease to be present in a single senior dog or cat.[1] Because of this variability, each older animal should be assessed as an individual, using functional changes in body systems rather than chronological age to assess old age changes.[1]

The three leading causes of non-accidental death in dogs and cats are cancer, kidney disease and heart disease.[6]

The objectives for the nutritional management of old dogs and cats are:

o Enhancing the quality of life.
o Delaying the onset of aging.
o Extending life expectancy.
o Slowing or preventing the progression of the disease.
o Eliminating or relieving clinical signs of disease.
o Maintaining optimal body condition.[3,6,7]

Metabolism

Dog and cat metabolism naturally slows as they age, causing a reduction in their resting and maintenance energy requirements. This decline is due primarily to the loss of lean body mass, even without subsequent loss of body weight.[1] There also tends to be a decrease in activity level as animals age, decreasing their energy output and muscular activity.[3] It has been estimated that the total DER may decrease as much as 30–40% during the final third of an animal's lifespan. This can be due to reduced activity and decreased metabolic rate.[1]

The degree to which these changes occur appears to be breed and size related in dogs. In cats, maintenance energy requirements remain relatively constant throughout their lives.[2] Recent studies have documented a decreased energy requirement in mature adult cats but an increased energy requirement when these cats reached 10–12 years of age. These changes were not linear but continued to rise between 12–15 years of age. It has also been reported that loss of lean body mass, body fat and bone mass put an older cat at increased risk of early death, with significant changes occurring within the last year of life.[2]

Physical activity can help to offset age-associated losses of lean body mass. The basal metabolic rate in older dogs and cats who are very active may not decrease significantly.[1]

The minimum nutrient requirements for older animals are probably similar to those of young to middle-aged animals.[8] Because of this, nutritional recommendations for these animals are based on risk factor management, information obtained from other species and good sense.[8] To date, the only nutritional modification known to slow aging and increase life span is reduced caloric intake over the animal's life to maintain a lean BCS.[7,8] Reducing caloric intake by 20–30% of normal while meeting essential nutrient needs reduces the aging process, cancer incidence, renal disease and immune-mediated disease.[7,8] This means that animals should be maintained with a BCS of 3/5 or 4/9, significantly lower than what we usually see in our companion animals.

Digestion

There is little to no evidence that healthy older animals are less able to digest their food than younger animals.[3] Changes in the digestive tract may contribute to inadequate food intake, decreased appetite and systemic disease.[2] Structural changes in the canine digestive tract are not evident during aging, and atrophy and fibrosis of the intestinal villi are seldom seen.[2] Despite histologic changes in older dogs, there does not appear to be any apparent loss in nutrient digestibility.[2]

Similar changes have not been well studied in cats, though several studies have demonstrated reductions in protein, fat and carbohydrate digestibility in older cats. A study by Carolyn Cupp et al. demonstrated that significant increases were seen in the average life span in cats fed a diet supplemented with increased levels of antioxidants, prebiotic fibers and a blend of oils over those not receiving the supplemented foods.[9]

The nutrient requirements for elderly dogs and cats are the same as for their younger counterparts. There may be changes in the volume consumed to maintain their body weight and some adjustments needed in how these nutrients are provided in the diet.[2] There is no evidence that "geriatric diets" are necessary if the animal is healthy and eating a sufficient amount of a good quality diet to maintain body weight and body mass.[10]

Many senior diets are reduced in fat and caloric density to help prevent weight gain as activity level reduces with age. While this may benefit many animals, some have difficulty maintaining their weight due to decreased caloric intake or decreased appetite secondary to various disease processes.[2] It would be prudent to switch these animals to a higher calorie diet, be it a kitten, puppy or recovery diet, or in the case of dogs, a performance diet to enable them to meet their caloric requirements.[2]

Protein

There are no actual protein reserves in the body. All protein found in the body, except for a small amount of amino acids found within each cell, is functional and plays a role in maintaining that body. When protein reserves are reduced, that decreases the actual functional proteins found in the body. Due to the lack of actual protein reserves in older animals, avoidance of negative nitrogen balance is important as this indicates an additional loss of functional tissue within the body.[3] These "reserves" are used by the body to help combat stress and disease.[2]

Dietary protein should not be reduced in apparently healthy older dogs and cats. Adequate protein and energy intake are needed to sustain lean body mass, protein synthesis and immune function.[7] An additional benefit to maintaining moderate protein concentration in foods for older animals is an increase in palatability, which may help maintain an adequate caloric intake.[7]

Evidence exists that feeding reduced protein diets to animals already showing signs of renal failure will improve clinical signs. But there is no evidence to suggest that feeding reduced protein diets to otherwise healthy animals provides any renal protection or prevents the development of chronic kidney disease.[2]

In animals with chronic kidney disease, a reduction in dietary protein may be needed to help decrease the serum/plasma urea nitrogen (BUN/SUN). The kidneys are responsible for the excretion of the end products of protein catabolism. With impaired function, these end products can accumulate in the bloodstream and cause problems for the animal through the development of uremia.[3,7] Feeding a protein source with high biologic value will help decrease the accumulation of these by-products. The higher the biological value, the greater the efficiency of the protein in replenishing or maintaining tissue protein. In proportion to intake, the less excreted in the urine as urea.[3] A reduction of protein intake without evidence of chronic renal failure has not been shown to prevent the occurrence of renal failure and may cause more problems such as decreased lean body mass and decreased body weight due to decreased energy intake and increased protein catabolism or body tissues to meet the animals' protein requirements.[1,2]

Healthy older animals should receive sufficient protein to meet their protein needs and avoid protein-calorie malnutrition adequately.[7] With decreased energy intake, if these older animals are fed a diet that meets the minimum protein requirements for adult animals, they may be in a protein deficit situation (protein-calorie malnutrition).[1] Therefore, older animals should be fed diets with a percentage of calories from protein slightly higher than the minimum recommended for adult maintenance.[1]

Fat

Fats provide energy and essential fatty acids (EFAs), act as a carrier for fat-soluble vitamins, and improve the palatability of foods.[3] Because of their high energy density (8.5 kcal/g), the diet's most effective way to affect caloric intake is to modify the fat content. Although weight loss can be seen in some older animals, obesity is the most common problem. It has been theorized that the increase in the percentage of body fat that occurs with aging is partially due to an impaired ability of the body to metabolize lipids.[1] There is also evidence that aging is associated with a gradual decline in the ability to desaturate EFAs.[1]

Supplementing foods with antioxidants to support immune function has become commercially popular. The implication is that the supplements will slow down the aging process and reduce the likelihood of disease development.[2] It has been shown that certain of these supplements, such as omega-3 fatty acids and beta-carotene, can improve the immune response in young animals, but few studies have been done on older animals to evaluate their response to these supplements.[2] The exception to this would be the previously mentioned study done by Dr. Cupp, where using older cats, they evaluated the effects of antioxidants vitamin E and beta-carotene and a blend of omega-3 and omega-6 fatty acids on the overall life spans of cats.[9] The positive effects were statistically significant between the control and those fed the enhanced diet.

Certain diseases associated with obesity are also commonly seen in older animals, primarily diabetes mellitus, hypertension and heart disease, as well as pancreatitis and arthritis.[3,7] The risk of death also increases significantly in older obese animals.[3,7]

Moderate- to low-fat levels in the diet is indicated to reduce the risk of obesity or treat obesity that already exists.[7] These very same animals may also have impaired fat digestion and fat metabolism. Fats included in foods for older animals should be highly digestible and contain high levels of EFAs. Foods with lower fat levels are recommended for those animals that are obese or obese-prone, while foods with higher fat levels should be fed to thin animals (BCS <3/5, 4/9).[2]

Fiber

Dietary fiber can promote gastrointestinal health by aiding normal motility and providing fuel for colonocytes through the production of then fatty acid, butyrate. Not all dietary fibers act the same way in the intestines. Some are highly digestible and can cause diarrhea (i.e., lactulose), some allow the colonic bacteria to make the SCFA butyrate (i.e., beet pulp), and some are nondigestible and act as bulking agents (i.e., cellulose).[3,7]

Many older animals have problems with constipation; this can be treated in one of two ways: by increasing the bulk of the stool to increase the frequency of defecation or by feeding low-fiber food to increase digestibility and decrease stool volume, therefore colonic distention.[1,7] In refractory cases, lactulose may be added to the diet to increase the amount of water pulled into the colon, keeping the stool moister and making it easier to defecate. As it is difficult to tell which method will work best for any individual animal, all three methods may need to be tried.

Taste

As dogs and cats age, their food preferences may become pickier. Their willingness to try new foods may also decrease. This may make it necessary for owners to resort to strong-smelling or highly-palatable foods. Options can often include using baby food meats as a top dressing for required diets, mixing in various broths or adding clam or tuna juice into the food. Older animals may develop fixed taste preferences and only accept one particular flavor or type of food. If possible, owners should try to accommodate these preferences, though various disease processes may make this accommodation more challenging.[1]

Conclusion

Many older animals become very particular about their eating habits. There may be a decreased willingness to eat new foods, and it may be necessary for the owners to provide especially strong-smelling or highly-palatable foods.[1] The animals may also develop very fixed food preferences; if possible, owners

Table 31.3 Practical feeding tips for senior dogs and cats.

- o Provide regular health exams at least twice yearly.
- o Avoid sudden changes in daily routine or diet.
- o Feed a diet that contains high-quality protein formulated for adult animals.
- o Use measured feedings to help prevent obesity and maintain ideal body weight.
- o Provide a moderate amount of regular exercise.
- o Maintain proper dental health with home care and regular dental cleanings.
- o If needed, provide a therapeutic diet to help manage or treat a disease.[1]

should accommodate these provided the food provides adequate nutrition to the animal to ensure continued food intake and help prevent loss of lean body mass and weight.[1]

If a chronic disease is present that requires specific nutrient alterations, such as diabetes, renal disease, arthritis or obesity, the animal should be fed a diet that is appropriate for the management of that disorder. If multiple diseases are present, feed for the most life-threatening disease.[1]

Proper care of teeth and gums is critical as animals age; if their mouths hurt or are a source of bacteria, this can negatively affect their overall health. As animals age, there is also a decrease in the amount of saliva produced, which can contribute to a decrease in food intake.[2] If owners are unable or unwilling to provide at-home dental care, yearly to bi-yearly oral health care should be done through the veterinarian.[1]

Exercise is also important in the older animal to help maintain muscle tone, enhance circulation, improve gastrointestinal motility and prevent excess weight gain. The level and intensity of the exercise should be adjusted to an individual animal's physical and medical condition.[1] Keeping an animal active will help to preserve lean body mass, engage the brain to maintain mental acuity and prevent the development of obesity. (see Table 31.3).

References

1 Case LP, Daristotle LD, Hayek MG, Foess Raasch M (2011) Geriatrics. In *Canine and Feline Nutrition* (3rd edn), pp. 261–72, St Louis, MO: Mosby.

2 Delaney S, Fascetti A (2012) Feeding the healthy dog and cat. In S Delaney, A Fascetti (eds), *Applied Veterinary Clinical Nutrition*, vol. 2012, pp. 85–6, Ames, IA: Wiley-Blackwell.

3 Anderson RS (1996) Feeding older pets. In N Kelly, J Wills (eds), *Manual of Companion Animal Nutrition and Feeding*, pp. 93–8, Ames, IA: Iowa State University Press.

4 Healthy Ageing. Nestle Purina PetCare Communications Principles (2015) pg 26–27. https://vetcentre.purina.co.uk/sites/default/files/2018-07/Meet_Purina_Book_230x230.pdf

5 Gross KL, Becvarova I, Debraekeleer J (2010) Feeding mature adult cats: middle aged and older. In MS Hand, CD Thatcher, RI Remillard *et al.* (eds), *Small Animal Clinical Nutrition* (5th edn), p. 394, Marceline, MO: Walsworth Publishing.

6 Gross KL, Debraekeleer J, Zicker SC (2000) Normal dogs. In MS Hand, CD Thatcher, RI Remillard, P Roudebush (eds), *Small Animal Clinical Nutrition* (4th edn), pp. 229–32, Marceline, MO: Walsworth Publishing.

7 Gross KL, Debraekeleer J, Zicker SC (2000) Normal cats. In MS Hand, CD Thatcher, RI Remillard, P Roudebush (eds), *Small Animal Clinical Nutrition* (4th edn), pp. 314–20, Marceline, MO: Walsworth Publishing.

8 Kealy RD, Lawler DF, Ballam JM *et al.* (2002) Effects of diet restriction on life span and age-related changes in dogs. *JAVMA* **220**(9) May 1, 2002:1315–1320.

9 Cupp C, Jean-Phillipe C, Wendell KW *et al.* (2006) Effect of nutritional interventions on longevity of senior cats. *International Journal of Applied Research in Veterinary Medicine* **4**(1): 34–50 https://www.purinainstitute.com/science-of-nutrition/extending-healthy-life/longevity-study-in-cats.

10 Buffington CA, Holloway C, Abood SK (2004) Normal dogs. In *Manual of Veterinary Dietetics*, pp. 21–3, St. Louis, MO: Saunders.

32

Performance and Dogs

Introduction

Over the years, people have spent much time and energy molding dogs into various shapes to suit our needs. The American Kennel Club recognizes 31 working breeds, 32 sporting breeds, 31 hound breeds, 31 terriers, 22 toy breeds, 30 herding and 20 nonsporting breeds.[1] Due to our changing lifestyle, many of these breeds are no longer needed for what they were bred. However, these breeds still contain the genetic makeup for their original activities; this means that many of our companions have much more energy than is needed for a couch potato, leading to the development of many behavioral problems if they are not given an appropriate outlet for all this energy. Genetics can determine an individual's mental, anatomic and metabolic characteristics; training can alter some of these characteristics and enhance exercise and scent detection.[2]

Working dogs are still found in many areas, though. The federal, local and state governments employ dogs in national defense, customs service, drug reinforcement and border patrol. Dogs are trained as service animals for the deaf and blind and the physically and mentally disabled. They are also used for hunting, racing, endurance sled pulling and other athletic competitions. Canine agility competitions, Frisbee competitions and herding competitions are found in many parts of our country. These provide an excellent opportunity for humans and dogs to work together again, as they were originally trained

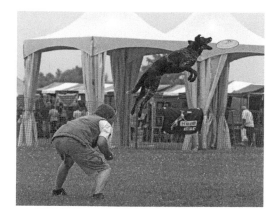

Figure 32.1 An owner and his dog competing in a Frisbee competition. *Source*: Courtesy of Heidi Reuss-Lamky LVT, VTS (Anesthesia/analgesia, Surgery).

without having to maintain a herd of sheep (see Figure 32.1).

Just like people who are athletes, training and nutrition can play a significant role in the canine athletes' success. But nutrition cannot overcome deficits in genetics and training. Matching nutrition to exercise type allows a canine athlete to perform to its genetic potential and level of training.[3] In general, all working dogs have increased energy requirements over those of an adult dog during a time of regular activity.[4] The type of work being done and the intensity of work may require modifications in the food's nutrient composition and the feeding schedule.[4] Individual variations in energy requirements exist, and calculation of metabolizable energy

Nutrition and Disease Management for Veterinary Technicians and Nurses, Third Edition. Ann Wortinger and Kara M. Burns.
© 2024 John Wiley & Sons, Inc. Published 2024 by John Wiley & Sons, Inc.
Companion Website: www.wiley.com/go/wortinger/3e

(ME) requirement based on daily energy requirements DERs provides no more than an estimate of their actual requirements.[5] Let the animal dictate if they are receiving enough energy for their activity level and adjust intake as required to meet these needs.

An ideal BCS for performance dogs has not been determined, but studies have shown that dogs live longer, perform better when fed less food and weigh slightly less than typically seen as "normal."[5] Racing greyhounds trained to run a 500 m race were on average 0.7 km/h faster if they weighed 6% less and were fed 15% less food than when they were fed free-choice.[5] These dogs had a BCS of 3.5/9 when fed the lesser amount of food, and when fed free-choice, had a BCS of 3.75/9.[5]

Most of our performance dogs typically are "weekend athletes." For optimal performance, their training should match the intensity, duration and frequency of the desired level of performance.[2] It is unrealistic to expect a dog that has not done any work since last season to go out on the first day of duck season and work for 6–8 hours.

The work performed by most intermediate athletes (hunting dogs, field trials, Frisbee trials, agility, service work, police work, search and rescue, livestock management and exercise with people) resembles that done by endurance athletes (sled pulling) but is of shorter duration. The muscle-fiber type profile of intermediate athletes should resemble that of an endurance athlete over that of a sprint athlete (sight hounds).[4] In general, endurance athletes have more well-developed slow-twitch fiber muscles; athletes involved in high-speed sprinting have increased numbers of fast-twitch muscles.[4] Slow-twitch muscles have a high oxidative capacity and endurance, with a higher capacity for aerobic metabolism.[2] They primarily use fat in the form of free fatty acids for energy. Fast-twitch muscles can use both aerobic and anaerobic pathways in that they can use both carbohydrates in the form of glycogen and glucose for immediate energy and fat for longer-term energy use.[3,4]

Fiber composition can vary between muscles and between individual dogs. Muscle fiber type is a function of genetics and can determine the type of exercise for which an individual dog is best suited. Training makes some changes possible, but you cannot turn a bulldog into an endurance athlete or have a Saluki run the Iditarod.[2]

Exercise requires the transfer of chemical energy into physical work. ATP (adenosine triphosphate) is the sole energy source for muscle contraction.[3] ATP is formed from metabolic fuels stored in muscle (endogenous) and from other body stores (exogenous). The energy is converted to ATP using either aerobic pathways using oxygen or anaerobic pathways that can work without oxygen.[3] The proportion of each pathway used is determined by the animal's duration and intensity of exercise, conditioning and nutritional status.[3]

Training and conditioning result in adaptive physiological changes, facilitating the efficient delivery of oxygen and other nutrients to the working muscles. These changes include increased blood volume, red blood cell mass, capillary density, mitochondrial volume, bone mass, muscle hypertrophy, activity level and total mass of metabolic enzymes.[2,4]

Fats

Fats, on average, provide 8.5 kcal of ME per gram of dry matter. Carbohydrates and proteins provide 3.5 kcal of ME per gram of dry matter. The easiest and quickest way to increase the energy density of a food is to increase the fat content in the diet.

The two primary fuels used by the body for working muscles are muscle glycogen and free fatty acids. An intermediate athlete would receive ~70–90% of their energy from fat metabolism and only a small amount from carbohydrate metabolism.[4] Dogs rely more heavily on free fatty acids for energy generation at all exercise levels than people.[3] Feeding a higher-fat diet to endurance and intermediate-trained athletes prepares the muscles to mobilize and use free fatty acids for energy efficiently. It also exerts a glycogen-sparing effect that can help prolong glycogen use during work.[4] By increasing dietary fat concentration, the energy intake is increased and stressed dogs are encouraged to increase food intake due to the increased palatability of fat in the diet.[3] Increased dietary fat levels may enhance free fatty acid availability.[3] As the duration of the event performed by the dog increases, so should the dietary fat intake. Fatigue and dehydration may decrease appetite, making intake of adequate amounts of energy even more challenging.[2]

Carbohydrate

Provided sufficient gluconeogenic precursors are available in the diet, no dietary requirements for carbohydrates exist for dogs except during gestation and neonatal development.[3] Gluconeogenesis (formation of glucose from noncarbohydrate sources) is done by the liver and kidneys using glycerol, lactate and glucogenic amino acids.[3] Stored fat in adipose tissue supplies glycerol for glucose production by breaking down triglycerides and fatty acids for oxidation to supply energy, whereas muscle catabolism releases glucogenic amino acids, lactic acid and pyruvate for glucose production by the liver.[3]

Since digestible carbohydrates contain only 3.5 kcal of ME per gram of dry matter, adding additional carbohydrates to a diet will not increase the caloric density and will not provide additional energy.[4] Dogs at rest obtain energy equally from the oxidation (aerobic metabolism) of fat and glucose. When trained dogs begin to walk and run, glucose oxidation increases only slightly, with most of the increased energy obtained is from fat oxidation.[2] As exercise intensity increases, oxygen supply becomes limited, and metabolic acid is produced. The increased levels of lactic acid further decrease the use of fat for energy.[2]

Aerobic metabolism generates ATP by combusting carbohydrates and fats into CO_2 and water. Lactate or lactic acid is the endpoint of anaerobic metabolism. Muscle enzyme activity is highly sensitive to pH levels, and if energy metabolism and muscle contraction continue at their optimal rates, muscle pH must be tightly regulated.[2]

Intracellular buffers can moderate some of the increased CO_2 and lactic acid concentrations. Remember that CO_2 acts like an acid in these situations. Ultimately, the elimination of the intracellular acids is the primary strategy for avoiding decreases in muscle pH. Carbon dioxide can be removed through respiration and renal excretion as bicarbonate (HCO_3-). With aerobic activity, significant acid-base changes are not seen, as the respiratory system can excrete (blow off) CO_2 as quickly as it is produced. With anaerobic activity, lactate is the primary acid produced and is more challenging for the body to neutralize. Lactate can be oxidized by muscle or converted back into glucose. It cannot be removed through respiration or the kidneys.[2]

Even though fat provides more energy than carbohydrates, the inclusion of carbohydrates in performance diets has decreased the incidence of "stress diarrhea" in endurance athletes. With sprinting athletes, the onset of fatigue can be delayed with the inclusion of carbohydrates, which work at or above their anaerobic threshold.[2] Despite this, carbohydrate loading of canine athletes is probably not as beneficial for dogs as a steady diet of foods with higher fat levels. The exception to this would be sprinting greyhounds. Since they do not have dramatically increased energy needs (small bursts of energy for less than 60 seconds), rely primarily on glycogen for energy and seldom get to the point of utilizing free fatty acids, and would not appreciate the value of a higher-fat diet other than for the provision of additional energy in the diet.[2]

Carbohydrates fed to athletes should be highly digestible to decrease fecal bulk in the colon. Excessive amounts of undigested carbohydrates reaching the colon can also increase water loss through the stool, increase colonic gas production and increase overall fecal bulk, adding unneeded weight.[3] Adding moderately fermentable fibers may benefit racing dogs, especially those fed raw food diets. Rapid fermentation of these fibers to oligosaccharides may decrease colonic pH and inhibit clostridial bacteria growth.[2]

Protein

Endurance training results in increased protein needs through increased protein synthesis (anabolism – the building up of muscle), protein degradation (catabolism – the breaking down of muscle), and gluconeogenesis.[3,4] Catabolism is only a small portion of the overall protein needs; the primary use is anabolism.[4] Increased tissue mass associated with training must be supplied by increased protein in the diet.[4] Amino acids are used to form new muscle and repair muscle and connective tissue damage during intensive conditioning; exercise increases amino acid catabolism.[3] Dogs initially use glycogen as a source of glucose during submaximal exercise, but gluconeogenesis from protein increases after about 30 minutes.[5] Because of this, dogs running for longer than 30 minutes require more protein in their diets than dogs that only do short bursts of activity, such as Greyhounds.[5]

Amino acids provide ~5–15% of the energy used during exercise; most of this energy comes from the metabolism of gluconeogenic amino acids.[3] All of these are essential amino acids and cannot be synthesized from other amino acids; they must be included in the diet.

A protein's "biologic value" indicates the amount of essential amino acids in that product. Egg has the highest biological value, followed closely by casein and whey, both milk-based proteins. Muscle and organ meat-based proteins have the next highest level of essential amino acids and are also highly digestible and bioavailable.[2,3]

An optimal protein concentration of 30–40% ME is recommended. However, excessive protein intake may predispose an athlete to increased amino acid catabolism.[3] Amino acids are not stored as proteins in the body but are deaminated (broken down) to ketoacids. These ketoacids are either oxidized for energy or converted to fatty acids and glucose and stored as adipose tissue (fat) or glycogen.[3] The diet fed should supply adequate calories, such as fat and carbohydrate, so that the protein fed can be used primarily for tissue synthesis, not energy.[4] During long periods of exercise, DER may increase 2–3 times over resting energy requirements (RERs), while protein requirements only increase slightly.[2]

Water

Water is a solvent for biological solutes; it is a transport medium for nutrients, wastes, and heat, absorbs physical shock, and lubricates various internal and external surfaces.[3] Heat is the primary byproduct of muscle contraction, and the respiratory tract, through panting, is responsible for the dissipation of this heat.[3] As much as 75–80% of the energy used during muscular activity is converted to heat.[2]

Because evaporative heat loss is the primary way dogs dissipate heat, ensuring adequate hydration is crucial for maintaining a normal body temperature.[3] Depending on the type of work done and environmental conditions, water losses can increase by 10–20 times normal during exercise.[4] Even mild dehydration can lead to decreased performance, strength and hyperthermia.[3] Water should be offered in small amounts frequently throughout the exercise period. If an insufficient amount is consumed, the dog might benefit by having water added to its food.[3]

While dogs require unlimited and frequent water supplies before, during and after exercise, they do not require additional electrolytes, including sodium or vitamins.[5] As dogs do not sweat, they do not lose electrolytes during exercise as do humans. Sports drinks designed for humans are not recommended for dogs and could decrease performance.[5] Any salt consumed in the drinking water will have to be excreted in the urine, increasing the rate of water loss and may exacerbate dehydration.[5]

Supplements

Many breeders, exhibitors and trainers believe stressed dogs must also receive specific vitamins and minerals supplements. There is no evidence to suggest that working dogs have increased requirements for these nutrients.[4] If a diet is nutritionally balanced and the dog is consuming enough to meet its energy requirements during work, then additional supplements should not be necessary.[3]

Requirements for antioxidant vitamins such as vitamin E increase as the diet's fat level increases, especially with higher levels of polyunsaturated fatty acids (PUFAs).[5] Research has not determined if exercising dogs require more antioxidants than sedentary dogs. But antioxidant requirements for moderately active dogs may be less than for sedentary dogs. It is better to exercise the dogs more frequently than to increase the antioxidants in the diet over recommended levels.[5] Oxidative stress can be decreased through adequate pre-exercise training.[2]

The addition of glucosamine/chondroitin may be of benefit for dogs with existing osteoarthritis, but there is no evidence that the inclusion of these supplements in the diet prevents the occurrence of osteoarthritis.[5]

Diet Requirements

A diet needs to be highly digestible to limit the total volume of food consumed at each meal. Some maintenance diets may supply enough energy if consumed in large quantities but may become bulk-limiting, thereby limiting performance in hard-working dogs (too much stool production due to low digestibility).[4] By increasing digestibility, fecal bulk is reduced. Decreased fecal water loss may decrease the incidence of "stress diarrhea."[4]

An ideal diet would provide increased levels of high-quality protein (high biological value) to meet anabolic requirements and enough nonprotein energy nutrients (fats and carbohydrates) to meet energy requirements. By doing this, the diet provides sufficient calories with fat to limit the use of amino acids for energy, leaving them available for muscle repair and replacement.[4] Dogs doing short-duration, maximal-intensity exercise may benefit from a lower fat, higher carbohydrate diet to increase available glycogen stores for immediate use.[2]

The food needs to be calorically dense and palatable, highly digestible and practical so that the dog can physically consume enough to meet their caloric requirements.[3] The price of the food, the form it is available in, storage conditions required and the number of animals being fed also need to be considered. What may be practical for 1 dog may be impractical for a kennel of 15 dogs.[3]

Most intermediate athletes are fed commercial diets, while many elite sprint and endurance athletes are fed homemade diets or a mixture of commercial diets with additional ingredients added in.[2] It is important to compare the nutritional content of the current food to the key nutritional factors (protein, fats, carbohydrates) to determine the adequacy of food for that dog. If the current food contains appropriate levels to meet that dog's needs, it can continue to be fed. If discrepancies are found, a more balanced diet would be recommended.[2] Determining the nutrient content for homemade and supplemented diets is difficult at best, and digestibility can only be determined using feeding trials. Consulting a veterinary nutritionist to formulate a homemade diet would be recommended to ensure nutritional adequacy for those clients who do not want to feed commercially available balanced diets.

Energy Considerations

DERs can be highly variable and are directly related to the amount of work being done and the condition and training of the dog. Most dogs fall between the extremes of endurance work, as seen with sled dogs, and the short bursts of activity seen with the sighthounds. Hunting and herding dogs may work for extended periods, but most of their activity is at a suboptimal level, with short bursts of activity. Service dogs work at relatively low activity levels but can do so for extended periods.[3]

Ambient temperature, psychological stress and geography are all environmental factors that may influence the nutritional needs of the canine athlete.[3] Of these, ambient temperature can exert the greatest effect; with an increased environmental temperature, you get increased work and increased water loss. Lower environmental temperature increases energy expenditure for thermogenesis; this may be as much as a 50% increase over DER.[3,4]

Stress in the form of intense physical exertion, weather extremes and psychological strain may negatively affect food intake, and an adequate amount of energy may not be available for the work required.[3,4] Geographical factors such as elevation above sea level, changing elevations throughout a course and working in sand or tall grass may increase the workload and energy expenditure.[3]

The goal for the nutrition and feeding of all working dogs is to maintain an ideal body condition and weight, support performance and prevent fatigue and injury.[3] All working dogs will have energy needs above those of house dogs living a sedentary lifestyle. For dogs working at prolonged, low-level activities, a consistent increase in caloric intake may be needed to maintain their weight.[3] For hunting and herding dogs, an increase may only be needed during the training period and their working season, but not during times they are not working.[3] For service dogs and police dogs, a high-fat, highly digestible diet is ideal and may require an increased caloric intake to maintain their weight and body condition.[3]

Dogs require time to adapt to diet changes. When these changes are dramatic, as with significant fat or protein increases, gastrointestinal and metabolic adaptations need to occur. GI adjustments can happen throughout a few days, whereas metabolic adjustments can take longer. Allowing adequate time for the body to adjust to a diet change is important to optimize the desired result. This can be especially important for seasonal athletes such as hunting dogs.[2] These dogs may be fed a maintenance diet during the nonhunting season, transitioning to a performance diet during the hunting season. This should not be done on opening weekend.

Diet Calculations

The energy required depends on the total work done: intensity × duration × frequency. DER is ~1.6 × RER for the average canine athlete. Sprinters may require 1.6–2 × RER, and endurance or other high-end athletes may require 2–5 × RER.

RERs can either be figured using $(70 \times \text{body weight in kilograms})^{0.75}$, or $70 + (30 \times \text{body weight in kilograms})$. From there, you can calculate the DER. Maintenance is typically 1.0–1.6 × RER depending on activity.

Feeding Plan

Look at where the dog is housed (inside/outdoors), medications or supplements they may be taking, dietary history, amount fed, type of food fed and timing of meals in relation to exercise/training, the nutrient profile of the diet and exercise and training history (amount of exercise done, frequency and performance of exercise).[3]

Compare the current diet's key nutritional factors to the recommended levels; determine the amount to be fed and the timing of the meals. Estimate energy expenditure using body condition scoring and exercise level.

Table 32.1 This list represents products with the largest market share, and for which published information is available. Values are expressed on a percentage of metabolizable energy. Information collected June 2022.[3,6,7]

Food	Caloric density (kcal)	ME protein (%)	ME fat (%)	ME carbohydrate (%)	Feeding trials
Diamond Performance, dry	439/cup	26	42	32	No
Eagle Pack Power pack, dry	445/cup	27	41	32	No
Kinetic Performance 30k, dry	462/cup	26	42	32	No
Eukanuba Premium Performance 30/20, dry	447/cup	26	42	31	Yes
Victor Performance, dry	399/cup	23	39	38	No
Purina Pro Plan Performance 30/20, dry	527/cup	26	43	31	Yes

Source: Adapted from a table in Small Animal Clinical Nutrition 4th Edition.

Table 32.2 Total calories in 100 g of food

Protein = 3.5 kcal/g × g in food

Fat = 8.5 kcal/g × g in food

Carbohydrate = 3.5 kcal/g × g in food

Total calories/100 g = protein calorie + fat calorie + carbohydrate calorie

Percentage of ME contributed by each nutrient (caloric distribution)

Protein = (protein calories/100 g ÷ by total calories/100 g) × 100 = % ME

Fat = (fat calories/100 g ÷ by total calories/100 g) × 100 = % ME

Carbohydrate = (carbohydrate calories/100 g ÷ by total calories) × 100 = % ME

Timing of the meals is important to allow the most availability of nutrients to the athlete. A recommended feeding schedule would be: 1 meal at least 4 hours before exercise, 1 meal within 2 hours after exercise, and if necessary, due to the duration of exercise, small amounts during exercise. After the dog has calmed down, the largest meal should be given postexercise.[2] Eating a meal directs blood to the intestinal tract for digestion. If fed soon before exercise or a large meal during exercise, this could compromise performance and digestion.[2] It is also important to allow

access to plenty of fresh, clean water to prevent dehydration.[3]

For optimal performance and long-term health, exercising dogs should not be fed free-choice but instead should receive measured feeding based on the volume of food required to maintain their desired level of activity and BCS.[5]

Reassess your plan based on body condition scoring, weight, hydration and performance. Adjust as needed to get the results that you want from your canine athlete (see Table 32.1).

To express nutrients as a percentage of metabolizable energy (see Table 32.2).

Comparing products using ME gives a better idea of caloric distribution and allows you to compare canned and dry diets accurately. This does not take into account digestibility. It is also important when comparing foods to see if feeding trials have been done on the product and look at digestibility if given. If you choose a food that has not had feeding trials done by the manufacturer, then you are doing the feeding trials for them (see Table 32.3).

Table 32.3 Recommended caloric distribution for Canine Athletes

Calories from protein: 30–35% ME

Calories from fat: 50–65% ME

Calories from carbohydrates: 10–15% ME[3]

References

1 American Kennel Club. Dog breeds. https://www.akc.org/dog-breeds. Accessed 7/30/22.

2 Toll P, Gillette R, Hand M (2010) Feeding working and sporting dogs. In MS Hand, CD Thatcher, RI Remillard *et al.* (eds), *Small Animal Clinical Nutrition* 5th edn, pp. 321–52, Marceline, MO: Walsworth Publishing.

3 Toll PW, Reynolds AJ (2000) The canine athlete. In MS Hand, CD Thatcher, RL Remillard, P Roudebush (eds), *Small Animal Clinical Nutrition* (4th edn), pp. 261–83, Marceline, MO: Walsworth Publishing.

4 Case LP, Daristotle LD, Hayek MG, Raasch F (2011) Melody. Performance. In *Canine and Feline Nutrition* 3rd edn, pp. 243–56, St Louis, MO: Mosby.

5 Richard H (2012) Nutritional and energy requirements for performance. In S Delaney, A Fascetti (eds), *Applied Veterinary Clinical Nutrition*, pp. 47–55, Ames, IA: Wiley-Blackwell.

6 Chewy.com for nutritional information.

7 Balanceit.com for GA to ME conversion. https://balance.it/convert

33

Feeding Requirements of Cats

Introduction

In their natural environment, cats are obligate carnivores, meaning their nutritional needs can only be met by eating a diet consisting of animal-based proteins (i.e., mice and birds). How have our efforts to domesticate cats been affected by this dietary requirement?

Cats and dogs are members of the order *Carnivora* and are therefore classified as carnivores. From a dietary perspective, dogs are omnivores, and cats and other members of the suborder *Felidae* are obligate carnivores. Domesticated cats (*Felis catus*) have evolved unique anatomic, physiologic, metabolic and behavioral adaptations consistent with eating a strictly carnivorous diet.[1,2]

By recognizing and addressing these special nutritional requirements for cats, we can help to ensure they have the best chance at a long, healthy life. As veterinary nutrition evolves, we will continue updating our feline nutrition information.

Feeding Behaviors

The evolutionary history of the cat indicates that it has eaten a purely carnivorous diet throughout its entire development.[2] Feeding behaviors that have evolved to fit this lifestyle include searching, hunting and caching of prey and postprandial behaviors such as grooming and sleeping.[3] Feral or outdoor cats feeding primarily on mice, voles and insects tend to live solitary lives when food is scarce and spread over a large area, but when food is plentiful and concentrated, as with households, dumps and farms, cats can be found living in large groups.[3]

Cats typically eat 10-20 small meals throughout the day and night. This eating pattern reflects the relationship between cats and their prey. Small rodents make up ~40% or more of the feral domestic cat's diets, with small rabbits, insects, frogs and birds making up the remainder. The average mouse provides ~30 kcal or an estimated 8% of a feral cat's daily energy requirements (DERs). Repeated cycles of hunting throughout the day and night are required to provide sufficient food for the average cat.[1,2] House cats typically continue this pattern by eating 10-20 small meals throughout the day and night, with each meal having a caloric content of ~23 kcal, remarkably close to the caloric value of one average mouse.[1,2]

For thousands of years, the primary economic value of cats has been their hunting skills.[3] Until recently, there has been little or no selective breeding to alter their behavior or looks. The predatory drive is so strong in cats that they will stop eating to make a kill. This behavior allows for multiple kills, which optimizes food availability.[1] From their viewpoint, the dead meal is not going anywhere, and they have no assurance that another prey will show up within the next 2-3 hours when they are due for their next meal. Many owners will feed outdoor cats, thinking this will decrease their

Nutrition and Disease Management for Veterinary Technicians and Nurses, Third Edition. Ann Wortinger and Kara M. Burns.
© 2024 John Wiley & Sons, Inc. Published 2024 by John Wiley & Sons, Inc.
Companion Website: www.wiley.com/go/wortinger/3e

hunting, especially of small songbirds. Unfortunately, supplemental feeding may reduce the time spent hunting but otherwise will not alter hunting behavior.[1]

Cats are extremely sensitive to food's physical form, odor and taste. They consume live prey beginning at the head. This head-first consumption is dictated by the direction of hair growth on the prey.[1] Food temperature also influences acceptance by cats. They do not readily accept food served at either extreme temperature but prefer food near body temperature (~38°C, 101.5°F) as found with freshly killed prey.[1,3] House cats accustomed to a specific texture or type of food may refuse foods with different textures. An individual cat's preferences are often influenced by early experiences (good or bad). Many cats will choose a new food over a diet that is currently being fed. The reverse is true in new or stressful situations, such as illness or hospitalization, where cats tend to refuse novel foods. This can be important when trying to switch foods or forms of food fed, especially in hospitalized or sick animals.[1]

Anatomic Adaptations

Cats have adapted physiologically to the life of a hunter. Their visual acuity is greater than that of dogs. In addition, their sense of hearing is well developed- their ears are upright, face forward and have 20 associated muscles to help them precisely locate a sound. Their sensitive facial whiskers and widely dispersed tactile hairs are thought to help them hunt in dim light and to protect their eyes.[1] Sharp and dagger-like, their retractable claws are ideal for capturing and securing prey, yet they are easily retracted to decrease noise when stalking.[1]

The scissor-like carnassial teeth are ideal for delivering the cervical bite used to sever the spinal cord and immobilize or kill prey.[1] Kittens can taste foods as early as 5 days before they are born, with continued improvement in their taste sensitivity as they age.

They can taste 4 of the 5 main flavor classes: acid > bitter > salty > sweet. Cats do not have active sweet receptors in their tongues, do not appear to taste or appreciate sweet tastes, and lack receptors for savory or umami tastes.[4] Cats have the receptors to detect sweet tastes, but they appear to have been switched off and have instead become a pseudogene. When synthetic sweeteners such as saccharine or cyclamates are used to flavor medications, cats detect a bitter, not a sweet taste.[4] An important fact to remember when administering liquid human medications is that use sweeteners to cover up the taste of the medication.

Their stomachs are smaller than dogs and simpler in structure. Because cats do not consume large meals, the stomach is less important as a storage reservoir.[1]

Intestinal length, as determined by the ratio of the intestine to body length, is markedly shorter in cats than in omnivores and herbivores. The ratio for cats is 4 : 1, meaning that the intestinal length is 4 times longer than the length of the cat. For dogs, this is 6 : 1, and for pigs, 14 : 1.[1] Cats have greater villus height in their intestinal lining, improving their absorptive capacity over dogs, so overall, they are only ~10% less efficient in digestion, especially with complex starches or fibers, even with their shorter intestinal length.[1] The bacterial populations in the feline small intestine are higher than those in dogs and other omnivores.[5] These additional bacteria may be needed to increase the digestive process due to their shorter intestinal length. The bacteria may also be beneficial in protein and fat digestion.[5]

Physiologic Adaptations

Cats cannot adapt to varying carbohydrate levels in their diets due to various changes in the digestive and absorptive functions of the intestine. Salivary amylase, the enzyme used to initiate the digestion of dietary starches, is absent in cats, and intestinal amylase appears to be exclusively derived from the pancreas. These enzymes were not necessary for a prey-based diet with minimal starch content.[1] The level of pancreatic amylase is only 5% of that found in dogs. The sugar transporter in the intestine is nonadaptive to changes in dietary carbohydrate levels. Disaccharide activity (i.e., the brush border enzymes responsible for sugar digestion) is also nonadaptive, with only ~40% found in dogs.[1,6] These changes evolved because cats had little natural carbohydrate intake, and it was not necessary to have systems intact that were of little use to the animal.

Despite these adaptive changes, cats can still use carbohydrates in their diets, with a sugar digestibility of ~94%, with a few exceptions. Lactose digestion declines sharply in kittens after 7 weeks of age. This is due to a decrease in intestinal lactase activity typical in mammals. Most adult cats can consume small amounts of milk without problems, but larger amounts (>1.3 mL/kg of body weight) can lead to signs of bloating, diarrhea and gas.[1]

High amounts of dietary carbohydrate levels can negatively impact diet digestibility. With high levels of dietary carbohydrates, decreases in protein digestibility are seen due to a combination of factors, including reduced fecal pH caused by incomplete carbohydrate digestion and increased microbial fermentation in the colon with increased production of organic acids.[1,6] Cats have a vestigial cecum and short colon, which limits their ability to use poorly digestible starches and fiber for energy through bacterial fermentation in the large bowel.[1]

Metabolic Adaptations

Energy

The liver of most animals has two active enzyme systems for converting glucose to glucose-6-phosphate (the first step to forming glycogen-the storage form of glucose within the cells); hexokinase and glucokinase.[7] The glucokinase system is used primarily when the liver receives a large glucose load, as seen with a high carbohydrate meal. Cats have very low liver glucokinase activity and, therefore, limited ability to metabolize large amounts of simple carbohydrates by this route. Blood glucose levels in carnivores are more consistent with less postprandial fluctuations because glucose is released in small continuous boluses over a more extended period due to the gluconeogenic catabolism of proteins.[1] If sufficient protein is not included in the diet (exogenous source), body muscle and organ tissue will be used to meet the cat's protein requirements (endogenous source). If fed according to their nutritional requirements, cats did not need to handle large carbohydrate loads and only used the hexokinase system for glucose metabolism.

Cats can often be seen eating grass or grazing on house plants. This is a natural phenomenon that makes vomiting easier, helping with the expulsion of hairballs.[4] This is not a dietary requirement but a behavior. As cats can become quite destructive if allowed unlimited access to house plants, and many house plants pose a poisoning hazard to cats when consumed, this behavior should be discouraged by owners.[4] Plants can be placed in areas inaccessible to the cat, removed from the house, or sprayed with hot pepper spray or other noxious-tasting sprays to make them taste bad.[4]

Water

Domestic cats are thought to have descended from the small African wildcat (*Felis silvestris lybica*); a cat naturally found in the deserts of Africa. Due to their limited water availability, *F. lybica* evolved to conserve water by concentrating their urine to reduce water loss.[4] Because of this ancient relationship, cats today maintain this adaptation to a dryer environment. Cats seem less sensitive to the stimulus of thirst and can survive on less water than dogs.[1,2,6] Average water requirements for cats vary from 55-70 mL/kg/day. This requirement is related to the dry matter intake in the diet.

With this decreased response to thirst, cats may ignore minor levels of dehydration (up to 4% body weight). They can compensate for this reduced water intake by forming highly concentrated urine.[6] Cats adjust their water intake based on the dry matter content of their diet rather than the moisture content. They consume 1.5-2 mL of water/g of dry matter. This 2 : 1 ratio of water to dry matter is like that of their typical prey.[1,4,6]

This means that cats consuming a dry diet will consume more water through drinking compared to cats eating a canned diet.[1,6] For us, if increased water turnover is necessary, as with FLUTD or the formation of urinary calculi, feeding a canned food diet can increase water intake without any additional work by the client or cat.

Protein

Protein metabolism in cats is unique; this is apparent because of their unusually high maintenance requirement for protein in the diet compared to dogs or other omnivores. Cats have both a higher basal requirement for protein and an increased requirement for essential amino acids.[6] Cats depend on protein not only for structural and synthetic purposes but also for energy. They will continue to use protein in the form of gluconeogenic amino acids to produce energy, even when inadequate protein is consumed in the diet.[1] The hepatic enzymes that catabolize amino acids for energy are always active and cannot be downregulated in times of decreased intake. Because of this, a fixed level of protein in the diet is always required for catabolism to provide energy.[5] Although these changes impair the cat's ability to conserve protein when dietary sources are limited, their natural diet conserves energy by eliminating the cost of enzyme synthesis and degradation.[1] There are four essential amino acids that are especially important for cats.

They are arginine, taurine, methionine and cysteine.[5]

In 1986, National Research Council recommended a minimum of 240 g of protein/kg in the diets of growing kittens and 140 g of protein/kg in the diets of adult cats. This is equivalent to 26% of metabolizable energy in the diet for kittens and 23% of metabolizable energy for adult maintenance. These are minimum recommendations, and they assume a highly digestible protein source is provided in the diet. Optimal results cannot be expected when feeding to meet minimal requirements.

Taurine

Taurine, an essential amino acid for cats, is not incorporated into proteins or degraded by mammalian tissues but is essential for the conjugation of bile salts, vision, cardiac muscle function, and the proper function of the nervous, reproductive and immune systems.[3,6,8] Taurine is a free amino acid in the natural diet of cats (i.e., rodents and small birds), but is found in lower concentrations in large animals such as cattle.[5]

Cats can only conjugate bile acids with taurine to make bile salts. Taurine continues to be lost in the gastrointestinal tract through this conjugation with bile. This, coupled with a low rate of synthesis, contributes to the obligatory requirement for cats.[1,3,6,8] A carnivorous diet supplies abundant taurine; however, cereal and grains supply only marginal or inadequate taurine levels for cats.[3] Therefore, diets based on these protein sources may be lacking or limited in taurine.

Taurine is either more available or better retained by cats fed dry food diets. Because of the widespread use of taurine within the body, changes from deficiency can be seen in virtually all body systems.[3] Three syndromes have been identified related strictly to taurine deficiency: feline central retinal degeneration, reproductive failure, impaired fetal development and feline dilated cardiomyopathy.[1]

Clinical signs of taurine deficiency occur only after prolonged periods of depletion (from 5 months to 2 years).[1]

Methionine and Cystine

Methionine is an essential amino acid for cats; this species has a higher requirement than dogs or other omnivores. Methionine and cystine are sulfur-containing amino acids and are considered together because cystine can replace up to half of the requirement for methionine.[5] Cystine is also required to produce hair and feline, an amino acid found in cat urine. Feline is found in the most significant amounts in intact male cats and is thought to be used for territorial marking.[1,6] Methionine tends to be the first limiting amino acid in many food ingredients.[1] This means that when breaking down proteins for use into their various amino acid components, methionine would "run out" first, limiting the number of proteins made in the body that need methionine for formation.

Nutritional deficiencies are possible, especially in cats fed homemade, vegetable-based or human enteral diets. Clinical signs of methionine deficiency include poor growth and crusting dermatitis at the mucocutaneous junctions of the mouth and nose.[1,6]

Arginine

Arginine deficiency in cats can be one of the most dramatic responses seen. Cats cannot synthesize sufficient ornithine or citrulline for conversion to arginine. Arginine is required for the urea cycle to work properly.[5] After consuming a meal, their highly active hepatic protein catabolism enzymes produce ammonia. Without sufficient arginine in the diet, the urea cycle cannot convert the ammonia to urea, resulting in ammonia toxicity. This hyperammonemia can result within 1 hour of consuming a deficient meal.[5]

Signs consistent with ammonia toxicity include vocalization, emesis, ptyalism, hyperactivity, hyperesthesia, ataxia, muscle rigidity and spasms, apnea and cyanosis. Death may ensue within 2-5 hours of ingesting a deficient meal.[5] Luckily, meat-based diets are high in arginine, and deficiencies have only been reported in cats fed experimental foods designed to be arginine deficient or in cats fed casein-based human enteral diets.[5]

Fats

Cats can digest high-fat levels, as found in meat-based diets. Like other obligate carnivores, cats have a dietary requirement for arachidonic acid, an essential fatty acid. They have limited ability to convert linoleic acid to arachidonic acid, as do dogs and other omnivores.[5] A preformed, exogenous source of arachidonic acid is vital during the more stressful stages of a cat's life, such as gestation and lactation. Arachidonic acid is abundant in animal tissues, especially organ and neural sources, but is absent in plant-based proteins.[5]

Vitamin Metabolism

The cat is unable to convert beta-carotene to retinol (vitamin A) because of a lack of intestinal enzymes necessary for the conversion, and therefore cats require a dietary source of preformed vitamin A. Vitamin A is necessary for the maintenance of vision, bone, muscle growth, reproduction and healthy epithelial tissues.[1] Because vitamin A is a fat-soluble vitamin and is stored in the liver, deficiencies are slow to develop and are only seen in cats with severe liver failure or gastrointestinal disease, resulting in fat malabsorption.[6]

Cats also lack sufficient enzymes to meet the metabolic requirements for vitamin D photosynthesis in the skin; therefore, they require a dietary source of vitamin D.[1] For indoor cats, this conversion of D2 to the active form D3 requires direct exposure to the sun, this cannot happen through a window. The primary function of vitamin D is calcium and phosphorus homeostasis, with particular emphasis on intestinal absorption, retention and bone deposition of calcium.[6] As with vitamin A, deficiency is rare and slow to develop.[1,6]

Vitamin A, vitamin D and arachidonic acid are found in plentiful amounts in animal fats and the liver. Dietary fat is important for providing fuel for energy, increasing palatability and acceptance of food and providing fat-soluble vitamins.[6]

Cats require increased amounts of many dietary water-soluble B vitamins, including thiamin, niacin, pyridoxine (vitamin B6), and in certain circumstances, cobalamin (vitamin B12). The requirement for niacin and pyridoxine is four times higher than that for dogs.[1,6] Cats cannot convert enough tryptophan to niacin to meet their physiologic requirements. Although cats have the metabolic pathway necessary to convert tryptophan to niacin,

their requirement exceeds the synthesis rate.[5] Because most water-soluble B vitamins are not stored (except cobalamin, which is stored in the liver), a continually available dietary source is required to prevent deficiencies.[6] Deficiencies in cats eating appropriate diets are rare because each B vitamin is found in high concentrations in animal tissue.[6]

Conclusion

The cat may be one of our most visible "specialists." As obligate carnivores, they have evolved to such a point that many of the redundant metabolic systems are no longer required. Instead of seeing cats as "inferior," we need to acknowledge that they have surpassed humans and dogs and streamlined their lives. We must appreciate this unique and wonderful creature that continues to enrich our lives and protect our houses and yards.

References

1 Kirk CA, Debraekeleer J, Armstrong PJ (2000) Normal cats. In MS Hand, CD Thatcher, RI Remillard, P Roudebush (eds), *Small Animal Clinical Nutrition* (4th edn), pp. 291–337, Marceline MO: Walsworth Publishing.

2 Case LP, Daristotle LD, Hayek MG, Raasch F (2011) Melody. Nutritional idiosyncrasies for cats. In *Canine and Feline Nutrition* 3rd edn, pp. 57–8, St Louis MO: Mosby.

3 Voith V (1994) Feeding behaviors. In J Wills, KW Simpson (eds), *The Waltham book of Clinical Nutrition of the Dog and Cat*, pp. 119–27, Tarrytown NY: Elsevier.

4 Horwitz D, Soulard Y, Junien-Castagna A (2008) The feeding behavior of the cat. In P Pibot, V Biourge, D Elliott (eds), *Encyclopedia of Feline Clinical Nutrition*, pp. 440–67, Aimarges, France: Aniwa SAS.

5 Armstrong J, Gross K, Becarova I, Debraekeleer J (2010) Introduction to feeding normal cats. In MS Hand, CD Thatcher, RI Remillard *et al.* (eds), *Small Animal Clinical Nutrition* 5th edn, pp. 321–52, Marceline, MO: Walsworth Publishing.

6 Zoran DL (2002) *The Journal of the American Veterinary Medical Association* **221**(11): 1559–66 https://avmajournals.avma.org/view/journals/javma/221/11/javma.2002.221.1559.xml. Accessed 9/5/22.

7 Welborn MB, Moldawer LL (1997) Glucose metabolism. In JL Rombeau, RH Rollandelli (eds), *Clinical Nutrition Enteral and Tube Feeding*, pp. 61–80, Philadelphia, PA: WB Saunders.

8 Wills JM (1996) Adult maintenance. In N Kelly, J Wills (eds), *Manual of Companion Animal Nutrition and Feeding*, pp. 44–6, Ames, IA: Iowa State Press.

34

Nutrition Myths

Introduction

With the ready availability of the internet, clients have even greater access to information. Where previously they had relied on information from their friends, breeders and news sources, now they can Google their source network. Unfortunately, they do not tend to "filter" the information, taking everything in their source network as gospel and do not look at the source or references. Many clients feel uncomfortable talking to their veterinary team about nutrition questions or feel that they know as much as the veterinarian and technicians do. This has led many good-intentioned clients to follow poor recommendations. Some of the more common "myths" are presented below, followed by the truth.

Myth: Meat By-Products are Inferior in Quality Compared to Whole Meat in a Diet

When listed on an ingredient label, meat is defined by the American Association of Feed Control Officials (AAFCO) as "any combination of skeletal striated muscle or that muscle found in the tongue, diaphragm, heart, esophagus with or without the accompanying and overlying fat, and the portions of the skin, sinew, nerve and blood vessels which normally accompany the muscle derived from part of whole carcasses".[1] It also must be suitable for use in animal foods. This definition **excludes** feathers, heads, feet and entrails.[2] Meat by-products are defined as "non-rendered, clean parts of the carcass which may contain lungs, spleen, kidneys, brain, liver, blood, bone, heads, feet (of poultry), partially defatted fatty tissue, stomach and intestines emptied of their contents." It does not include hair, horns, teeth or hooves.[2] Depending on the supplier and the type of refining process that the manufacturer uses, by-products can vary greatly in the amount of nondigestible material they contain.

The ash content can give you an idea of the quality of the by-products. High ash content is an indicator of a poorer quality protein with lower digestibility. The presence of by-products does not indicate a poor-quality diet, a higher ash-to-protein ratio would. Feeding trials evaluating nutrient content and digestibility will help in evaluating the quality of the ingredients. Feeding trials can establish digestibility levels. The higher the digestibility, the better the quality of the ingredients found in the diet. This information is available in most product reference guides, online references and by contacting the manufacturer.

An additional benefit to using by-products is that more of the animal carcass is used, and less is wasted. This is "greener" as less usable, nutritious product is left unused or sent to landfills.

Foods that have not undergone feeding trials will not have digestibility information available. Knowing the reputation of the

Nutrition and Disease Management for Veterinary Technicians and Nurses, Third Edition. Ann Wortinger and Kara M. Burns.
© 2024 John Wiley & Sons, Inc. Published 2024 by John Wiley & Sons, Inc.
Companion Website: www.wiley.com/go/wortinger/3e

manufacturer is your best indicator of a good quality diet.

Myth: Feeding Trials are not Necessary

The feeding trial protocol as established by the AAFCO for adult maintenance lasts 6 months, requires only 8 animals per group, and monitors a limited number of parameters. These parameters are set at the minimum nutrient requirements as defined by the National Research Council (NRC).[1,2] These levels tend to be lower than the recommended daily intake (RDI). Requirements are the minimum level of a nutrient, which over time, is sufficient to maintain the desired physiological functions of the animals in the population. RDI is the level of intake of a nutrient that is adequate to meet the known nutritional needs of practically all healthy individuals. The NRC recommendations are to serve as a guide to diet formulations, but they do not account for digestibility or nutrient availability. AAFCO feeding trials provide reasonable assurance of nutrient availability and sufficient palatability to ensure acceptability. They also provide some assurance that the product will support certain functions such as gestation, lactation and growth.[2]

A feeding trial is also the only way to accurately access the quality of the protein in a diet, as this is the only valid way to determine the digestibility of a protein, and therefore its quality. Passing a feeding trial does not ensure that the food will be effective in preventing long-term nutrition/health problems or detecting problems with a low prevalence in the general population. A feeding trial is also not designed to ensure optimal growth or maximize physical activity.

If a diet has not gone through a feeding trial by the manufacturer, you will be conducting the feeding trial for them using your patients and pets. While feeding trials especially on therapeutic diets cannot be expected to detect all deficiencies or excesses (which may also be due to disease processes, malabsorption or maldigestion) they provide an added advantage of having someone else evaluate the diets before they are fed to our patients.

Feeding trials are conducted on healthy dogs and cats, with controls that are of the same breed and gender. During the trials, the animals must receive the test food as their only source of nutrition. The same formula must be fed throughout the entire trial. The trials are conducted by measuring the daily food consumption, weekly body weight measurement, stated lab parameters measured at the end of the trial and a complete physical exam by a veterinarian at the beginning and end of the trial. A number of animals, not to exceed 25% can be removed for non-nutritional reasons or poor food intake, with a necropsy conducted on any animal which dies during the trial with findings recorded. Reproducing animals need the additional following information recorded: body weight within 24 hours of delivery, offspring's body weight within 24 hours of birth, litter size at birth, 1 day later and at end of the study, as well as a recording of any stillborn or congenital abnormalities.[1,2]

At the end of the feeding trial, the results obtained are compared to the results from a control group, a historical colony average or reference values published by the AAFCO.[1,2]

Manufacturers who follow the World Small Animal Veterinary Association (WSAVA) Nutritional Guidelines conduct feeding trials on their foods and continue to conduct them as the foods are changed and updated both for palatability and as new evidence is discovered regarding nutritional requirements.[3] Unfortunately, this is only a small segment of the pet food manufacturers.

To verify if feeding trials have been conducted on food, check the product label to find the source of AAFCO certification: if feeding trials have been done, it will be stated on the label as such. Feeding trials are designed to ensure the food meets the minimal requirements, not to ensure they are able to provide optimal results. Therefore, the quality of a diet should not be based solely on the presence of feeding trials.

Myth: Pet Food Preservatives are Bad

Preservatives are defined as any substance that is capable of inhibiting or retarding the growth of microorganisms or of masking the evidence of such deterioration.[2,4] The primary nutrient requiring protection from preservatives during storage is dietary fat. These fats can be in the form of vegetable oils, animal fats or the fat-soluble vitamins A, D, E and K. These nutrients have the potential to undergo oxidative destruction, called lipid peroxidation, during storage. Antioxidants are included in foods to prevent this lipid peroxidation.[2,4] Oxidation of fats in pet foods also results in loss of calorie content and the formation of toxic forms of peroxides that can be harmful to the health of the pets.

The Food and Drug Administration (FDA) defines an antioxidant as any substance that aids in the preservation of foods by retarding deterioration, rancidity or discoloration as the result of oxidation processes.[2,4] Various types of antioxidants have been accepted for use in human and animal foods since 1947. Antioxidants do not reverse the oxidative effects on foods once they have started, but rather retards the oxidative process and prevent the destruction of the fats in the food. Because of this, for antioxidants to be fully effective they must be included in the food when it is initially mixed and processed. This inclusion helps prevent rancidity, maintains the food's flavor, odor and texture, and prevents the accumulation of the toxic end products of lipid degradation.[2,4]

Antioxidants can be divided into two basic types-natural derived products and synthetic products. Natural-derived products are commonly found in certain grains, vegetable oils and some herbs and spices. While these products do exist in nature, all of these compounds are processed in some way to make them available for use in commercial foods. The most common naturally derived antioxidants include mixed tocopherols (vitamin E compounds), ascorbic acid (vitamin C), rosemary extract and citric acid.[2,4]

Alpha-tocopherol has the strongest biological function on tissues but is a poor antioxidant in foods. Delta and gamma-tocopherols both have low biologic activity but are more effective than alpha-tocopherol as antioxidants. Tocopherols used in foods are obtained primarily from the distillation of soybean oil residue. Tocopherols are rapidly decomposed as they protect the fat from oxidation, for this reason, food preserved with mixed tocopherols has a shorter shelf life than food preserved with a mixture of antioxidants.[4]

Ascorbic acid (vitamin C) is a water-soluble antioxidant and is not easily soluble with the fatty portion of foods. It does work synergistically with other antioxidants, such as vitamin E and butylated hydroxytoluene (BHT). Ascorbyl palmitate is similar in structure to ascorbic acid, though it is not normally found in nature. When hydrolyzed, it yields ascorbic acid and the free fatty acid (FFA) palmitic acid, both of which are natural compounds.[4]

Rosemary extract is obtained from the dried leaves of the evergreen shrub, *Rosmarinus officinalis*. It is effective as a natural-derived preservative in high-fat diets and has been shown to enhance antioxidant efficiency when combined with mixed tocopherols, ascorbic acid and citric acid. Much processing of the plant oil is needed before adding it to foods due to the taste associated with the oil affecting the taste of the food.[4]

Citric acid is found in citrus fruits such as oranges and lemons and is often included in combination with other naturally derived antioxidants.[4]

Due to the high cost of using these compounds, they are usually used in conjunction with synthetic antioxidants as preservatives in pet foods. It is difficult to attain the necessary level of naturally derived antioxidants without the food becoming cost prohibitive to the client.[4]

Synthetic antioxidants are more effective than naturally derived antioxidants and better withstand the heat, pressure and moisture during food processing, this is called "carry through." By being more effective, they better preserve the fat-soluble vitamins A, D and E for activity in the body rather than being used in food as antioxidants.[2,4]

Synthetic antioxidants include butylated hydroxy anisole (BHA), BHT, tertiary butyl-hydro quine (TBHQ) and ethoxyquin. BHA and BHT are approved for use in both human and animal foods and have a synergistic antioxidant effect when used together. BHA and BHT also have good carry-through and high efficiency in the protection of animal fats but are slightly less effective when used with vegetable oils. TBHQ is an effective antioxidant for most fats and is approved for use in human and animal foods in the United States, but is not approved for use in Canada, Japan or the European Union. Because of this, it is not usually used in pet foods sold in the international market.

Ethoxyquin has been approved for use in animal feeds for more than 40 years and has been used in pet food manufacturing for more than 25 years. It is approved for both human and animal foods, has good carry-through, and has especially high efficacy in the protection of fats in foods. Ethoxyquin is more efficient as an antioxidant than BHA or BHT, which allows lower levels to be used. It is especially effective in the protection of oils that contain elevated levels of polyunsaturated fatty acids (PUFA).[2,4]

If the use of synthetic antioxidants has clients concerned, they should be made aware that most canned foods do not contain antioxidants, and that many commercially prepared dry foods use naturally derived antioxidants. There are no studies that support the contention that synthetic antioxidants in general or ethoxyquin, in particular, are responsible for the variety of health problems reported by owners to the FDA.

The proper use of antioxidants prevents the occurrence of rancidity and the production of toxic peroxide compounds in foods. In most cases, synthetic antioxidants are the best choice because of their efficacy, good carry-through and cost. In contrast, poor carry-through, instability and the elevated levels needed for effective protection make natural-derived antioxidants difficult to use as the sole source of pet foods.[2,4]

Myth: All Foods are Created Equally

Food quality cannot be determined by the label, the commercial or the celebrity endorsement. When trying to compare two different foods whether they are canned, dry or somewhere in between, comparing products using metabolizable energy (ME) gives a better idea of caloric distribution, and allows you to accurately compare dissimilar diets. ME does not consider the digestibility of the diet in the animal; this can only be determined using feeding trials (see Table 34.1).

If the grams of nutrients/100 g of food are not given, then using the guaranteed analysis and kilocalories/100 g the following formula can be used. Remember that the guaranteed analysis only provides minimums and maximums of a small number of nutrients and is used as a reference only. Because you are not accounting for metabolic or fecal/urine losses, these values are not as accurate as the ME values (see Table 34.2).

As with human-grade foods and products, the same factory can produce multiple foods of varying quality. Factories may also produce food for multiple pet food companies. The food manufacturer does not necessarily determine the quality of the food any more than a parts manufacturer for a car determines the quality of the final product. It is also important when comparing foods to see if feeding trials

Table 34.1 To determine ME

Total calories in 100 g of food

Protein grams × 3.5 kca × l/g = protein kilocalories in food

Fat grams × 8.5 kcal/g = fats kilocalories in food

Carbohydrate grams × 3.5 kcal/g = carbohydrate kilocalories in food

Total calories/100 g – protein calorie + fat calorie + carbohydrate calorie

Percentage of ME contributed by each nutrient (caloric distribution)

Protein = (protein calories/100 g ÷ by total calories/100 g) × 100 = %ME

Fat = (fat calories/100 g ÷ by total calories/100 g) × 100 = %ME

Carbohydrate = (carbohydrate calories/100 g ÷ by total calories) × 100 = %ME

Table 34.2 Energy density from guaranteed analysis

Percentage in the diet of nutrient × modified Atwater factor = kcal/100 g of food

Divide % nutrient by total calories to get nutrient distribution

Modified Atwater factors are the amounts of energy/g of nutrient

Protein and carbohydrates are 3.5, fats are 8.5

If the kilocalories/100 g are not given, a rough estimate of the ME can be determined from the Guaranteed Analysis. This is also called a "proximate analysis" and is the same as "percent as fed."

% in diet of protein × 3.5 = protein/100 g of food

% in diet of fat × 8.5 = fat/100 g of food

To find carbohydrates: (100%−(% protein- % fat- % crude fiber- % moisture- % ash)) × 3.5 = carbohydrate/100 g of food.

Add these three numbers together to get an estimate of total calories/100 g. Calculate percent ME as above.

have been done on the product and look at digestibility if given. If a food that has not had feeding trials done by the producer is fed, then you are doing the feeding trials for them. ☺

Myth: Corn is just Filler

Botanically speaking, corn is a grain and as such can provide carbohydrates, proteins and fats to whatever animal is consuming it. The corn used in most pet foods is a type called dent corn. On average dent corn contains 70% carbohydrates, 9% protein and 4.5% oil. According to Penn State's Agronomy Guide, approximately 38.7% of the corn grown in the United States is used as livestock feed, 17.5% is exported and 34% is used to produce ethanol for energy. The remaining 9.8% is used for food.[5]

As a protein source, it has a biologic value of ~59. This means that corn contains 59% of the essential amino acids required for dogs and cats. When compared with egg (BV 100) corn is a less complete protein. Plant-based proteins typically have lower biologic values than

meat-based proteins and corn is no exception. For comparison, skeletal meat regardless of animal source has a BV of ~74, soybean meal BV of ~73, wheat BV of ~65 and white rice BV of ~64.

Biologic value is determined by the first limiting amino acid found in a food, this is the first essential amino acid that the food "runs out of" after being digested. The first limiting amino acid found in corn is lysine, the second is histidine and the last is valine.[1] A limiting amino acid just indicates that plant-based proteins need to be combined with a complementary protein to provide all the essential amino acids. This concept is not a new one and one that is used daily by many healthy human vegetarians. Many foods use multiple protein sources to improve the overall quality and amino acid profile of the final food product. Corn and soybean meal are often combined to take advantage of protein complementation.[6]

When digesting food, the animal is concerned with amino acids profile and nutrients, not with protein source or type. If all the amino acids are provided for, it makes no difference to the animal where that protein source came from.

Meat-based proteins tend to be more digestible since they lack the outside cellulose layer found in most plants, but they are more expensive to produce since the animal whose meat is being eaten must consume the plant-based protein and reassemble it into an animal protein.[6]

The time to harvest for most types of corn is 65–90 days. For most meat-based protein sources, who eat corn to obtain their amino acids to make their protein the time to harvest can be as low as 16–20 weeks for chickens to as long as 2 years for cattle. Obviously, the longer it takes to obtain the final product, the more expensive the protein source will become.

As a "green-conscious" and economical protein, carbohydrate and fat source, corn is hard to beat. Corn also contains high levels of PUFA, B vitamins, minerals and natural antioxidants that can benefit the animal consuming it; this is hardly the description of a "filler."[6]

Conclusion

Once clients are given the facts regarding pet foods, all our jobs should become easier! A well-informed client is our best friend. With the proper information, they will be able to pick a pet food that contains quality ingredients, has undergone feeding trials, and is properly preserved so that all the ingredients are available to their pet. They may also learn that their veterinary team is the best source for nutrition information.

References

1 Case LP, Carey DP, Hirakawa DA, Daristotle L (2011) Digestion and absorption. In *Canine and Feline Nutrition* (3rd edn), pp. 45–52, St Louis, MO: Mosby.

2 Gross K, Wedekind KJ, Cowell CS *et al.* (2000; pp 58–60, 140–146, 167–169) Nutrients. Making commercial pet foods. Making pet foods at home. In MS Hand, CD Thatcher, RL Remillard, P Roudebush (eds), *Small Animal Clinical Nutrition* (4th edn), Marceline, MO: Walsworth Publishing.

3 WSAVA 2011. Nutritional Guidelines. https://wsava.org/global-guidelines/global-nutrition-guidelines/. Accessed 9/5/22.

4 Case LP, Carey DP, Hirakawa DA, Daristotle L (2011) Nutrient content of pet foods. In *Canine and Feline Nutrition* (3rd edn), pp. 141–60, St Louis, MO: Mosby.

5 Penn State Agronomy Guide (2021). Part 1, Section 4: Corn. http://agguide.agronomy.psu.edu/cm/sec4/sec41.cfm. Accessed 9/5/22.

6 Gross Kathy L, Jewell Dennis E, Yamka Ryan M *et al.* (2010) Macronutrients. In MS Hand, CD Thatcher, RI Remillard *et al.* (eds), *Small Animal Clinical Nutrition* (5th edn), pp. 89–96, Marceline, MO: Walsworth Publishing.

35

Cost of Feeding

Introduction

The cost of feeding a specific food can be determined by the cost per bag or can, the cost per day to feed or the cost per meal to feed. These will depend on the animal's individual daily energy requirements (DER) requirements, and any disease processes that may or may not be present.

Cost per Bag-Dry Food

Clients will often look only at the cost per bag to determine the best value or quality of the food. This can be misleading because the caloric content and the nutritional value may not be the same between products. Canned foods tend to be higher cost per meal because of the added water, and the cost associated with canning the food. Foods that need to be kept in the refrigerator, also accrue additional, unseen costs due to the energy needed to keep the food cold.

While the 46# bag that is only $27 may seem like a good value, when you look at the AAFCO certification, you may find that no feeding trials have been done and that the food only contains 340 kcal/cup.

If we have a 25# active, *m/n* Beagle, his RER would be:

25# ÷ 2.2 = 11.36 kg
RER = (wt in kg × 30) + 70 = 411 kcals
(wt in kg)$^{0.75}$ × 70 = 433 kcals
Moderately active = DER of 1.3
DER = RER × 1.3 =

411 × 1.3 = 534 kcals/day
433 × 1.3 = 563 kcals/day
Kcals/day ÷ kcals/cup of food =
534/340 = 1.57 cups/day
563/340 = 1.65 cups/day

Interestingly, the package feeding directions recommend that a 26# dog be fed 1.75 cups of food, above what we have calculated, and if our dog was inactive, this would be too much food fed daily, contributing to the potential for obesity.

Alternatively, we can determine the cost/ pound of food by dividing the number of pounds by the cost.

46#/$27 = $1.70/pound of food
46#/2.2 = 20.9 kg/$27 = $0.77/kg of food

Many times, a client will want to know how many meals can be fed from each bag.

There is approximately 4 cups/ pound of dry dog food.

46# × 4 = 184 cups/46# bag of food

Our Beagle needs between 1.57 – 1.65 cups/day.

184/1.57 = 117 days/30 days = 3.9 months
184/1.65 = 111 days/ 30 days = 3.7 months

The daily cost to feed this diet can be determined by taking the $27 and dividing this by the 184 cups/bag.

$27/184 = $0.15/cup =

We know our Beagle should be fed 1.57 – 1.63 cups/day

1.57 cups × 0.15 = $0.24/day
1.63 cups × 0.15 = $0.24/day

Let's calculated the cost to feed an 8# intact female cat, with a DER of 1.4.

Nutrition and Disease Management for Veterinary Technicians and Nurses, Third Edition. Ann Wortinger and Kara M. Burns.
© 2024 John Wiley & Sons, Inc. Published 2024 by John Wiley & Sons, Inc.
Companion Website: www.wiley.com/go/wortinger/3e

8#/2.2 = 3.6 kg

RER

Wt in kg × 40 = 3.6 × 40 = 144 kcals

$(\text{Wt in kg})^{0.75} \times 70 = 183$ kcals

DER 144 – 183 × 1.4 = 202 – 256 kcals/day

A dry diet has also been selected for this 8# cat. The food is available in an 8# bag, that costs $25/bag. Each cup of food is 375 kcals/cup.

DER = 202 – 256 kcals/day

Cups/day = 202 – 256 ÷ 375 kcals/cup = 0.54 – 0.68 cups/day

An 8# bag of food will have approximately 32 cups.

Each cup of food would cost:

$25/32 cups = $0.78/cup

For our 8# cat, who is fed 0.54 – 0.68 cups/day would cost

0.54 cups × $0.78 = $0.42/day

0.68 cups × $0.78 = $0.53/day

These estimates only work if no other food or treats are being fed, including table scraps.

By using the cost of the food, and the volume of food fed, the cost per meal can be determined for any dry food.

Cost per Can

Our Beagle client has picked a canned diet that costs $42.00/12 can case. Each can is 13.5 oz, and 386 kcals/can.

Keeping with our Beagle, with a DER of 534 – 563 kcals/day.

534 kcals/386 kcals/can = 1.38 cans/day

563 kcals/386 kcals/can = 1.45 cans/day

Cost/can is: $42/12 = $3.5/can

Cost/day = 1.38 × $3.5 = $4.83/day

1.45 × $3.5 = $5.07/day

Our client with the 8# cat would like to feed a food that is $2 for each 3.5 oz can, and each can contains 100 kcals.

202 – 256 = 2 – 2.5 can/day

2 – 2.5 cans × $2 = $4 – 5/day

As previously stated, we can see that feeding a canned food diet is more expensive than feeding a bargain brand dry food.

Conclusion

These calculation techniques can be used for both OTC foods and therapeutic diets, and can be used to demonstrate to the client that a therapeutic diet may not be as expensive to feed as the client thought. I will often let clients know, that by utilizing a therapeutic diet, we may be able to use fewer prescription medications, further decreasing the client's overall cost to treat their pet.

Section IV

Nutritional Disease Management for Dogs and Cats

36

Nutritional Management of Gastrointestinal Disorders

In veterinary hospitals around the world, gastrointestinal (GI) problems are one of the most common reasons that pet parents bring their pets to the hospital. The main challenge to the veterinary healthcare team presented with a pet that has GI dysfunction is to determine whether an emergency situation exists or is the presentation leading to a potentially serious problem versus a chronic or intermittent problem. The GI tract is known for its resiliency, and the veterinary healthcare team has seen numerous pets with clinical signs of acute vomiting and/or diarrhea resolve uneventfully, sometimes without any supportive care. However, this is not true of all acute GI events as some may be life-threatening disorders, which if not identified and treated, could lead to poor patient management and/or death of the pet.

Vomiting is a clinical sign seen frequently in small animals, and vomiting is associated with GI disorders; however, vomiting may occur with nongastrointestinal conditions as well. Thus, it is difficult to identify the etiology of the vomiting and may require extensive diagnostic workup in some dogs and cats. Vomiting is the forceful discharge of ingested material from the stomach and sometimes proximal small intestines. Vomiting consists of three stages: nausea, retching, and subsequently vomiting. Nausea is the first stage. Outward signs of nausea for which the healthcare team should be aware may include depression, shivering, hiding, yawning, and licking of the lips. Increased salivation and swallowing occur, subsequently lubricating the esophagus. Retching often helps distinguish the episode from regurgitation, gagging, or coughing. Retching is the forceful contraction of the abdominal muscles and diaphragm. Negative intrathoracic pressure and positive abdominal pressure changes cause the movement of gastric contents into the esophagus and out of the mouth. This vomiting process is initiated by the central nervous system.

In addition to vomiting, diarrhea is one of the most common reasons owners bring their pets to the veterinary hospital. Diarrhea is the passage of feces containing an excessive amount of water thus resulting in an abnormal increase in stool liquidity and weight. Patients may also experience an increase in the frequency of their defecation. This would lead to the broad description of too rapid evacuation of too loose stools. It is important for the veterinary technician to gain a thorough understanding of the owner's definition of diarrhea as it may not be as accurate as the healthcare team's definition. This would incorporate a very involved discussion with the owner while gathering the history. Diarrhea is the trademark sign of intestinal dysfunction. It is important for healthcare team members to determine acute from chronic problems when assessing animals with diarrhea. Acute diarrhea is typically the result of diet, parasites, or infectious diseases (e.g., parvovirus, coronavirus, etc.). Diarrhea is termed chronic when it has not responded to conventional therapy within a two to three week time frame.

Nutrition and Disease Management for Veterinary Technicians and Nurses, Third Edition. Ann Wortinger and Kara M. Burns.
© 2024 John Wiley & Sons, Inc. Published 2024 by John Wiley & Sons, Inc.
Companion Website: www.wiley.com/go/wortinger/3e

Table 36.1 Identifying small and large intestine signs in gastrointestinal disease.

Sign	Small intestine	Large intestine
Feces volume	Normal to ↑	↓
Blood in feces	Dark, black/tarry (if present)	Frank blood (if present)
Mucus in feces	Not common	Common
Tenesmus	Absent	Present
Dyschezia	Not common	Present
Urgency of defecation	Normal	↑
Frequency of defecation	Normal to ↑	↑
Concurrent vomiting	May be present	Not common
Concurrent weight loss	Common	Not common
Status of appetite	Normal or altered	Generally normal

The next step is to determine the origination of the diarrhea – small intestine or large intestine (see Table 36.1). A thorough history by the veterinary technician is again the best tool. Increased frequency of defecation resulting in larger than normal amounts of soft-to-watery stool is often seen in small bowel diarrhea. Failure to lose weight or body condition is typically indicative of large bowel disease. Weight loss usually indicates small bowel disease although severe large bowel diseases such as malignancy, histoplasmosis, and pythiosis may result in weight loss. Animals with weight loss from severe large bowel disease usually have signs associated with colonic involvement such as fecal mucus, marked tenesmus, and hematochezia. Fresh blood (bright red in color) in the stool or evidence that the pet is straining to defecate is indicative of a large bowel disorder. Hematochezia (bright-red blood) typically originates in the anus, rectum, or descending colon. Melena is described as coal tar black stools that result from digested blood. Melena may originate from the pharynx, lungs (coughed up and swallowed), esophagus, stomach, or upper small intestine. Tarry stools are the result of bacterial breakdown of hemoglobin. Dyschezia is difficult and/or painful defecation. Tenesmus refers to persistent and/or prolonged straining, typically with no effect. Owners may mistake tenesmus for constipation, so it is important to question the owner further to determine which clinical sign truly is manifesting in their pet. Dyschezia and tenesmus are most often associated with large bowel disorders.

Assessment

A complete history is the first step (and it is a crucial step) in trying to establish a cause for vomiting and diarrhea. The signalment and history, as well as a description of the vomiting and/or diarrhea episodes, are important. Figure 36.1 Fecal scoring chart. This chart aids owners in describing their pet's stool form. When inquiring about the patient's vomiting status, first, one must determine whether the animal truly is vomiting. The healthcare team should differentiate the owner's report of vomiting from gagging, coughing, dysphagia, or regurgitation. The description of retching is characteristic of vomiting. Signalment may also be helpful. For example, young, unvaccinated pets are more susceptible to infectious diseases, such as parvovirus. Vaccination status, travel history, previous medical problems, and medication history should be determined. Many drugs can result in vomiting, such as nonsteroidal anti-inflammatory drugs (NSAIDs), which are known to cause GI ulceration and vomiting. The healthcare team member should also explore the possibility of toxin or foreign body ingestion and of other

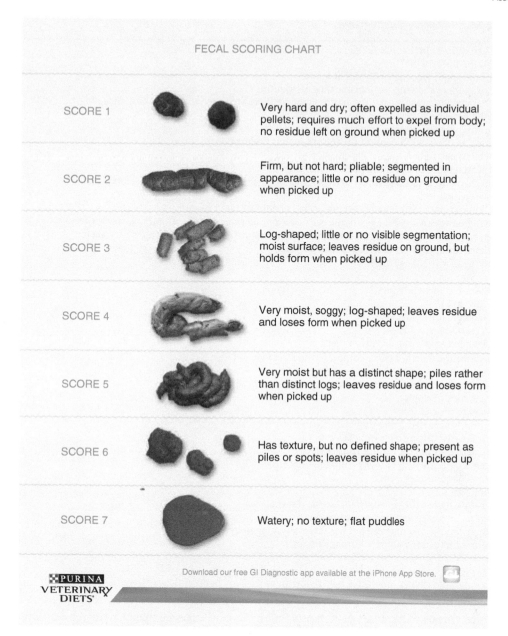

FECAL SCORING CHART

SCORE 1 — Very hard and dry; often expelled as individual pellets; requires much effort to expel from body; no residue left on ground when picked up

SCORE 2 — Firm, but not hard; pliable; segmented in appearance; little or no residue on ground when picked up

SCORE 3 — Log-shaped; little or no visible segmentation; moist surface; leaves residue on ground, but holds form when picked up

SCORE 4 — Very moist, soggy; log-shaped; leaves residue and loses form when picked up

SCORE 5 — Very moist but has a distinct shape; piles rather than distinct logs; leaves residue and loses form when picked up

SCORE 6 — Has texture, but no defined shape; present as piles or spots; leaves residue when picked up

SCORE 7 — Watery; no texture; flat puddles

Download our free GI Diagnostic app available at the iPhone App Store.

PURINA VETERINARY DIETS

Figure 36.1 Fecal scoring chart. (Permission from Nestlé Purina).

concurrent signs that often arise with systemic or metabolic disease. For example: polydipsia, polyuria, and weight loss are typical of vomiting associated with diabetic ketoacidosis or chronic kidney failure.

The history should then focus on the actual vomiting episodes. The duration, frequency, and relationship of the episodes to eating or drinking should be ascertained. Table 36.2 GI history questionnaire. A complete physical description of the vomited material should be documented. A dietary history, including the type of diet or recent dietary changes, is important because vomiting may

Table 36.2 GI history questionnaire.

- When did you first notice GI signs/issues?
- Was the onset acute?
- Tell me about any other animals at home.
  - Are others showing signs of diarrhea or vomiting?
- Tell me about areas the patient has been where there are other animals? Obedience, dog parks, pet stores, pet shows, etc.
- Has there been access to drinking from a pond or streams?
- Describe the environment where the pet spends their time.
- Breed of pet.
- Typical temperament of the pet?
- Did the pet get into/ingest any of the following: trash, toxins, other pet foods, foods that have spoiled, etc.
- Tell me of any medications been prescribed or administered recently.
- Have there been any changes in the pet's environment that may be stressful to the pet? New pet, change in family dynamics, alteration in home environment, boarding, daycare, etc.
- Tell me what your pet eats in a 24 hour period.
- Tell me of any change in diet.
  - Dry to can?
  - New bag or case of food?
  - Raw food?
  - Homemade food?
  - Treats? Be specific
  - People foods? Added? Part of diet?
- Describe the diarrhea (size, volume of the feces)
- Consistency of stool? Watery? Soft, formed
- Are there any normal stools passed during the day?
- Frequency of stools?
- Blood or mucus seen?
- Timing? Increased defecation? Unable to make it outside?
  - Increased during nighttime? Urgency?
  - If feline – does the cat use litterbox?
- Does it defecate near or away from the litterbox?
- Other symptoms present?
- Vomiting
- How often does the pet vomit? Describe the vomitus?
- Can the pet keep any food or water down?
- When was the last time the pet has taken anything in by mouth?
- Other family in the home – human, animal?

be associated with an adverse reaction to food. Vomiting of an undigested or a partly digested meal more than 6–8 hours after eating, a time at which the stomach should normally be empty, suggests a gastric outflow obstruction or gastric hypomotility disorder. The description of the vomit should include the volume, color, consistency, odor, and the presence or absence of bile or blood. Undigested food suggests a gastric origin, whereas vomit-containing bile makes a gastric outflow obstruction unlikely. Vomit having a fecal odor is suggestive of a low-intestinal obstruction or bacterial overgrowth in the small intestine. Hematemesis (either as fresh, bright-red blood or as digested blood with the appearance of coffee grounds) is indicative of GI erosion or ulceration. Gastric ulceration is caused by metabolic conditions such as hypoadrenocorticism, reaction to certain drugs, clotting abnormalities, gastritis, or neoplasia.

A complete physical examination should begin with an evaluation of the mouth and oral cavity. The presence of a fever is suggestive of an infectious or inflammatory process. Bradycardia or cardiac arrhythmias in a vomiting animal may be a sign of a metabolic disturbance, such as hypoadrenocorticism. Careful palpation of the abdomen should be part of the physical examination to rule out; distention or tympany (e.g., gastric dilatation–volvulus [GDV] syndrome), effusion (e.g., peritonitis), masses or organomegaly (e.g., neoplasia, intussusception, or foreign body), and pain (e.g., peritonitis, pancreatitis, or intestinal obstruction). Obstruction is suggested when there are gas- and fluid-filled intestines, whereas, bunching of the bowel is characteristic of intestinal plication from a linear foreign body obstruction. A rectal examination provides characteristics of colonic mucosa and feces. Melena suggests upper-gastrointestinal bleeding while the presence of foreign material in the feces supports a possible foreign body etiology.

Performing a complete blood count (CBC) is extremely important for GI patients, especially in those animals at risk for neutropenia (e.g., parvoviral enteritis), infection, and anemia (e.g., melena and hemataemesis). Patients should also have a serum chemistry profile performed upon presentation. A serum biochemistry profile, especially in patients presenting with severe vomiting, diarrhea, ascites, unexplained weight loss, and/or anorexia should include alanine transaminase, alkaline phosphatase, blood urea nitrogen, creatinine, total protein, albumin, total CO_2, cholesterol, calcium, phosphorous, magnesium, bilirubin, and glucose concentrations, along with electrolytes; sodium, chloride, and potassium.

Vomiting may result in significant fluid, electrolyte, and acid–base alterations. The most common electrolyte disturbance in vomiting cats and dogs is hypokalemia. Acid–base changes generally are minimal or, if abnormal, tend toward acidosis. If metabolic alkalosis is identified and is associated with hyponatremia, hypochloremia, and hypokalemia, the most likely cause will be gastric outflow or high-duodenal obstruction. Rarely animals with gastrinomas or with frequent and unrelenting vomiting have metabolic alkalosis. When routine diagnostic testing fails to identify an obvious etiology, additional tests may be necessary. Additional tests may include viral or heartworm serology, thyroid hormone testing, adrenocortical testing for hypoadrenocorticism, bile–acid determination for liver disease, toxicologic testing (e.g., lead poisoning), and a neurologic examination.

When testing fails to identify a nongastrointestinal cause for the vomiting, the focus should move to an investigation of GI disease as a possible etiology. The diagnostic approach includes contrast radiography, ultrasonography, endoscopy, or laparotomy. Frequently, inflammatory GI lesions are a cause of chronic vomiting; these conditions include chronic gastritis, *Helicobacter* gastritis, inflammatory bowel disease (IBD), and chronic colitis. Cats with IBD often have vomiting as the main clinical sign and diarrhea as a minor clinical component. Conditions such as gastric antral pyloric mucosal hypertrophy, antral polyps, foreign bodies, or neoplasia can cause gastric outflow obstruction. These conditions cause gastric retention and vomiting. Such gastric lesions can be easily identified endoscopically or using contrast radiography.

Nutritional Factors

Following a diagnosis by the veterinarian, the vomiting and/or diarrhea will need to be managed. The healthcare team should be cognizant of key nutritional factors and their impact when managing a patient nutritionally. Nutritional management of patients suffering from vomiting and/or diarrhea should consider the following nutritional factors:

Water

Water is extremely important when working with patients with acute vomiting and diarrhea due to the potential for life-threatening dehydration from excess fluid loss and inability of the patient to replace the lost fluid. Patients with persistent nausea and vomiting should be supported with subcutaneous or intravenous rather than oral fluids. Where applicable, moderate to severe dehydration should be corrected with appropriate parenteral fluid therapy.

Electrolytes

Gastric and intestinal secretions differ from extracellular fluids in electrolyte composition, so their loss can result in systemic electrolyte abnormalities. Dogs and cats presenting with vomiting and diarrhea may have abnormal serum potassium, chloride, and sodium concentrations. Serum electrolyte concentrations are useful in tailoring appropriate fluid therapy and nutritional management for these patients. Mild hypokalemia, hypochloremia, and either hypernatremia or hyponatremia are the electrolyte abnormalities most commonly associated with acute vomiting (and diarrhea). Initially, electrolyte disorders should be addressed and corrected with appropriate parenteral fluid and electrolyte therapy. Patients experiencing vomiting and/or diarrhea should begin nutritional therapy ideally containing levels of potassium, chloride, and sodium above the minimum allowances for normal dogs and cats. Recommended levels of these nutrients are 0.8%–1.1% potassium (dry matter [DM]), 0.5%–1.3% DM chloride, and 0.3%–0.5% DM sodium).

Protein

Protein and amino acids are essential for synthesis and repair of tissue. Additionally, they play a role in energy metabolism. Although all proteins are functional, protein is the second largest potential store of energy in the body following adipose tissue. Energy and protein needs are tied together. Amino acids from protein can be converted to glucose by gluconeogenesis; thus, serving as a continuing supply of glucose after consumption of glycogen during fasting. The main route in which

protein enters the body is through the GI tract. The availability of dietary protein and the ability of the GI tract to digest and absorb protein are the two factors that maintain protein balance in the body. Subsequently, disorders which affect protein absorption can quickly deplete protein stores in the body and lead to protein malnutrition. Protein malnutrition has harmful effects on numerous body functions, including muscle strength, organ function, and immune function. Protein malnutrition can also result in mucosal atrophy in the GI tract; this further impairs protein absorption.

Nutritional therapy for patients exhibiting vomiting and/or diarrhea should probably not provide excess protein (no more than 30% for dogs and 40% for cats). Products of protein digestion (peptides, amino acids, and amines) increase gastrin and gastric acid secretion. "Hypoallergenic" or elimination foods for patients with vomiting/diarrhea have been recommended as dietary antigens are suspected to play a role in the etiopathogenesis.

Ideal elimination foods should: (1) avoid protein excess (16%–26% for dogs; 30%–40% for cats), (2) have high protein digestibility (≥87%), and (3) contain a limited number of novel protein sources to which the patient has never been exposed. Additionally, a food containing a protein hydrolysate may be utilized in nutritional management of the patient.

Glutamine

Glutamine is considered a conditionally essential nutrient under stress conditions, such as starvation, infection, injury, and recovery from surgery. Glutamine fuels enterocytes lining the small intestinal epithelium, providing as much as 40% of the energy needed for enterocytes. Glutamine is also used by white blood cells and contributes to normal immune system function. Additionally, this amino acid is involved in essential processes such as nucleotide synthesis, protein synthesis, and gluconeogenesis. Dietary glutamine supplementation reduces enterocyte and lymphocyte susceptibility to apoptosis while concurrently improving antioxidative function and cell proliferation in the small intestine.

Arginine

Arginine is another important amino acid which plays an important role in promoting immune system function. Arginine also serves as a precursor for nitric oxide (NO), polyamines, and creatine and plays a major role in cell growth and proliferation.

Arginine stimulates intestinal fluid secretion through a NO-mediated mechanism. Inhibition of NO synthase (NOS) leads to decreased intestinal secretion and intestinal ischemia. Arginine supplementation is also effective in improving intestinal barrier function and vascular development.

Rats fed an arginine-enriched diet have seen:

– increased protection of the gut mucosa from injury caused by radiation-induced enteritis
– accelerated healing ability
– prevention of translocation of bacteria.

Remember, the beneficial effects of arginine may be dose-dependent. In fact, higher doses of dietary arginine ($\sim$1.2%) can cause adverse effects such as gut dysfunction.

Fat

Dietary fat is one of the most complex nutrients to process in the GI tract. Dietary fat can play a very important role in the management of GI disorders. Some disorders respond best to low-fat diets, whereas others respond best to medium- or high-fat diets. Not only is the amount of fat in the diet important, but the type of fat is also important in determining its effect in the GI tract. Solids and liquids higher in fat empty more slowly from the stomach than comparable foods with less fat. Fat in the duodenum stimulates the release of cholecystokinin, which delays gastric emptying. Foods with less than 15% DM fat for dogs and less than 25% DM fat for cats are appropriate for dietary management.

Carbohydrates

Dogs and cats do not have a definitive dietary requirement for carbohydrates. However, carbohydrates are a major part of most diets for dogs and cats. Mainly, the carbohydrate found in pet food is starch. The storage form of carbohydrates in plants is starch, while the storage form in animals is glycogen. Digestibility is key when discussing dietary starch and digestibility is dependent upon the carbohydrate source, the degree of processing, and the type of processing. Properly processed, corn, wheat, rice, and barley can be extremely digestible (>90%). Other starches, such as potato and tapioca, are less digestible, especially if undercooked.

Fiber

Although not digestible, dietary fiber is considered to have nutritional value due to its importance in maintaining the functional integrity of the GI tract. Specific fiber types can be utilized for specific effects on the GI tract. Major components of dietary fiber include:

– non starch polysaccharides
– cellulose
– hemicellulose
– mixed-linkage β-glucans
– pectins
– gums
– mucilages.

Lignins are also included in total dietary fiber as they are plant cell wall constituents that can greatly affect the digestibility of plant-derived foods. Categorizing fiber types based on fermentability describes specific fiber sources for dogs and cats because the capacity for fiber breakdown by intestinal bacteria is a more accurate assessment of fiber's potential beneficial effects in the GI tract.

Foods containing gel-forming soluble fibers should be avoided in vomiting and/or diarrhea patients as these fibers increase the viscosity of ingesta and slow gastric emptying. These fibers include pectins and gums (e.g., gum arabic, guar gum, carrageenan, psyllium gum, xanthan gum, carob gum, gum ghatti, and gum tragacanth). Overall, the crude fiber content should not exceed more than 5% DM.

Food Form and Temperature

Moist foods are considered to be the best form since they reduce gastric retention time. For the same reason, the veterinary health-care team should educate clients to warm foods between room and body temperature (70–100°F (21–38°C)).

Vitamins and Trace Minerals

Vitamin abnormalities may be associated with GI disorders, including alterations in metabolism of folate and cobalamin (vitamin B12). Decreases in serum folate concentrations can be associated with proximal small intestinal disorders. Decreases in serum cobalamin concentrations may be associated with distal small intestinal disorders and exocrine pancreatic disease. In diffuse small intestinal disease, serum folate and cobalamin may be decreased. Thus, the veterinary team should keep these two vitamin abnormalities in mind for patients with chronic diarrhea and an unthrifty, unkempt appearance – especially cats.

Iron, copper, and B vitamins may benefit patients with gastroduodenal ulceration and GI blood loss. Hematinics should be used in patients with nonregenerative, microcytic/hypochromic anemias attributable to iron deficiency. However, they probably are not necessary in most animals that have received a blood transfusion.

GI Bacterial Ecosystem

Companion animals have vast GI bacterial ecosystems. A mammal's digestive system has more than 500 different species of bacteria. The overall health of the animal is affected by the balance between beneficial and pathogenic bacteria. Thus, the microbial population in the GI tract is acknowledged to play a significant role in the health of animals, and its role appears to extend beyond the GI tract. Many of the extragastrointestinal effects appear to be related to alterations in the immune system. Enteric bacteria also influence the patient's resistance to infectious disease. A healthy gut bacterial flora is critical for overall health, and this flora is often disrupted during illnesses and may, in some cases, be a precipitating factor.

Acid Load

Alkalemia should be expected if vomiting patients lose hydrogen and chloride ions in excess of sodium and bicarbonate. Hypochloremia perpetuates the alkalosis by increasing renal bicarbonate reabsorption. A common finding is mild alkalemia in vomiting patients; however, profound alkalemia is more likely to occur with pyloric or upper duodenal obstruction. Acidemia may occur in vomiting patients if the vomited gastric fluid is relatively low in hydrogen and chloride ion content (e.g., during fasting) or if concurrent loss of intestinal sodium and bicarbonate occurs. It is best to correct severe acid–base disorders with parenteral fluid and electrolyte therapy. Foods for patients with acute vomiting and diarrhea should avoid excess dietary acid load. Foods that normally produce alkaline urine are less likely to be associated with acidosis.

Summary

GI disorders are a common reason for pet parents to bring their pets to the hospital. It is essential for the veterinary healthcare team to identify these clinical signs and perform a complete history and evaluation regarding these frequent signs when pets present. Nutritional management is a crucial part of therapy in the management of vomiting and/or diarrhea. Certain key nutritional factors play a role in managing vomiting and diarrhea in cats and dogs – through enteral and parenteral nutrition – and veterinary technicians should recognize the circumstances and reasoning for the key nutritional factors (KNFs) to ensure a positive outcome for the vomiting and diarrheic patient.

Further Reading

Allenspach K, Gaschein FP (2008) Small intestinal disease. In JM Steiner (ed.), *Small Animal Gastroenterology*, pp. 187–202, Germany: Schlutersche.

Burns KM (2012) Gastrointestinal disorders. In L Merrill (ed.), *Internal Medicine for Veterinary Technicians*, Ames, IA: Wiley-Blackwell.

Chandler ML (2013) Nutritional approach to gastrointestinal disease. In RJ Washabau, MJ Day (eds), *Canine and Feline Gastroenterology*, pp. 386–444, St. Louis: Elsevier.

Davenport DJ, Remilliard RL (2010a) Introduction to small intestinal disease. In MS Hand, CD Thatcher, RL Remilliard *et al.* (eds), *Small Animal Clinical Nutrition* (5th edn), pp. 1047–9, Marceline MO: Walsworth Publishing, Mark Morris Institute.

Davenport DJ, Remillard RL (2010b) Acute gastroenteritis and enteritis. In MS Hand, CD Thatcher, RL Remilliard *et al.* (eds), *Small Animal Clinical Nutrition* (5th edn), pp. 1053–61, Marceline MO: Walsworth Publishing, Mark Morris Institute.

Grimble GK (2007) Adverse gastrointestinal effects of arginine and related amino acids. *J Nutr.* **137**: 1693S–701S.

Hall EJ, German AJ (2010) Diseases of the small intestine. In SJ Ettinger, EC Feldman (eds), *Textbook of Veterinary Internal Medicine* (7th edn), pp. 1526–72, St Loius, MO: Elsevier.

Lenox CE (2021) Nutritional management for dogs and cats with gastrointestinal diseases. *Veterinary Clinics of North America: Small Animal Practice* **51**(3): 669–84.

Rudinsky AJ, Rowe JC, Parker VJ (2018) Nutritional management of chronic enteropathies in dogs and cats. *J Am Vet Med Assoc.* **253**: 570–8.

Sanderson SL (2013) Gastrointestinal Tract. In RJ Washabau, MJ Day (eds), *Canine and Feline Gastroenterology*, pp. 409–28, St. Louis: Elsevier.

Tams TR (2003) Chronic diseases of the small intestine. In TR Tams (ed.), *Handbook of Small Animal Gastroenterology* (2nd edn), pp. 211–50, St Louis, MO: Saunders.

Toresson L, Burns KM (2018) Nutritional assessment in a dog with chronic enteropathy. *Clinician's Brief*, April: 26–9.

Willard MD (2009) Disorders of the intestinal tract. In *Small Animal Internal Medicine* (4th edn), pp. 441–76, St Louis, MO: Mosby.

Witzel A (2018) Diarrhea, vomiting, and food, oh my! Nutritional management for gastrointestinal disease. *Today's Vet Pract.* **8**: 18–20.

37

Critical Care Nutrition

Historically, nutritional support of critically ill patients has been considered a supportive measure of low priority. However, advances in both human and veterinary medicine have demonstrated that nutritional support is an important therapeutic modality and can aid in the management of diseases. In diseased states, the inflammatory response triggers alterations in cytokines and hormone concentrations and shifts metabolism toward a catabolic state. With insufficient food intake, the predominant energy source is derived from accelerated proteolysis, which in itself is an energy-consuming process. Thus, critically ill animals may preserve fat deposits in the face of lean muscle tissue loss. The goal of nutritional support in these catabolic patients is to feed the catabolism with exogenous sources of protein and fat thus sparing endogenous protein which is critical to recovery.

Malnutrition in veterinary patients is believed to increase morbidity and mortality. In the gastrointestinal (GI) tract, transit times increase, absorptive capabilities decrease, villi atrophy, and there is an increased risk of bacterial translocation. In the kidneys, excretion of urinary calcium and phosphorus increases, ability to excrete acid decreases, gluconeogenesis increases, and glomerular filtration rate decreases. Malnutrition has been documented to decrease humoral immunity and barrier function (skin and mucosal surfaces), inflammatory response, leukocyte motility, and bactericidal activity. Patients are at risk for pulmonary complications as a result of decreased response to hypoxia, decreased lung elasticity, and secretion production, altered permeability, and decreased tidal volume. Cardiovascular complications include increased incidence of arrhythmias and decreased weight of the heart muscle. Protein malnutrition may also alter the normal or expected metabolism of certain drugs, which may increase or decrease their therapeutic effect even when given at recommended dosages.

What Patients Should be Fed?

In the past, nutritional support was not considered necessary until animals had inadequate intake for 10 days. This concept currently is outdated and unfounded. Evidence suggests a more appropriate goal in most cases is to initiate nutritional support within three days of hospitalization (at the latest). Evaluating nutritional status may be challenging for healthcare team members. Historical weight loss may provide some evidence of inadequate intake and body condition scoring may be helpful to assess fat loss but is not as sensitive for muscle wasting. Laboratory abnormalities may not be present or may be nonspecific. Because of the limitations in assessing nutritional status, early risk factors must be identified that predispose patients to malnutrition. The risk factors to consider are:

- a history of inadequate nutritional intake lasting more than five days

Nutrition and Disease Management for Veterinary Technicians and Nurses, Third Edition. Ann Wortinger and Kara M. Burns.
© 2024 John Wiley & Sons, Inc. Published 2024 by John Wiley & Sons, Inc.
Companion Website: www.wiley.com/go/wortinger/3e

- serious underlying disease (e.g., severe trauma, sepsis, peritonitis, acute pancreatitis, and major GI surgery)
- large protein losses (e.g., protracted vomiting, diarrhea, protein-losing nephropathies, draining wounds, and burns).

Patients with these risk factors are candidates for nutritional support.

As with any intervention in critically ill animals, nutritional support may pose some risk. The risk of complications increases with disease severity. To minimize risks, patients must be cardiovascularly stable before nutritional support begins. If the patient is found to be in shock, perfusion of the GI tract is reduced in favor of maintaining adequate perfusion of heart, brain, and lungs. With reduced perfusion, processes such as GI motility, digestion, and nutrient assimilation are altered, increasing the chance of complications. In addition, feeding should be delayed until preexisting fluid and electrolyte abnormalities are corrected to avoid exacerbating GI hypoxia secondary to increasing cellular metabolism and to prevent hypophosphatemia and hypokalemia related to refeeding syndrome (see Chapter 44 Refeeding Syndrome).

How Should the Patient be Fed?

The GI tract needs to be fed. The gut receives an overwhelming percentage of its nutrition from the chyme passing through it. In the small intestine, enterocytes utilize luminal glutamine preferentially as their source of metabolic fuel. The colonocytes prefer butyrate, a short-chain fatty acid formed by fermentation of luminal carbohydrates. In the absence of these fuel sources, the gut epithelium slows growth and replication resulting in atrophy, necrosis, and increased risk of bacterial translocation across the now abnormal gut barrier. A key to prevention of this potentially serious problem is providing nutritional support to the gut. The rule of nutritional support is "if the gut works use it."

Force-feeding sick, hospitalized animals is not ideal and is the best way to create food aversions. Force feeding is an inefficient feeding method resulting in more nutrients on the patient and the healthcare team member rather than in the patient. Typically force feeding will not provide a significant percent of needed calories and will lead to a false sense of accomplishment and continued inadequate intake. Similarly, appetite stimulants are seldom successful in causing meaningful increases in food intake. Pharmacologic stimulation of appetite is often short-lived and only delays true nutritional support. Appetite stimulants should not be used to manage hospitalized animals when more effective measures of nutritional support, such as placement of feeding tubes, are more appropriate. Appetite stimulants may be considered in recovering animals once they are home in their own environment because the primary reason for loss of appetite should ideally be reversed by discharge. As with many drugs, appetite stimulants also have negative side effects, such as behavioral changes associated with cyproheptadine and sedation associated with diazepam, and therefore should be used with caution.

An indwelling feeding tube is the method of choice if enteral-assisted feeding is necessary for more than two days. After an indwelling tube has been placed, feeding is easier and less stressful. Nasoesophageal (NE), esophagostomy, gastrostomy, and jejunostomy feeding tubes are the most commonly used. In animals undergoing laparotomy, placing gastrotomy or jejunostomy feeding tubes should be considered. The decision to use one tube over another is based on the anticipated duration of nutritional support (e.g., days versus months), the need to circumvent certain segments of the GI tract (e.g., oropharynx, esophagitis, and pancreatitis), clinician experience, and the patient's ability to withstand anesthesia (very critical animals may only tolerate placement of NE feeding tubes). See Chapter 38 Assisted Feeding for further feeding tube details.

Feeding Tube Options

- NE tubes are generally used for three to seven days. Polyurethane tubes and silicon tubes may be placed in the caudal esophagus or stomach. An eight Fr tube will pass through the nasal cavity of most dogs. A five Fr tube is more comfortable in cats. Anesthesia or tranquilization is not necessary (use topical ophthalmic anesthetics to numb the nasal cavity). These tubes can be used in patients considered anesthetic risks.
- Pharyngostomy and esophagostomy tubes vary from 8 to 16 Fr and may be placed in patients with disease or trauma to the nasal or oral cavity. These tubes can be used for long-term in hospital or home feedings. Gastrostomy (mushroom-tipped, 16–22 Fr) can be placed either intraoperatively or percutaneously.
- Any tube that has been placed in the esophagus or stomach generally allows for bolus-type meal feeding except in patients who vomit after each feeding. These patients will benefit from a slow continuous drip administered by a pump or gravity.
- Jejunostomy tubes (J-tubes, 5–8 Fr) are placed within the small intestine either surgically or endoscopically and are appropriate for cases where the stomach and proximal duodenum must be bypassed. Ideally, food is administered at a slow, continuous drip delivered by a pump.

What Should the Patient be Fed?

Nutritionists debate the exact formula for determining daily energy requirements in critically ill patients. A good starting point is to calculate the resting energy requirements for the patient's current weight. If a patient's ideal weight is used, underweight animals may be at greater risk for complications from overfeeding. Resting energy requirements (RER) can be calculated using the following equations:

- $RER = 70 \times (\text{current body weight in kg})^{0.75}$

or

- $RER = (kg \times kg \times kg, \sqrt{}, \sqrt{}) \times 70$.

It is imperative that the nutritional status of the patient be monitored carefully as caloric intake may need to be adjusted to prevent weight loss or unintended weight gain. Food selection depends on tube size and location within the GI tract, the availability and cost of products, and the experience of the clinician.

Diets for tube feeding of critical veterinary patients should be energy and nutrient-dense (1–2 kcal/mL) and highly digestible, thus allowing for minimal feeding volumes to be used. Feeding smaller volumes of an energy-dense diet helps to prevent gastric distention. Additionally, lower food volumes may alleviate GI discomfort and stress on the respiratory system (i.e., pressure on the diaphragm). When considering diets for tube feeding, they should be easy to administer either as a bolus or as a constant rate infusion (CRI) (where applicable) and should be specifically formulated for dogs and cats.

Commercial enteral diets formulated for tube feeding of small animal patients include "recovery-type diets" (e.g., semiliquid canned diets) and veterinary liquid diets. Semiliquid diets can also be prepared with a household blender through blenderization of canned foods with water or with liquid diet.

Commercial foods available for enteral use in veterinary patients can be divided into two major types: (1) liquid or modular products and (2) blended pet foods. Nasal and jejunostomy tubes usually have a small diameter (<8 Fr.), which requires the use of liquid foods. Orogastric, pharyngostomy esophagostomy, and gastrostomy tubes have large diameters (>8 Fr.) and are suitable for blended pet foods.

It is important to note that there are commercial human liquid diets available from pharmacies and grocery stores. These human liquid diets' cost vary, but the important point to remember is that these diets are nutritionally inadequate and may contain inappropriate ingredients for dogs and/or cats, such as cocoa powder, a source of toxic methylxanthines.

While canine patients tolerate short-term feeding of human liquid diets without adverse effects, their use is inappropriate for cats because they are often too low in protein and lack adequate taurine, arginine, and arachidonic acid. In addition, they can be too low in protein for puppies and adult dogs with increased protein losses (e.g., protein-losing enteropathies, drains). It is recommended that veterinary liquid products be used when managing veterinary patients.

Liquid foods are of two basic types: (1) elemental or monomeric and (2) polymeric. Foods said to be "elemental" are not truly elemental; rather they are "semi-elemental" and contain nutrients in small hydrolyzed absorbable forms and are best described as monomeric. The proteins are usually present as free amino acids, small dipeptides or tripeptides, or larger hydrolyzed protein fractions. The fat source is often an oil of mixed (medium- and long-chain) fatty acids and the carbohydrate sources are mono-, di- and trisaccharides. Semi-elemental nutrition provides easier digestion and rapid absorption of nutrients, designed to support the critical systems of the body.

The GI tract is lined with cells called enterocytes, which aid in digestion, absorption, and transportation of nutrients into the body. Vital nutrients absorbed by enterocytes include amino acids and peptides, carbohydrates (complex and simple saccharides), lipids, water, vitamins, and ions (or minerals). Enteral nutrition is preferred whenever possible because enterocytes undergo atrophy without luminal nutrient stimulation. By focusing on the nutritional needs of the enterocyte, semi-elemental diets provide the maximum amount of nutrition that can be absorbed with the least energy expenditure.

In critically ill patients, the body's main goal is to support key organs like the heart, brain, liver, and lungs. Blood flow to the GI tract is reduced thus slowing GI motility. As enterocytes form a tight seal to protect the body from harmful bacteria or toxins, digestion, and absorption of nutrients are similarly altered. Unfortunately, these physiologic changes make it difficult for nutrients to be absorbed when the body needs nutrition the most. Thus, weakened, and debilitated patients benefit from a predigested or a semi-elemental diet.

Semi-elemental diets contain ingredients that are purified and hydrolyzed and are usually combined with a small amount of complex highly digestible ingredients. Semi-elemental diets that nourish the enterocytes of the GI tract help to maintain an osmotic balance which minimizes the risk of diarrhea by preventing the loss of water and other vital nutrients from the GI tract. At this time, EmerAid produces species-specific semi-elemental diets which have been shown to be beneficial to the GI tract and to the management of the critically ill and/or recovering patient (https://emeraid.com/vet/). This product is aimed at bolus feeding of the critical patient.

There are several liquid foods on the human medical market that are positioned as monomeric or hydrolyzed diets and are suitable when **initially** refeeding dogs and cats. These monomeric products are homogenized liquids that can be fed through any feeding tube including a J-tube. Monomeric foods are indicated in disease conditions such as inflammatory bowel disease, lymphangiectasia, refeeding parvoviral enteritis and pancreatitis cases, and any other condition in which a patient's digestive capabilities are questionable. Still, the author recommends feeding a monomeric/semi-elemental diet specific to the cat or dog species versus a human formulation.

Polymeric products contain mixtures of more complex nutrients. Protein is supplied in the form of large peptides (e.g., casein or whey). Carbohydrates are usually supplied as corn starch or syrup, and fats are provided by medium chain triglycerides (MCT) or vegetable oil. These foods require normal digestive processes and are appropriate for most veterinary clinical situations, especially when a small tube (<8 Fr.) has been placed and specific nutrient profiles are needed (e.g., low sodium, high protein, and soluble fiber).

Several liquid milk replacer products are available; however, these products are not appropriate to feed to adult dogs and cats. They typically contain lactose, have high osmolarity, are lower in caloric density, and do not meet Association of American Feed Control Officials (AAFCO) nutrient allowances for adult animals.

Module products are concentrated powdered or liquid forms of nutrients and are primarily supplemental. These products may be added to a liquid product to increase the concentration of a specific nutrient. There are protein, fat, and carbohydrate modules (e.g., casein powder, vegetable oil, or corn syrup). For example, a protein modular product may be added to a human liquid product for an animal with high protein requirements. Soluble fiber can be added to these foods using psyllium husk fiber or pectin; however, these fibers may block the small side ports in 8 Fr. and smaller tubes.

Blended pet foods refer to commercial products nutritionally complete and balanced according to AAFCO allowances for dogs and cats. These products can easily be blended with a liquid to make a consistency that flows through a feeding tube. Some products have a blended texture, a high water content, and very small particle size, whereas others are products that must be blenderized with water and may have to be strained to remove particulate matter.

The best recommendation when using the blended pet food method is to use a product that has been tested in feeding trials and is proven to be balanced and complete for dogs or cats. These products are more readily available, better tolerated, and often less expensive than human liquid foods. These pet food products contain essential amino acids and essential micronutrients properly balanced to the caloric density of the food. Fewer medical complications (e.g., diarrhea) are likely to result. However, blended products are more likely to clog the feeding tube if the tube is not properly flushed after feeding. Patients may later consume the pet food orally, eliminating a diet change when the patient's appetite returns and the tube has been removed. These products are appropriate for patients in catabolic states who are using fat and protein substrates from body stores. When using small-diameter (<8 Fr.) feeding tubes, it will be necessary to dilute the pet food with water, which dilutes the caloric density. Blenderized moist veterinary therapeutic foods may have a place in assisted feeding of patients with specific disease conditions.

Veterinarians have fed human baby food packed in jars because some canine and feline patients would voluntarily eat these products. The meat and/or egg baby foods are high in protein (30–70% DM) and fat (20–60% DM), which compares favorably with blended pet food products. However, baby foods are more costly, contain only one or two food types (protein, protein/grain), and do not contain a balanced mixture of other essential nutrients (amino acids, vitamins, and minerals). For example, many of these products contain only 10% of the calcium required by dogs and cats and, therefore, have a large inverse calcium-phosphorus ratio. Some products contain onion powder, which may result in Heinz body formation in cats. These products will flow through 8 Fr. or larger feeding tubes and may be used on a very limited, short-term basis only when appropriate pet food is unavailable. Human and veterinary liquid products have a better nutritional profile and thus should be used versus human baby food products.

The feeding schedule is often determined by the patient's ability to tolerate food and the logistics of feeding. Feeding an amount equal to the patient's RER during the first 24 hours of food reintroduction, if physically tolerated, is recommended. Feeding one-third of the RER and then increasing the amount by one-third every 24 hours is a more cautious approach to initial feeding but is not always necessary. Foods should be warmed to room temperature, but not higher than body temperature before feeding.

Food boluses must be infused slowly (over approximately one minute per bolus) to allow gastric expansion. Daily food dosage should be divided into several meals according to the expected stomach capacity. Capacities for cats and dogs are 5–10 mL/kg body weight during initial food reintroduction. Maximum capacities as high as 45–90 mL/kg body weight have been measured in cats and dogs when fully re-alimented. Most often, meeting the patient's RER can be done in volumes far less than these maximums. Salivating, gulping, retching, and even vomiting may occur when too much food has been infused or when the infusion rate is too fast.

Research in people has demonstrated that the stomach does not "shrink" during a prolonged fast, but rather the stretch receptors are more sensitive and stimulated by a smaller volume when refeeding occurs. Feeding should be stopped at the first sign of retching or salivating, the meal size reduced by 50% for 24 hours, and then increased by 25% gradually. Foods provided via J-tubes must be infused slowly and often in either very small quantities or by a slow gravity drip or enteral pump with an hourly rate equal to RER/24 hours because the jejunum is volume-sensitive.

Remember to follow each meal with water flush to clear the feeding tube of food residue. When the patient is volume sensitive, it is important to know the minimum volume required to flush the tube. The patient's daily fluid requirement must also be met, and additional tap water may be administered through the feeding tube to meet that requirement. Liquid oral medications may also be administered easily through feeding tubes. Plugged feeding tubes can be cleared by filling the tube with water or a nonalcoholic carbonated beverage and allowing time for the food plug to dissolve. In general, end port tubes are easier to maintain than side port tubes because food tends to become trapped in the blind end of side port tubes. All tubes except orogastric and NE tubes require standard every-other-day bandage care.

Summary

The consequences of malnutrition in all patients, especially critically ill patients, are decreased immunocompetence, decreased tissue synthesis and repair, and altered drug metabolism. Nutritional management in patients with critical illness requires constant monitoring and careful calculations by the veterinary technician to address malnutrition. Constant vigilance and exceptional nursing care will help the patient to manage their malnutrition and facilitate healing and recovery.

Further Reading

Becvarova I (2015) Tube feeding in small animals: diet selection and preparation. In D Chan (ed.), *Nutritional Management of Hospitalized Small Animals*, pp. 80–90, Ames, IA: Wiley Blackwell.

Burns KM. *Semi-Elemental nutrition in Critical Care Patients*. Proceedings of NAVC, 2016.

Chan D. Nutritional Support of Critically Ill Patients. Vol **16**, No 3, 2006. *WALTHAM Focus*

Chan DL, Freeman LM (2015) Parenteral nutrition in small animals. In *Nutritional Management of Hospitalized Small Animals*, Ames, IA: Wiley Blackwell;36(6):100–116.

Chandler ML *et al.* (2000) Use of peripheral parenteral nutritional support in dogs and cats. *Journal of the American Veterinary Medical Association* **216**: 669–73.

Eirmann L, Michel K (2009) Enteral nutrition. In *Small Animal Critical Care Medicine*, pp. 53–8, St. Louis: Saunders.

Kerl ME, Johnson PA (2004) Nutritional plan: matching diet to disease. *Clinical Techniques in Small Animal Practice* **19**(1): 9–21.

Larsen J (2012) Enteral nutrition and tube feeding. In J Andrea, AJ Fascetti, SJ Delaney (eds), *Applied Veterinary Clinical Nutrition*, pp. 329–52, Ames, IA: Wiley Blackwell.

Latimer-Jones K. The role of nutrition in critical care. *The Veterinary Nurse*. May, 2020. https://www.theveterinarynurse.com/review/article/the-role-of-nutrition-in-critical-care# Accessed August 19, 2023

Liu DT, Brown DC, Silverstein DC (2012 Aug) Early nutritional support is associated with decreased length of hospitalization in dogs with septic peritonitis: a retrospective study of 45 cases (2000-2009). *Journal of Veterinary Emergency and Critical Care (San Antonio, Tex.)* **22**(4): 453–9.

Perea SC (2012) Pareneral feeding. In AJ Fascetti AJ, SJ Delaney (eds), *Applied Veterinary Clinical Nutrition*, pp. 353–73, Ames, IA: Wiley Blackwell.

Perea SC (2015) Routes of nutritional support in small animals. In D Chan (ed.), *Nutritional Management of Hospitalized Small Animals*, pp. 14–20, Ames IA: Wiley Blackwell.

Proulx J (2000) Nutrition in critically Ill animals. In *The Veterinary ICU Book*, pp. 202–17, Jackson Hole, WY: Teton NewMedia.

Remillard RL, Saker K (2010) Parenteral-assisted feeding. In *Small Animal Clinical Nutrition* (5th edn), pp. 477–98, Topeka, KS: Mark Morris Institute.

Saker K, Remillard RL (2010) Critical care nutrition and enteral assisted feeding. In *Small Animal Clinical Nutrition* (5th edn), pp. 439–76, Topeka, KS: Mark Morris Institute.

Thomovsky E *et al.* (2007) Parenteral nutrition: uses, indications, and compounding. *Compendium: Continuing Education For Veterinarians* **29**(76-8): 80–5.

Thomovsky E *et al.* (2007) Parenteral nutrition: formulation, monitoring, and complications. *Compendium: Continuing Education For Veterinarians* **29**: 88–102.

Wortinger A, Burns KM (2015) *Nutrition and Disease Management for Veterinary Technicians and Nurses*, Ames, IA: Wiley-Blackwell.

38

Assisted Feeding in Dogs and Cats

Introduction

Addressing the nutritional needs of our hospitalized and critically ill patients can dramatically improve their outcomes and allow them to return home sooner. Oral enteral nutrition is the ideal route. However, if the patient is unable or unwilling to consume at least 85% of their calculated resting energy requirements (RER) another route must be utilized.

Routes of nutritional support are broadly grouped into enteral and parenteral routes. Enteral routes (other than the patient eating on its own) to be considered include the following feeding tubes:

- Nasoesophageal
- Esophagostomy
- Gastrostomy
- Jejunostomy

Parenteral nutrition routes include peripheral and central venous catheters.

The route or combination of routes selected for a specific patient is dependent upon the patient's medical and nutritional status, the anticipated length of required nutritional support, and the nutritional needs and diet limitations and advantages presented by each route.[1]

The first step would be to calculate the RER for the individual patient. The most widely used formula is (weight in kilograms $\times 30) + 70 =$ RER. This formula can be utilized in both cats and dogs over 2–45 kg.[2–4]

For animals outside this range, RER can be calculated by the following:

- $\text{RER} = 70 \times (\text{current body weight in kg})^{0.75}$

or

- $\text{RER} = (\text{kg} \times \text{kg} \times \text{kg}, \sqrt{}, \sqrt{}) \times 70$.

Feeding Tube Materials

The best feeding tubes for prolonged use are made of polyurethane or silicone. For short-term feeding, usually less than 10 days, polyvinylchloride (PVC) tubes can be used. These are not appropriate for long-term feeding because they tend to become stiff with prolonged use causing additional discomfort for the patient. Silicone is softer and more flexible than other tube materials and has a greater tendency to stretch and collapse. Polyurethane is stronger than silicone, allowing for thinner tube walls and a greater internal diameter, despite the same French size. Both the silicone and polyurethane tubes do not disintegrate or become brittle in situ, providing a longer tube life. Latex (rubber) feeding tubes are soft and comfortable for the patient, but due to their composition, tend to have larger tube wall thicknesses, decreasing the internal diameter of the tube. They also tend to become brittle in situ and will undergo significant material disintegration ~12–16 weeks after placement. If the anticipated length of use is less than this period of time, this would not pose a significant problem. Latex is inexpensive, nonirritating to the animal, and comfortable for long-term use.[5]

Nutrition and Disease Management for Veterinary Technicians and Nurses, Third Edition. Ann Wortinger and Kara M. Burns.
© 2024 John Wiley & Sons, Inc. Published 2024 by John Wiley & Sons, Inc.
Companion Website: www.wiley.com/go/wortinger/3e

The French unit measures the outer lumen diameter of a tube and is equal to 0.33 mm. Because the outer diameter is being measured, a thinner tube wall can produce a larger internal lumen making feeding easier on the nursing staff or owner.[3] The type of material the feeding tube is composed of can also affect the ease of passage for the food. Silicon and polyurethane are "slick" and offer less resistance to food passage, latex offers slightly more resistance, and PVC tubes can offer more resistance than latex.[5]

While force-feeding can be used to provide the necessary nutrition, it has not proven to be a method to truly get enough nutrients into the patient. Syringe or force-feeding is extremely stressful to the patient, the healthcare team, and the owner. Seldom is this method able to deliver the volume of nutrients necessary to meet the patients' needs. Often, food aversion is created due to the stress and anxiety of the force-feeding method. Additionally, more product ends up on the team member, the pet itself, and hospital walls than what goes into the pet.

Enteral feeding tubes include tubes that enter through a natural opening (the nares) to those where surgical openings are made, such as esophagostomy, gastrostomy, and jejunostomy tubes. They may terminate anywhere from the mid-esophagus to the jejunum, depending on what type of tube is being placed and the desired placement site (Table 38.1).

Nasoesophageal/Nasogastric Tube

Nasoesophageal (NE) tubes are useful for providing short-term nutritional support, usually less than five days. They can be used in patients with a functional esophagus, stomach, and intestines. NE tubes are contraindicated in patients who are vomiting, comatose, or lack a gag reflex.[2,6] Because of the requirement of passage through the nose, they are typically a smaller diameter tube (3.5–5 Fr in cats and 6–8

Fr in dogs).[1] These tubes offer the advantage of placement without general anesthesia (topical is recommended in the nose), and no specialized equipment is required. NE tubes can also be of benefit for those animals with confirmed or suspected coagulopathies, as no incisions are needed for placement.[4]

Conversely, NE tubes can be quite irritating to the patient due to the facial sutures, the sight line of the tube on the animal's face, and the potential need for an Elizabethan collar to ensure the tube is not "accidentally" removed.[5] As a result of the requirement for a liquid diet being fed frequently, NE/NG tubes are not the most practical for owners to use at home, and are considered mainly for short-term use.[5]

Complications include epistaxis, rhinitis, lack of tolerance of the procedure, and inadvertent removal by the patient. These tubes should not be used in vomiting patients or those with respiratory disease, as the potential exists that the tube can be vomited up from the esophagus and displaced into the trachea, causing aspiration pneumonia during feeding.[2–4,6]

Removal of the feeding tube secondary to sneezing, coughing, or vomiting, despite the continuous use of Elizabethan collars, is also a common complication with NE feeding in cats.[7] Radiographic confirmation of NE tube placement is necessary to minimize risks associated with inappropriate placement of the feeding tube prior to implementation of feeding.

Liquid enteral diets or diluted critical care or recovery diets can be used and the patient is bolus fed. Tube clogging may be a problem; flushing well before and after bolus feeding will aid in mitigating tube clogging. If the tube becomes clogged, replacement may be necessary. Diluting the liquid with water may also help, though this further decreases the caloric concentration of the diet, increasing the volume necessary to meet the caloric needs.

Nasogastric (NG) tubes are placed in the same manner as a NE tube, but the terminal

Table 38.1 Tube feeding comparisons.

Type of tube	Condition	Disease	ICU costs	Food type used	Length of time
Nasoesophageal/ nasogastric	Not recommended for patients who are vomiting or those with respiratory disease	Short-term anorexia, supplement oral intake	$	Liquid +/− thinning required; CRI or bolus	Short-term, in-hospital use only (3–7 days)
Pharyngostomy/ esophagostomy	Not recommended for patients that are vomiting or those with respiratory disease	Hepatic lipidosis, anorexia, oral surgery or trauma, cancer	$$	Liquid, recovery diet, or gruel commercial diet based on tube size; CRI or bolus	Long-term, in-hospital, and at-home use (1–20 weeks, depending on tube type used)
Gastrostomy	Can be used on patients who are vomiting or who have respiratory disease	Pancreatitis, hepatic lipidosis, anorexia, esophageal strictures, oral surgery or trauma, cancer	$$$	Liquid, recovery diet, or gruel commercial diet based on tube size; CRI or bolus	Long-term use, can be permanent, depending on tube type used
Jejunostomy	Can be used on patients who are vomiting or who have respiratory disease	Pancreatitis, intestinal anastomosis, coma	$$$$	Liquid diet; CRI or bolus	Short-term, in-hospital use only (3–10 days)

end is located in the stomach rather than the distal esophagus. By passing through the cardiac sphincter into the stomach, the risk of gastroesophageal reflux increases, therefore, increasing the incidence of esophageal strictures.[5]

The patient's food can continue to be offered with an NE/NG feeding tube, as its presence is unlikely to cause any difficulty to the patient's appetite or swallowing.

Esophagostomy Tube Placement

An esophagostomy feeding tube allows delivery of nutrients to patients with inadequate intake who cannot prehend, masticate, or swallow food in a normal or safe manner. It can be used to meet the nutritional needs of anorexic patients, such as cats with hepatic lipidosis. Esophagastomy tubes are indicated in patients with nasal, oral, or pharyngeal disease since the midcervical placement of the tube bypasses these anatomic regions.[8] Patients with oropharyngeal neoplasia, mandibular or maxillary trauma, oronasal fistulas, or dysphagia are potential candidates for an esophagostomy feeding tube.

General anesthesia is required for placement of the feeding tube, so the anesthetic risk to the specific patient must be considered. Sedation alone for placement of an esophagostomy tube is not recommended because suppression of the gag reflex is not achieved, thus making placement very challenging.[8] Esophagostomy tube placement is contraindicated in patients with coagulopathy due to the risk of bleeding. The esophagus and more distal gastrointestinal tract need to be functional to allow for nutrition through an esophagostomy tube to be successful. Therefore, patients with megaesophagus, esophagitis, or esophageal strictures are not considered good candidates for an esophagostomy tube.[8] Rather, these patients would benefit from a more distally placed feeding tube (gastrostomy tube).

Esophagostomy tubes are generally well tolerated by the patient. The biggest advantages of these tubes include the large size that can be placed (12–14 Fr for cats and 14 Fr or higher for dogs), and the ability to discharge the animal with the tube in place for continued care with the owner at home. Polyethylene tubes appear to be quite irritating and should be avoided, as should PVC tubes if long-term use is anticipated.[5] If clogging of the tube occurs or if the patient experiences other tube failures, a new tube can be placed through the existing stoma site if nutritional support is still needed.[5]

Complications include tube displacement due to vomiting or removal by the patient, skin infection around the exit site, and biting off the tube end by the patient after vomiting. There may be some signs of discomfort seen with the neck bandage, and many softer, long-term bandages are commercially available for use.[5]

The large bore of these catheters allows for feeding of a gruel recovery diet, sometimes without dilution with water. These catheters are also easy for clients to use and maintain at home as long as vomiting is not a problem. Since the incision is located in the neck, feeding can begin immediately after recovery from anesthesia with no additional time needed for a temporary stoma to form.[5,8]

When removing, the tube may be simply pulled out after the sutures are removed. The exit hole is allowed to heal by the second intention. A light bandage may be applied for the first 12 hours (Figure 38.1).

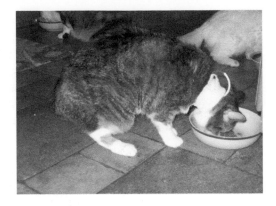

Figure 38.1 Neck wrap being used at home on an esphagostomy tube.

Gastrostomy Tube

Gastrostomy tubes are well tolerated, can be placed with less invasive techniques (i.e., percutaneously placed with endoscopy), and are highly effective as a means of providing nutritional support. They also permit bolus meal feeding and can be used for long-term feeding at home.

Gastrostomy tubes can be placed either endoscopically, blindly, or surgically. All three techniques require general anesthesia. Endoscopic placement allows for visualization of the esophagus and stomach as well as biopsy collection from the stomach and proximal duodenum and foreign body removal. While the blind placement technique exists, it is not recommended. Surgical placement is useful during surgical exploratory or when the scope cannot be passed through the esophagus due to trauma or esophageal strictures.

A minimum of 12 hours is needed for a temporary stoma to form before feeding can begin. The feeding tube should be left in place for a minimum of 7–10 days to allow a permanent stoma to form before removal. The tubes can be left in long-term (1–6 months) without replacement. When replaced with another PEG tube, low-profile silicone tube, or foley-type feeding tube, the stoma can be used for the rest of the patient's life.

Complications associated with PEG tubes include those seen from tube placement such as splenic laceration, gastric hemorrhage, and pneumoperitoneum. Delayed complications can also be seen such as vomiting, aspiration pneumonia, tube removal, tube migration, and peritonitis and stoma infection.[3]

Blind percutaneous gastrostomy tube placement involves basically the same technique as endoscopic placement, but a large plastic or steel tube is used instead of the endoscope and a firm wire is used instead of the suture. The catheter is the same as in the endoscopic insertion technique. Reported complications are the same as for PEG tubes, though the risk of splenic, stomach, or omental laceration is greater. Contraindications to using the blind technique include severe obesity that would make palpation of the end of the tube difficult and esophageal disease.

Surgical placement has been largely superseded by endoscopic placement because of the ease and speed of placement, lower cost, and decreased morbidity. A surgical approach may be indicated in obese animals, those with esophageal disease, or when laporatomy is already scheduled. To place a surgical gastrostomy, a larger incision is needed into the stomach, and the exit location is sometimes hard to locate because of the position on the surgical table. Surgical placement involves placing purse string sutures around the catheter to secure it as well as attaching the stomach to the body wall.

Gastrostomy tube placement is the technique of choice for long-term enteral support. These tubes are well tolerated by the patient, produce minimal discomfort, allow feeding of either gruel recovery diets or blenderized commercial foods, and can be easily managed by owners at home.[6] Patients are able to eat normally with gastrostomy tubes in place and can easily be used as a nutritional supplement until the patient is totally self-feeding. For patients who are difficult to medicate and require long-term medications, many medicines can also be given through the feeding tube. The major disadvantage of gastrostomy tubes is the need for general anesthesia and the risk of peritonitis.[6]

For animals requiring long-term management, the initial Pezzer catheter can be replaced with either low-profile silicone tubes or with foley-type gastrostomy tubes. Both of these types can be placed through the external stoma site without the endoscope. Sedation or anesthesia may be necessary based on the individual patient.

For removal, if the tube has been in place for 16 weeks or less the tube may be simply removed. This is best accomplished by placing the patient in the right lateral recumbency. The tube is grasped with the right hand close to the body wall, with the left hand holding the animal. Pull firmly and consistently to the right in an upward motion. Some force may be required for this. It is also helpful to ensure that the patient has been fasted, and placing a towel over the tube site to catch any "stuff." If the tube has been in longer than 16 weeks, the incidence of tube breakage is much higher. Depending on where the breakage occurs, the remaining tube pieces may need to be endoscopically retrieved. Larger patients can easily pass retained parts; smaller patients may need to have them retrieved.

The exit hole is allowed to heal by second intension. A light bandage may be applied for the first 12 hours.

Jejunostomy Tube

Jejunostomy feeding is indicated when the upper gastrointestinal tract must be rested or when pancreatic stimulation must be decreased. Jejunal tubes can be placed either surgically or threaded through a gastrostomy tube for transpyloric placement. Standard gastrojejunal tubes designed for humans are unreliable in dogs due to frequent reflux of the jejunal portion of the tube back into the stomach. Investigation is ongoing involving endoscopic placement of transpyloric jejunal tubes through PEG tubes.

Due to the small diameter of these tubes (typically 5–8 Fr) and the location, liquid enteral diets are recommended. Because the jejunum has minimal storage capacity compared to the stomach, continuous rate infusion using a syringe pump is the preferred method of delivery. If using a syringe pump, completely change the delivery equipment every 24 hours to help prevent bacterial growth within the system.

Common complications include osmotic diarrhea, vomiting, premature removal of the tube, retrograde tube movement out of the jejunum, focal cellulitis, leakage of gastrointestinal contents, and tube obstruction.

It is recommended that the jejunal tube be left in place for 7–10 days to allow adhesions to form around the tube site and prevent leakage back into the abdomen.[2,6] Completely changing the delivery equipment every 24 hours will help prevent bacterial growth within the system. Clogging is a common problem; a syringe pump may help to decrease the incidence as will flushing well every 4 hours.

When removing, the tube may be simply pulled out after the sutures are removed. The exit hole is allowed to heal by the second intension. A light bandage may be applied for the first 12 hours.

Beginning Enteral Feeding

Tube placement is only the beginning of the feeding for these animals. Next, we have to start feeding and be able to maintain it for the length of time the animal requires to recover or begin eating on their own again. Initially, we will start feeding a liquid or gruel recovery diet at a consistency that will easily pass through the feeding tube. With NE or NG tubes, feeding can begin immediately after tube placement. For esophagostomy tubes, feeding can begin after anesthetic recovery. For gastrostomy and jejunostomy tubes, feeding must be delayed for 12 hours post placement to allow a temporary

Table 38.2 Feeding schedule for a 12# cat with a DER calculated at 280–303 kcal/day. The food has 2.1 kcal/ml.

Total feeding volume will be 280–303/2.1 = 133–144 ml/day

- Day 1 – 1.8 ml/h CRI (30%)
- Day 2 – 3 ml/h CRI (50%)
- Day 3 – 3.6 ml/h CRI (60%)
- Day 4 –14 ml q 4 h (60%)
- Day 5 –18 ml q 4 h (75%)
- Day 6 – 27 ml q 6 h (75%)
- Day 7 – 36 ml q 6 h (100%)
- Day 8 – 48 ml q 8 h (100%)

Feedings are only increased in volume or time between feedings if the patient tolerates the schedule without vomiting.
Typically, either the volume is increased or the time between feedings is increased but not both.

stoma to form around the tube placement site.[5]

Depending on the physical condition of the patient and the disease processes being addressed, feeding frequency and volumes may need to be adjusted. For animals who are at a normal body condition score (BCS) and do not have concurrent disease processes (i.e., hit by car [HBC], postsurgical) feeding can be started at 50% RER, divided into 3–4 equal feedings. For those that are physically debilitated or have significant disease processes (i.e., hepatic lipidosis, diabetes mellitus, and renal failure), feedings can be started at 25–30% RER with frequency of q 4 h or as a CRI.[5]

As the recovery progresses, the feeding volume can be increased while the feeding frequency decreases (Table 38.2).

This is a typical feeding schedule for a moderately severe hepatic lipidosis cat from the time of the initial feeding until it is ready for discharge from the hospital.

Diet Choices

There are many diet options for enteral tube feeding.[5] When looking for a diet you need to evaluate the disease process you are treating, the size of the tube you wish to use, and the cost and availability of the food, especially if used by the owners at home.

Gruel, liquid, canned, and dry foods can all be used for enteral feeding, but not every food can be used with every tube. Liquid diets can usually go through tubes larger than 5 Fr, gruel diets need a 10–12 Fr tube, and may still have some clogging problems with this size. For blenderized diets, whether they are canned or dry food a 14 Fr or larger is usually advised.[5] The finer the diet can be processed, the less chance of tube clogging. Ideally, recovery diets do not need additional processing, but if using a canned or dry diet additional processing will be needed.

For canned diets, they are usually processed in a food blender with a ratio of 1 can of food to 1 can of water, mix well. You need to get the particles fine enough to pass easily through the feeding tube and have a consistency that can be drawn up and administered with a feeding syringe.[5]

For a dry diet add the dry food to the blender dry, pulverize the food well then add an equal amount of water. Mix well again. Due to the dry carbohydrates found in this type of diet, allow the food to site for 20–30 min to allow the carbohydrates to soak up the water. Additional water may need to be added to thin out the consistency to allow passage through the syringe.

When blenderizing foods, the calories will not be calculated on a per mL amount, as we may not know what the final volume will be as the amount of water to add may vary. We will know what the calorie content will be on a per can or per cup basis and will need to figure out our volumes from there.

Example

Our patient needs 1 can of Dog Gruel/day through their feeding tube divided into 3 equal meals. Each can is 13.5 oz. When we blenderize 1 can of food with 1 3/4 cup of water we get a final mixture of ~3.5 cups. If we divide 3.5 cups/3 meals we get 1.16 cups/meal. There are 240 ml in a cup. 1.16 cup × 240 ml = 278 ml/meal. 278 ml/meal × 3 meals = 835 ml/day.

The higher the caloric density of the food, the lower the volume that must be fed to reach their daily energy requirement (DER). When using over the counter (OTC) foods (canned or dry), the caloric density will be inherently lower than that found in therapeutic recovery diets, necessitating feeding of higher volumes of food. In the long run, feeding a commercial diet to a feeding tube animal may not be less expensive or easier on the owner.

Mechanical Complications

Mechanical complications include both tube obstruction and premature removal of the tube or dislodgement from the site of placement.[8] The most common problem, tube obstruction, can be prevented in most cases by proper tube maintenance. Food should never be allowed to sit in the tube. The tube should be flushed with warm water after *every* feeding and whenever gastrointestinal contents aspirated through the tube are seen when checking residuals. When using the feeding tube to administer medications, administer one medication at a time through the tube, and ensure the medication is given separately from the food.[8] This will help to prevent drug-to-drug interactions as well as drug-to-food interactions as not all medications and enteral foods are compatible with one another.

If the feeding tube becomes clogged either from insufficient flushing after feeding, or from hair accumulation through the holes in the end of the tube, try to flush the clog out using warm water and the feeding syringe.[3] Hold the tube firmly and push the water with force. If the clog is not bad, this may work. If it is still clogged, try switching to a carbonated cola beverage in the feeding tube, and allow this to sit for a period of time. Some practitioners have suggested the use of pancreatic enzymes mixed with water and various other mixtures instilled into the tube to break up the clog.[8,9]

Premature tube removal or dislodgement is best prevented by choosing the most appropriate tube for the animal and using Elizabethan collars and wraps when appropriate.[3] Whenever the location of the tube is in doubt, it should be checked radiographically. While most tubes are radiopaque, a sterile contract media (i.e., Omnipaque) can be infused through the tube to check for leaks into the peritoneal or thoracic cavity.[9]

Gastrointestinal Complications

Some of the gastrointestinal complications seen with tube feeding are related to the feeding itself. Food that is administered too quickly, in too large an amount or at the wrong temperature can all cause nausea, vomiting, or abdominal discomfort.[8] These signs can also be related to the patient's underlying disease process or a complication of medications the patient is receiving.

Liquid enteral diets are typically very low residue and are likely to cause a soft stool if not actual diarrhea in a normal animal let alone one who is already ill. Likewise, most recovery diets, both liquid and gruel forms, are high in fat; thus, a patient with impaired fat digestion and absorption may develop steatorrhea when fed these diets.[5]

One cause of diarrhea not typically thought of is the medications that we are giving to the animals, whether they are administered orally or through the feeding tube. Many liquid oral forms of medications are hypertonic or contain sorbitol, a nonabsorbable sugar, and may cause, at least in part diarrhea.[6] We also need to remember that a number of commonly used antibiotics, analgesic agents, and other drugs can cause nausea, vomiting, and gastrointestinal ileus and might contribute to the discomfort our patients are feeling. Canned pumpkin, 5–15 mL per feeding, aids in resolving diarrhea. Since canned pumpkin is typically sold in large cans, you can recommend the client measure the volume of pumpkin needed for each meal, place this in an ice cube tray, and freeze it. Once frozen they can be removed from the ice cube trays, placed in a plastic freezer bag, and stored until needed. The amount used at each feeding will need to be adjusted for the individual animal.

Constipation is not an unusual complication seen in patients with feeding tubes. Patients can be weak from muscle loss and metabolic derangement; thus the development of constipation is not unexpected.[9] Adding lactulose to the diet will often solve this problem, 1–2 mL per meal, adjusted as needed to maintain stool consistency.

Metabolic Complications

There are two types of metabolic complications that our patients can develop. The first is the result of the patient's inability to assimilate certain nutrients.[3] This can best be anticipated by doing a proper nutritional assessment of the patient before developing the nutritional plan. The other type is seen with refeeding syndrome (See Chapter 57 – Refeeding Syndrome).

Keeping in mind the changes the body has undergone while in starvation, when reintroducing food several areas need to be monitored closely to prevent refeeding syndrome. During recovery, excessively rapid refeeding (or hyperalimentation) can overwhelm the patient's already limited functional reserves.[5,8]

Refeeding or reintroduction of nutrition causes a shift in the body from a catabolic state where protein is the primary energy source to an anabolic state where carbohydrates are the preferred energy source. Administration of enteral or parenteral nutrition stimulates the release of insulin; this causes dramatic shifts in serum electrolytes from the extracellular space to the intracellular space, primarily phosphorus, potassium, and to a lesser degree magnesium.[5,9] Insulin promotes intracellular uptake of glucose and phosphorus for glycolysis. These electrolyte shifts can have a profound impact on metabolic functions within the body; phosphorus is used by the red blood cells as their primary source of energy in the form of 2,3 DPG. Without this, the red blood cells (RBCs) have a higher risk of mortality resulting in hemolysis. Phosphorus is integral in the formation of adenosine triphosphate (ATP). ATP is the power source for most cells within the body and without it, cells cannot function properly. Potassium is involved in the sodium/potassium pump and is needed for muscle contraction and relaxation.

Serum cobalamin (B12) is often low in cats that have small intestinal disease, pancreatic disease, and hepatic lipidosis. Supplementation may be necessary even before enteral nutrition is started to allow adequate assimilation of nutrients within the intestine.

Serum electrolytes, phosphorus, and packed cell volume should be monitored closely. A baseline value should be established prior to treatment and then once daily thereafter unless dramatic changes are seen. If changes are seen in any values, supplementation needs to be started immediately. This can either be done intravenously or through the feeding tube. Refeeding syndrome is one of the most dramatic "side-effects" and can lead very quickly to death.[9]

Metabolic complications of any type are less likely to occur if estimated caloric needs are conservative. Current recommendations are to initiate feeding at caloric amounts equal to the patient's calculated RERs without the addition of any "illness requirements." As recovery progresses, we can increase the amount to DER.

Infectious Complications

The types of infectious complications that can occur in tube-fed patients include contamination of the enterally fed formulas, peristomal cellulitis, septic peritonitis, and aspiration pneumonia.[8]

Microbial contamination of the food is easily avoided by following basic hygiene in preparation and storage of the food. Blenderized foods should be prepared daily, and opened commercial liquid diets should be kept refrigerated and discarded after 48 hours. When food is being delivered via syringe pump, no more than six hours' worth of food should be setup at a time. One of the biggest sources of contamination is inadequate cleaning of equipment used for preparation and delivery of food. Syringes, containers, and tubing used for preparing, storing, and delivering food should be discarded after use.[8] Things that are reused, such as blenders and storage containers, should be cleaned thoroughly and preferably sterilized each time they are used. The equipment used to deliver the food should also be replaced every 24 hours; this includes the syringes and delivery tubes and if the food is suspended, the administration bag.

Peristomal cellulitis can be seen with esophagostomy, gastrostomy, and jejunostomy tubes. This complication can typically be avoided by: (1) ensuring the tube is not secured too tightly to the body wall, and (2) by keeping the site clean and protected.[9] Septic peritonitis can develop in patients where the gastrostomy or jejunostomy tube has become dislodged or removed before a permanent stoma has formed.[4] Proper tube selection can help prevent this problem; button or balloon size should be large enough to secure the tube in the stomach lumen. Wraps or Elizabethan collars may be necessary to prevent the patient from accidentally or intentionally removing the tube. Ensuring that a mature stoma has formed prior to tube removal can help to prevent peritonitis. Patients that are malnourished (hypoalbunemic) or are receiving medications that impair wound healing may take longer to develop a mature stoma than would healthy patients.

Aspiration pneumonia can be seen with patients especially if that patient has a history of developing aspiration pneumonia. Additionally, patients with impaired mental status, neurologic injuries, reduced or absent cough or gag reflexes, and those on mechanical ventilation, are at increased risk for aspiration pneumonia. Feeding patients in any of these categories pre-pylorically puts them at risk of aspiration of food.[6] Viable alternatives would include jejunostomy tubes and parenteral nutrition. Lastly, caution should be used when feeding patients with NE or esophagostomy tubes using constant rate infusion. These types of tubes can be vomited up and the tip of the tube could relocate in the pharynx and place the patient at risk for pulmonary aspiration.

Hospital Management

Patients should be allowed to exercise for 20–30 minutes, approximately 1 hour before feeding, 2–3 times daily. This can be started even while the CRI feedings are being done. The team member should remember to disconnect the syringe pump, flush the line with water, and cap. Exercise has been found to greatly enhance both gastric motility and patient attitude.[4]

Potential Post-discharge Complications

Most patients do very well after discharge, particularly if good communication is established with the owners and regular rechecks are scheduled. Recheck frequency should be based on the type of tube being used, the condition of the patient, and how their recovery is going. It may be as frequent as every 2 weeks or as long as every quarter for long-term tube usage (Figure 38.2).

Granulation tissue normally forms around the tube site on the outside and may be quite pink and can even bleed when handled.[4] It is important to let clients know this is normal and to expect it; granulation tissue allows the hole to close after the tube is removed. It has been found in cats with dark hair coats (including tabbies) that the hair will grow in a dark ring around the tube site. It will

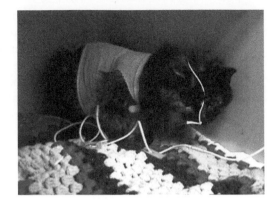

Figure 38.2 Example of an in-hospital "t-shirt" using tube gauze. Be sure to place 1″ tape folded over the neck edge to keep the shirt from sliding down the cat's torso.

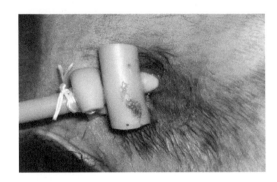

Figure 38.3 Hair regrowth around a tube site.

also regrow thicker than the surrounding hair regrowth.[5] Many clients will think that this is necrosis and become very concerned, thus a quick warning to expect this will greatly ease their minds (Figure 38.3).

What do you do about the patient who insists on chewing on their tube? A simple solution is to place a baby's t-shirt on a cat, usually an infant's size 6–9 months works well for most. For large patients, larger shirts can be used. Use a t-shirt that has a fitted neck, not fitted shoulders. Once the t-shirt is on, place a piece of 1″ porous tape near the end of the feeding tube, tuck the tube up under the t-shirt, and use a safety pin to pin the tape to the t-shirt. This makes removal easier for feeding and decreases the risk of pinning through the tube and damaging it.

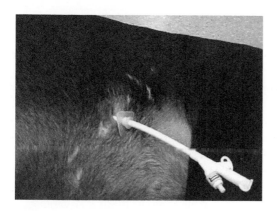

Figure 38.4 This stoma hole is almost 3 years old. The Great Dane developed esophageal strictures when she was 8 years old. She was managed for over 3 years with a gastrostomy tube and eventually died of heart failure.

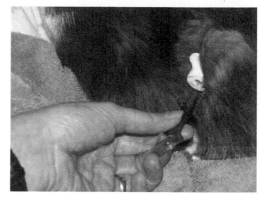

Figure 38.5 An example of a low-profile feeding tube being used in an oral cancer patient. Placement of this type of feeding tube requires a mature stoma hole.

Once the patient goes home, tube feedings are continued – even after the patient begins self-feeding. Owners are given instructions to always have fresh food and water available for the convalescing patient and when the desired weight is reached, tube feedings are decreased by 25–50% (depending on the oral intake). The tube can be removed after the patient has reached its desired weight, has recovered from the trauma, has finished chemotherapy treatment, and has been totally self-feeding for 2 weeks without signs of weight loss. Many feeding tubes can be maintained long term, and if needed the same stoma hole can be used for repeated tube placements (Figures 38.4 and 38.5).

Summary

The enteral route is the preferred method of nutritional support for patients with a functional gastrointestinal tract. Many tube and food choices are available and can be tailored to fit the individual patient and condition.

Typically, owners are very happy with the results when using a feeding tube and the animal feels much better. Feeding tubes do require routine daily care such as cleaning around the tube site and flushing the feeding tube with water; even if the tubes are not being used every day to feed the patient. The use of feeding tubes can give many clients the benefit of enjoying their pets for a longer period of time and providing a better quality of life for both.

References

1 Perea SC (2015) Routes of nutritional support in small animals. In D Chan (ed.), *Nutritional Management of Hospitalized Small Animals*, pp. 14–20, Ames, IA: Wiley Blackwell.

2 Nelson RW Digestive system disorders, general therapeutic principles. In RW Nelson, CG Couto (eds), *Small Animal Internal Medicine* (6th edn), pp. 432–46, St Louis, MO: Elsevier.

3 Marks SL (2015) The principles and implementation of enteral nutrition. In SJ Ettinger, EC Feldman (eds), *Textbook of Veterinary Internal Medicine* (7th edn), vol. **1**, pp. 715–7, St. Louis: Saunders/Elsevier.

4 Saker KE, Remillard RL Critical care nutrition and enteral-assisted feeding. In MS Hand, CD Thatcher, RL Remillard *et al.* (eds), *Small Animal Clinical Nutrition* (5th edn), pp. 439–76, Topeka, KS: Mark Morris Institute.

5 Larsen J (2012) Enteral nutrition and tube feeding. In S Delaney, A Fascetti (eds), *Applied Veterinary Clinical Nutrition*, pp. 329–48, Ames, IA: Wiley-Blackwell.

6 Marks S (2013) Enteral and parenteral nutrition. In RJ Washabau, MJ Day (eds), *Canine and Feline Gastroenterology*, pp. 429–44, St. Louis: Elsevier.

7 Abood SK, Buffington CAT (1992) Enteral feeding of dogs and cats: 51 cases (1989–1991). *Journal of the American Veterinary Medical Association* **4**: 619–22.

8 Eirmann L (2015) Esophagostomy feeding tubes in dogs and cats. In D Chan (ed.), *Nutritional Management of Hospitalized Small Animals*, pp. 29–40, Ames IA: Wiley Blackwell.

9 Michel K (2006) Monitoring the enterally fed patient to maximize benefits and minimize complication. In *IVECCS Proceedings*, pp. 495–8.

39

Liver Disease

The liver is the central metabolic organ of the body. The liver is the second largest organ in the body and is responsible for approximately 1500 essential biochemical functions. The liver's main responsibility is maintaining homeostasis and removing waste products that have accumulated within the body. The liver also plays a key role in digestion and metabolism of food and nutrients. The liver has a large storage capacity as well as functional reserve and regenerative capability. Hepatic disease is typically severe before clinical signs and/or laboratory tests reveal/confirm the disease. Consequently, the patient is often suffering significant metabolic alterations by the time an appropriate feeding plan is implemented by the healthcare team. Nutritional management of liver disease usually is directed at the clinical manifestations of the disease as opposed to the specific cause of the disease. There are five goals for nutritional management of hepatic disease[1]:

(1) maintaining normal metabolic processes,
(2) correction of electrolyte disturbances,
(3) providing substrates to support hepatocellular repair and regeneration,
(4) avoiding toxic by-product accumulation,
(5) and avoiding and managing hepatic encephalopathy (HE).

In most liver disease cases, protection of animals from HE is not as important as providing adequate dietary energy intake and preserving body mass through adequate caloric intake and provision of adequate protein intake, as it is believed that animals with hepatic disease are frequently in a catabolic state.[1,2]

Regardless of the primary liver disease, the hepatic reaction pattern is similar; thus, most of these disorders, if severe and/or longstanding, often lead to a few syndromes with potentially serious metabolic consequences (e.g., cholestasis, icterus, portal hypertension, ascites, and HE).[1,2]

Assessment of the patient with hepatic disease includes a history and physical examination (including a nutritional history, body weight, body condition scoring, and muscle condition scoring), laboratory evaluation, and imaging of the liver. There is a wide range of hepatobiliary diseases which differ in severity, therefore, making it difficult to recommend one nutrient profile for all liver patients. However, general recommendations of key nutritional factors can be made to benefit most patients with hepatic disease. The foundation of adequate nutritional management in hepatic patients is the provision of adequate calories. Veterinary nurses/technicians should think first about the total caloric need of the patient and then consider protein requirements.

All breeds are susceptible to liver disease with Yorkshire Terriers, Cairn Terriers, Scottish Terriers, Malteses, Golden and Labrador Retrievers, Schnauzers, Poodles, Dobermann, Cocker Spaniel, and German Shepherds at an increased risk.[3] No breed predisposition was observed in cats; however, obese cats are more prone to hepatic lipidosis (HL).[3] Younger animals are predisposed to portosystemic shunt

Nutrition and Disease Management for Veterinary Technicians and Nurses, Third Edition. Ann Wortinger and Kara M. Burns.
© 2024 John Wiley & Sons, Inc. Published 2024 by John Wiley & Sons, Inc.
Companion Website: www.wiley.com/go/wortinger/3e

(PSS) which may result in nervous signs in severe cases.

Key Nutritional Factors in Hepatobiliary Diseases

General recommendations of key nutritional factors can be made to benefit the majority of patients with hepatic disease. However, key nutrients in managing HL in cats will be discussed separately toward the end of this chapter. The foundation of adequate nutritional management in hepatic patients is the provision of adequate calories. It is prudent to think first of the total caloric need of the patient and then consider protein requirement.

Malnutrition is a very common feature of chronic hepatic disease, and correct nutrition should be evaluated in each individual patient. Protein malnutrition is seen in patients with hepatic disease, manifesting clinically as weight loss, muscle atrophy, and hypoalbumineria. The amount of protein fed to hepatic patients must be finely balanced. The biological value or digestibility of the proteins should be increased. Proteins with higher biological value help to fulfill the patient's needs while producing minimally nitrogenous waste.[1,4,5] Small frequent meals help the patient optimize blood flow through the liver, manage fasting glucose, and minimize HE.

Hepatic disease is often accompanied by disorders which predispose animals to malassimilation. One example is cholestasis, which is associated with decreased ability to digest and absorb fat due to reduced intestinal availability of bile acids. Cats with cholangitis/cholangiohepatitis often have gastrointestinal (GI) comorbidities, such as pancreatic disease or inflammatory bowel disease (IBD). These may further compromise nutrient absorption through a decrease in digestive enzyme activity or mucosal dysfunction.

Common symptoms in liver disease patients are significant nausea and anorexia. As hepatic functional mass declines, less glycogen storage capacity is accessible within the liver; thus requiring the use of lean muscle glycogen stores and protein as substrates for gluconeogenesis to maintain blood glucose concentrations. Subsequently, reduced voluntary intake due to nausea and anorexia coupled with increased muscle protein mobilization to provide substrates for gluconeogenesis, result in rapid weight loss in patients with hepatic disease.[6] Muscle tissue is also a storage site for a large proportion of the total ammonia amount in the body, which is a major encephalopathic toxin. Failure to meet the patient's metabolic energy requirements and maintain a positive nitrogen balance through provision of sufficient dietary protein and fat can promote the development of HE through release of muscle ammonia stores. Given the difficulty of detecting HE in more mildly affected animals, many veterinary team members will recommend protein-restricted diets in the early stages of liver disease. If low-protein diets have decreased palatability, this may result in insufficient caloric intake, which in turn can worsen the clinical state of the patient. The first aim of nutritional support for most animals with hepatic disease should be to ensure adequate caloric intake to meet metabolic energy requirements.

Additionally, there are a number of other key nutritional factors to consider when managing patients with hepatic disease. The liver plays an important role in the regulation of carbohydrate homeostasis and serum glucose levels through its ability to remove glucose from and release glucose into the circulation. Therefore, it is important to have highly digestible carbohydrate sources.[1,4] This will reduce protein breakdown and the resulting gluconeogenesis. Vitamin K and zinc are recommended in dietary management of liver disease to help avoid deficiencies commonly found in patients suffering from hepatic disease. Soluble fiber is essential to help promote colonic evacuation and to encourage nitrogen fixation by enteric bacteria thus reducing the amount of ammonia production and absorption.

Chronic Hepatitis and Cirrhosis

Chronic hepatitis in dogs is a poorly defined group of clinicopathologic entities characterized by parenchymal necrosis with associated lymphoplasmacytic inflammation. Chronic hepatitis may result from a myriad of causes including copper accumulation, infectious diseases, drugs, breed-associated hepatitis, and possibly autoimmune disease. Unfortunately, the majority of the time a cause is never determined. Lymphoplasmacytic inflammation suggests an immune-mediated mechanism. Autoantibodies have been recognized in dogs with chronic hepatitis but it is unknown if such an immune reaction is the cause or result of the disease. The subtle onset contributes to the poor understanding of the pathogenesis because most patients have an advanced stage of the disease when it is recognized. Hepatic fibrosis is an accumulation of extracellular collagen and connective tissue within the liver and is a sequela to hepatic inflammation. Fibrosis not only results in distortion of normal hepatic structural design but also becomes a barrier to movement of substances back and forth between blood and hepatocytes. Cirrhosis is defined as fibrosis with loss of normal acinar liver design and with regenerative nodules. The architectural changes in cirrhosis impair blood and bile flow and nutrient exchange, thus perpetuating hepatocellular injury.

Canine Copper Associated Hepatotoxicosis

Hepatic copper storage disease is an inherited autosomal recessive trait that impairs biliary excretion of copper. Veterinary medicine sees this disease most prevalently in the Bedlington terrier breed. Affected dogs progressively accumulate copper. Evidence of hepatic necrosis is observed when copper concentrations exceed approximately 2000 ppm (μg/g) dry weight (DW) liver (normal copper concentrations are <400 μg/g DW). As copper concentrations

increase, damage progresses to chronic hepatitis and ultimately cirrhosis. Rarely, massive widespread hepatic necrosis can result in some dogs presenting with acute liver failure. Without appropriate treatment with dietary management and copper chelation, affected dogs usually do not live longer than 7–10 years of age.[1-3] The gene responsible for this defect has been identified and it has become possible to distinguish affected, homozygous normal and carrier Bedlington terrier dogs using DNA markers. It was once estimated that about 25% of Bedlington terriers were affected with copper toxicosis and another 50% were carriers.[3,4] Now, through genetic testing and responsible breeding programs, the incidence of this disease is significantly lower.

Hepatic mitochondria are important intracellular targets of copper toxicosis. Functional abnormalities of mitochondria associated with oxidative injury (i.e., lipid peroxidation) have been documented to occur in people, rats, and Bedlington terriers with copper-induced hepatic injury. Oxidative injury and abnormal hepatic mitochondrial respiration may be involved in the pathogenesis of copper toxicosis. This theory forms the basis for using vitamin E and other antioxidants as potential therapeutic agents in addition to chelation therapy.

The role of copper in hepatic diseases observed in other dog breeds is less clear.[3] Abnormal concentrations of copper in the liver can result secondary to cholestatic liver disease or as a primary defect in hepatic copper excretion resulting in hepatic injury. Breeds that are currently thought to have primary copper-associated hepatopathies include Skye terriers, West Highland white terriers, Doberman pinschers, Dalmatian dogs, and Labrador retrievers.[3] The liver diseases in these dogs differ from copper toxicosis in Bedlington terriers in that hepatic copper concentrations are generally lower and do not always increase with age. Other factors may be responsible for hepatic damage in some breeds. The exceptions might be Doberman pinschers and Dalmatian dogs because they tend to accumulate hepatic copper in concentrations similar to Bedlington terriers, suggesting defects in hepatic copper excretion.

Cholangitis

Cholangitis (i.e., inflammation of the biliary ducts, especially the intrahepatic ducts and the surrounding liver tissue) is the most common feline inflammatory liver disease. The World Small Animal Veterinary Association Liver Pathology Standardization Working Group categorized the two most common forms of cholangitis into neutrophilic and lymphocytic forms.[7] Bacterial infection from enteric bacteria (especially *Escherichia coli*) ascending through the bile ducts is thought to be the cause of most neutrophilic forms, whereas immunologic mechanisms may be involved in the lymphocytic type. Chronic cholangitis may progress to biliary cirrhosis.[7] Many cats with cholangitis develop significant cholestasis and may have sludged or inspissated bile, causing partial or complete biliary obstruction. Concurrent cholecystitis, pancreatitis, and IBD are common in feline cholangitis patients.

Portosystemic Shunts

PSS are vascular communications between the portal and systemic venous circulation. PSS can be either congenital or acquired and is seen in both dogs and cats. Congenital shunts can be further subdivided into intrahepatic shunts, occurring mostly in large-breed dogs or extrahepatic shunts, occurring mostly in smaller dog breeds and cats. Intrahepatic shunts are the remnant of a ductus venosus that did not completely close after birth. Extrahepatic shunts are seen as anomalous embryonic vessels between the portal vein and the systemic circulation. A hereditary basis for congenital shunts has been established in Irish wolfhounds and a number of other breeds have a significant risk for development of congenital shunts, again

supporting a hereditary cause.[3] Acquired PSS may develop as multiple shunts in response to portal hypertension caused by cirrhosis or other causes (e.g., tumors or portal vein thrombosis). Both congenital and acquired PSS are seen more often in dogs than in cats.

Primary portal vein hypoplasia (also referred to as microvascular dysplasia) is a second congenital vascular anomaly occurring in dogs, but rarely in cats. This anomaly is a consequence of portal vein hypoperfusion that results in hepatic arterialization in the portal triad and the development of microscopic intrahepatic shunts. Commonly affected breeds include cairn terriers, Yorkshire terriers, and Maltese.[3] Affected dogs have abnormal bile acid concentrations and variable liver enzymes but rarely have clinical signs. A less common variant of portal vein hypoplasia associated with fibrosis in the portal triads results in portal hypertension, ascites, and PSS.

Polydipsia and polyuria are commonly seen in patients with PSS.[1,2] Ammonium urate and other purine uroliths occur in some animals because of high urinary excretion of ammonia and uric acid. Stunted growth or failure to gain weight may occur in young animals with congenital shunts. Surgical closure is the treatment of choice for congenital PSS but not for acquired PSS. Dietary management is the cornerstone of successful case management and prevention of HE in the pre- and immediate postoperative phase and in partially closed shunts.

Neoplasia

The most commonly encountered hepatic malignancies in dogs and cats are metastases, lymphoma, hemangiosarcoma, hepatocellular carcinoma, and cholangiocarcinoma. The appearance may be localized or diffuse. Due to the liver's tremendous reserve capacity, tumors (especially localized malignancies) may go undetected for long periods. In advanced stages, tumors may be visible or palpable during physical examination. Severe liver dysfunction with icterus, coagulopathies, and portal hypertension may occur especially in diffusely distributed malignancies (e.g., malignant lymphoma and hemangiosarcoma).

Hepatic Lipidosis

In felines, HL is a well-recognized syndrome. HL is characterized by the accumulation of excess triglycerides in hepatocytes resulting in choleostasis and hepatic dysfunction. It occurs when there is an increase in peripheral lipolysis with decreased export of very low-density lipoproteins (VLDL) from the liver. It is believed that protein deficiency from decreased intake impairs creation of apolipoproteins, thus limiting transport. Intrahepatic fat collects and if not treated results in distended canaliculi and pronounced intrahepatic cholestasis and hepatic failure.

Lipidosis may occur secondary to diabetes mellitus, diseases resulting in anorexia and weight loss (e.g., pancreatitis or IBD), or as an idiopathic disorder of unknown etiology. Cats with idiopathic HL often present with a history of prolonged anorexia after a stressful event. The biochemical mechanisms responsible for causing HL during fasting are not completely understood. Potential causes include protein deficiency, excessive peripheral lipolysis, excessive lipogenesis, inhibition of lipid oxidation, and inhibition of the synthesis and secretion of VLDL. The prognosis for this life-threatening disorder has improved dramatically during the past several years as a result of long-term enteral feeding (i.e., three to eight weeks or longer). HL is considered a reversible process but resolution of HL secondary to pancreatitis, infection, or other causes depends on the success of treating the underlying disorder and providing appropriate nutritional support. It is important for the veterinary healthcare team to remember that success may take weeks to months and consistency and patience are assets to managing HL.

HL is a serious and life-threatening disorder. Patient outcome has improved dramatically over the past decade due to long-term enteral feeding (i.e., 3–8 weeks or longer).[1,2,8] HL is a reversible process. However, resolution of HL secondary to pancreatitis, infection, or other causes is dependent upon two factors: the success of managing the underlying disorder and the ability to provide appropriate nutritional support. Veterinary nurses/technicians play an integral role in the successful treatment of HL and must remember that success may take weeks to months.

Initial management should be directed toward correcting complications such as dehydration, electrolyte abnormalities, HE, and infection. Resolution of HL associated with pancreatitis, infections, and drugs is dependent on the success in treating the underlying disorder.

Nutrition is the cornerstone to managing HL patients. There are a number of key nutritional factors to consider when managing patients with hepatic disease. The liver plays an important role in the regulation of carbohydrate homeostasis and serum glucose levels through its ability to remove glucose from and release glucose into the circulation. Therefore, again it is important to have highly digestible carbohydrate sources. This will reduce protein breakdown and the resulting gluconeogenesis. Vitamin K and zinc are recommended in dietary management of liver disease to help avoid deficiencies commonly found in patients suffering from hepatic disease. Soluble fiber is necessary to help promote colonic evacuation and to encourage nitrogen fixation by enteric bacteria thus reducing the amount of ammonia production and absorption.

Primary nutritional therapy must be aimed at meeting the patient's resting energy requirement. Typically, this consists of rapid replenishment with a high protein (if there is no evidence of encephalopathy), moderate carbohydrate, and moderate fat. When assessing nutrient utilization, protein in the diet improves the disease process making feeding a priority – especially, given that most cats are severely jaundiced and anorexic at presentation. Early tube feeding via esophagostomy or gastrostomy tubes remains the cornerstone of therapy.[9,10] If the cat cannot be safely anesthetized for placement of an enteral feeding tube, a nasoesophageal tube should be placed, and a liquid, enteral formula should be administered until the cat is stabilized for placement of a longer-lasting esophagostomy or gastrostomy tube.

As soon as the diagnosis of HL has been made a tube should be placed and the cat fed through this tube versus offering several commercial diets to which the cat can develop an aversion. Cats should not be offered any food by mouth for approximately 10 days following placement of a feeding tube. Cats that express an interest in eating can then be presented with a novel diet that they have not been fed before. The prognosis for HL is influenced to a large degree by the ability of the veterinary team and subsequently, the pet owner to aggressively meet the cat's caloric requirements via enteral feeding.

The GI tract needs to be fed. The gut receives an overwhelming percentage of its nutrition from the chyme passing through it. In the small intestine, enterocytes utilize lumenal glutamine preferentially as their source of metabolic fuel. The colonocytes prefer butyrate, a short-chain fatty acid formed by fermentation of lumenal carbohydrates. In the absence of these fuel sources, the gut epithelium slows growth and replication resulting in atrophy, necrosis, and increased risk of bacterial translocation across the now abnormal gut barrier. A key to prevention of this potentially serious problem is providing nutritional support to the gut. The rule of nutritional support is "if the gut works use it."

Force-feeding sick, hospitalized animals is **contraindicated** and is the best way to create food aversions. Force feeding is an inefficient feeding method resulting in more nutrients on the patient and the healthcare team member rather than in the patient. Typically, feeding will not provide a significant percentage of needed calories and will lead to a false sense of accomplishment and continued inadequate intake.

Similarly, appetite stimulants are seldom successful in causing meaningful increases in food intake. The use of appetite stimulants such as diazepam, oxazepam, cyproheptadine, and mirtazapine can be attempted but is not recommended as the typical result is failure to meet the cat's caloric requirement and frustration for the owner and most importantly, the cat. Caution should be noted when using diazepam in cats with hepatic disease as fulminant hepatic failure may ensue.

Pharmacologic stimulation of appetite is often short-lived and only delays true nutritional support. Appetite stimulants should not be used to manage hospitalized animals when more effective measures of nutritional support, such as placement of feeding tubes, are more appropriate. Appetite stimulants may be considered in recovering animals once they are home in their own environment because the primary reason for loss of appetite should ideally be reversed by discharge. As with many drugs, appetite stimulants also have negative side effects, such as behavioral changes associated with cyproheptadine and sedation associated with diazepam, and therefore, should be used with caution.

How Much to Feed?

A good starting point is to calculate the resting energy requirements for the patient's current weight. If a patient's ideal weight is used, underweight animals may be at greater risk for complications from overfeeding. Resting energy requirements can be calculated using the following equation: RER = 70 × (current body weight in kg)$^{0.75}$. Another equation that may be used is RER = (kg × kg × kg, $\sqrt{}$, $\sqrt{}$) × 70.

Initiate refeeding slowly – typically over a 3 day period. Start with $\frac{1}{3}$ RER on day one. If tolerated, increase to $\frac{2}{3}$ RER on day 2, and again if tolerated with no complications, provide full RER on day three.

This gradual transition will be less likely to lead to hyperammonemia and reduce the possibility of refeeding syndrome. It is of utmost importance to monitor electrolytes in HL cats as hypophosphatemia has been observed during enteral feeding of cats with various hepatopathies including HL.[1] Switching to a lower protein diet and beginning lactulose or soluble fiber therapy[6] is recommended if hyperammonemia is suspected by the presence of signs of encephalopathy or confirmed by measuring blood ammonia.

The use of L-carnitine is prudent as it has been shown that L-carnitine may improve whole-body fat metabolism and help prevent HL and ketosis.[1,2,4] This is true even though liver and serum carnitine concentrations in HL are not depleted.[1,4,7] Although not fully understood, it is suggested that carnitine may help peripheral tissues use ketones and fatty acids for energy or decrease hepatic ketone production. Supplementation of L-carnitine is recommended at a dose of 250 mg/day.[1,9]

Storage and utilization of water-soluble vitamins are altered in HL; therefore, vitamin B levels should be monitored, and if needed supplementation at two times maintenance should be initiated. If clinical signs of thiamine deficiency, such as neck ventroflexion, are present, supplementation at a dose of 50–100 mg/cat each day in the food for one week is recommended.[1]

Testing for serum folate and vitamin B12 is commonly performed in HL cats as they are often low or normal. Vitamin B12 at 1mg every 7–28 days has been successfully used to replenish B12 serum concentrations in cats.[8] The liver produces vitamin K-dependent clotting factors which are often reduced in patients with chronic hepatic disease. Therefore, the veterinary team may need to administer vitamin K to offset poor production of clotting factors in HL. Dosages of 0.5–1.5 mg/kg IM or SC every 12 hours for 3 doses and then once weekly for two weeks is recommended.[1,9]

Protein

Do not restrict dietary protein in cats with HL unless the cat is showing signs of encephalopathy. Protein restriction for cats with HE should not fall below minimum protein requirements. Commercial veterinary diets containing between 25% and 30% protein on an ME basis and 60–68% fat on an ME basis have been well tolerated in most cats with HL that are not encephalopathic. The feeding of human liquid enteral formulas should be avoided as they are often deficient in the essential amino acids arginine and taurine and contain inadequate levels of protein.

Sodium and Chloride

Excessive dietary sodium chloride should be avoided in liver disease patients with ascites, portal hypertension, and/or significant hypoalbuminemia. Dietary sodium chloride should be offered at levels recommended for patients with renal and cardiac failure. Thus, sodium levels should be 0.07%–0.3% DM for cats. Recommended DM chloride levels are typically 1.5 times sodium levels.

Potassium

Hypokalemia is A relatively common finding in HL cats is hypokalemia which can lead to inadequate potassium intake, vomiting, magnesium depletion, and concurrent renal failure.

Hypokalemia is detrimental because it can prolong anorexia and exacerbate HE. Thus, diets for cats with HL should be contain potassium (0.8–1% potassium on a DM basis, or 1.5 g/Mcal). Additionally, potassium can be orally supplemented at 2 to 6 mEq potassium gluconate per day.

Successful treatment of feline HL involves veterinary team knowledge, active owner involvement, and education. Treatment may require weeks or months of assisted enteral feeding and the success depends upon the communication and education of the cat owner.

The veterinary team plays a crucial role in monitoring, reassessing, and overall management of the hepatic patient. Therefore, It is important to remember that hepatic disease is typically severe before clinical signs and/or laboratory tests reveal/confirm the disease. Consequently, the patient is often suffering significant metabolic alterations by the time an appropriate feeding plan is implemented by the healthcare team. It is imperative that nutritional management of liver disease be directed at the clinical manifestations of the disease as opposed to the specific cause of the disease. Proper nursing care and nutritional management of hepatic patients will help to reduce patient suffering and provide a better quality of life for these patients.

References

1 Meyer HP, Twedt DC, Roudebush P and Dill-Macky E (2010) Hepatobiliary disease. In In MS Hand, CD Thatcher, RL Remillard *et al.* (eds), *Small Animal Clinical Nutrition* (5th edn), pp. 1155–92, Topeka, KS: Mark Morris Institute.

2 Norton RD, Lenox CE, Manino P, Vulgamott JC (2016) Nutritional Considerations for Dogs and Cats with Liver Disease. *J Am Anim Hosp Assoc.* Jan-Feb; 52(1): 1–7.

3 Watson P (2017) Canine breed-specific hepatopathies. *Veterinary Clinics: Small Animal Practice.* 47(3): 665–82.

4 Michel KE (1995) Nutritional management of liver disease. *Vet Clin North Am Small Anim Pract* 25(2): 485–502.

5 Ruaux CG (2010) Nutritional management of hepatic conditions. In *Textbook of Veterinary Internal Medicine* (7th edn), pp. 682–7, St Louis: Elsevier.

6 Bagavan RP, Sonali N, Vaani ST, et al. (2023) Nutritional management of liver diseases in dogs and cats. *The Pharma Innovation Journal* 12(1): 1352–1359.

7 Rothuizen J, Bunch SE, Charles JA, *et al.* (2006) *WSAVA Standards for Clinical and Histological Diagnosis of Canine and Feline Liver Disease.* Oxford, UK: Saunders.

8 Negasee KA (2021) Hepatic diseases in canine and feline: A review. *Vet Med Open Jl.* 6(1): 22–31.

9 Streeter RM, Wakshlag JJ (2015) Nutritional support in hepatic failure in dogs and cats. In *Nutritional Management of Hospitalized Small Animals.* Daniel L. Chan, ed. Wiley Blackwell, Ames, IA. pp. 199–221.

10 Burns KM (2022) Critical Cases Benefit from Specialized Nutrition. *Veterinary Practice News* March.

40

Dermatology

The management and treatment of skin disorders rely heavily on nutritional management. The use of dietary fatty acids, antioxidants, and novel and hydrolyzed proteins can be beneficial in managing inflammatory skin problems.[1] Additionally, zinc, vitamin A, and vitamin E are also utilized for their effects on skin and haircoat.[2] The veterinary healthcare team plays a large role in improving patient care through understanding of inflammatory skin diseases in dogs and cats, the application of nutritional therapy in managing these disorders, client communication, and enhanced compliance.[3]

The skin, which is the largest organ of the body, protects the animal against water loss as well as physical, chemical, and microbiologic injury. The skin is also a sensory organ and can perceive temperature, pain, touch, pruritus, and pressure. Skin disorders are among the most common conditions treated in veterinary hospitals.[3] Surveys indicate that approximately 15–25% of small animal practice involves the diagnosis and treatment of skin and haircoat disorders.[1,3–5]

Patient History

Obtaining an adequate patient history is the first step in evaluating patients with skin disorders. This must be done every time the pet visits the hospital. A complete history should include signalment (i.e., species, breed, age, gender, reproductive status, and hair color), presenting complaint, weight and body condition score, nutrition regimen, medical history, and home environment.

A complete nutritional history should also be performed on every visit to determine the quality and adequacy of the food being fed to the pet, the feeding protocol (e.g., meal fed, free choice, amount, and family member responsible for the feeding), and a thorough history of the types of foods fed, including access to treats, supplements, and/or other foods. All members of the health care team should be familiar with taking a nutritional history.[3,4] The questions should be asked in an open-ended manner, allowing the pet owner to discuss and expand upon their pet's nutrition. A nutritional history should include all of the following (Figure 40.1):

Remember, it is imperative that the healthcare team learn everything that enters the pets' mouths. For instance, a dog may be eating dry commercial food as its main source of nutrition but may also receive pig ears, dog biscuits, flavored monthly oral heartworm prophylactic medication, and table scraps. If the family also includes cats, the dog may have access to commercial food fed to the family cats. Each of these items could be sources of adverse food reactions. Consequently, the pet owner should document everything that enters their pets' oral cavity on a daily basis. This diary should be kept for several weeks prior to the pets' appointment. During the appointment, the pet's nutritional history should be reviewed carefully for allergens or

Nutrition and Disease Management for Veterinary Technicians and Nurses, Third Edition. Ann Wortinger and Kara M. Burns.
© 2024 John Wiley & Sons, Inc. Published 2024 by John Wiley & Sons, Inc.
Companion Website: www.wiley.com/go/wortinger/3e

- Tell me everything that your pet eats in a day. _____
- Tell me the brand of food do you feed your pet (try to get specific name or a picture) _____
- Tell me how you give food to your pet. _____
- Tell me how you feed your pet _____
    ° How much? _____
    ° How often? _____
        o Canned food _____
        o Dry Food _____
        o Both _____
- What snacks or treats are provided? _____
    ° What treats? _____
    ° How often? _____
- What supplements does your pet receive? _____
- Tell me the medications, including chewable medications, you give to your pet.
    ° Medication name _____
    ° Dosage _____
- Tell me about the toys your pet enjoys _____
- Do you feed your pet any foods or treats not specifically designated for pets? _____
    ° Human foods? _____
    ° Others? _____
    ° How often? _____
- To what other food does your pet have   access? _____
    ° Neighbor? _____
    ° Trash? _____
    ° Compost? _____
    ° family member (e.g., baby in house, grandparents in house)? _____

Figure 40.1 Nutritional History Questionnaire.

ingredients believed to be commonly associated with adverse food reactions.

Physical Examination

The comprehensive physical examination should include a nose-to-tail evaluation of the pet's skin and hair condition. Any evidence of parasites as well as signs of excessive scratching or licking should be noted in the patient's medical record. The overall health of the patient should be assessed and documented in the medical record.

Common Skin Disorders in Dogs and Cats

Inflammatory skin diseases are typically an allergic (atopy or hypersensitivity) response or an adverse reaction to foods, and the resulting clinical signs often are similar. Clinical signs associated with inflammatory skin diseases include redness, edema, excoriation, hair loss, ulceration, lichenification, pruritus, and dry, flaky skin. The response by the pet is often self-trauma from chronic licking, rubbing, chewing, and scratching of the affected area. Because signs of internal disease may be manifested in skin and haircoat changes, these differentials should not be overlooked because of external lesions. A series of diagnostic tests should be conducted to pinpoint the cause of the skin disorder so that the most effective treatment can be recommended.

Inflammatory skin diseases define a broad range of skin disorders. The most commonly diagnosed inflammatory skin disorders in dogs include allergies, bacterial infections, parasite infestations, and adverse reactions to food. The list is similar in cats, except cats also develop miliary dermatitis and eosinophilic granuloma complex.

Allergic Dermatitis

Canine atopic dermatitis is a multifactorial disease process. Dogs and cats may be sensitive to allergens in the environment. These allergens are proteins which cause an allergen-specific IG-E production leading to allergy symptoms, such as inflammation when inhaled or absorbed through the skin, respiratory tract, or gastrointestinal (GI) tract.[6–11]

Canine research suggests dermal barrier defects contribute to environmental allergens and microbes penetrating the skin, thus stimulating the epidermal immune system. The immunologic response results in release of inflammatory mediators.[6,7] As cats have increased in popularity, the recognition of atopy in this species has increased. The estimated prevalence of canine atopic dermatitis is approximately 10–15%.[11,12]

Even though the pathogenesis is not understood fully, evidence supports genetic abnormalities, an altered immune system with cutaneous inflammation, and a skin barrier defect.[13]

Atopic dermatitis is the top claim submitted by canine Nationwide policyholders in 2022. It ranked #8 with feline policyholders. Among Nationwide-insured dogs in 2022 skin allergies were the most common health issue, with more than 373,000 individual claims received (up from 335,000 in 2021).[14] This marks the 11th year in a row that skin allergies were the top claim for canine policyholders. Additionally, one single dog residing in New York came in with the highest cost with a skin allergy diagnosis at ∼ $9,480. In addition, this dog has multiple chronic conditions. His regimen includes monthly Cytopoint injections, daily oral Atopica, and weekly at-home allergen injections.[14]

The predisposition of German shepherds for allergic dermatitis (AD) is likely due to a risk haplotype in combination with multiple variants resulting in a changed expression of the plakophilin 2 gene and nearby genes.[11,15] In the United Kingdom the risk of Labrador and Golden retrievers to develop AD was almost 50% due to the genetic background.[11] Multiple breeds including Boxer, Westhighland White Terrier, French bulldog, Bullterrier, American cocker spaniel, English springer spaniel, Poodle, Chinese Sharpei, Dachshund, Collie, Miniature schnauzer, Lhasa apso, Pug, and Rhodesian ridgeback are also predisposed[16,17] and breed predispositions vary with geographic location.[18]

In cats any breed can be at risk; however, the Devon rex, purebred cats in general, and orange cats or cats with orange color in their coats seem to be more predisposed than other breeds and colors.[19] Most dogs are diagnosed with atopy from 6 months to 3 years of age. Cats diverge from dogs and the range is 6 months to 14 years.[19]

Allergic skin diseases include atopy and flea-bite hypersensitivity. Allergic dermatitis might be the cause if the pet has seasonal pruritus, lichenification (thickening of the skin which indicates chronic inflammation), and hyperpigmentation. The feet, face, ears, flexural surfaces of the front legs, axilla, and abdomen are most affected. Lesions can develop due to self-trauma. Also, otitis, pyoderma, or Malassezia dermatitis are seen secondary to atopy.[9] Diagnosis for atopy involves eliminating other conditions with similar symptoms.[6,9] Thus, diagnosis includes appropriate control for external parasites, and potentially elimination food trials. Intradermal skin testing or serologic testing can also be performed to identify possible antigens, but they are not a definitive diagnosis of atopy. Skin testing or serological testing is only used to guide immunological therapy after a diagnosis of atopy is made.

Flea-bite hypersensitivity is typically characterized by pruritic, papular dermatitis with lesions in the dorsal lumbosacral area, caudomedial thighs, ventral abdomen, and flanks. Lesions involving the ears, footpads, or face strongly suggest a concurrent atopy or adverse food reaction. Secondary bacterial infections, hot spots, and seborrhea are common in chronic hypersensitivity cases.[2,20]

The development of hypersensitivity reaction(s) and ensuing skin lesions accompanied by variable pruritus in response to exposure to flea salivary antigens is known as flea allergy dermatitis (FAD).[2,20] Pet owners often describe this as a flea bite allergy. It is reasonable to assume there is high variability within individual patients as to the amount of flea salivary antigen necessary to induce clinical flea allergic dermatitis. Flea allergies are the most common type of allergic skin diagnosed in dogs. It is also one of the most commonly diagnosed skin disorders in cats.[1,4] Specific breed of gender predilection has not been seen in patients with fleabite hypersensitivity. Dogs that are predisposed to flea allergy and live in a flea-endemic area typically show clinical signs by five years of age.[2,4] However, clinical signs can develop at any age, especially if animals move from a low-exposure area to an area where fleas are widespread. Flea allergies typically present as pruritic papular dermatitis, concentrated on the rump, dorsal thorax, flanks, tail, and perineal area.[1,4] Pruritus occurs on the caudal areas and tail, although generalized pruritus may be seen. Papules in the umbilical area are also very suggestive of flea hypersensitivity. Front limb "corn cobbing" is another characteristic behavior seen in flea-allergic dogs. Cats are more prone to miliary dermatitis lesions on the back, neck, and face, although lesions may be found anywhere. It is important to obtain a history, including clinical signs and diet history. When diagnosing flea allergies, look for the presence of live fleas or flea dirt. Diagnosis may start simply with a thorough combing of the patient's coat with a flea comb. However, further diagnostics including intradermal testing, may be warranted.[4]

Adverse Reactions to Food

Adverse reactions to food often imitate allergic diseases. An adverse reaction to food is an abnormal response to an ingested food or food additive. Adverse food reactions in dogs typically occur as nonseasonal pruritic dermatitis, occasionally accompanied by GI signs.[4,21,22] The pruritus varies in severity. Lesion distribution is often indistinguishable from that seen with atopic dermatitis; feet, face, axillae, perineal region, inguinal region, rump, and ears are often affected. One-fourth of dogs with adverse food reactions have lesions only in the region of the ears.[4,23] Therefore, adverse food reactions should always be suspected in dogs with pruritic, unilateral, or bilateral otitis externa, even if accompanied by secondary bacterial or *Malassezia* infections.

Adverse food reactions often mimic other common canine skin disorders, including pyoderma, pruritic seborrheic dermatoses, folliculitis, and ectoparasitism.[21] Concurrent allergic diseases, such as flea-allergic dermatitis and atopic dermatitis, may be present in 20–30% or more of dogs with suspected adverse food reactions (Table 40.1).[23]

Table 40.1 Skin lesions in dogs caused by adverse food reactions.

- Epidermal collarettes
- Erythroderma
- Excoriations
- Hyperpigmentation
- Otitis externa
- Papules
- Pododermatitis
- Seborrhea sicca

Miliary dermatitis in cats' results in numerous small, red papules capped with brownish crusts and associated with varying degrees of hair loss and pruritus. The lesions are typically located in the dorsal lumbar and cervical lesions and are a common response to flea allergy. Miliary dermatitis may also be associated with adverse food reactions and atopy.[24]

Feline eosinophilic granuloma complex describes a skin disorder that involves several syndromes, including indolent ulcers, eosinophilic plaques, and linear granulomas. *Indolent ulcer* is the term used to describe raised, ulcerated lesions in cats seen most commonly on the upper lip and in the mouth. An eosinophilic plaque describes reddened, raised, flat, and firm lesions commonly seen on the abdomen or inner thigh regions. A linear granuloma is a series of raised plaques in a linear configuration often seen on the caudal aspect of a cat's thighs. Feline eosinophilic granuloma complex has been associated with underlying allergies such as flea-bite hypersensitivity, food allergy, and atopy.[25]

Nutritional Management

Key Nutritional Factors

The skin is a metabolically active organ affected by the nutritional status of the animal. Inflammatory skin disorders result in inflammation and infection and require additional nutritional support. An adverse food reaction is an abnormal response to an ingested protein or food additive. Therefore, it is important to ensure that essential nutrients to support normal skin and hair as well as reparative functions are available to the pet. Also, in patients with adverse food reactions, the offending ingredients must be eliminated. Key nutritional factors that help maintain healthy skin and aid in the management of skin disorders are protein, energy, essential fatty acids (EFAs), minerals (copper and zinc), and vitamins (A, E, and B-complex). The pet's food should include optimal levels of these nutrients and the nutrients should be highly digestible and available to the pet.[1]

Protein and energy are essential for the development of new hair and skin. It is important that the pet's food provides optimal protein quality with appropriate levels of essential amino acids, adequate protein quantity, and digestibility. Growth, gestation, lactation, and illness require increased protein and energy; abnormal skin and hair may be noted if nutritionally inadequate foods are fed during these life stages. Inadequate intake of protein and energy may result in depigmentation, dry, dull haircoat, and hair loss. Changes in lipid content of the epidermis may affect the protective barrier function of the skin, thereby predisposing the pet to secondary bacterial or yeast infection. Inadequate protein and energy are also associated with impaired wound healing. Pets with severe seborrhea have increased epidermal cell turnover and may have increased protein and other nutrient requirements.

Because most food allergens are thought to be glycoproteins, protein in food is the nutrient of most concern in patients with suspected adverse food reactions. The following should be considered:

- types and numbers of diverse proteins in the food
- protein sources
- amount of protein
- digestibility of the protein
- previous exposure to the protein.

Pet food additives, such as antimicrobial preservatives, colorants, antioxidant preservatives, and emulsifying agents, rarely cause either food intolerance or food allergy.

EFAs are polyunsaturated fatty acids found in phospholipids. They are important in structural function of the lipoproteins of cell membranes allowing conformational responses during temperature fluctuations and providing a barrier function to prevent the loss of water and other nutrients.[26] EFAs are also a source of energy for the skin and are precursors to a variety of important molecules involved in the inflammatory response. EFA deficiencies may result in scaly skin, matting of hair, loss of skin elasticity, alopecia, dry and dull haircoat, erythroderma, hyperkeratosis, interdigital exudation, otitis externa, and poor hair regrowth. These changes affect transepidermal water loss, epidermal cell turnover, poor wound healing, and increased susceptibility to infection. Another important role of EFAs is as antipruritic agents. The inflammation and dermatitis associated with allergic skin disease may be partially caused by abnormal EFA metabolism. The presence of EFA in the cellular membranes may decrease inflammation through competition with arachidonic acid for metabolic enzymes or by anti-inflammatory properties.[27] Several studies have looked at the effect of EFAs on pruritus, and on average, 50% of dogs and cats with allergic pruritus improve with modification in EFA intake as long as secondary bacterial and yeast infections are also controlled.[27,28]

Mineral and vitamin imbalances are often associated with skin lesions. Copper deficiency can lead to loss of normal hair coloration, lack of hair, and a dull or rough coat. Zinc is an important enzyme cofactor and modulator of many biological functions. Zinc deficiency can lead to a dull, rough coat, skin ulcerations, hyperkeratosis, and other dermatoses. Vitamin A, E, and B-complex imbalances are associated with different skin disorders; therefore, foods should be evaluated for appropriate quantity and balance of these vitamins. In general, most commercial pet foods contain excessive vitamins; therefore, skin disorders caused by vitamin deficiencies are rare. However, vitamin deficiency should be considered in animals being fed homemade, noncommercial, or species-generic pet foods.

Nutritional Protocol

A complete nutritional protocol in the management of inflammatory skin disorders includes an assessment of the current foods being fed, an assessment of the feeding method, identification of an appropriate feeding plan, and reassessment of the feeding plan.

The pet's food should contain optimal levels of protein, energy, EFAs, minerals, and vitamins for the appropriate life stage of the pet. The nutrients should be high quality to ensure digestibility and availability to meet the pet's nutritional requirements. Assessment of nutritional supplements is also important to identify potential interference with key nutrients or unnecessary supplementation.

The feeding method includes the feeding route, quantity fed, how the food is offered, access to other food, and who is responsible for feeding the pet. This information was gathered when the nutritional history was obtained. It is extremely important when verifying an appropriate feeding method with the pet owner. It is important to thoroughly evaluate the feeding method, although it may not always be necessary to change the nutritional protocol when managing a patient with an inflammatory skin disorder.[3,5]

Selecting appropriate foods is an important consideration in the nutritional management of patients with inflammatory skin disorders. There are a number of influences which must be considered when treating skin conditions. The patient's access to treats, table scraps, and flavored medicines are a few of the factors which healthcare team members should be mindful of when managing skin conditions. For generalized nutritional skin disorders, the diet should be transitioned to a highly digestible food with increased levels of protein and EFAs and an appropriate balance of minerals and vitamins. Oftentimes, the following indications signal a need for change in the pets' diet:

- abnormal hair growth
- abnormal hair regrowth
- loss of normal haircoat color
- adverse reaction to food
- widespread scaling, crusting
- dull haircoat or hair loss
- hyperproliferative skin disorders
- poor/delayed wound healing
- decubital ulcers
- severe and/or generalized inflammatory skin disorders.

The same nutritional management that works for dietary-related skin problems may also help with inflammatory skin disorders and dermatologic signs associated with metabolic diseases in dogs and cats. Research has demonstrated that the use of novel protein foods with enhanced levels of omega-3 fatty acids and antioxidants is warranted to aid in management of pets with chronic, nonseasonal pruritic dermatitis caused by suspected atopic dermatitis and/or adverse food reactions. Improvements in itchy skin, otitis externa, skin redness, and hair loss were noted by pet owners. Veterinarians recognized the overall improvement in skin and coat condition in the majority of dogs. Novel protein foods with enhanced levels of omega-3 fatty acids and antioxidants should be considered in managing dogs with suspected allergic dermatitis.[29]

Skin disorders caused by nutrient deficiencies usually respond quickly when the pet's diet is changed to a high-quality, highly digestible food. Patient improvement is relatively quick – a few days to a couple of weeks. The healthcare team should closely monitor and document any food and supplement changes. The patient should be examined on a weekly to monthly basis, depending on the diagnosis and severity of the lesions.

A diagnosis of adverse food reaction is more complex and involves a series of elimination trials with novel protein foods or protein hydrolysate foods. Dietary elimination trials are the main diagnostic method used in dogs and cats with suspected adverse food reactions. Ingredients in an ideal elimination food should provide a limited number of highly digestible protein sources, preferably a protein hydrolysate or one to two different types of intact protein to which the animal has not been previously exposed. This recommendation often includes commercial or homemade food with one animal and one vegetable protein source. An alternate strategy is to use a food containing protein hydrolysate(s). Protein hydrolysates have molecular weights below levels that commonly elicit an allergic response.[30] Caution should be used when recommending homemade food because most homemade foods fail to meet nutritional requirements because they are made from a minimum of ingredients.[31] If a homemade diet is warranted, this should be done in cooperation with a board-certified veterinary nutritionist. It is important to assess the patient for concurrent allergic skin diseases, particularly atopy and flea allergy hypersensitivity because these patients may only partially respond to an elimination trial.

As with any therapeutic protocol, client compliance is critical to a successful outcome. Managing inflammatory skin disorders properly is a long-term investment by the veterinary health care team and the client. Management frequently involves a combination of symptomatic treatment until a definitive diagnosis and appropriate treatment protocol are determined. The technician has a great opportunity to provide vital client support by reinforcing the veterinarian's diagnosis and treatment protocol, educating the client about the importance of and proper application of nutritional protocols and adjunctive therapies, and monitoring patient care through follow-up communications, including callbacks and rechecks.

Skin disorders are one of the most common conditions treated in veterinary hospitals. Owners of pets with chronic skin problems often seek veterinary help for symptomatic relief for their pet, resolution of chronic inflammation, and an improvement in the quality and appearance of their pet's haircoat.

Allergic inflammatory skin disorders and adverse reactions to foods are often concurrent and have similar presenting clinical signs. Symptomatic treatment may be necessary while differential diagnoses and appropriate treatment protocols are determined. Nutrition can play an important role in helping to manage and treat skin disorders. The role of the veterinary technician is crucial to optimal patient care through reinforcement of the veterinarian's diagnosis and treatment protocol enhancing client communication and compliance. By encouraging compliance, technicians can help ensure successful patient care, client satisfaction, and improved quality of life for the pet.

References

1 Roudebush PR, Guilford WG, Jackson HA (2010) Adverse reactions to food. In MS Hand, CD Thatcher, RL Remillard *et al.* (eds), *Small Animal Clinical Nutrition* (5th edn), pp. 609–33, Marceline, MO: Walsworth Publishing, Mark Morris Institute.

2 Miller WH, Griffin CE, Campbell K (eds) (2013) Nutrition in skin disease. In *Muller and Kirk's Small Animal Dermatology* (7th edn), pp. 685–94, St. Louis: Elsevier.

3 Burns KM (2019) Nutrition and adverse reactions to food. *The NAVTA Jl.* February/March: 25–9.

4 Ograin VL, Burns KM (2016) Nutritional considerations in allergic skin disease. *The NAVTA Jl* Convention Issue: 12–9.

5 Burns KM (2005) *Nutritional management of inflammatory skin disorders, Veterinary Technician,* November, pp. 794–800.

6 Olivry T, Deboer D, All E, Treatment of Canine Atopic Dermatitis (2010) Clinical practice guidelines from the international task force on canine atopic dermatitis. *Veterinary Dermatology* **2010**(21): 233–48.

7 Inman AO, Olivry T, Dunston SM *et al.* (2001) Electron microscopic observations of stratum corneum intercellular lipids in normal and atopic dogs. *Veterinary Pathology* **38**(6): 720–3.

8 Bizikova P, Pucheu-Haston CM, Eisenschenk MNC *et al.* (2015) Review:

role of genetics and the environment in the pathogenesis of canine atopic dermatitis. *Veterinary Dermatology* **26**: 95–e26.

9 Diaz S. Atopic Dermatitis. *The Merck Veterinary Manual.* October, 2022. https://www.merckvetmanual.com/integumentary-system/atopic-dermatitis/atopic-dermatitis-in-animals. Accessed June 1, 2023.

10 Halliwell R (2006) Revised nomenclature for veterinary allergy. *Veterinary Immunology and Immunopathology* **114**(3–4): 207–8.

11 Gedon NKY, Mueller RS (2018) Atopic dermatitis in cats and dogs:a difficult disease for animals and owners. *Clinical and Translational Allergy* **8**: 41.

12 Hillier A, Griffin CE (2001) The ACVD task force on canine atopic dermatitis (I): incidence and prevalence. *Veterinary Immunology and Immunopathology* **81**(3–4): 147–51.

13 Marsella R, De Benedetto A (2017) Atopic dermatitis in animals and people: an update and comparative review. *Veterinary Sciences* **4**(3): 37.

14 Dermatitis, otitis externa continue to top common conditions that prompt veterinary visits. *Nationwide Pet Insurance* April 2023. https://news.nationwide.com/dermatitis-otitis-externa-top-common-conditions-vet-visits/ Accessed 6/29/2023.

15 Tengvall K, Kierczak M, Bergvall K *et al.* (2013) Genome-wide analysis in German

shepherd dogs reveals association of a locus on CFA 27 with atopic dermatitis. *PLoS Genetics* **9**(5): e1003475.

16 Verlinden A, Hesta M, Millet S, Janssens GP (2006) Food allergy in dogs and cats: a review. *Critical Reviews in Food Science and Nutrition* **46**(3): 259–73.

17 Picco F, Zini E, Nett C *et al.* (2008) A prospective study on canine atopic dermatitis and food-induced allergic dermatitis in Switzerland. *Veterinary Dermatology* **19**(3): 150–5.

18 Jaeger K, Linek M, Power HT *et al.* (2010) Breed and site predispositions of dogs with atopic dermatitis: a comparison of five locations in three continents. *Veterinary Dermatology* **21**(1): 118–22.

19 Jeromin AM. Feline atopy—are you seeing more cases in your veterinary clinic lately? DVM360. June 2012. Accessed November 2015.

20 Banovic F (2018) Canine atopic dermatitis: updates on diagnosis and treatment. *Today's Veterinary Practice*. January/February: 43–58.

21 MacDonald JM (1993) Food allergy. In CE Griffin, KW Kwochka, JM MacDonald (eds), *Current Veterinary Dermatology*, pp. 121–32, St Louis, MO: Mosby.

22 Roudebush P, Schick RO (1994) Evaluation of a commercial canned lamb and rice diet for the management of adverse reactions to food in dogs. *Veterinary Dermatology* **5**: 63–7.

23 Rosser EJ (2001) Evaluation of a novel carbohydrate and hydrolyzed protein containing diet in previously confirmed food allergic dogs [abstract]. *Veterinary Dermatology* **12**: 230.

24 Sousa CA (1995) Exudative, crusting and scaling dermatoses. *The Veterinary Clinics of North America. Small Animal Practice* **25**: 813–32.

25 Campbell KL (2004) *Small Animal Dermatology Secrets*, pp. 220–4, Philadelphia: Hanley and Belfus Medical Publishers.

26 Roudebush PR, Schoenherr WD (2010) Skin and hair disorders. In MS Hand, CD Thatcher, RL Remillard *et al.* (eds), *Small Animal Clinical Nutrition* (5th edn), pp. 638–65, Marceline, MO: Walsworth Publishing, Mark Morris Institute.

27 Miller WH, Scott DW, Wellington JR (1992) Investigation on the antipruritic effects of ascorbic acid given alone or in combination with a fatty acid supplement to dogs with allergic skin disease. *Canine Practice* **17**: 11–3.

28 Harvey RG (1991) Management of feline miliary dermatitis by supplementing the diet with essential fatty acids. *The Veterinary Record* **128**: 326–9.

29 Fritsch DA, Roudebush PR, Allen TA *et al.* (2010, 2010) Effect of two therapeutic foods in dogs with chronic non-seasonal pruritic dermatitis. *International Journal of Applied Research in Veterinary Medicine* **8**(3): 146–54.

30 Loeffler A, Lloyd DH, Bond R *et al.* (2004) Dietary trials with a commercial chicken hydrolysate diet in sixty-three pruritic dogs. *The Veterinary Record* **154**(17): 519–22.

31 Roudebush P, Cowell CS (1992) Results of a hypoallergenic diet survey of veterinarians in North America with a nutritional evaluation of homemade diet prescriptions. *Veterinary Dermatology* **3**: 23–8.

41

Fatty Acids in Disease Management

Osteoarthritis (OA), cardiac disease, feline lower urinary tract disease, dermatological conditions, and cancer are a few of the conditions that have been found to be aided by the addition of fatty acids in nutritional management. This chapter will focus on fatty acids, especially omega-3 fatty acids, and their role in inflammatory processes and managing disease conditions.

Cardiovascular disease is a common disorder in dogs and cats, with 11% of canines and up to 20% of feline populations affected by cardiac disease.[1,2] Chronic valvular disease (CVD) has been found to be the most common acquired heart disease in dogs with an overall incidence greater than 40%.[3] The most common acquired cardiac abnormality in dogs is chronic mitral valvular disease, affecting more than one-third of patients over 10 years of age.[4] In approximately 30% of cases the tricuspid valve is involved. However, disease of the tricuspid valve is usually less severe. Valvular disease is more prevalent in small-breed dogs. In cats, acquired valvular disease is rare. Following the discovery that taurine deficiency was the principal cause of dilated cardiomyopathy (DCM) in cats in 1987, the prevalence of this disease has decreased significantly.[3,4] Today, hypertrophic and restrictive cardiomyopathies are more prevalent causes of myocardial failure in cats.[5]

In human medicine, there is extensive evidence supporting the positive effects of omega-3 fatty acids in primary and secondary prevention of cardiac disease. Recent, evidence in veterinary medicine has been supportive of the use of omega-3 fatty acids in dogs with cardiac disease. The benefits of omega-3 fatty acids include anti-inflammatory effects and antiarrhythmic effects which help in managing the patient's lean body mass and arrhythmias, two problems associated with cardiac disease.

Dietary fat is important for energy, as a carrier of fat-soluble vitamins, and is a source of essential fatty acids (EFA). Although the term "fat" suggests negative connotations in today's society, dietary fat is essential for life. Dietary fat is the most concentrated form of energy in pet foods, providing 2.25 times (9 kcal/g) the metabolizable energy of proteins and carbohydrates. Fats affect immune function, inflammation, and hemodynamics. Fat, especially omega-3 fatty acids, has also been shown to affect the cardiovascular system.[6-8]

Fatty Acids

Lipid structure ranges from simple to complex. Hydrocarbon molecules are basic subunits of lipids and are linked by covalent bonds in various manners to themselves and to other molecules, thus resulting in the numerous functions and structures occurring in the animal.[9]

Nutrition and Disease Management for Veterinary Technicians and Nurses, Third Edition. Ann Wortinger and Kara M. Burns.
© 2024 John Wiley & Sons, Inc. Published 2024 by John Wiley & Sons, Inc.
Companion Website: www.wiley.com/go/wortinger/3e

The functions of distinct fatty acids are dependent upon their structure and composition. The classification of fatty acids is based on[10]:

1. Length of the hydrocarbon chain
2. Number of double bonds present in the chain
3. Location of the first double bond relative to the methyl (or omega) end of the hydrocarbon chain

Fatty acids in the omega-3 fatty acid family have the first double bond between the third and fourth carbon; omega-6 fatty acids have the first double bond between the sixth and seventh carbon; and the omega-9 fatty acids have the first double bond between the ninth and tenth carbon.[6–9] The omega-3 and omega-6 fatty acid families are EFA because they cannot be synthesized in animals. Members of the omega-6 family include linoleic acid (18:2n-6), g-linolenic acid (18:3n-6), and arachidonic acid (20:4n-6). Dogs are able to synthesize linoleic acid to form arachidonic acid. Subsequently, linoleic acid is customarily listed as an EFA for dogs. However, in cats, both linoleic acid and arachidonic acid are EFAs. Omega-6 fatty acids are necessary for growth, reproduction, and precursors of eicosanoid and prostaglandin synthesis. Omega-3 fatty acids include α-linolenic (18:3n-3), eicosapentaenoic (20:5n-3) (EPA), and docosahexaenoic (22:6n-3) (DHA) acids. Omega-3 fatty acids are needed for proper brain and retinal function. Omega-3 and omega-6 fatty acids are responsible for cell membrane fluidity and skin health.

The makeup of the diets for dogs, cats, and humans is primarily omega-6 fatty acids. Nevertheless, dietary adaptation or supplementation of omega-3 fatty acids can significantly increase omega-3 fatty acid concentrations in the blood and tissues as omega-3 and omega-6 fatty acids compete with one another for enzymes required for their metabolism. As a result, the higher the amount of omega-3 fatty acids in the diet, the more omega-3 fatty acids will be utilized and incorporated into cells.[6,8,9]

Nutrition is an important part of management of cardiac disease and each cardiac patient should have a nutritional assessment and specific dietary recommendation by the veterinarian and the veterinary technician as part of their overall management. The goals of nutritional management of cardiac patients include: (1) maintaining the pets' ideal body condition, (2) maintaining appropriate balance of nutrients, and (3) receiving benefits from pharmacologic doses of certain nutrients. It is exciting to note that omega-3 fatty acids play a role in each nutritional goal.[6] Although cardiac cachexia is prevalent in cardiac disease, this discussion will review the role of omega-3 fatty acids in cardiac disease with respect to arrhythmias, valvular disease, etc. Cardiac cachexia and the role of nutrition and fatty acids specifically deserve their own presentation and discussion.

Fatty Acid Deficiencies and Cardiac Disease

It has been noted that when compared to normal dogs, dogs diagnosed with heart failure had a deficiency of plasma EPA and DHA.[6,11] It was also shown that in dogs with heart failure secondary to DCM, the supplementation of fish oil for eight weeks stabilized plasma fatty acid abnormalities.[6,10] Although the use of omega-3 fatty acids helps to improve myocardial energy metabolism and mitochondrial function is in its infancy, the results thus far have been promising. Therefore, in an attempt to correct deficiencies in cardiac patients and to benefit energy metabolism, omega-3 fatty acids may be supplemented.[6–8]

Arrhythmia

To date, studies in humans have correlated the benefits of fish consumption with the reduction in risks for developing coronary heart disease and subsequent death from myocardial infarction.[6–8] Human studies historically have looked at fatty acids and ventricular arrhythmias. However, recent studies have looked at and have shown benefits of omega-3 fatty acids on atrial fibrillation. Results suggest that omega-3 fatty acids reduce atrial fibrillation. Human populations which eat higher amounts of fish or have higher omega-3 fatty acid concentrations were linked to a lower incidence of atrial fibrillation.

There has only been one study reported to date that looked at the effect of omega-3 fatty acids on naturally occurring diseases in dogs. In this study, the number of ventricular arrhythmias in Boxers was reduced. This reduction was noted after six weeks of fish oil supplementation as compared to the control – sunflower oil. Obviously, more research will need to be done as this is only one study and with only one breed of dog. Therefore, although the results of omega-3 fatty acids on arrhythmias have been positive, at this point, omega-3 fatty acids should only be considered as an addition to medical therapy for dogs with significant arrhythmias.

Omega-3 Fatty Acids and the Overall Effect on the Cardiac Patient

Omega-3 fatty acids have been shown to have a significant effect on survival times when used in dogs diagnosed with DCM or CVD.[12] The effect of the omega-3 fatty acids may be attributed to anti-inflammatory effects, cachexia prevention, improved appetite, or anti-arrhythmic effects. The veterinary healthcare team should also be aware of further effects of omega-3 fatty acids on the patient. The healthcare team must be mindful of the fact that omega-3 fatty acids have the potential to alter immune function. This alteration in immune function may contribute to the cardiovascular effects of omega-3 fatty acids. Also, omega-3 fatty acids reduce platelet aggregation

resulting from the production of thromboxane B5. The reduction in platelet aggregation might be of benefit to cats with cardiac disease and at risk for thrombus formation. However, this effect is also important to be mindful of when using omega-3 fatty acids in animals with coagulopathies.

The discussion has only touched the tip of the research of the effects of fatty acids and cardiac disease. While more studies and discussion are needed in the long term, it is believed that dogs and cats with cardiac disease may benefit from omega-3 fatty acid supplementation. However, the healthcare team must consider a number of factors: (1) dose, (2) timing, and (3) omega-3 fatty acid form.

At this point in time, no optimal dose of omega-3 fatty acids has been established for humans, cats, or dogs. The current recommendation from nutritionists studying fatty acids and cardiac disease is a dose of 40 mg/kg EPA and 25 mg/kg DHA for both dogs and cats.[6]

Timing also needs to be taken into consideration when supplementing omega-3 fatty acids. The healthcare team should remember and educate owners that most omega-3 fatty acid benefits occur after peak plasma and tissue concentrations have been achieved. Although plasma concentrations may increase significantly in the first week of omega-3 fatty acid supplementation, typically 4–6 weeks are required to reach peak plasma concentrations.

EPA and DHA can be provided via the diet or as a dietary supplement. There are a few therapeutic pet foods with high levels of EPA and DHA, but many foods manufactured today do not achieve the recommended level of EPA and DHA. The current recommended dose is 40 mg/kg EPA + 25 mg/kg DHA. Therefore, a manufactured commercial food would need to contain between 80 and 150 mg/100 kcal EPA + DHA.[6–8] Other factors that would need to be taken into consideration would be the size of the pet and the amount of food consumed. If the pet is not prescribed one of the high-fatty acid foods, a recommendation of fish oil supplementation would be necessitated. However, caution must be given when making a supplement recommendation, as fish oil supplements vary widely in the amount of EPA and DHA they contain. The healthcare team should be familiar with various brands of fish oil supplements and plan to make a recommendation based on a specific brand with which the concentrations of EPA and DHA have been researched and confirmed.

Fatty acids – especially omega-3 fatty acids – have been shown to provide benefits to dogs and cats suffering with cardiac disease. Although more research is needed, omega-3 fatty acids should and have been recommended – not only for dogs and cats but also to a large degree in humans with cardiac disease as well. Following the correct dose and timing of omega-3 fatty acids and being cognizant of the risks (such as the potential reduction in platelet aggregation) is beneficial to overall patient care.

Omega-3 Fatty Acids and Osteoarthritis

OA is the most common form of arthritis recognized in humans and in veterinary species. Typically, OA is a slowly progressive condition characterized by two main pathologic processes: degeneration of articular cartilage with a loss of both proteoglycan and collagen; and proliferation of new bone. In addition, there is a variable, low-grade inflammatory response within the synovial membrane.

In North America, age-specific prevalence values range from 20% in dogs older than 1 year to 80% in dogs older than 8 years, based on radiographic and clinical data from referral settings.[13–15] In adult cats, the prevalence of OA is 33%, rising to 90% in senior cats.[15,16] The objectives of treatment for OA are multifaceted; reduce pain and discomfort, decrease clinical signs, slow the progression of the disease, promote the repair of damaged tissue, and improve the quality of life.

OA is initiated by damage to chondrocytes. Damaged chondrocytes produce inflammatory mediators. Inflammatory cytokines contribute to the perpetuation and progression of arthritis by sustaining catabolic processes.[15,17] Arachidonic acid and EPA act as precursors for the synthesis of these inflammatory cytokines. The amounts and types of eicosanoids synthesized are determined by the availability of the fatty acid precursor and by the activities of the enzyme systems, which synthesize them. In most conditions, the principal precursor for these compounds is arachidonic acid, although EPA competes with arachidonic acid for the same enzyme systems. The eicosanoids produced from arachidonic acid are proinflammatory. In contrast, eicosanoids derived from EPA promote minimal to no inflammatory activity. Ingestion of oils containing n-3 fatty acids results in a decrease in membrane arachidonic acid levels. This produces an accompanying decrease in the capacity to synthesize eicosanoids from arachidonic acid. Studies have documented that inflammatory eicosanoids produced from arachidonic acid are depressed when dogs consume foods with high levels of n-3 fatty acids.[18]

Reducing the production of proinflammatory mediators is only one mechanism by which n-3 fatty acids promote the termination of inflammation and return to homeostasis. In people, failure of resolution of inflammation has emerged as a central component of many diseases in modern Western civilization (e.g. arthritis, periodontal disease, cardiovascular disease, cancer, and Alzheimer disease).[15,19] Recent work has demonstrated that resolution of inflammation is an active endogenous process aimed at protecting the individual from an excessive inflammatory response. The first endogenous local counter-regulatory mediators recognized were the lipoxins, which are derived from arachidonic acid.[20] More recently, two new families of lipid mediators derived from omega-3 fatty acids, resolvins, and protectins, have been identified. These bioactive mediators have potent anti-inflammatory; neuroprotective, and pro-resolving properties.[8,18] Further elucidation of the molecular actions of these previously unappreciated families of lipid-derived mediators may shed light on the clinically recognized beneficial effects of omega-3 fatty acids. Although the molecular mechanisms for controlling the resolution of inflammation through resolvins and protectins have not been fully elucidated, it is conceivable that omega-3 fatty acids modulate this process at the level of the genome or proteome providing another example of how nutrigenomics can aid in the control of clinical signs of disease.

High levels of n-3 PUFAs control inflammation in cats as in dogs. Unlike dogs, in cats DHA rather than EPA inhibits the aggrecanase enzymes responsible for cartilage degradation.[15,21]

FLUTD

Inflammation in the urinary bladder is typical in the majority of lower urinary tract disorders. This includes feline idiopathic cystitis (FIC) and urolithiasis. Consequently, a key nutritional factor for managing cats with FLUTD includes omega-3 fatty acids, such as EPA and DHA, which are known to have potent anti-inflammatory effects. These dietary fatty acids are absorbed and assimilated into cell membranes, including those of the urinary bladder, thus altering production of inflammatory mediators.[8]

The recommended range of dietary total omega-3 fatty acids, DHA, and/or EPA, for the management of inflammation concomitant with lower urinary tract diseases, is 0.35 – 1.0% DM.[22,23]

Cancer

Tumor cells use carbohydrates and proteins as a fuel source, but find it more difficult to use lipids. Therefore, lipids are available as an energy source for the body. Omega-3 fatty acids EPA and DHA generally have an inhibitory effect on tumor growth, while omega-6(n-6) fatty acids such as linoleic acid or g-linolenic acid enhance metastases. In fact, studies done in vivo have shown EPA to have selective tumoricidal action without producing harm to normal cells.[8,20] Comparable findings have been reported in dogs with lymphoma and non-hematopoietic malignancies. Dogs receiving chemotherapy for lymphoma and being fed a nutritional formula supplemented with arginine and omega-3 fatty acids were found to have elevated levels of plasma arginine, EPA, and DHA. Additionally, the plasma levels of arginine and omega-3 fatty acids were connected to increased survival time. Another study found that dogs with nasal carcinomas who were undergoing radiation therapy had plasma levels of arginine, EPA, and DHA, linked to improved quality of life, and decreased inflammatory mediators and mucositis in irradiated areas.[8]

In both cardiac disease and cancer, cachexia is a concern. Omega-3 fatty acids provide an anticachectic effect and contribute to decreased blood lactate levels. EPA has been found to decrease protein degradation, but not alter protein synthesis. The result is an anticachectic effect.[24]

In patients with cancer, omega-3 fatty acids have epidemiological evidence supporting their use, due to low cancer rates found in populations with high dietary omega-3 fatty acid consumption. Omega-3 fatty acids in humans reportedly reduce the risk of colorectal, prostate, and mammary cancer. Omega-3 fatty acids increase the immunologic response against tumor cells, increase tumor susceptibility to oxidative stress, decrease TNF-α production, and reduce metastases. In patients with cancer, a high level of omega-3 fatty acids has many clinical benefits, including reduced tumorigenesis, tumor growth, and metastasis, as well as anticatabolic effects.[23–25]

High levels of the omega-3 fatty acids EPA and DHA, in addition to arginine in food have been shown to benefit dogs with lymphoma, nasal carcinomas, hemangiosarcomas, and osteosarcomas. Additionally, a double-blind, placebo-controlled clinical trial with chemotherapy found that food with high levels of omega-3 fatty acids and arginine (test food) was shown to reduce lactic acid consistently over a 12-week period versus dogs fed food without the fatty acids and arginine (control food). Omega-3 fatty acids in conjunction with arginine were shown to improve clinical signs, increase survival time, provide longer remission time, and improve quality of life.[24,25]

Nutrition must be part of the management of disease conditions. OA, cardiac disease, feline lower urinary tract disease (FLUTD),

and neoplasia are a few of the conditions that are supported with nutritional management, specifically by the addition of fatty acids. Omega-3 fatty acids and their anti-inflammatory properties help in the management of a number of different disease conditions. Registered veterinary technicians have the critical role of educating pet owners about the importance of nutrition in managing disease. Pet owners want to know that nutrition may help their pets live longer and feel better. Pet owners also want to be involved in their pets' care and treatment. Nutrition, specifically fatty acids, not only helps pets to live longer with a better quality of life but also allows for the pet owner to play a role in the disease management of their pet.

References

1 Freeman LM, Rush JE (2012) Nutritional management of cardiovascular diseases. In AJ Fascetti, SJ Delaney (eds), *Applied Veterinary Clinical Nutrition*, pp. 301–13, Ames, IA: Wiley Blackwell.

2 Paige CF, Abbott JA, Elvinger F, Pyle RL (2009) Prevalence of cardiomyopathy in apparently healthy cats. *Journal of American Veterinary Medical Association* **234**: 1398–403.

3 Rush JE (2009) Chronic Valvular Disease in Dogs. In JD Bongura, DC Twedt (eds), *Kirk's Current Therapy XIV* (14th edn), St. Louis, MO: Suanders Elsevier.

4 Roudebush P, Keene BW (2010) Cardiovascular disease. In M Hand, C Thatcher, R Remillard *et al.* (eds), *Small Animal Clinical Nutrition* (5th edn), Topeka, KS: Mark Morris Institute.

5 Fox PR, Keene BW, Lamb K *et al.* (2018) International collaborative study to assess cardiovascular risk and evaluate long-term health in cats with preclinical hypertrophic cardiomyopathy and apparently healthy cats: The REVEAL Study. *J Vet Intern Med.* **32**: 930–43.

6 Freeman LM (2010) Beneficial effects of omega-3 fatty acids in cardiovascular disease. *Journal of Small Animal Practice.* **51**. September: 462–70.

7 Lunn J, Theobald HE (2006) The health effects of dietary unsaturated fatty acids. *British Nutrition Foundation Nutrition Bulletin* **31**: 178–224.

8 Burns KM (2017) Fatty acids in disease management. *The RVT Journal.* Winter: 34–7.

9 Gross KL, Yamka RM, Khoo C *et al.* (2010) Macronutrients. In M Hand, C Thatcher, R Remillard *et al.* (eds), *Small Animal Clinical Nutrition* (5th edn), Topeka, KS: Mark Morris Institute.

10 Lenox C (2016) *Role of Dietary Fatty Acids in Dogs & Cats*, September/October: Today's Veterinary Practice.

11 Freeman LM, Rush JE, Kehayias JJ *et al.* (1998) Nutritional alterations and the effect of fish oil supplementation in dogs with heart failure. *Journal of Veterinary Internal Medicine* **12**: 440–8.

12 Slupe JL, Freeman LM, Rush JE (2008) Association of body weight and body

condition with survival in dogs with heart failure. *Journal of Veterinary Internal Medicine* **22**: 561–5.

13 Johnston SA (1997) Osteoarthritis—joint anatomy, physiology, and pathobiology. *Vet Clin North Am Small Anim Pract* **27**: 699–723 https://doi.org/10.1016/S0195-5616(97)50076-3.

14 Anderson KL, O'Neill DG, Brodbelt DC *et al.* (2018) Prevalence, duration, and risk factors for appendicular osteoarthritis in a UK dog population under primary veterinary care. *Sci Rep* **8**: 5641.

15 Burns KM (2021) Osteoarthritis: getting patients moving through nutrition. *Today's Veterinary Nurse.* Winter: 35–43.

16 Lascelles BD, Robertson SA (2010) DJD-associated pain in cats: what can we do to promote patient comfort? *J Feline Med Surg* **12**: 200–12.

17 Curtis CL, Rees SG, Cramp J *et al.* (2002) Effects of n-3 fatty acids on cartilage metabolism. *Proceeding of the Nutrition Society* **61**: 381–9.

18 Wander RC, Hall JA, Gradin JL *et al.* (1997) The ratio of dietary (n-6) to (n-3) fatty acids influences immune system function, eicosanoid metabolism, lipid peroxidation and vitamin E status in aged dogs. *Journal of Nutrition.* **127**(6): 1198–205.

19 Schwab JM, Serhan CN (2006) Lipoxins and new lipid mediators in the resolution of inflammation. *Current Opinions in Pharmacology* **6**(4): 414–20.

20 Serhan CN (2005) Novel omega–3-derived local mediators in anti-inflammation and resolution. *Pharmacology and Therapeutics* **105**(1): 7–21.

21 Innes *et al.* (2008) *Proceedings Hill's Global Mobility Symposium*, pp. 22–6.

22 Forrester SD, Kruger JM, Alen TA Feline lower urinary tract disease. In MS Hand, CD Thatcher, RL Remillard *et al.* (eds), *Small Animal Clinical Nutrition* (5th edn), pp. 925–76, Topeka, KS: Mark Morris Institute.

23 Burns KM (2010) Therapeutic foods and nutraceuticals in cancer therapy. *Veterinary Technician.* April. Vetlearn.com: E1–7.

24 Saker KE, Selting KA (2010) Cancer. In MS Hand, CD Thatcher, RL Remillard *et al.* (eds), *Small Animal Clinical Nutrition* (5th edn), pp. 587–607, Topeka, KS: Mark Morris Institute.

25 Forrester SD, Roudebush P, Davenport DJ (2010) Supportive care of the cancer patient: nutritional management of the cancer patient. In CJ Henry, ML Higginbotham (eds), *Cancer Management in Small Animal Practice*, pp. 167–87, Maryland Heights, MO: Saunders Elsevier.

42

Endocrinology

Diabetes Mellitus

Diabetes mellitus (DM) is a disorder of the endocrine system that is seen in both dogs and cats. DM describes an alteration in cellular transport and metabolism of glucose, lipids, and amino acids due to insufficient amounts of insulin released from the pancreas, a lack of insulin receptors, or an inability of the receptors to transduce the signal. The outcome is an elevated glucose level and an inability of the tissues to obtain the glucose they need.[1]

DM is a syndrome associated with prolonged hyperglycemia because of loss or dysfunction of insulin secretion by pancreatic beta cells, diminished insulin sensitivity in tissues, or both. In the dog, beta-cell loss tends to be fast and ongoing and is usually due to immune-mediated destruction, vacuolar degeneration, or pancreatitis.[2] In the cat, loss or dysfunction of beta cells is the result of insulin resistance, islet amyloidosis, or chronic lymphoplasmacytic pancreatitis.[2]

Most dogs with diabetes are classified as Type 1 or insulin dependent diabetes mellitus (IDDM). Cats can be diagnosed with either Type 1 (IDDM) or Type 2, noninsulin dependent diabetes mellitus (NIDDM) and may have one form and then over time may revert to the other. The theory is that beta cell function in cats can fluctuate, moving them from one category into the next.[3] Nutritional management in animals with DM is essential. Although nutritional management of IDDM does not eliminate the need for insulin replacement,

it may be used to improve glycemic control. In NIDDM patients, nutritional therapy can also improve glycemic control and in some cases may eliminate the need for exogenous insulin therapy. Whether the patient is Type 1 or Type 2, the following factors should be considered in every patient[3]:

- overall health and body condition,
- presence of other diseases,
- type of diet,
- nutrient composition of the diet,
- nutritional adequacy of the diet,
- the animal's caloric requirement,
- and feeding schedule.

Risk factors for developing DM in both dogs and cats include[2]:

- insulin resistance caused by obesity,
- specific diseases (e.g., acromegaly and kidney disease in cats; hyperadrenocorticism [HAC], hypertriglyceridemia, and hypothyroidism in dogs),
- medications (e.g., steroids, progestins, and cyclosporine).
- genetics
  - certain breeds of dogs (Australian terriers, beagles, Samoyeds, and keeshonden)
  - certain breeds of cats (Burmese)

Dogs and cats with DM typically present to the veterinary hospital with the following signs, regardless of the underlying etiology: polydipsia, polyphagia, weight loss, and lethargy. Weight loss results from protracted hyperglycemia and glucosuria. Increased fat mobilization leads to hepatic lipidosis, hepatomegaly, hypercholesterolemia, hypertriglyceridemia, and increased catabolism. If the patient's DM is not treated or adequately controlled, ketonemia, ketonuria, and ketoacidosis develop resulting in advancing compromise of the patient's health.

If the patient is suffering from diabetic ketoacidosis (DKA), the healthcare team will see signs of anorexia, vomiting, diarrhea, weakness, and an overall state of decline. DKA may be brought on by many things including infection, severe stress, hypokalemia, hypomagnesemia, renal failure, drugs that decrease insulin secretion, drugs that cause insulin resistance, or inadequate fluid intake. A thorough history and physical examination by the healthcare team, including a nutritional assessment is crucial for developing an appropriate management protocol for dogs and cats diagnosed with DKA.

The foundation of treatment for DM in dogs and cats is insulin along with nutritional management. Controlling the patient's blood glucose below the renal threshold for as much of a 24-hour period as possible is a major goal of managing DM. This will result in improved clinical signs of DM and help to avoid clinically significant hypoglycemia.

Key Nutritional Factors

In DM patients, nutritional management goals are aimed at optimizing body weight with appropriate protein and carbohydrate levels, fat restriction, and calorie and portion controls. Weight loss in obese patients and stopping DM-associated weight loss are treatment goals for diabetic canine and feline patients. The veterinary healthcare team should approach DM management by instituting the following:

- Calculate the patient's daily caloric requirements.
- Obtain body weight 1–2×/month
- Obtain BCS 1–2×/month

- Adjustments of the daily calories based on BW and BCS should be made to maintain optimal weight.
- Ensure safe weight loss goals:
  - obese cats = 0.5–2% reduction/week
  - dogs = 1–2% reduction/week.
- Reduce postprandial hyperglycemia by managing protein and carbohydrate intake.

Water

Water is one of the key nutrients for all animals. Water is of the utmost importance in animals with diabetes. Patients with DM have increased water losses associated with an osmotic diuresis secondary to glucose and ketone bodies if DKA is present. Clean, fresh water should be available at all times.

Energy

Many cats and dogs with diabetes exhibit polyphagia. Despite this, many patients with DM suffer from weight loss. The overall nutritional management of cats and dogs with DM is dependent upon how well the primary DM is controlled. Another consideration is the presence of concurrent diseases. Weight loss in DM patients may be the result of poorly controlled diabetes or an underlying infection. Weight gain in DM patients may be due to the presence of concurrent diseases such as a thyroid disorder or Cushing disease.

Studies have shown a correlation between obesity and NIDDM in cats. In fact, obesity is well-documented as a significant risk factor for DM in cats. Approximately 80% of cats are overweight when diagnosed. Additionally, overweight cats have been found to have a fivefold risk increase of developing DM versus cats that are at their optimal weight.[4] The development of feline obesity was accompanied by a 52% decrease in tissue sensitivity to insulin and diminished glucose effectiveness.[4] Studies have also shown that baseline insulin levels and insulin response to a glucose load increase in dogs as their weight increases.[3]

A classification system for food based on its effects on blood glucose levels is referred to as "glycemic index." As a general rule, complex carbohydrates (i.e., barley) have a lower glycemic index than simple carbohydrates (i.e., potatoes) because they are digested and absorbed more slowly.

Fiber

In discussing proper nutritional management of diabetic patients, the amount and type of dietary fiber is often brought up. Dietary fiber is generally classified into two categories: insoluble and soluble. Soluble fibers, such as pectins, gums, mucilages, and fructooligosaccharides (FOS) have great water-holding capacity, delay gastric emptying, slow the rate of nutrient absorption across the intestinal surface, and are highly fermentable by intestinal bacteria. Whereas insoluble fibers such as cellulose, lignin, and most hemicelluloses have less initial water-holding capacity, decrease gastrointestinal transit time, and are less efficiently fermented by gastrointestinal bacteria. Fiber is believed to slow digestion and absorption of dietary carbohydrates as well as decrease insulin peaks after meals. Soluble fibers are thought to form gels in aqueous solutions, resulting in glucose and water binding; thus, preventing their transfer to the intestine's absorptive surface.[1,3]

Although the ideal fiber percentage has not been established, evidence suggests that moderate amounts (approximately 7–18% dry matter basis (DMB)) of insoluble or mixed insoluble and soluble dietary fiber in high-carbohydrate foods benefits nutritional management of type I and type II DM in dogs and cats. Low carbohydrate/high-protein foods intended for diabetic cats usually contain lower levels of fiber – between 2% and 7% DM.[3]

The amount and structure of carbohydrates used in the nutritional management of DM are different for dogs and cats; mainly due to the fact that dogs are omnivores and tolerate digestible (soluble) complex carbohydrates

better than diabetic cats. Foods containing 55% or less digestible carbohydrate (dry matter basis [DMB]) are suitable for dogs with DM, especially when the food also contains an increased amount of dietary fiber. Conversely, we recognize that cats are carnivores and have higher dietary protein requirements. The low activity of hepatic enzymes in cats suggests that they generally use gluconeogenic amino acids and fat for energy. It also suggests that diabetic cats may be predisposed to developing higher postprandial blood glucose concentrations following consumption of foods containing a high carbohydrate load and vice versa. Therefore, it is recommended that digestible carbohydrates be less than 20% DMB in low-carbohydrate/high-protein foods for diabetic cats and increased-fiber/high-carbohydrate foods for diabetic cats should contain less than 40% digestible carbohydrates DMB.[1,3,6] Digestible carbohydrate content in increased-fiber/high-carbohydrate foods for dogs should not exceed 55% DMB. When owners want to provide foods and snacks containing simple sugars, the healthcare team should dissuade them as simple sugars rapidly increase blood glucose concentrations and should be avoided in diabetic pets. Also, in cats, fructose is contraindicated as cats do not seem to metabolize fructose. This leads to fructose intolerance, polyuria, and possible damage to the kidneys.[1,3,7] Semimoist foods and high-fructose corn syrup should be avoided.

Fat

Diabetic animals will often present with abnormalities in lipid metabolism (i.e., hypertriglyceridemia, hypercholesterolemia, etc.). Foods that are high in fat may also lead to insulin resistance and the promotion of hepatic glucose production. Pancreatitis occurs often in many diabetic animals. Pets with alterations in their lipid metabolism or with concurrent pancreatitis should have limited fat in their diet. The amount of fat restriction will be dependent upon the diet history of the pet and the current fat consumption at the time of concurrent disease diagnosis. It is recommended that the fat content be relatively low in fat content, i.e., less than 25% DM. Feeding lower-fat foods will help minimize the risk of pancreatitis, control some aspects of hyperlipidemia, and reduce overall caloric intake to favor weight loss or maintenance. Foods with a greater fat content may be considered in diabetic dogs and cats when the patient presents as thin or emaciated.

Protein

Diabetic animals may have increased amino acid losses through their urine. Poorly controlled diabetic patients may experience muscle wasting as protein is catabolized to meet energy needs.[1,3] It is important to provide protein quantity and quality that will meet the requirements of diabetic animals in the face of increased amino aciduria while avoiding excess protein content that may enhance renal damage or contribute to excessive insulin secretion. Currently, there are two basic approaches to managing diabetes in dogs and cats, high-carbohydrate/moderate-protein foods or low carbohydrate/"high-protein" foods (in some cases "high protein" often only translates into the same amount of protein found in typical maintenance diets). We recognize that as true carnivores, cats primarily use gluconeogenic amino acids rather than dietary carbohydrates for energy.

Currently, the recommendation for diabetic cats is that they be fed a high-protein diet (defined as ≥40% protein metabolizable energy). The benefits of this feeding regimen are:[2,8]

- maximizing metabolic rate,
- limiting the risk of hepatic lipidosis during weight loss,
- improving satiety,
- and preventing lean muscle-mass loss.
- Preventing protein malnutrition
- and preventing loss of lean body mass.

High-protein diets typically provide the lowest amount of carbohydrates without impacting palatability. The following dietary principles for diabetic cats should also be considered:

- Protein normalizes fat metabolism and provides a consistent energy source.
- Arginine stimulates insulin secretion.
- Carbohydrate intake should be limited because carbohydrates may contribute to hyperglycemia and glucose toxicity.

It is also beneficial to feed portioned meals to cats as it is easier for the owner to monitor the cat's appetite and amount eaten, along with portion control being facilitated.

For dogs with DM, it is recommended to utilize diets which contain increased amounts of soluble and insoluble fiber or use foods designed for weight maintenance or weight loss in diabetics as these lead to improved glycemic control (by reducing postprandial hyperglycemia). These also aid in restricting calories in obese dogs undergoing weight reduction. Remember the importance of regular and appropriate exercise in the diet based weight-loss program.

If the diabetic dog is underweight, the goal is to normalize body weight, increase muscle mass, stabilize metabolism, and level insulin requirements. Underweight DM dogs should be fed a high-quality maintenance diet or a diabetic diet that has both soluble and insoluble fiber and is not designed for weight loss. Increased palatability is necessary to ensure caloric intake when fed at consistent times and in consistent amounts. Remind owners it is OK to give treats, as long as the treats are taken into consideration when calculating daily caloric intake.

Hyperthyroidism

Hyperthyroidism is known as the most common endocrinopathy diagnosed in older cats and is seen in cats all over the world. Hyperthyroidism is a clinical condition that results from excessive production and secretion of thyroxine (T4) and triiodothyronine (T3) by the thyroid gland. Management of feline hyperthyroidism has traditionally included thyroidectomy, antithyroid medications, and radioactive iodine. Surgery and radioactive iodine therapy are intended to provide long-term solutions, whereas oral antithyroid drugs are used to control hyperthyroidism and must be given daily to achieve and maintain their effect. The healthcare team should be familiar with these modalities as well as nutritional management – a new way to manage hyperthyroidism in cats. Studies reveal that feeding a limited-iodine food normalizes thyroid hormone concentrations and alleviates clinical signs in hyperthyroid cats.[9–12] Now, veterinary healthcare teams have a nutritional tool in their toolbox to aid in the management of feline hyperthyroidism.

Feline hyperthyroidism is the result of excessive thyroid hormone production. Thyroid hormone production requires the thyroid gland to take up sufficient amounts of iodine provided by dietary intake.[13] The idea that feline hyperthyroidism could be managed nutritionally through limiting the amount of dietary iodine available for production of thyroid hormone was investigated and introduced to the veterinary profession.[14,15]

Nutritional management of feline hyperthyroidism has been evaluated for over 15 years.[11] Three published studies have documented the safety and effectiveness of therapeutic nutrition when used as the only management for cats with naturally occurring hyperthyroidism.[9–11] These studies investigated the magnitude of iodine limitation necessary to return newly diagnosed cats to a euthyroid state;[8] the maximum level of dietary iodine that will maintain cats in a euthyroid state[9]; and the effectiveness of a therapeutic food formulated to control naturally occurring hyperthyroidism in cats.[11] The results of these studies support that feeding ≤ 0.32 ppm iodine on a DMB provides a safe and effective therapy for cats with naturally occurring

hyperthyroidism. Serum total thyroxine concentrations decreased within 3 weeks and returned to the reference range within 8–12 weeks of initiating nutritional therapy. When fed ≤ 0.32 ppm iodine DMB as the sole source of nutrition, 90% of hyperthyroid cats remained euthyroid. In all studies to date, indicators of renal function (blood urea nitrogen and serum creatinine) remained stable and no other biochemical abnormalities were observed.[14,15]

Water

Cats with hyperthyroidism often exhibit polydipsia and polyuria. Thus, it is important to remind owners to provide fresh, clean water at all times.[1,3]

Energy/Fat

Hyperthyroid patients are typically in an increased metabolic, energy-deficit state. Often, this results in decreased fat stores because of the increased metabolic state. Treatment of the primary disease and use of food that meets AAFCO nutrient allowances for the desired physiologic state should result in rapid normalization of body weight. If severe wasting of body mass has occurred, the fat content of foods may be increased to achieve higher energy density and enhance weight gain.

Protein

Hyperthyroid cats are in a hypercatabolic state and often present with signs of protein/muscle wasting and protein deficiency.[1,3] Increased protein intake may be needed during the recovery period to replenish body protein. Remember, hyperthyroidism is frequently concomitant with renal failure. Thus, a complete evaluation of renal function should be completed before feeding a higher protein food. Provide increased dietary protein for underweight animals. The following protein levels are adequate unless renal function is compromised: 28–45% DMB. The digestibility of the protein should be greater than 85%.[3]

Fiber

Avoid food with fiber levels greater than 8% DMB in patients with poor body condition.

Nutritional management of feline hyperthyroidism is applicable to cats that are newly diagnosed, currently being managed with antithyroid medications, or with recurrence of hyperthyroidism post-thyroidectomy. It is important that healthcare teams educate pet owners regarding the benefits of this new management option. Appropriate and ongoing monitoring of the cat is necessary, especially with concurrent diseases (e.g., kidney disease). If patients are newly diagnosed or not currently receiving other therapy for hyperthyroidism, nutritional management may be implemented. As with any new food, transitioning to the limited-iodine therapeutic food is crucial and it is important to educate owners about transition options.[14,15] While the majority of cats require less than 7 days to transition from their current food to a new food, veterinary healthcare team members must educate owners that a longer transition (e.g., several weeks) may be necessary for some cats. The end goal is to have the cat eat the recommended food long-term, therefore, a little time spent initially ensuring a gradual transition is worth the effort. It is important to review each cat's situation and individualize treatment for patients based on all factors, including T_4 concentration and the period of time needed to transition to the therapeutic food.

It is imperative that all hyperthyroid cats nutritionally managed with limited-iodine food do not have access to any other food sources. When utilizing the therapeutic food as the sole source of nutrition, 90% of hyperthyroid cats have become and remained euthyroid as long as the cat had no access to other sources of dietary iodine. Should the veterinary healthcare team find persistently increased T_4 in a feline patient prescribed the therapeutic food, concerns of poor adherence to dietary recommendations should be considered.[14,15] Discovering the source of dietary iodine intake can be a challenge for the veterinary health care team. Sources of dietary iodine that may alter the response to this therapy include treats, flavored or compounded medications, access to "people food," consumption of wild caught prey, and access to other pet foods. The veterinary technician must perform an in-depth nutritional history to determine exposure to other food sources. The iodine content of compounded medications is of particular concern as many use fish flavoring which may be high in iodine. The iodine content of many over-the-counter supplements may not be known. Therefore, any supplement, treatment, homeopathic/holistic therapy, or food additive that is fish flavored or derived from ingredients from the sea (fish, shellfish, seaweed, etc.) should be questioned and discontinued. Iodine content of water may be considered if all other sources of iodine have been eliminated through a thorough history taken by the technician. This is unlikely if cats are supplied water from municipal water sources. However, it is possible if well water or natural sources of water are available. If iodine in water is suspected, the owner should be counseled to switch to distilled water for one month to assess the response.[14,15]

Hyperthyroidism is a common disease in older cats and thus is seen frequently in veterinary hospitals. While the pathogenesis of feline hyperthyroidism remains unclear, a variety of therapeutic options are available. It is important that veterinary technicians be familiar with all modes of therapy so they can answer questions for pet owners, including advantages and disadvantages of all options. Methods of managing feline hyperthyroidism traditionally have included thyroidectomy, antithyroid medications, and radioactive iodine. Nutritional management of hyperthyroidism helps cats return to a euthyroid state and control their clinical signs. Veterinary teams now have a nutritional tool to help manage feline hyperthyroidism.

References

1 Fascetti AJ, Delaney SJ (2012) Nutritional management of endocrine diseases. In AJ Fascetti, SJ Delaney (eds), *Applied Veterinary Clinical Nutrition*, Ames, IA, Wiley Blackwell.

2 Behrend E, Holford A, Lathan P *et al.* (2018) 2018 AAHA diabetes management guidelines for dogs and cats. *J Am Anim Hosp Assoc* **54**: 1–21.

3 Zicker SC, Nelson RW, Kirk CA, Wedekind KJ (2010) Endocrine disorders. In M Hand, C Thatcher, R Remillard *et al.* (eds), *Small Animal Clinical Nutrition* (5th edn), Topeka, KS: Mark Morris Institute.

4 Case LP, Daristotle L, Hayek MG, Raasch MF (2011) Diabetes mellitus. In *Canine and Feline Nutrition* (3rd edn), St Louis, MO: Mosby.

5 Appleton DJ, Rand JS, Sunvold GD (2001) Insulin sensitivity decreases with obesity, and lean cats with low insulin sensitivity are at greatest risk of glucose intolerance with weight gain. *Journal of Feline Medicine and Surgery* **3**: 211–28.

6 Bennett N, Greco DS, Peterson ME *et al.* (2006) Comparison of a low carbohydrate–low fiber diet and a moderate carbohydrate–high fiber diet in the management of cats with diabetes mellitus. *Journal of Feline Medicine and Surgery* **8**(2): 73–84.

7 Kienzle E (1994) Blood sugar levels and renal sugar excretion after the intake of high carbohydrate diets in cats. *Journal of Nutrition* **124**(12 Suppl): 2563S–7S.

8 Zoran DL, Rand JS (2013) The role of diet in the prevention and management of feline diabetes. *Vet Clin North Am Small Anim Pract* **43**(2): 233–43.

9 Melendez L, Yamka R, Forrester S *et al.* (2011) Titration of dietary iodine for reducing serum thyroxine concentrations in newly diagnosed hyperthyroid cats. *J Vet Intern Med* **25**: 683 (abstract).

10 Melendez L, Yamka R, Burris P (2011) Titration of dietary iodine for maintaining normal serum thyroxine concentrations in hyperthyroid cats. *J Vet Intern Med* **25**: 683 (abstract).

11 Yu S, Wedekind K, Burris P *et al.* (2011) Controlled level of dietary iodine normalizes serum total thyroxine in cats with naturally occurring hyperthyroidism. *J Vet Intern Med* **25**: 683–4 (abstract).

12 Data on file, Hill's Pet Nutrition, 2011.

13 Mooney CT (2010) Hyperthyroidism. In SJ Ettinger, EC Feldman (eds), *Textbook of Veterinary Internal Medicine: Diseases of the Dog and Cat* (7th edn), pp. 1761–79, St Louis, MO: Saunders.

14 Burns KM (2012) Managing feline hyperthyroidism: As safe and easy as feeding your cat. *NAVTA Journal*, Jan./Feb.: 36–40.

15 Burns KM (2011) A team approach to managing feline hyperthyroidism. *Canadian Vet.* Nov./Dec.: 16–8.

43

Cancer Nutrition

Veterinary healthcare teams realize that cancer is a disease which evokes a great deal of emotion. Pet owners are acutely aware of the term "cancer" and conjure images and notions of how their neoplasia-diagnosed pet should be managed. Therefore, as healthcare team members, we need to remember to approach pets with cancer and their owners in a positive, compassionate, and knowledgeable fashion.

Cancer in companion dogs and cats is common, although it is somewhat less common in cats as compared to dogs. Neoplastic disease has been found to be the most common deadly pathological process in ~90% of canine breeds. It has also been reported to be the most common cause of death in dogs >1 year of age, with an incidence >3 times that of traumatic injury.[1,2]

Nutritional management of dogs and cats with cancer is part of a multimodal approach to therapy that the veterinary team should consider when initiating treatment. Providing appropriate nutrition may improve quality of life, enhance the effectiveness of treatment, and increase survival time. Nutrition also allows the pet owner to be involved in the management of their beloved family member.[3]

Nutritional Assessment

Nutritional status should be assessed with every cancer patient. The nutritional assessment should include at the very least:

- the type of diet,

- the feeding method,
- the patient's appetite,
- the client's attitude in relation to the patient's current nutritional regimen.

It is important to note the patient's current and past body weights, body condition score, and muscle condition score.[4] These tools will aid in the identification of patients who may be malnourished and/or inappetent. In human cancer patients, nutritional assessments have found 40–80% experience varied degrees of malnutrition. This malnutrition is dependent upon type of tumor, location, stage, and treatment plan.[4,5] The same can be said of veterinary cancer patients, thus the importance of a nutritional assessment.

Metabolic Alterations in Patients with Cancer

Veterinary healthcare teams must remember that patients with cancer may lose weight and have a decrease in body condition due to the location of the tumor (e.g., oral mass); complications due to cancer treatment (e.g., radiation of an oral mass); and cancer cachexia.

Veterinary healthcare teams must be vigilant to help identify cancer cachexia.

Cancer cachexia is a paraneoplastic syndrome manifested by weight loss and a decrease in body condition despite adequate nutritional intake.[6] The numbers of dogs and cats with cancer cachexia are not fully known – but it is imperative for veterinary nurses to remember

Nutrition and Disease Management for Veterinary Technicians and Nurses, Third Edition. Ann Wortinger and Kara M. Burns.
© 2024 John Wiley & Sons, Inc. Published 2024 by John Wiley & Sons, Inc.
Companion Website: www.wiley.com/go/wortinger/3e

cachexia when obtaining a patient history and body condition score for pets with cancer.

The metabolic alterations described below have been identified in human and canine cancer patients and have been associated with cachexia, a decreased response to therapy, a decreased remission rate, and an increased mortality rate.[3]

Alterations in Carbohydrate Metabolism

Studies have shown that dogs with lymphoma and many other malignant diseases have a significant alteration in carbohydrate metabolism.[7,8] Tumors preferentially metabolize glucose (carbohydrates) for energy and form lactate (lactic acid) as an end product. Therefore, the host must expend energy to convert lactate back to glucose. This results in a net energy gain by the tumor and a net loss by the animal. As a result, dogs with cancer lose energy to the tumor and have elevated blood lactate and insulin levels (e.g., laboratory evidence of altered carbohydrate metabolism). Additionally, it is important that healthcare team members avoid administering fluids that contain glucose or lactate to pets with cancer.

Alterations in Protein Metabolism

Patients with cancer and weight loss experience a decrease in body muscle mass and an alteration in protein synthesis.[3,9] Simultaneously, to support tumor growth, cancer patients experience increased skeletal muscle protein breakdown, liver protein synthesis, and whole-body protein synthesis.[3] Thus, if protein intake does not keep pace with use, immune response, gastrointestinal function, and wound healing are affected.

Cytokines such as tumor necrosis factor-α (TNF-α) are also involved in protein catabolism. An increased level of TNF-α does not induce muscle protein catabolism directly but adversely affects important pathways that replenish lost muscle tissue.

Findings suggest that compared with normal control dogs, dogs with cancer had altered plasma amino acid profiles.[10] Interestingly, these altered profiles did not return to normal after surgically removing the tumors. This outcome suggests that cancer induces long-lasting changes in canine protein metabolism.

Fat Metabolism Alterations

Catabolism of adipose tissue is the second major feature of cachexia in a variety of chronic diseases, including cancer.[3,9-11] A decrease in fat synthesis or an increase in lipolysis can deplete fat stores. Studies in animal models suggest that production of lipid-mobilizing factors by tumors may account for loss of body fat, especially when this is combined with decreased food intake.

Several cytokines are responsible for altering lipid metabolism. TNF-α is the major cytokine involved in the catabolism of adipose tissue during cachexia in rodents. Altered lipid profiles in dogs with lymphoma suggest that similar changes may occur in pets with cancer.

Unlike host tissues, some tumor cells have difficulty using lipids as a fuel source compared with soluble carbohydrates and protein.[3,12,13] This finding has led to the hypothesis that foods relatively high in fat, particularly omega-3 fatty acids, may benefit dogs with cancer compared with foods relatively high in carbohydrates.[13]

Pets in North America receive most of their nutrient intake from commercial dry pet foods. These foods are usually high in soluble carbohydrates (25–60%) and relatively low in fat (7–25%). These characteristics may make most commercial dry foods unsuitable for nutritional management of dogs with cancer.

Starvation versus Cachexia

Weight loss associated with cancer differs from that seen with simple starvation. In cachexia, there is an equal loss of muscle and fat characterized by increased catabolism of skeletal muscle. During starvation, fat is mobilized first sparing muscle proteins, resting energy expenditure is decreased and glucose metabolism is reduced. In contrast, patients with cancer cachexia have normal or elevated resting energy expenditures and glucose turnover. Adequate nutrition will halt and reverse the metabolic alterations that accompany simple starvation but will not completely reverse the metabolic disturbances associated with cancer cachexia.

Prevalence and Diagnosis

Cancer cachexia has been reported to affect 30–85% of human cancer patients. Cachexia is reported as the cause of death in approximately 20% of human patients with cancer.[3,10] Similar data are not available for veterinary patients. However, one study did document clinically relevant muscle wasting in 15% of dogs presented to a veterinary oncology service. In addition, 4% exhibited cachexia as defined by a body condition score of ≤3/9 and 68% had documented weight loss of 5% to >10%.[10] There are no specific criteria for diagnosis of cachexia in humans but the clinical features which characterize the syndrome include progressive involuntary weight loss with depletion of lean body mass, muscle wasting and weakness, edema, and declines in motor and mental function. There are no specific criteria for diagnosis of cancer cachexia

in veterinary patients except weight loss. The diagnosis of cachexia in both human and veterinary patients is complicated by the fact that malnutrition occurs long before clinical signs are evident. Veterinary technicians should suspect cancer-associated malnutrition in all tumor-bearing animals even in the absence of documented weight loss.

Pathophysiology

Cancer-associated malnutrition occurs as a consequence of an imbalance between the nutritional needs of the patient, the demands of the tumor, and the availability of nutrients in the body. The competition for nutrients between the tumor and the host promotes a variety of metabolic disturbances including alterations in carbohydrate, lipid, and protein metabolism. Cytokines play a key role as the main humoral and tumor-derived factors involved in cancer cachexia and may be responsible for the majority of metabolic changes associated with cancer cachexia. Table 43.1 summarizes the effects of cytokines on nutrient metabolism in patients with cancer cachexia.

Nutritional management of dogs and cats with cancer is part of a multimodal approach to therapy that the veterinary team should consider when initiating treatment. Providing appropriate nutrition may improve quality of life, enhance the effectiveness of treatment, and increase survival time. Alterations in carbohydrate, protein, and fat metabolism precede obvious clinical disease and cachexia in

Table 43.1 Effects of cytokines on nutrient metabolism in patients with cancer cachexia.

Carbohydrate	Increased resistance to insulin
	Increased glucose synthesis
	Increased Cori cycle activity (lactate recycling; net energy loss to tumor)
Protein	Increased protein breakdown (catabolism)
	Increased liver (acute phase proteins) and tumor protein synthesis
Fat	Increased lipid mobilization
	Elevated levels of triglycerides

dogs with cancer and may persist in animals with clinical remission of, or apparent recovery from, cancer. Until research results show differently, pathophysiologic and therapeutic principles for cats with cancer should follow those of people and dogs with cancer.[12]

Key nutritional factors in animals with cancer include soluble carbohydrates, fiber, protein, arginine, fat, and omega-3 fatty acids (Table 43.1). These factors should be incorporated in the nutritional management of every patient with cancer.

Nutrients to Consider in Cancer Management

Soluble Carbohydrates and Fiber

Soluble carbohydrates may be poorly used by animals with cancer and can contribute to increased lactate production. Historically, it was suggested that soluble carbohydrates should make up less than 25% dry matter basis (DMB) of a cancer patient's food. However, the concept of a low or no carbohydrate diet has been recommended recently based on the Warburg effect. Warburg reported that compared with normal tissue, tumors showed unusually high rates of glucose uptake and lactate production even in the presence of oxygen.[4] This resulted in the concept of low- or no-carbohydrate diets recommended to "starve" cancer cells. Interestingly, further cancer research on cell metabolism revealed that not all cancer cells survive by employing aerobic glycolysis only; in fact, they have metabolic flexibility.[14–17] This flexibility involves adaptively upregulating and downregulating carbohydrate, fat, and protein metabolism as needed in response to nutrient availability, tumor microenvironment, and even cancer treatments.

The veterinary team must also remember that soluble and insoluble fiber sources are important to help maintain intestinal health, especially in animals undergoing chemotherapy, radiation therapy, or surgery. Increased dietary fiber may help prevent and resolve abnormal stool quality (soft stools and diarrhea) encountered when changing from a high-carbohydrate commercial dry food to a high-fat commercial or homemade food.

Protein

Because patients with cancer experience altered protein metabolism, resulting in loss of lean muscle mass (cachexia), dietary protein should be highly digestible, and exceed the level normally used for maintenance of adult animals.

Arginine is an essential amino acid that may have specific therapeutic value in pets with cancer. The minimum effective level of dietary arginine for animals with cancer is unknown; however, a positive correlation between plasma arginine concentrations and survival in dogs with lymphoma receiving chemotherapy suggests that it is appropriate to provide more than 2.5% arginine on a dry matter basis.[12] Arginine has also been shown to improve immune function in cancer patients, promote wound healing, and inhibit tumorigenesis.[3,12] Cats should receive foods with a similar level of arginine (i.e., >2%). L-arginine can be included in the diet by providing a supplement or a high level of good-quality protein.

Glutamine is an essential precursor for nucleotide biosynthesis and is an important oxidative fuel for enterocytes. Glutamine has recently been recognized as a conditionally essential amino acid in certain physiologic states, including stress. Cancer would be considered to elicit a stressful physiologic response. Glutamine has several important biochemical roles and is a preferred source of energy for cells with rapid turnover, such as lymphocytes, enterocytes, and cancer cells. Glutamine has been shown to stabilize weight loss, improve protein metabolism, improve immune response, and improve gut barrier function in rodent cancer models and in human clinical trials.[3,12] Glutamine is best provided by high-quality, high-protein pet foods.

Fat and Omega-3 Fatty Acids

Omega-3 fatty acids may have a preventive and therapeutic role in cancer therapy. There is epidemiologic evidence supporting the use of omega-3 fatty acids in human patients with cancer. Low cancer rates have been recognized in populations with high dietary intake of omega-3 fatty acids, which have been shown to reduce the risk of colorectal, prostate, and mammary cancer.[3,12,18] Omega-3 fatty acids increase the immunologic response against tumor cells, increase tumor susceptibility to oxidative stress, and decrease TNF-α production. In patients with cancer, a high level of omega-3 fatty acids has many clinical benefits, including reduced tumorigenesis, tumor growth, and metastasis as well as anticatabolic effects.[19,20] Omega-3 fatty acids in combination with arginine were shown to influence clinical signs, increase survival time, provide longer remission time, and improve quality of life.[16]

Antioxidant

The use of antioxidants in cancer patients is somewhat controversial. Some veterinary professionals think that antioxidants improve the efficacy of cancer therapy, improve immune function, decrease toxicity to normal cells, and reverse metabolic changes contributing to cachexia. Others think that dietary antioxidants may protect cancer cells against damage from chemotherapy or radiation therapy.

Vitamins

It has been reported that many human cancer patients use vitamin supplements as complementary therapy, usually without the recommendation or knowledge of their physician.[21-23] It is assumed that owners of pets with cancer may also commonly provide vitamin supplementation; however, this has not been studied. The need for vitamin E in the diet is influenced by composition of the food. The vitamin E requirement increases with increasing levels of polyunsaturated fatty acids (including omega-3 fatty acids), oxidizing agents, and trace minerals and decreases with increasing levels of fat-soluble vitamins, sulfur-containing amino acids, and selenium. Many specialty-brand pet food manufacturers have increased levels of antioxidant vitamins such as vitamins E and C since they appear to improve immune function and reduce cell damage in normal animals. However, the role of antioxidant vitamins in animals with cancer is far more complex. Additional studies are needed to determine optimal antioxidant nutrient intake for pets with cancer. At the present time, if the animal is fed a complete and balanced commercial food, megadose vitamin therapy does not appear to be indicated. The levels of vitamin E and other antioxidant nutrients should be appropriate in regard to the levels of polyunsaturated fatty acids, trace minerals, and oxidants in the food.

Trace Minerals

Serum zinc, chromium, and iron concentrations are lower in dogs with lymphoma and osteosarcoma than in normal dogs.[24] The clinical significance of these abnormalities is unknown, especially given that serum levels may or may not correlate with tissue levels of trace minerals. Additional studies are warranted to determine the optimal trace mineral intake for cats and dogs with cancer. Currently, trace mineral supplementation does not seem to be indicated if the pet is fed a complete and balanced commercial food, but is very important if the owner plans to feed home-prepared food.

Tea Polyphenols

Tea polyphenols, found in the leaves of the tea plant *Camellia sinensis* protect against cancers induced by chemicals or ultraviolet radiation. Tea polyphenols have also been found to increase chemotherapy efficacy in animal cancer models.[18,25] Although green tea supplements are available, proper dosage has not been established for cats and dogs.

Vitamin A

Natural and synthetic vitamin A derivatives, also known as retinoids, are currently being studied for their effects on cancer. The functions of vitamin A include growth promotion, differentiation and maintenance of epithelial tissues, and maintenance of normal reproductive and visual functions. Retinoic acid affects differentiation and proliferation of epithelial cells by binding to and activating specific cell nuclear receptors that can modify rates of gene transcription. Human and veterinary studies suggest that retinoids, alone or with other agents, may be effective in treating certain types of malignancies. Retinoids promote cellular differentiation and may enhance the susceptibility of cancer cells to chemotherapy and radiation therapy.[12]

Pet owners want to be actively involved in the care of their pets with cancer. Veterinary patients living with cancer are often reported to have reduced appetite and poor nutritional intake, which is accompanied by weight loss or cachexia. When managing cancer-related cachexia in pets, it is important to maintain adequate nutritional and energy intake.[26] Thus, having clients involved in the nutritional management of their pet benefits both pet and owner. A recent study looked at the acceptance and eating enthusiasm in dogs with cancer fed a new therapeutic, nutritionally balanced, and calorically dense food designed for canine cancer patients.[27] Findings showed high food acceptance in dogs with cancer within the first day, in addition to exhibiting enthusiastic eating through the study's entirety.

As healthcare team members, veterinary nurses need to approach pets with cancer and their owners in a positive, compassionate, and knowledgeable fashion, and remember that owners want to be part of the overall management of their pets. Educating clients on the important role of nutrition in cancer management not only involves the client but also helps to improve the pet's appetite and well-being. It is imperative that veterinary healthcare teams remember that nutritional management may help pets live longer and feel better and involving pet owners in their pets' care and treatment helps family members to feel a part of their pets' treatment.

Nutritional therapy can influence remission time, survival time, and quality of life. As healthcare team members, we must ensure the client understands the diagnosis, what this means for their pet, and accepts the recommendation being made. Nutrition is one therapy that can be offered to clients to involve them in the treatment process and help this special member of the family lengthen their survival time and feel better overall.

References

1 Biller B, Berg J, Garrett L *et al.* (2016) 2016 AAHA oncology guidelines for dogs and cats. *Jl Am Anim Hosp Assoc* **52**: 181–204.

2 Fleming JM, Creevy KE, Promislow DE (2011) Mortality in North American dogs from 1984 to 2004: an investigation into age-, size- and breed related causes of death. *J Vet Intern Med* **25**(2): 187–98.

3 Burns KM (2015) Cancer. In A Wortinger, KM Burns (eds), *Nutrition and Disease Management for Veterinary Technicians and Nurses* (2nd edn), pp. 202–7, Ames, IA: Wiley Blackwell.

4 Raditic D, Gaylord L (2021) Nutrition for small animal cancer patients. *Today's Veterinary Practice* January/February: 16–21.

5 Lach K, Peterson SJ (2017) Nutrition support for critically ill patients with cancer. *Nutr Clin Pract* **32**(5): 578–86.

6 Fearon KC, Voss AC, Hustead DS (2006) Definition of cancer cachexia: effect of weight loss, reduced food intake, and

systemic inflammation on functional status and prognosis. *Am J Clin Nutr* **83**: 1345–50.

7 Ogilvie GK, Walters L, Salman MD *et al.* (1997) Alterations in carbohydrate metabolism in dogs with non-hematopoietic malignancies. *Am J Vet Res* **56**: 277–81.

8 Mazzaferro EM, Hackett TB, Stein TP *et al.* (2001) Metabolic alterations in dogs with osteosarcoma. *Am J Vet Res* **62**: 1234–9.

9 Costelli P, Baccino FM (2000) Cancer cachexia: from experimental models to patient management. *Curr Opin Clin Nutr Metab Care* **3**: 177–81.

10 Ogilvie GK, Vail DM, Wheeler SL (1988) Alterations in fat and protein metabolism in dogs with cancer [abstract]. *Proc Vet Cancer Soc* **31**.

11 Langhans W (2002) Peripheral mechanisms involved with catabolism. *Curr Opin Clin Nutr Metab Care* **5**: 419–26.

12 Saker KE, Selting KA (2010) Cancer. In MS Hand, CD Thatcher, RL Remillard *et al.* (eds), *Small Animal Clinical Nutrition* (5th edn), pp. 587–607, Topeka, KS: Mark Morris Institute.

13 Burns KM (2010) Therapeutic foods and nutraceuticals in cancer therapy. *Veterinary Technician*. April. Vetlearn.com.: E1–7.

14 Ogilvie GK, Ford RB, Vail DM *et al.* (1994) Alterations in lipoprotein profiles in dogs with lymphoma. *J Vet Intern Med* **8**(1): 62–6.

15 Munir R, Lisec J, Swinnen JV, Zaidi N (2019) Lipid metabolism in cancer cells under metabolic stress. *Br J Cancer* **120**(12): 1090–8.

16 Rodríguez-Enríquez S, Marin-Hernandez A, Gallardo-Perez JC *et al.* (2009) Targeting of cancer energy metabolism. *Mol Nutr Food Res* **53**(1): 29–48.

17 Boroughs LK, DeBerardinis RJ (2015) Metabolic pathways promoting cancer cell survival and growth. *Nat Cell Biol* **17**(4): 351–9.

18 Michel KE, Sorenmo K, Shofer FS (2004) Evaluation of body condition and weight loss in dogs presented to a veterinary oncology service. *JVIM* **18**: 692–5.

19 Forrester SD, Roudebush P, Davenport DJ (2010) Supportive care of the cancer patient: nutritional management of the cancer patient. In CJ Henry, ML Higginbotham (eds), *Cancer Management in Small Animal Practice*, pp. 167–87, Maryland Heights, MO: Saunders Elsevier.

20 Roudebush P, Davenport DJ, Novotny BJ (2004) The use of nutraceuticals in cancer therapy. *Vet Clin North Am Small Anim Pract* **34**: 249–9.

21 Bougnoux P (1999) Omega-3 polyunsaturated fatty acids and cancer. *Curr Opin Clin Nutr Metab Care* **2**: 121–6.

22 Zhou J-R, Blackburn GL (1999) Dietary lipid modulation of immune response in tumorigenesis. In D Heber, GL Blackburn, VLW Go (eds), *Nutritional Oncology*, pp. 195–213, San Diego, CA: Academic Press.

23 Ross JA, Moses AGW, Fearon KCH (1999) The anti-catabolic effects of omega-3 fatty acids. *Curr Opin Clin Nutr Metab Care* **2**: 219–26.

24 Kazmierski KJ, Ogilvie GK, Fettman MJ *et al.* (2001) Serum zinc, chromium and iron concentrations in dogs with lymphoma and osteosarcoma. *J Vet Intern Med* **15**: 585–8.

25 Sandler RS, Halabi S, Kaplan EB *et al.* (2001) Use of vitamins, minerals, and nutritional supplements by participants in a chemoprevention trial. *Cancer* **91**: 1040–5.

26 Saker KE (2021) Nutritional concerns for cancer, cachexia, frailty, and sarcopenia in canine and feline pets. *Vet Clin North Am Small Anim Pract.* **51**(3): 729–44.

27 Anthony RM, Amundson MD, Brejda J, Becvarova I (2023) Acceptance of a novel, highly palatable, calorically dense, and nutritionally complete diet in dogs with benign and malignant tumors. *Vet Sci.* **10**(2): 148.

44

Refeeding Syndrome

Refeeding syndrome (RS) refers to the metabolic alterations that occur after nutritional support is started in a severely malnourished, underweight, and/or starved patient. These metabolic changes include severe hypophosphatemia, hypomagnesemia, hypokalemia, hyponatremia, hypocalcemia, hyperglycemia, and vitamin deficiencies.[1,2] Clinical manifestations of these abnormalities include peripheral edema, hemolytic anemia, cardiac failure, neurological dysfunction, and respiratory failure.

When a patient is in a starved state, the body maintains extracellular concentrations of electrolytes at the expense of intracellular concentrations. This may then result in inward restructuring when glucose and insulin are introduced to the patient with refeeding. The result of this shift is critical decreases in vital serum electrolyte concentrations which may be life-threatening. When food is reintroduced to the patient, the blood glucose rises and the body releases insulin which pumps glucose and potassium intracellularly. Consequently, a profound hypokalemia may result. This can occur rather quickly in patients being fed parenterally but may take days to appear when feeding enterally. In general, RS occurs within the first 2–5 days after initiation of feeding[2]; however, signs can be detected within hours of refeeding or even delayed up to 10 days. The patient may also experience hypomagnesemia and hypophosphatemia. Hypophosphatemia has also been associated with hemolysis and may lead to additional cardiac and neurologic complications. Hypophosphatemia is the most common and consistent abnormality seen in RS and results in many of the complications observed.[2] Malnourished patients, especially those experiencing RS, may also have a thiamine deficiency, so it is imperative to monitor thiamine levels in malnourished patients.[3–5]

RS occurs in disease conditions such as starvation from feline hepatic lipidosis, overall malnutrition, and prolonged diuresis as ensues in uncontrolled diabetes renal failure. Again, the greatest risk is seen in patients who are severely malnourished and experiencing significant loss of lean body mass.[6] RS includes a variety of fluid and electrolyte abnormalities affecting multiple organ systems, including neurologic, cardiac, hematologic, neuromuscular, and pulmonary function which is especially prevalent in humans. In cats, RS effects are mainly seen in the hematologic and neurologic systems. In canines, the effects seen are typically in the hematologic, cardiac, and neurologic systems. It is believed that cats are more susceptible to RS as opposed to dogs because cats' hepatic glycogen stores are low and gluconeogenesis is accelerated within the first day of malnutrition. Veterinary technicians must be familiar with the risks that may lead to RS in both cats and dogs in addition to how to manage RS in all patients.

An in-depth history from the owner is critical when determining whether a patient is suffering from RS. If the patient has been hospitalized attentive nursing care and constant monitoring must be performed to

Nutrition and Disease Management for Veterinary Technicians and Nurses, Third Edition. Ann Wortinger and Kara M. Burns.
© 2024 John Wiley & Sons, Inc. Published 2024 by John Wiley & Sons, Inc.
Companion Website: www.wiley.com/go/wortinger/3e

watch for signs and laboratory evidence of RS. Oftentimes, the owner will communicate the following signs upon history and physical examination of the patient: anorexia, weight loss, lethargy, weakness, nausea and/or vomiting, diarrhea, pigmenturia, restlessness, seizures, and coma.

The physiology of starvation helps to provide a clearer understanding of the development of clinical signs associated with refeeding a severely malnourished patient. Initially during the period of starvation (24–72 h), the liver uses glycogen stores for energy and skeletal muscle to provide amino acids as a source for new glucose production (i.e., gluconeogenesis) for glucose-dependent tissues, such as the brain and red blood cells. After 72 h of starvation, metabolic pathways shift and take energy from ketone production as a result of free fatty acid oxidation while sparing protein utilization from skeletal muscle. Also, the body's adaptive mechanisms include; an overall decrease in liver gluconeogenesis, a decline in basal metabolic rate, reduction in the secretion of insulin, and an increased use of free fatty acids by the brain as the primary energy source in place of glucose.[7,8]

In critically ill patients, endogenous protein catabolism is accelerated beyond the requirement of gluconeogenesis. The key to survival is whether the animal can recover from the underlying disease or injury. Amino acids are needed not only for gluconeogenesis but also for the synthesis of new proteins (e.g., clotting factors, immunoglobulins, and granulation tissue). Consequently, endogenous proteins are reallocated from less essential tissues to tissues critical for survival, thus leading to the extreme catabolic response that is seen in the sickest patients. In stressed starvation, the hormones and peptides are released in response to tissue injury and inflammation, not simply due to a deficit of nutrient intake. Therefore, the effects will not be simply reversed through feeding. Subsequently, while the goals of nutritional support should be to provide enough energy and protein to the patient to sustain the increased nutrient demands of critical illness and preserve the patient's endogenous tissues, the catabolic response will be, at best, blunted by the provision of nutrients in the face of ongoing disease.[9–11] Veterinary technicians must also remember that nutrients given in excess of the patient's needs will not be utilized in a critically ill patient, as they would in a healthy patient. Thus, overfed patients are at increased risk of developing hepatic lipidosis, hypercapnia, and a multitude of metabolic abnormalities.

The literature shows that metabolic disturbances of any type are less likely to occur if estimates of caloric needs are conservative. Current recommendations for feeding critically ill patients are to begin feeding equal to the patient's estimated resting energy expenditure. To cover all sizes of canines and felines the following calculation is recommended: RER $= (kg \times kg \times kg, \sqrt{}, \sqrt{}) \times 70$. Make sure you do not use any stress/illness factors in your initial energy calculation. Particularly with critically ill patients, starting with an estimate of the patient's RER and making adjustments based on response is the safest course of action.

Electrolytes

Potassium

Hypokalemia is probably the most commonly detected electrolyte disturbance when providing nutritional support to a patient. Typically, patients who are receiving nutritional support are also receiving intravenous fluids; thus the patients' serum sodium and potassium levels should be constantly monitored. Potassium is also affected by resumption of exogenous carbohydrate metabolism. With refeeding, glucose is absorbed, insulin is secreted, and potassium is taken up by cells along with glucose. Veterinary technicians should look for the following clinical signs that may accompany hypokalemia: glucose intolerance, muscle weakness, ileus, respiratory depression, cardiac arrhythmias, and ECG changes.

Phosphorus

Hypophosphatemia has been reported as a consequence of enteral nutrition in veterinary patients and of insulin administration in diabetic patients. Hypophosphatemia is actually an uncommon condition in dogs in cats. However, in RS, it is the most significant disturbance. Chan Serum phosphorus levels are not as likely to be routinely monitored as serum potassium levels. Therefore, it is important that the healthcare team recognizes "at-risk" patients so that they can be monitored more closely. The healthcare team should look for the following clinical signs associated with severe hypophosphatemia: hemolytic anemia, muscle weakness, acute ventilatory failure, and altered myocardial function. Liquid enteral diets may not contain maintenance quantities of phosphorus. This is not a problem for patients who are not phosphorus depleted but will be for those who become hypophosphatemic on feeding. Phosphorus can be supplemented in liquid diets by adding potassium phosphate. Dogs and cats that develop hypophosphatemia on enteral and parenteral feeding will require additional supplementation in their fluid therapy.

Magnesium

Magnesium abnormalities are being detected more often in critically ill dogs and cats, especially in patients suffering from prolonged starvation, diabetes mellitus, or renal disease. The clinical signs of hypomagnesemia include tetany and other neurological abnormalities, cardiac arrhythmias, ECG changes, and secondary effects on the homeostasis of other electrolytes. Magnesium is a cofactor in many enzyme systems including the ATPase associated with membrane-bound sodium–potassium pumps. It is the dysfunction in the sodium–potassium pump in the renal tubules that is believed to be the mechanism for refractory hypokalemia that can be seen concurrent with hypomagnesemia. Hypocalcemia is another secondary electrolyte effect of hypomagnesemia. Magnesium is necessary for both parathyroid hormone (PTH) secretion and the actions of PTH on bone. Hypocalcemic patients will respond to parenteral calcium supplementation but will rapidly become hypocalcemic again once calcium infusion is ceased unless serum magnesium levels are also corrected. Magnesium can be supplemented parenterally with magnesium sulfate in patients who have severe clinical signs and good urine output. Oral magnesium supplementation is not recommended in these patients as most oral magnesium preparations are cathartic and are poorly absorbed. Patients are able to better tolerate magnesium gluconate or amino acid chelates of magnesium.

Managing Refeeding Syndrome

When RS is suspected in a patient or to prevent RS in critically ill patients, begin feeding the patient *very* slowly. Also, as discussed above, with RS patients, it is best to begin nourishment at a portion of the RER, with increasing amounts as tolerated, over the course of 3–5 days. Consideration should be given to starting nutrition at 25–30% of the calculated RER for the first 24 h (small frequent meals) working up to 100% of the RER after 5 days. This should be done regardless of oral, other enteral, or parenteral feeding.[5,9,11,12]

Veterinary healthcare team members must monitor patients considered at risk for developing RS daily as successful treatment may be dependent on identifying this condition in the early stages. The following must be monitored closely:

- body weight,
- urine output,
- serum electrolytes (i.e., phosphorus, potassium, magnesium, and calcium),
- electrocardiography,
- hematocrit,
- presence of hemolysis,

- serum glucose,
- cardiovascular function,
- and respiratory function.

Any metabolic abnormalities detected should prompt adjustments of nutritional therapy along with further correction of serum electrolyte concentrations. Phosphate supplementation is justified in patients at risk for development of hypophosphatemia, patients with clinical signs resulting from hypophosphatemia, and patients with hypophosphatemia. When formulating enteral or parenteral nutrition solutions for patients with normal serum phosphorus levels, phosphates should be added to the solution to meet the patient's estimated daily requirements. The estimated daily phosphorus requirement is 200–400 mg in cats and 75 mg/kg in dogs. Patients with severe hypophosphatemia and patients exhibiting hemolytic anemia, IV potassium, or sodium phosphate should be administered at 0.01–0.06 mmol/kg/h until the patient is no longer severely hypophosphatemic or until serum phosphorus is >2 mg/dL.

If patients develop hypokalemia, potassium supplementation should begin. Potassium chloride or potassium phosphate may be added to parenteral fluid therapy depending upon the level of hypokalemia. Patients with severe hypokalemia can be given a KCl IV infusion at 0.5 mEq/kg/h for 6 h. The KCl should be diluted in an equal volume of normal saline. The overall potassium infusion should *not* exceed 0.5 mEq/kg/h. The veterinary healthcare team must be cognizant of the contribution of potassium phosphate to the overall potassium supplementation especially if this solution is being used to correct hypophosphatemia.

In patients that develop hypomagnesemia, supplementation of magnesium should be started by the healthcare team. Magnesium chloride or sulfate may be added to parenteral fluid therapy at 1 mEq/kg/day for the first 24 h. If further magnesium supplementation is needed past the initial 24 hours, decrease the rate to 0.5–0.75 mEq/kg/day.

Remember to monitor the patients' thiamine levels as thiamine supplementation is recommended in all malnourished patients. This is especially important when beginning to reintroduce nutrition to the patient. Cats and dogs should receive 10–100 mg/day SQ during the refeeding period.

The veterinary healthcare team should assess the patient's food intake or administration of nutritional support every day and often assessment multiple times a day is warranted. The patient's body weight and body condition score should be recorded in the medical record at least once a day. Depending upon the amounts of fluids going into the patient, their weight may change numerous times throughout the day. Patients undergoing treatment with IV phosphates, serum phosphorus, and serum calcium concentrations should be evaluated every 6–12 h. Serum phosphate, glucose, potassium, and magnesium levels should be monitored at least once a day during the refeeding period (≥5 days) or more frequently for patients receiving potassium, magnesium, or insulin supplementation. Packed cell volume (PCV) and hematocrit (HCT) should be monitored for evidence of anemia, and serum should be monitored for evidence of hemolysis in animals with hypophosphatemia. Nursing care should also include monitoring patients frequently for signs of fluid overload and congestive heart failure.

Summary

RS is a serious condition that may develop in underweight, severely malnourished, or starved patients during nutrition repletion. RS involves significant electrolyte, fluid, and vitamin abnormalities that can lead to significant illness and possibly death. The veterinary healthcare team should be aware of RS, identify patients at risk of developing RS, learn how to manage RS should it develop in patients, and most importantly, take steps to prevent RS. Patients who develop signs and symptoms of RS require aggressive electrolyte supplementation, vitamin supplementation, supportive care, and nutrition support should be restarted, but with great caution.

References

1 Skipper A (2012) Refeeding syndrome or refeeding hypophosphatemia: a systematic review of cases. *Nutrition in Clinical Practice* **27**: 34–40.

2 Chan D DL Chan (ed.) *Nutritional Management of Hospitalized Small Animals* (1st edn) © 2015 John Wiley & Sons, Ltd. Published 2015 by John Wiley & Sons, Ltd.

3 Lippo N, Byers CG (2008) Hypophosphatemia and refeeding syndrome. *Standards of Care: Emergency and Critical Care Medicine* **10**(4): 6–10.

4 Saker K, Remillard RL (2010) Critical care nutrition and enteral-assisted feeding. In MS Hand, CD Thatcher, RL Remillard *et al.* (eds), *Small Animal Clinical Nutrition* (5th edn), pp. 439–76, Marceline, MO: Walsworth Publishing, Mark Morris Institute.

5 Larsen JA (2012) Enteral nutrition and tube feeding. In A Fascetti, S Delaney (eds), *Applied Veterinary Clinical Nutrition*, pp. 328–52, Ames, IA: Wiley Blackwell.

6 Wortinger A (2007) Nutritional support. In *Nutrition for Veterinary Technicians and Nurses*, pp. 211–20, Ames, IA: Wiley-Blackwell.

7 Chandler ML, Guilford WG, Payne-James J (2000) Use of peripheral parenteral nutritional support in dogs and cats. *J Am Vet Med Assoc* **216**: 669–73.

8 Proulx J (2000) Nutrition in critically ill animals. In *The Veterinary ICU Book*, pp. 202–17, Jackson Hole, WY: Teton New Media.

9 Eirmann L, Michel K (2009) Enteral nutrition. In *Small Animal Critical Care Medicine*, pp. 53–8, St Louis, MO: Saunders.

10 Michel K (2011) Metabolic complications of nutritional support: prevention and troubleshooting. In *Proceedings 17th IVECCS*, San Antonio, TX.

11 Chan DL, Freeman LM (2006) Nutrition in critical illness. *Veterinary Clinics of North America Small Animal Practice* **36**(6): 1225–41.

12 Delaney SJ, Fascetti AJ, Elliott DA (2006) Critical care nutrition of dogs. In P Pibot, V Biourge, D Elliot (eds), *Encyclopedia of Canine Clinical Nutrition*, pp. 426–51, Aniwa SAS, France: Royal Canin.

45

Cardiac Disease

Cardiovascular disease is a common disorder in dogs and cats, with 11% of canines and up to 20% of feline populations affected by cardiac disease.[1,2] Chronic valvular disease has been found to be the most common acquired heart disease in dogs with an overall incidence greater than 40%.[3] Chronic mitral valvular disease is the most common acquired cardiac abnormality in dogs, affecting more than one-third of patients over 10 years of age.[4] Approximately 30% of cases involve the tricuspid valve but disease of the tricuspid valve is usually less severe. Valvular disease is more prevalent in small-breed dogs. Acquired valvular disease is rarely seen in cats. Taurine deficiency was discovered to be the principal cause of dilated cardiomyopathy (DCM) in cats in 1987, and since this time the prevalence of this disease has decreased significantly.[3,4] Today, hypertrophic and restrictive cardiomyopathies are more prevalent causes of myocardial failure in cats.

Several types of myocardial disease not recognized 40 years ago now appear commonly in dogs. Large-breed dogs, especially males, are predisposed to DCM, and the Doberman pinscher breed seems to stand out as the predisposed breed. Hypertrophic cardiomyopathy in dogs is rarely seen. Arrhythmogenic right ventricular cardiomyopathy is common among boxer dogs.

Pulmonary vascular disease with secondary cor pulmonale is most often seen with *Dirofilaria immitis* infection (heartworm disease). This disease is more widespread in areas with higher mosquito and heartworm populations and is worsened when the dog does not receive appropriate preventive medication. Pulmonary hypertension appears to be more common than previously believed with diagnosis of pulmonary hypertension increasing due to heightened awareness. Pulmonary thromboembolism is most commonly associated with renal disease, hyperadrenocorticism, corticosteroid therapy, neoplasia, nephrotic syndrome, pancreatitis, and immune-mediated hemolytic anemia. Primary systemic vascular disease is uncommon. Secondary aortic thromboembolism in cats may occur with any of the forms of cardiomyopathy and is the most frequently acquired feline vascular abnormality. Systemic hypertension in dogs and cats now appears to be more common than believed 40 years ago.

Dogs and cats with hypertension may present at any age, but typically, hypertension is seen in middle-aged to geriatric patients. The mean age of dogs with hypertension is nine years and the mean age of cats is 15 years. The strength of the peripheral pulses does not help detect systemic hypertension. Retinal hemorrhages and detachments are common end-organ changes in patients with moderate to severe hypertension. These ocular signs are frequently the first signs seen associated with hypertensive disease. A fundic examination should be part of the routine evaluation of all dogs and cats. Other clinical signs of hypertension are most often related to the underlying disease that causes systemic hypertension. The effects of long-term or severe systemic hypertension may cause significant heart disease (e.g., left ventricular concentric hypertrophy), and hypertension may complicate the treatment of chronic mitral valvular disease in dogs by worsening valvular regurgitation. The healthcare team should screen dogs and cats with significant heart disease for the presence of systemic hypertension. The healthcare team should also search for underlying heart disease in patients with known hypertension, especially those exhibiting clinical signs that may be indicative of heart disease.

The most frequently encountered problems associated with cardiovascular disease that require nutritional modification are fluid retention states associated with chronic congestive heart failure (CHF), primary or secondary hypertension, obesity, cachexia, and myocardial diseases related to a specific nutrient deficiency (taurine and carnitine) and electrolyte disorders that may predispose to cardiac dysrhythmias.

Effective treatment requires a multifaceted approach, of which nutritional management is an important component. Foods designed for patients with cardiovascular disease should supply age-appropriate nutrition and specific nutrients that may help manage hypertension, decrease fluid retention, control the signs associated with ascites, maintain heart muscle function, help slow the progression of concurrent kidney disease, and help counter the loss of nutrients in the urine of pets prescribed diuretics.

Heart failure is characterized by inadequate cardiac output and insufficient delivery of nutrients relative to tissue metabolic needs. Heart failure is a clinical syndrome which results from a variety of structural and functional disorders of the heart or great vessels. Clinical manifestations of heart failure are due to reduced cardiac output (weakness, exercise intolerance, and syncope), pulmonary congestion (dyspnea, orthopnea, cough, and abnormal breath sounds with crackles and wheezes), systemic fluid retention (jugular venous distention, hepatomegaly, ascites, and pleural effusion), or a combination of these conditions. Obesity and chronic bronchitis often occur in dogs and cats with heart disease and cause clinical manifestations similar to those of heart failure, which can further complicate the diagnosis. Obesity can also exacerbate previously existing cardiac conditions.

Key Nutritional Factors

Sodium and Chloride

Sodium, chloride, and water retention are linked with CHF. Subsequently, the healthcare team should focus on these nutrients in patients with cardiovascular disease. A few hours after the ingestion of high levels of sodium, healthy dogs and cats easily excrete any excess in their urine. However, patients in early cardiac disease may lose this ability to excrete excess sodium. As heart disease worsens and CHF arises, the ability to excrete excess sodium worsens. Historically, sodium retention was primarily implicated in the pathogenesis of CHF and some forms of hypertension. A number of studies have examined the interaction of sodium with other ions, including chloride. Chloride may also act as a direct renal vasoconstrictor. According to the National Research Council (NRC), the minimum recommended allowance for sodium and chloride in foods for adult dogs is 0.08% and 0.12% dry matter (DM), respectively. In foods for adult cats, it is 0.068% for sodium and 0.096% for chloride (DM). When dealing with patients with cardiovascular disease the sodium levels in foods designed to manage these patients should be limited to 0.08–0.25% DM for dogs and 0.07–0.3% DM for cats. Recommended chloride levels are typically 1.5 times sodium levels.

Avoiding excess sodium chloride in cat foods is more difficult than in dog foods as ingredients used to meet the higher protein requirement of cats also contain sodium and chloride, thus increasing the sodium chloride content of cat food.

Taurine

Taurine is an important amino acid in dogs and cats with myocardial failure. The mechanism of heart failure in taurine-deficient cats and dogs is not well understood. Taurine may function in inactivation of free radicals, osmoregulation, and calcium modulation. Taurine is also known for its direct effects on contractile proteins. Additionally, there may be other factors responsible for contributing to the development of myocardial failure in patients with taurine deficiency. DCM and heart failure may result from an inciting or contributing factor combined with taurine deficiency. As we know, taurine is an essential amino acid in cats, therefore, a minimum recommended allowance for taurine is necessary in cat foods. Taurine should be 0.04% DM. Taurine content of foods for cats with cardiovascular disease should contain at least 0.3% DM. Levels of taurine typically recommended for supplementation of feline cardiovascular patients (250–500 mg taurine/day) provide approximately twice that much.

Taurine is not an essential amino acid for dogs. Nevertheless, an association between DCM and plasma taurine deficiency and low myocardial taurine concentrations has been observed. The association between taurine deficiency and DCM is strongest in American cocker spaniels and Golden retrievers. An association between taurine deficiency and DCM has also been shown in Newfoundlands, Labrador retrievers, Dalmatians, English bulldogs, Portuguese water dogs, and Irish wolfhounds. Even in canine DCM dogs with normal plasma and whole blood taurine levels, additional taurine may be warranted. Therefore, foods for management of cardiovascular disease in dogs should contain added taurine. The level of taurine in foods for canine patients can be lower than for cats due to the fact that dogs can synthesize taurine. The recommendation for taurine in foods for canine cardiovascular disease patients is at least 0.1% DM. This is somewhat lower than would be supplied by the typical recommendation for taurine supplementation of foods for dogs with DCM (500–1000 mg taurine/day). Studies support the fact that in dogs and cats, taurine is considered safe.

L-Carnitine

Deficiency of L-carnitine in dogs has been linked to DCM in dogs. Cardiac muscle function benefits from carnitine because carnitine is a critical component of the mitochondrial membrane enzymes responsible for transporting-activated fatty acids in the form of acyl-carnitine esters. These are transported across the mitochondrial membranes to the matrix. From here, b-oxidation and high-energy phosphate generation occur. Free L-carnitine serves as a mitochondrial detoxifying agent.

Currently, the recommendation for carnitine supplementation in dogs with DCM is 50–100 mg L-carnitine/kg body weight three times daily. It is widely accepted that even if the cause of cardiomyopathy in a heart disease patient is not due to carnitine deficiency, supplementing dogs with carnitine does not appear to do any harm and may in fact be beneficial. Foods for heart disease patients should provide at least 0.02% DM of carnitine.

Phosphorus

Patients with cardiac disease are often suffering from concurrent disease conditions. It is understood that phosphorus is a nutrient of concern in patients with concurrent chronic kidney disease and that kidney disease is one of the more prevalent diseases seen concurrently with cardiac disease. Therefore, nutritional management should avoid excess phosphorus in patients with concurrent chronic kidney disease. The recommended amount of phosphorous in nutritional management of cardiac disease is 0.2–0.7% DM in dogs and 0.3–0.7% DM in cats.

Potassium and Magnesium

Another concern in cardiac disease patients is the metabolism of potassium and magnesium. Hypokalemia, hyperkalemia, and hypomagnesemia, all have the potential for complications when medication therapy is introduced in patients with cardiovascular disease. Veterinary technicians should be aware that potassium or magnesium homeostasis abnormalities can:

- cause cardiac dysrhythmias;
- decrease myocardial contractility;
- produce profound muscle weakness;
- and potentiate adverse effects from cardiac glycosides and other cardiac drugs.

The amounts of potassium and magnesium recommended for adult maintenance in dogs and cats (0.4% and 0.52% DM potassium, respectively, and 0.06% and 0.04% DM magnesium) should be the minimum amounts included in nutritional management of CHF. If abnormalities in these electrolytes occur, the healthcare team should consider supplementation or switching to a different food.

Protein

Cardiac cachexia is a major concern in patients with cardiac disease. The protein requirements of patients with cardiac cachexia have not been investigated extensively to date. The metabolic changes associated with cachexia and their effect on overall nutrient requirements are only recently being investigated. Many patients with cachexia present with concomitant disease (i.e., chronic kidney disease), which also significantly affects nutrient requirements. Nutritionists do know that profound anorexia enhances protein–energy malnutrition in patients with cachexia. Subsequently, patients with cachexia or exhibiting signs potentially leading to cachexia should be encouraged to eat a complete and balanced food that contains adequate calories and adequate high-quality, highly digestible protein.

Omega-3 Fatty Acids

In cardiac cachexia, tumor necrosis factor (TNF) and IL-1 cytokines have been implicated as pathogenic mediators. Fish oil (known to be high in omega-3 (n-3) fatty acids) has been shown to alter cytokine production. Early investigations involving fish oil suggest that fish-oil-mediated alterations in cytokine production may help dogs with CHF. Consequently, it is believed that heart failure patients with cachexia may benefit from the alterations of cytokine production through omega-3 fatty acid supplementation.

It is believed that omega-3 fatty acids electrically stabilize heart cells through modulation of the fast voltage-dependent $Na(+)$ currents and the L-type $Ca(2+)$ channels which results in the heart cells becoming resistant to dysrhythmias. Clinical studies of fish oil as a source of long-chain omega-3 fatty acids have confirmed the reduction in frequency of ventricular arrhythmia in boxer dogs.

Omega-3 fatty acids have been shown to have a significant effect on survival times when used in dogs diagnosed with DCM or chronic valvular disease. The effect of the omega-3 fatty acids may be attributed to anti-inflammatory effects, cachexia prevention, improved appetite, or antiarrhythmic effects. The veterinary healthcare team should also be aware of further effects of omega-3 fatty acids on the patient. The healthcare team must be mindful of the fact that omega-3 fatty acids have the potential to alter immune function. This alteration in immune function may contribute to the cardiovascular effects of omega-3 fatty acids. Also, omega-3 fatty acids reduce platelet aggregation resulting from the production of thromboxane B5. The reduction in platelet aggregation might be of benefit in cats with cardiac disease and at risk for thrombus formation. However, this effect is also important to be mindful of when using omega-3 fatty acids in animals with coagulopathies.

Additional studies and discussion are needed in the long term, but it is believed that dogs and cats with cardiac disease may benefit from omega-3 fatty acid supplementation. However, the healthcare team must consider a number of factors: (1) dose, (2) timing, and (3) omega-3 fatty acid form.

At this point in time, no optimal dose of omega-3 fatty acids has been established for humans, cats, or dogs. The current recommendation from nutritionists studying fatty acids and cardiac disease is a dose of 40 mg/kg eicosapentaenoic acid (EPA) and 25 mg/kg docosahexaenoic acid (DHA) for both dogs and cats.

Timing also needs to be taken into consideration when supplementing omega-3 fatty acids. The healthcare team should remember and educate owners that the majority of omega-3 fatty acid benefits occur after peak plasma and tissue concentrations have been achieved. Although plasma concentrations may increase significantly in the first week of omega-3 fatty acid supplementation, typically 4–6 weeks are required to reach peak plasma concentrations.

EPA and DHA can be provided through the diet or as a dietary supplement. There are a few therapeutic pet foods with high levels of EPA and DHA, but the majority of foods manufactured today do not achieve the recommended level of EPA and DHA. The current recommended dose is 40 mg/kg EPA + 25 mg/kg DHA. Therefore, a manufactured food would need to contain between 80 and 150 mg/100 kcal EPA + DHA. Other factors that would need to be taken into consideration would be the size of the pet and the amount of food consumed. If the pet is not prescribed one of the high-fatty acid foods, a recommendation of fish oil supplementation would be necessitated. However, caution must be given when making a supplement recommendation, as fish oil supplements vary widely in the amount of EPA and DHA they contain. The healthcare team should be familiar with various brands of fish oil supplements and plan to make a recommendation based on a specific brand with which the concentrations

of EPA and DHA have been researched and confirmed.

Water

With all patients, veterinary technicians must remember to talk with clients about the importance of water for pets. Veterinary technicians need to remind clients that pets should be offered water-free choices and they should be clean and fresh. Healthcare teams must also keep in mind that water quality varies considerably, even within the same community. We must be cognizant of the fact that water can be a significant source of sodium, chloride, and other minerals. Veterinary healthcare teams should be familiar with the mineral levels in their local water supply. Water samples can be submitted to state or other government laboratories for analysis. Also, municipal water companies can be contacted to ask about mineral levels in local water supplies. Distilled water or water with less than 150 ppm sodium is recommended for patients with advanced heart disease and failure.

Nutrition-Related Dilated Cardiomyopathy

While pet owners are focusing more on their pets' nutrition, they are often getting their information from non-veterinary personnel or from the internet. According to data from the US Bureau of Labor and Statistics, the pet food market is on a growth trajectory, with $31.1 billion spent on pet food in 2017,[5] and 36.9 billion in 2019,[6] including growing niche markets such as grain-free diets. Pet owners are looking to niche diets (e.g., grain-free) believing these are better for their pets. Owners assume these foods are more natural, carbohydrate-free, and less likely to result in health problems such as allergies, but this is not the case.[7,8]

To date, no credible evidence has been found showing grain-free diets are better for pets, nor do any nutritional foundations support this claim. In fact, to the contrary what is being investigated is a correlation between grain-free diets and cardiac disease. It is acknowledged that heart disease is not uncommon in companion animals; with prevalence rates reportedly 10–15% of all dogs and cats, and certain breeds seeing an even higher incidence. Frequently cardiac cases include a nutritional management component in treatment.[8,9]

However, an increase in heart disease in dogs eating certain types of diets has been observed and is being investigated, as it appears certain types of diets or specific ingredients in them, may increase dogs' risk for heart disease. The US Food and Drug Administration (FDA) first alerted the nation regarding this investigation in July 2018. An update was provided in February 2019, and a third status report in June 2019. Since then, the FDA's Center for Veterinary Medicine (CVM) has been collaborating with veterinarians, veterinary nutritionists, veterinary cardiologists, etc., to evaluate information about the DCM cases and the diets of those pets. Thus far, the FDA has not established why certain diets may be associated with the development of DCM in some dogs.

Most of the diets being looked at are boutique, exotic ingredient, and grain-free diets (BEG).[8,9] As owners investigate nutrition for their pets, they encounter and believe many of the myths and misperceptions that are circulating about pet food. Therefore, veterinary healthcare teams must educate pet owners about proper nutrition and the difference between nutrients and ingredients.

The Misperceptions

Pet owners hear misinformation about grains in pet foods. Some of the most common misperceptions are the following:

- **Whole grains are used as fillers in pet foods**: Filler implies the ingredient has little or no nutritional value,[7,8,10,11] but whole grains do contribute key nutrients such as vitamins, minerals, and essential fatty acids to pet foods.[7,12] Various grain products also provide protein, which may be easier for the pet to digest than some proteins from meat. Most dogs and cats (>90%) can utilize and digest nutrients from grains normally found in pet foods.[13-15]

- **Grain-free pet foods are carbohydrate-free**: Grain-free pet foods typically contain carbohydrates from other sources such as sweet potatoes, which have a higher carbohydrate level than corn. Grains are carbohydrates, which are an important energy source, and one of the 6 basic nutrients (i.e., water, protein, fat, carbohydrates, vitamins, and minerals). Veterinary teams must remember that the variety of grain-free diets on the market means a variety of nutritional profiles, which affect not only carbohydrates but also protein, fat, and other nutrients. Grain-free diets lower in carbohydrates may indicate a higher amount of fat and calories. Some grain-free diets merely substitute grain with highly refined starches (e.g., potatoes and cassava) that may deliver fewer nutrients and less fiber than whole grains and are not considered cost-efficient.[8,11] In other grain-free products, the grains are replaced with beans, peas, or lentils, which may provide carbohydrates but are not necessarily any better for pets than grains and may lead to gastrointestinal (GI) upset.

- **Grains cause food allergies**: Food allergies and insensitivities are abnormal responses to a normal food or ingredient.[16] Food allergies in pets are uncommon (i.e., <1% of skin disease, <10% of all allergies[13,14]), and allergies to grains are even more uncommon. The few pets diagnosed with a food allergy are probably eating animal protein such as chicken, beef, or dairy.[15] This is more a reflection of the commonality of ingredients in pet foods rather than their increased tendency to cause allergies.

- **Grains cause gluten intolerance**: Celiac disease is an inherited autoimmune disease seen in humans that has been associated with hypersensitivity to gluten proteins in wheat and related grains such as barley and rye. Gluten intolerance is extremely rare in dogs and nonexistent in cats. Only one inbred family of Irish Setters is known to have manifested GI signs from consuming gluten.[17]

DCM is a disease of the heart muscle characterized by heart enlargement resulting in improper cardiac function. Often seen in DCM cases are abnormal heart rhythms, congestive heart failure, and sometimes even sudden death. In dogs, DCM is typically diagnosed in large and giant breeds, where it is believed to have a genetic component. Over the past couple of years, veterinary cardiologists have been reporting increased rates of DCM in dogs – in both the "typical" breeds, as well as in small dog breeds not usually connected with DCM.[8,9,18] The thought in these dogs, is that the disease is associated with eating boutique or grain-free diets. What has also been documented is that both the typical and atypical breeds were more likely to be eating boutique or grain-free diets, and diets with exotic ingredients – kangaroo, lentils, duck, pea, fava bean, tapioca, salmon, lamb, barley, bison, venison, and chickpeas. This is further associated when improvement in the dogs' condition is seen upon diet change. As mentioned earlier, the US FDA's CVM, veterinary nutritionists, and veterinary cardiologists are investigating this issue.

What can be causing these DCM cases? A taurine deficiency was one of the first considerations. Historically, DCM was a common disease in cats. However, in the late 1980s, the cause of DCM in felines was found to be insufficient taurine amounts in the diet. With taurine supplementation in the diet, it was found that DCM in cats could be reversed. This led to reformulations of taurine levels in the diet and production of commercial cat foods containing enough taurine to prevent DCM.[19]

In the 1990s, Golden retrievers and American cocker spaniels were found to be at risk for DCM caused by taurine deficiency; and improvement was seen when American cocker spaniels with DCM were provided taurine supplementation.[20] Additional studies have since shown associations between dietary factors and taurine deficiency in dogs (e.g., lamb, rice bran, high fiber diets, and very low protein diets). Although the reasons for taurine deficiency in dogs are not completely understood, suggestions include reduced production of taurine due to dietary deficiency or reduced bioavailability of taurine or its building blocks, increased losses of taurine in the feces, or altered metabolism of taurine in the body.[9,18] Now, as mentioned earlier, higher rates of DCM are being seen in both Golden retrievers and some atypical dog breeds.

Again, many of these affected dogs were eating boutique, grain-free, or exotic ingredient diets. Some of the dogs had low taurine levels which improved with taurine supplementation. But even some of those dogs that were not taurine deficient improved with taurine supplementation and diet change.

In June 2019, the FDA issued an update to its ongoing investigation of the potential connection between certain diets and DCM in dogs.[21] The FDA continues to look at diets that list peas, lentils, other legume seeds, and potatoes within the first 10 ingredients on the label.

The FDA's most recent update provided good background information on this ongoing issue, addressing many of the common questions that veterinarians have been getting. Of most interest to those of us actively engaged in researching or following this issue was the update on the number of reports the FDA has *received*. As of November 1, 2022, approximately 1,390 dogs with DCM have been reported to the FDA (and over

20 cats). The amount of supporting scientific evidence published on diet-associated DCM since the FDA's first alert in July 2018 is significant. In the past 5 years, since the first FDA alert, 16 peer-reviewed research articles on the topic have been published (see compiled list at https://vetnutrition.tufts.edu/2023/02/diet-associated-dilated-cardiomyopathy-the-cause-is-not-yet-known-but-it-hasnt-gone-away/). The tireless effort of veterinarians and other scientists investigating this has resulted in more findings, and the profession is getting closer to an answer. This disease provides an excellent opportunity for scientists, industry, and trade organizations to collaborate to understand this current problem and to optimize our pets' nutrition and health.

It was identified early on that dogs with diet-associated DCM were eating diets with similar properties. Research has now shown that these "non-traditional diets" are commonly grain-free commercial dry diets that contain pulses and potatoes or sweet potatoes. Pulses are peas, lentils, chickpeas, and dry beans. While pulses are part of the legume family, soy (another legume) has not been associated with this problem. Pulses – and especially peas – seem to be the most likely culprits; however, we have a lot more to learn about their effects on dogs eating diets high in these ingredients.[22]

Grain-free diets have been connected to diet-associated DCM. However, the connection appears to be more closely associated with diets containing pulses, versus the presence or absence of grains in a diet. Historically, grain-free diets largely included high levels of pulses and potatoes as ingredients to replace grains; however, more recently some grain-inclusive diets containing pulses have been found to be associated with DCM as well.[22] Findings suggest that most dogs with diet-associated DCM have been eating non-traditional diets for over one year (or more). Thus, it appears that DCM does not develop immediately after eating these diets, nor does every dog that eats these nontraditional diets develop cardiac problems.

Where are we today with diet-associated DCM? It is believed that the ingredients most likely at the core of diet-associated DCM are peas and other pulses. Veterinary teams must recognize that the presence or absence of pulses cannot be predicted based solely on the name of the diet or whether the diet contains grains. Thus, the veterinary team must assess the full ingredient list of the product. If the diet contains pulses (e.g., peas, pea protein, lentils, chickpeas, etc.) in the top ten ingredients (or multiple pulses anywhere in the ingredient list), the product may put dogs at risk for heart problems.[22] Additionally, the current recommendation when pets are diagnosed with DCM, is a change in diet to a reduced sodium diet with no pulses or potatoes/sweet potatoes, in combination with appropriate medical treatment.

A number of questions remain unanswered. The veterinary profession can agree that more investigation is needed, as we do not have the whole picture as to why these pets are developing DCM. A great deal of work needs to happen to gain a better understanding of DCM, and the role nutrition may play in the development or exacerbation of this disease.

The growing grain-free category of the expanding pet food market is perpetuating the misperception that grain is bad for pets. Pet owners increasingly consider their pet's diet as important as their own. Consequently, various human food trends have found their way into the pet food market, especially those believed to center on pets' wellness. Remember, grain-free diets offer no more health benefits than a diet with grains, and each diet should be considered based on the overall nutrient profile rather than individual ingredients. However, some owners will adamantly believe their pet should eat only grain-free food; the veterinary team should follow pet food selection recommendations and apply the recommendations to the grain-free pet foods that are available.

References

1 Buchanan JW (1999) Prevalence of cardiovascular disorders. In PR Fox, D Sisson, NS Moise (eds), *Textbook of Canine and Feline Cardiology* (2nd edn), pp. 457–70, Philadelphia, PA: Saunders.

2 Paige CF, Abbott JA, Elvinger F, Pyle RL (2009) Prevalence of cardiomyopathy in apparently healthy cats. *Journal of American Veterinary Medical Association* **234**: 1398–403.

3 Rush JE (2009) Chronic valvular disease in dogs. In JD Bongura, DC TWedt (eds), *Kirk's Current Therapy XIV* (14th edn), St Louis, MO: Saunders Elsevier.

4 Roudebush P, Keene BW (2010) Cardiovascular disease. In M Hand, C Thatcher, R Remillard *et al.* (eds), *Small Animal Clinical Nutrition* (5th edn), Topeka, KS: Mark Morris Institute.

5 Phillips-Donaldson D. Pet food data: US spending up, pet owners turn to vets. PetFoodIndustry.com. https://www.petfoodindustry.com/blogs/7-adventures-in-pet-food/post/7720-pet-food-data-us-spending-up-pet-owners-turn-to-vets Published December 17, 2018. Accessed January 30, 2019.

6 Pet Industry Market Size & Ownership Statistics, U.S. Pet Industry Spending Figures & Future Outlook. American Pet Products Association. https://www.americanpetproducts.org/press_industrytrends.asp Accessed July 30, 2020

7 Burns KM (2017) Grain-free pet foods: fact vs fiction. *Veterinary Team Brief.* March: 28–30.

8 Burns KM (2020) Grain-free diets and dilated cardiomyopathy. *Today's Veterinary Nurse.* Winter: 2–9.

9 Freeman L (2018) A broken heart: risk of heart disease in boutique or grain-free diets and exotic ingredients. *Published June* 3 Accessed July 30, 2020.

10 Laflamme D, Izquierdo O, Eirmann L, Binder S (2014) Myths and misperceptions about ingredients used in commercial pet foods. *Vet Clin North Am Small Anim Pract.* **44**(4): 689–98.

11 Wortinger A, Burns KM (2015) Nutrition myths. In *Nutrition and Disease Management for Veterinary Technicians and Nurses*, pp. 255–63, Ames, IA: Wiley Blackwell.

12 Grain-free diets: big on marketing, small on truth. Cummings Veterinary Medical Center at Tufts University. http://vetnutrition.tufts.edu/2016/06/grain-free-diets-big-onmarketing-small-on-truth. Published June 14, 2016. Accessed December 16, 2016

13 Scott DW, Miller WH, Griffin CE (2001) *Muller & Kirk's Small Animal Dermatology* (6th edn), pp. 615–27, Philadelphia, PA: WB Saunders.

14 Outerbridge CA (2012) Nutritional management of skin diseases. In AJ Fascetti, SJ Delaney (eds), *Applied Veterinary Clinical Nutrition*, pp. 157–74, Ames, IA: Wiley Blackwell.

15 Roudebush P (2013) Ingredients and foods associated with adverse reactions in dogs and cats. *Vet Dermatol.* **24**(2): 293–4.

16 Ograin VL, Burns KM (2016) Nutritional considerations in allergic skin disease. *The NAVTA Journal. Convention Issue*: 12–9.

17 Garden OA, Pidduck H, Lakhani KH *et al.* (2000) Inheritance of gluten-sensitive enteropathy in Irish Setters. *Am J Vet Res.* **61**(4): 462–8.

18 Freeman LM, Stern JA, Fries R *et al.* (2018) Diet-associated dilated cardiomyopathy in dogs: what do we know? *JAVMA*, Dec 1 **253**(11): 1390–4.

19 Pion PD, Kittleson MD, Rogers QR *et al.* (1987) Myocardial failure in cats associated with low

plasma taurine: a reversible cardiomyopathy. *Science* **237**: 764–8.

20 Kittleson MD, Keene B, Pion PD *et al.* (1997) Results of the multicenter spaniel trial (MUST): taurine- and carnitine-responsive dilated cardiomyopathy in American Cocker Spaniels with decreased plasma taurine concentration. *J Vet Intern Med* **11**: 204–11.

21 FDA investigation into potential link between certain diets and canine dilated cardiomyopathy. June 29, 2019.

22 Freeman LM. Diet-associated dilated cardiomyopathy: The cause is not yet known but it hasn't gone away. https://vetnutrition.tufts.edu/2023/02/diet-associated-dilated-cardiomyopathy-the-cause-is-not-yet-known-but-it-hasnt-gone-away/ Accessed April, 2023.

Further reading

Freeman LM (2010) Beneficial effects of omega-3 fatty acids in cardiovascular disease. *Journal of Small Animal Practice* **51, September**: 462–70.

Lunn J, Theobald HE (2006) The health effects of dietary unsaturated fatty acids. *British Nutrition Foundation Nutrition Bulletin* **31**: 178–224.

Gross KL, Yamka RM, Khoo C *et al.* (2010) Macronutrients. In M Hand, C Thatcher, R Remillard *et al.* (eds), *Small Animal Clinical Nutrition* (5th edn), Topeka, KS: Mark Morris Institute.

Freeman LM, Rush JE, Kehayias JJ *et al.* (1998) Nutritional alterations and the effect of fish oil supplementation in dogs with heart failure. *Journal of Veterinary Internal Medicine* **12**: 440–8.

Slupe JL, Freeman LM, Rush JE (2008) Association of body weight and body condition with survival in dogs with heart failure. *Journal of Veterinary Internal Medicine* **22**: 561–5.

46

Musculoskeletal

Disrupting normal joint mechanics may lead to or result from injury to the various components of a joint. Frequently, this injury results in osteoarthritis (OA).[1] OA can result in physical incapacity and pain, which leads to a reduction in the pet's quality of life. OA is the most common form of arthritis recognized in humans and in all veterinary species. OA is often a slowly progressive condition characterized by two main pathologic processes: degeneration of articular cartilage with a loss of both proteoglycan and collagen; and proliferation of new bone. In addition, there is a variable, low-grade inflammatory response within the synovial membrane.[2]

In North America, OA prevalence is reported to range from 20% in dogs older than one year up to 80% in dogs older than eight years.[3] In adult cats, the prevalence of osteoarthritis is 33%, rising to 90% in senior cats.[4] The objectives of treatment for OA are multifaceted; reduce pain and discomfort, decrease clinical signs, slow the progression of the disease, promote the repair of damaged tissue, and improve the quality of life. It has been suggested that the best results in dogs with chronic pain due to OA include a combination of anti-inflammatory and analgesic medications, disease-modifying osteoarthritis agents (DMOA's), specific nutrients, nutraceuticals, weight reduction, exercise programs, physical therapy, and therapeutic foods. Applying an individualized combination of these management options to each patient will enhance quality of life which is the ultimate goal of therapy.[5]

Obesity as a Risk Factor

It is well-recognized that obesity is an epidemic in companion animals. In 2022, the Association for Pet Obesity Prevention estimates that 59% of dogs and 61% of cats in the United States were overweight or obese.[6] In addition, a long-term study has documented that the prevalence of OA is greater in overweight/obese dogs compared to ideal-weight dogs (83% versus 50%).[4-9] Given these data, it is reasonable to assume a significant portion of arthritic dogs will be overweight/obese, and vice versa. Managing these comorbid conditions presents a variety of challenges.

As disease entities, OA, and obesity present diagnostic challenges for very different reasons. Clinical signs of OA may not be obvious on examination, particularly early in the disease process. Although signs of pets being overweight or obese are readily apparent, these signs are often overlooked or dismissed as inconsequential. Diagnosis of OA generally requires a combination of history, physical examination findings, and radiographic evidence of degenerative joint disease. Although this seems straightforward, historical clues, which are vital to creating an index of suspicion, may be elusive, and clinical signs are often subtle and not evident on routine veterinary examination. Owners may attribute many signs of OA to normal aging and therefore fail to report them unless prompted.

Diagnosing overweight/obesity is of the utmost importance and leads to diagnostic,

Nutrition and Disease Management for Veterinary Technicians and Nurses, Third Edition. Ann Wortinger and Kara M. Burns.
© 2024 John Wiley & Sons, Inc. Published 2024 by John Wiley & Sons, Inc.
Companion Website: www.wiley.com/go/wortinger/3e

curative, and preventive strategies that may be lost in the absence of a diagnosis. The first step to diagnosing overweight/obesity is consistent recording of both body weight and body condition score (BCS). The BCS is a subjective assessment of an animal's body fat that takes into account the animal's frame size independent of its weight. In addition to body weight, BCS should always be documented at every exam. Body weight alone does not indicate how appropriate the weight is for an individual animal. A Labrador retriever weighing 30 kg may be underweight, optimal weight, or overweight. The BCS puts body weight in perspective for each individual patient. In both human and veterinary medicine timely identification of overweight/obesity by primary care providers remains the crucial initial step in their management.

Owners of dogs at risk for obesity and OA should be educated on the importance of lifelong weight management. The incidence and severity of OA secondary to canine hip dysplasia (CHD) can be significantly influenced by environmental factors such as nutrition and lifestyle.[3,5]

Risk factors for developing OA include age, large or giant breeds, genetics, developmental orthopedic disease, trauma, and obesity. Risk factors for overweight/obesity in dogs and cats include age, certain breeds, being neutered, consuming a semimoist, homemade, or canned food as their major diet source, and consumption of "other" foods (meat or other food products, commercial treats, or table scraps). The radiographic prevalence of CHD, a leading cause of OA in dogs, has been reported to be as high as 70% in Golden retrievers and Rottweilers.[10] Golden retrievers, Rottweilers, and Labrador retrievers are overrepresented in the population of overweight/obese dogs.

Dogs found to be overweight at nine to 12 months of age were 1.5 times more likely to become overweight adults.[11–14] Owners of dogs at risk for obesity and OA should be educated on the importance of lifelong weight management. The incidence and severity of

OA secondary to CHD can be significantly influenced by environmental factors such as nutrition and lifestyle.[15] One long-term study has documented that the prevalence and severity of OA is greater in dogs with BCSs above normal compared to dogs maintained at an ideal body condition throughout life. Over the lifespan of these same dogs, the mean age at which 50% of the dogs required treatment for pain attributable to OA was significantly earlier (10.3 years, $p < 0.01$) in the overweight dogs as compared to the dogs with normal BCSs (13.3 years). Obesity is also a risk factor for the most common traumatic cause of OA in dogs, ruptured cruciate ligaments. Overweight/obese dogs have a 2–3 times greater prevalence of ruptured cruciate ligaments compared to normal-weight dogs. Understanding the correlation between maintaining their dog at a healthy weight and decreasing the risk of disease may be a powerful motivator for many owners.

Clinical Signs

Clinical signs of arthritis include difficulty rising from rest, stiffness, or lameness. A thorough disease-specific history may reveal evidence of subtle changes early in the course of OA such as reluctance to walk, run, climb stairs, jump, or play. Signs may be as inconspicuous as lagging behind on walks. Additionally, veterinary teams must listen to owners when they are describing that their dog does not want to walk on tile or hardwood floors, and their pet no longer wants to go for rides in the vehicle – something that was once a favorite activity. Owners are often unaware of the correlation between behavior changes and arthritis. Yelping or whimpering and even personality changes such as withdrawal or aggressive behavior may be indicative of the chronic pain of OA. Additionally, the veterinary team may uncover subtle signs that the owner did not notice such as longer nails indicating the dog is not walking resulting in the nails not being "worn" by hard surfaces, or abnormal fur patterns over joints, indicating the dog has been licking the area – often due to OA pain. Consistent use of an owner questionnaire may facilitate early detection of OA.

Recognizing signs of OA in cats is much more difficult. Cats often suffer in silence and the veterinary healthcare team must rely upon the owner's evaluation and a thorough history to discover potential signs and symptoms of OA in cats. Oftentimes, the changes that may be noted by owners can be categorized into four groups: mobility, activity level, grooming, and temperament. Mobility changes include reluctance to jump; not jumping as high; and changes in toileting behavior due to inability to climb into the litter box. Activity level changes manifest in decreased playing and hunting and a change in sleep patterns. Grooming changes may be noticed when the cat is more matted or unable to groom certain areas, and the claws may be overgrown because they cannot stretch out to "scratch/sharpen" claws. Changes in temperament are demonstrated by the cat hiding from owners or other pets in the house and seeming "grumpy."[4,5] Many of these signs are again attributed to "old age" in the cat by the owner. Thus, it is important for the technician to take a thorough history and ask open-ended questions that may help uncover otherwise overlooked signs of OA in cats.

Stages of Canine Osteoarthritis

OA is a progressive disease consisting of four stages.[4]

- Stage 1: Patient experiencing early signs which are often difficult to identify. These signs are most likely to occur in growing dogs or young adult dogs. The signs are typically sporadic, lasting a few seconds/minutes
- Stage 2: Patient experiencing intermittent signs and are considered the first flare-ups. These signs are easy for owners to rationalize and ignore. This stage is typically seen in young adult dogs and these signs are intermittent and last a few hours

- Stage 3: Patient experiencing performance impairment involving progressive loss of the ability to perform activities of daily living. This stage is more impactful and recognizable by the owner. This stage is often seen in adult dogs and is evident through exercise intolerance and difficulties in the dog's performing activities of daily living.
- Stage 4: Patient experiencing loss of mobility along with loss of strength and fitness. The patient has lost the ability to walk and this stage is much harder for the owner to manage.

It is important to remember that both young and old dogs can be in any of these stages. Historically, most dogs with OA have been diagnosed in stage 3 or 4. Ideally, veterinary teams must be cognizant of the earlier stages and recognize the signs of OA in the earlier stages.

Nutrigenomics and Osteoarthritis

Nutritional supplementation of omega-3 fatty acids has been shown to aid in the management of dogs and cats with OA. Studies show feeding a diet with high levels of total omega-3 fatty acids and eicosapentaenoic acid (EPA) in dogs and docosahexaenoic acid (DHA) in cats, can improve the clinical signs of canine OA. The use of a therapeutic food (Hill's® Prescription Diet® j/d® canine mobility support) for the management of OA has been supported by four randomized, double-blinded, controlled clinical trials using client-owned dogs.[16–19] One 6-month study and two 3-month studies were conducted in US veterinary hospitals. Another 3-month prospective study was conducted in two veterinary teaching hospitals. Overall, more than 500 dogs with OA were studied. Participating dogs were diagnosed with OA based on history, clinical signs, and radiographic evidence. Dogs were fed either a typical commercial dog food or a test mobility food, which has higher concentrations of total omega-3 fatty acids and EPA and lower omega-6: omega-3 fatty acid ratios. At baseline and throughout the studies, subjective and objective veterinary evaluations were performed. Owners were also asked to subjectively evaluate their dogs throughout the studies.

These studies illustrate the benefits of incorporating a food with high levels of omega-3 fatty acids, into the management of the pain of OA in dogs. In normal canine cartilage, there is a balance between synthesis and degradation of cartilage matrix. In arthritic joints, damage to chondrocytes incites a viscous circle which culminates in the destruction of cartilage, inflammation, and pain. The mechanisms responsible for the demonstrated clinical benefits of omega-3 fatty acids include controlling inflammation and reducing the expression and activity of cartilage-degrading enzymes.

Cartilage degradation begins with loss of cartilage aggrecan and is followed by loss of cartilage collagens. This results in the loss of ability to resist compressive forces during movement of the joint. EPA is the only omega-3 fatty acid able to considerably decrease the loss of aggrecan in canine cartilage. EPA inhibits the up-regulation of aggrecanases by blocking the signal at the level of messenger RNA.[20,21]

Inflammation is a vital reaction, and it plays a fundamental role in the pathophysiology of OA. The polyunsaturated fatty acids are critical components in the initiation and mediation of inflammation. Arachidonic acid (AA, 20:4n-6) and EPA (20:5n-3) act as precursors for the synthesis of eicosanoids, a significant group of immunoregulatory molecules that function as local hormones and mediators of inflammation. The amounts and types of eicosanoids synthesized are determined by the availability of the fatty acid precursor and by the activities of the enzyme systems that synthesize them. In most conditions, the principal precursor for these compounds is AA, although EPA competes with AA for the same enzyme systems. The eicosanoids produced from AA are proinflammatory and when produced in excess amounts may result in pathologic conditions. In contrast, eicosanoids derived from

EPA promote minimal to no inflammatory activity.[22]

Ingestion of foods containing omega-3 fatty acids results in a decrease in membrane AA levels because omega-3 fatty acids replace AA in the substrate pool. This produces an accompanying decrease in the capacity to synthesize eicosanoids from AA. Studies have documented that inflammatory eicosanoids produced from AA are depressed when dogs consume foods with high levels of omega-3 fatty acids. In addition to their role in modulating the production of inflammatory eicosanoids, omega-3 fatty acids have a direct role in the resolution of inflammation. Resolution of inflammation is a progressive, active process involving a switch in the production of lipid-derived mediators over time. Pro-inflammatory products of omega-6 fatty acids metabolism (PGE2, PGE12, and LTB4) are thought to initiate this sequence. AA-derived mediators foster the extravasation of inflammatory cells. With time and in the presence of sufficient levels of omega-3 fatty acids, a class shift occurs toward production of pro-resolving omega-3-derived mediators (resolvins, protectins). These mediators serve as endogenous stop signals by preventing inflammatory cell recruitment, stopping "cell entry" and promoting resolution by removing inflammatory cells from the site. The identification of these two new families of omega-3-derived chemical mediators (resolvins and protectins) may clarify the mechanisms that underlie the many reported benefits of dietary omega-3 PUFAs. Absence of sufficient dietary levels of omega-3 fatty acids may contribute to "resolution failure" and perpetuation of chronic inflammation.

In cats with OA, high levels of n-3 polyunsaturated fatty acids (DHA), natural sources of glucosamine and chondroitin, methionine, and manganese, all aid in the management of OA. Just as in dogs, high levels of n-3 PUFAs control inflammation in cats. However, in cats DHA rather than EPA inhibits the aggrecanase enzymes responsible for cartilage degradation.[5,23] Natural sources of glucosamine and chondroitin increase proteoglycan production by chondrocytes and inhibit inflammatory mediators. Methionine and manganese enhance chondrocyte viability, provide building blocks, and act as a sulfur donor for the production of proteoglycans.

Studies suggest therapeutic nutrition provides an effective and safe way to manage both dogs and cats with OA. Foods with high levels of n-3 fatty acids have the dual value of controlling inflammation and pain while slowing progression of the disease by reducing cartilage degradation. Efficacy of therapeutic nutrition for OA is supported by multiple clinical trials in arthritic pets.

Managing Mobility Nutritionally

Dietary factors can potentially modify some of the underlying processes involved in arthritis, including modulation of the inflammatory response, provision of nutrients for cartilage repair, and protection against oxidative damage. Where effective, dietary management may help to reduce or eliminate the need for conventional drugs, some of which are associated with adverse secondary effects.

Key Nutrients

Amino acids, the building blocks of proteins, play a role in the makeup of the tissues and organs in the body. Methionine is a unique amino acid that produces several important molecules in your body which are essential for the proper functioning of cells. Methionine contains sulfur and can produce other sulfur-containing molecules in the joint and is involved in protein production. Manganese is an essential nutrient involved in many chemical processes in the body, including bone formation. Manganese plays a role in the health and maintenance of bone and cartilage in joints. In addition, manganese supports collagen formation for joint strength. Methionine and manganese are building blocks for cartilage in joints.

Carnitine is an amino acid which enables the body to turn fat into energy. Carnitine aids in muscle maintenance and transports long-chain fatty acids and their derivatives into the mitochondria of cells. By strengthening skeletal muscle and turning fat into energy, the severity of OA may be lessened.

Hyaluronic acid is a principal component of synovial fluid and works in the joint to maintain joint viscosity, aid in lubrication of the joint, and aid in shock absorption. Additionally, vitamins C and E are antioxidants which neutralize free radicals to maximize mobility. *N*-acetyl D-glucosamine "shortcuts" the glycosaminoglycan pathway to maintain healthy joint structure and function.

Omega-3 fatty acids have been shown to aid in the management of dogs with OA. Studies show foods with high levels of total omega-3 fatty acids and EPA, can improve the clinical signs of canine OA.[5,10–13]

In normal canine cartilage, there is a balance between synthesis and degradation of cartilage matrix. In arthritic joints, damage to chondrocytes incites a viscous circle which culminates in the destruction of cartilage, inflammation, and pain. The mechanisms responsible for the demonstrated clinical benefits of omega-3 fatty acids include controlling inflammation and reducing the expression and activity of cartilage-degrading enzymes.

Cartilage degradation starts with loss of cartilage aggrecan followed by loss of cartilage collagens, resulting in loss of ability to resist compressive forces during joint movement. EPA significantly decreases the loss of aggrecan in canine cartilage by inhibiting the up regulation of aggrecanases by blocking the signal at the level of messenger RNA.[5]

Omega-3 fatty acids results in a decrease in membrane AA levels because omega-3 fatty acids replace AA in the substrate pool. This produces an accompanying decrease in the capacity to synthesize inflammatory eicosanoids from AA. Studies have documented that inflammatory eicosanoids produced from AA are depressed when dogs consume foods with high levels of omega-3 fatty acids. In addition to their role in modulating the production of inflammatory eicosanoids, omega-3 fatty acids have a direct role in the resolution of inflammation.

Shellfish supplements have been used to manage arthritis in humans and, in recent years, interest has focused on the potential benefits of a nutritional supplement prepared from the New Zealand green-lipped mussel (GLM), *Perna canaliculus*.[24] GLM is known to contain anti-inflammatory components and other nutrients which benefit joint health. Heat processing of GLM has been shown to destroy its activity. Therefore, the processing of whole GLM and incorporation of the GLM product into food products requires special care and processing techniques to avoid destroying any efficacy of the final product.

GLM has been shown to contain a unique omega-3 fatty acid, eicosatetraenoic acid (ETA), which appears to act as a dual inhibitor of AA oxygenation by both the cyclooxygenase and lipoxygenase pathways.[25] GLM is a rich source of nutrients, including glycosaminoglycans (GAGs), such as chondroitin sulfates, vitamins, minerals, and omega-3 series PUFAs.

Nutrition, and specific nutrients, provide an effective and safe way to manage dogs with OA. Foods with high levels of n-3 fatty acids have the dual benefit of controlling inflammation and pain while slowing progression of the disease by decreasing cartilage degradation.

Successful treatment and prevention of obesity and OA requires a comprehensive approach which includes preventive measures and a multimodal treatment program. Documenting the presence of comorbid conditions is critical.

Clinical signs of OA are often not obvious on examination, particularly early in the disease process. Early diagnosis of OA facilitates early intervention which will likely improve the long-term outcome for the patient. Nutritional management should be part of the multimodal approach in dogs with joint disease. Mobility is powerful and allows humans and canines to live healthy and happily in body and mind.

Joint health is fundamental to moving in comfort and should be addressed with every dog that comes into the hospital.

Developmental Orthopedic Disease

The goal of a feeding plan for pediatric pets is to create a healthy adult. The specific objectives of a good feeding plan are to achieve healthy growth, optimize trainability and immune function, and minimize obesity and developmental orthopedic disease. Growth is a complex process involving interactions between genetics, nutrition, and other environmental influences. Nutrition plays a role in the health and development of growing pets and directly affects the immune system body composition, growth rate, and skeletal development.

Developmental orthopedic diseases (DOD) are a diverse group of musculoskeletal disorders that occur in growing puppies and may be related to nutrition. CHD and osteochondrosis are the most common musculoskeletal problems with nutrition-related etiology. Specific nutritional factors that are thought to increase the risk of DOD in young dogs include: (1) free choice feeding (excess energy consumption), (2) feeding high-energy foods (rapid growth), and (3) excessive intake of calcium from food, treats and or supplements (dietary imbalance).[26,27] OA secondary to DOD can be minimized by educating young dog owners to offer appropriate nutrition during the critical growth phase. All puppies whose adult weight is estimated to be ≥50 lbs should be fed a growth food specifically formulated for large breed dogs. As discussed earlier, maintaining an ideal BCS throughout life will decrease trauma to joints and the development of OA.

Patient Assessment

Pediatric patients should be assessed for risk factors before weaning to allow implementation of recommendations for appropriate nutrition. A thorough history and physical evaluation are necessary. Special attention should be paid to large- and giant-breed puppies, breeds, and genders (including intact and neutered) at risk for obesity. In addition, growth rates and BCSs provide valuable information about nutritional risks. Growth rates of young dogs are affected by the nutrient density of the food and the amount of food fed. It is important that puppies be fed to grow at an optimal rate for bone development and body condition rather than at a maximal rate. Growing animals reach a similar adult weight and size whether the growth rate is rapid or slow. Feeding for maximum growth puts puppies at increased risk for skeletal deformities and has been found to decrease longevity in other species.[26] In Labrador retrievers, even moderate overfeeding resulted in overweight adults and decreased longevity. The most practical indicator of whether a puppy's and kitten's growth rate is healthy is its BCS. Healthcare team members should be comfortable body condition scoring all patients; and with growing patients should reassess at least every two weeks to allow for adjustments in amounts fed and, thus, growth rates. Owners can and should be taught to assess body condition and are likely to become more aware of the appearance of a healthy growing puppy and kitten. Regularly assessing body condition provides immediate feedback about optimal nutrition.

Key Nutritional Factors

The requirements for all nutrients are increased during growth compared with requirements for adult dogs. Most nutrients supplied in excess of that needed for growth cause little to no harm. However, excess energy and calcium are of special concern; these concerns include energy for puppies of small and medium breeds (for obesity prevention) and energy and calcium for puppies of large and giant breeds (for skeletal health).

Also, essential fatty acids can affect the neural development and trainability of puppies.

Energy

Energy requirements for growing puppies consist of energy needed for maintenance and growth. During the first weeks after weaning body weight is relatively small and the growth rate is high; puppies use about 50% of their total energy intake for maintenance and 50% for growth. Gradually, the growth curves reach a plateau, as puppies become young adults. The proportion of energy needed for maintenance increases progressively, whereas the part for growth decreases. Energy needed for growth decreases to about 8% to 10% of the total energy requirement when puppies reach 80% or more of adult body weight. A puppy's daily energy requirement (DER) should be about 3× its resting energy requirement (RER) until it reaches about 50% of its adult body weight.[27] Thereafter, energy intake should be about $2.5 \times \text{RER}$ and can be reduced progressively to $2 \times \text{RER}$. When approximately 80% of adult size is reached, 1.8 to $2 \times \text{RER}$ is usually sufficient.

$$\text{RER}\,(\text{kcal/day}) = 70 \times \text{BW}\,(\text{kg})^{0.75}$$

$$\text{RER}\,(\text{kcal/day}) = \left(\text{BW}_{kg} \times \text{BW}_{kg} \times \text{BW}_{kg}, \sqrt{\,}, \sqrt{\,}\right) \times 70$$

These factors are general recommendations or starting points to estimate energy needs. Body condition scoring should be used to adjust these energy estimates to individual puppies.

Prevention of obesity is essential and should start at weaning. After puppies and kittens become overweight, it is challenging to return, and maintain normal weight. Too much food intake during growth may contribute to skeletal disorders in large- and giant-breed puppies. If the pet is overweight and/or obese and this is carried into adulthood, the risk for several important diseases is increased. These include hypertension, heart disease, diabetes mellitus, dyslipidemias, OA, heat, and exercise intolerance, and decreased immune function. Studies show that moderate energy and food restriction during the postweaning growth period reduces the prevalence of hip dysplasia in large-breed (Labrador retriever) puppies and increases longevity in rats without hindering adult size.[26,27] However, the pet may not receive enough energy and nutrients to support optimal growth if fed food with a very low energy density and low digestibility. This may lead to consumption of large quantities of food, which can overload the gastrointestinal (GI) tract resulting in vomiting and diarrhea. Healthcare team members should initiate monitoring of energy and food intake and body condition at an early age to help keep the pet at a healthy weight throughout life.

Protein

Protein requirements of growing dogs differ from the requirements of adult dogs. During puppyhood, protein requirements are highest at weaning and decrease progressively until adulthood. Puppies 14 weeks and older should receive at least the minimum recommended allowance for crude protein which is 17.5% DM. The recommended protein range in foods intended for growth in all puppies (small, medium, and large breeds) is 22–32% DM. Most dry commercial foods marketed for puppy growth provide protein levels within this range.[26]

Protein levels above the upper end of this range have not been shown to be detrimental but are well above the level in bitch's milk. Protein requirements of growing dogs differ from those of adults. An important difference is that arginine is an essential amino acid for puppies, whereas it is only conditionally essential for adult dogs. Foods formulated for adult dogs *should not* be fed to puppies.[26] Although protein levels may be adequate, energy levels and other nutrients may not be balanced for growth.

Fat

Dietary fat serves three primary functions:

1. a source of essential fatty acids
2. a carrier for fat-soluble vitamins
3. a concentrated source of energy.

Growing dogs have an estimated daily requirement for essential fatty acids (linoleic acid) of about 250 mg/kg body weight, which can be provided by food containing between 5% and 10% DM fat. Studies indicate that DHA is essential for normal neural, retinal, and auditory development in puppies. Inclusion of fish oil as a source of DHA in puppy foods improves trainability and should be considered essential for growth. The minimum recommended allowance for DHA plus EPA is 0.05% DM; EPA should not exceed 60% of the total. Thus, DHA needs to be at least 40% of the total DHA plus EPA, or 0.02% DM.[27]

When feeding young pets we must remember that fat contributes greatly to the energy density of a food and excessive energy intake can cause overweight/obesity and developmental orthopedic disease. The minimum recommended allowance of dietary fat for growth (8.5% DM) is much less than that needed for nursing but more than is needed for adult maintenance (5.5% DM). In order to deliver a DM energy density between 3.5 to 4.5 kcal/g; 10% to 25% DM fat is necessary. This range of dietary fat is recommended from postweaning to adulthood.[26,27]

Calcium and Phosphorus

Although growing dogs need more calcium and phosphorus than adult dogs, the healthcare team must remember and educate owners that the minimum requirements are relatively low. Puppies have been successfully raised when fed foods containing 0.37–0.6% DM calcium and 0.33% DM phosphorus.[26]

Foods for large- and giant-breed puppies should contain 0.7–1.2% DM calcium (0.6–1.1%

phosphorus). Foods with a calcium content of 1.1% DM provide more calcium to puppies just after weaning than if bitch's milk is fed exclusively. Small- to medium-sized breeds are less sensitive to slightly overfeeding or underfeeding calcium; thus the level of calcium in foods for these puppies can range from 0.7% to 1.7% DM (0.6–1.3% phosphorus) without risk. The phosphorus intake is less critical than the calcium intake, provided the minimum requirements of 0.35% DM are met and the calcium–phosphorus ratio is between 1:1 and 1.8:1. For large- and giant-breed dogs, the calcium/phosphorus ratio should be between 1:1 and 1.5:1.[26]

Digestibility

Puppies that are fed foods low in energy density and digestibility will need to eat larger amounts of food to achieve growth. This will increase the risk of flatulence, vomiting, diarrhea, and the development of a "pot-bellied" appearance. As a result, foods recommended

for puppies should be more digestible than typical adult foods. An indirect indicator of digestibility is energy density. Foods with a higher energy density are likely to be more digestible.[26,27]

Carbohydrates

While no specific level of digestible (soluble) carbohydrates exists for growing puppies, it is recommended that the level of digestible (soluble) carbohydrates around 20% (DM) may optimize health.

Successful treatment and prevention of musculoskeletal disease conditions require a comprehensive approach which includes preventive measures and a multimodal management program. Clinical signs of musculoskeletal diseases are often not obvious on examination, especially early in the disease process. Although signs of overweight/obesity are readily apparent they are often overlooked or dismissed as inconsequential. Documenting a diagnosis of overweight/obesity is critical to the management of these disease conditions. Diagnosing overweight/obesity requires consistent recording of both a body weight and BCS. Early diagnosis of OA and DOD enables early intervention which in turn often improves the long-term outcome for the patient. Consistent use of a thorough, disease-specific history may raise awareness of subtle changes early in the course of OA and DOD. Successful management of OA/DOD and obesity requires nutritional intervention.

References

1 CE DC, Johnston SA, Déjardin LM, Schaefer SL (2016) Arthrology. In J DeCamp, S Déjardin (eds), *Brinker, Piermattei, and Flo's Handbook of Small Animal Orthopedics and Fracture Repair* (5th edn), St. Louis, MO: Elsevier.

2 Anandacoomarasamy A, Caterson I, Sambrook P *et al.* (2008) The impact of obesity on the musculoskeletal system. *International Journal of Obesity* **32**: 211–22.

3 Anderson KL, O'Neill DG, Brodbelt DC *et al.* (2018) Prevalence, duration and risk factors for appendicular osteoarthritis in a UK dog population under primary veterinary care. *Scientific Reports* **8**(5641): 1–12.

4 Burns KM (2021) Osteoarthritis: getting patients moving through nutrition. *Today's Veterinary Nurse.* Winter: 35–43.

5 Burns KM (2011) Are your patients suffering in silence? managing osteoarthritis in pets. *The NAVTA Journal.* Convention Issue: 16–22.

6 Ward E (2022) State of US pet obesity. *Moving from Awareness to Treatment.*

https://petobesityprevention.org/ accessed May 10, 2022.

7 Burns KM (2020) Mobility matters: nutritional management of canine joint disease. *Vetted*: 8–11.

8 Burns KM (2021) Get them moving: Mobility management in dogs. *PetVet*, January: 18–21.

9 Kealy RD, Lawler DF, Ballam JM *et al.* (2000) Evaluation of the effect of limited food consumption on radiographic evidence of osteoarthritis in dogs. *Journal of the American Veterinary Medical Association* **217**: 1678–80.

10 Paster ER, LaFond E, Biery DN *et al.* (2005) Estimates of prevalence of hip dysplasia in Golden Retrievers and Rottweilers and the influence of bias on published prevalence figures. *Journal of the American Veterinary Medical Association* **226**(3): 387–92.

11 Eby J, Colditz G (2008) Obesity/overweight: prevention and weight management. In S Quah, K Heggenhougen (eds), *International Encyclopedia of Public Health*, pp. 602–9, St Louis: Elsevier.

12 Kienzle E, Bergler R, Mandernach A (1998) A comparison of the feeding behavior and the human-animal relationship in owners of normal and obese dogs. *The Journal of Nutrition* **128**: 2779S–82S.

13 Anandacoomarasamy A, Fransen M, March L (2009) Obesity and the musculoskeletal system. *Current Opinion in Rheumatology* **21**: 71–7.

14 Christensen R, Bartels EM, Astrup A, Bliddal H (2007) Effect of weight reduction in obese patients diagnosed with knee osteoarthritis: a systematic review and meta-analysis. *Annals of the Rheumatic Diseases* **66**: 433–9.

15 Impellizeri JA, Tetrick MA, Muir P (2000) Effect of weight reduction on clinical signs of lameness in dogs with hip osteoarthritis. *Journal of the American Veterinary Medical Association* **216**: 1089–91.

16 Roush JK *et al.* (2010) Multicenter practice assessment of the effects of omega-3 fatty acids on osteoarthritis in dogs. *Journal of the American Veterinary Medical Association* **236**(1): 59–66.

17 Fritsch D, Allen TA, Dodd CE *et al.* (2010) Dose-titration effects of fish oil in osteoarthritic dogs. *Journal of Veterinary Internal Medicine* **24**: 1020–6.

18 Roush JK *et al.* (2010) Evaluation of the effects of dietary supplementation with fish oil Omega-3 Fatty Acids on weight bearing in Dogs with Osteoarthritis, 3-month feeding study. *Journal of the American Veterinary Medical Association* **236**(1): 67–73.

19 Fritsch DA, Allen TA, Dodd CE *et al.* (2010) A Multi-Center Study of the effect of dietary supplemetation with fish oil omega-3 fatty acids on carprofen dosage in dogs with osteoarthritis. *Journal of the American Veterinary Medical Association* **236**: 535–9.

20 Caterson B, Flannery CR, Hughes CE *et al.* (2000) Mechanisms involved in cartilage proteoglycan catabolism. *Matrix Biology* **19**: 333–44.

21 Caterson G (2004) Omega-3 fatty acids-incorporation in canine chondrocyte membranes. Unpublished data. Cardiff University, Wales.

22 Wander RC, Hall JA, Gradin JL *et al.* (1997) The ratio of dietary (n-6) to (n-3) fatty acids influences immune system function, eicosanoid metabolism, lipid peroxidation and vitamin E status in aged dogs. *The Journal of Nutrition* **127**: 1198–205.

23 Innes J, Gabriel N, Vaughan-Thomas A *et al.* (2008) *Proceedings Hill's Global Mobility Symposium*, pp. 22–6.

24 Bui LM, Bierer TL (2001) Influence of green lipped mussels (*Perna canaliculus*) in alleviating signs of arthritis in dogs. *Veterinary Therapeutics* **2**: 101–11.

25 Treschow AP, Hodges LD, Wright PF *et al.* (2007) Novel anti-inflammatory omega-3 PUFAs from New-Zealand green-lipped mussels, *Perna canaliculus. Comparative Biochemistry and Physiology. Part B, Biochemistry & Molecular Biology* **147**: 645–56.

26 Burns KM (2014) Pediatric nutrition: Optimal care for life! *NAVC Proceedings.*

27 Richardson DC, Zentek J, Hazewinkel HAW *et al.* (2010) Developmental orthopedic disease in dogs. In M Hand, CD Thatcher, R Remillard (eds), *Small Animal Clinical Nutrition* (5th edn), pp. 667–93, Topeka, KS: Mark Morris Institute.

47

Weight Management

Pet obesity has reached epidemic proportions in North America as well as other industrialized countries. This mirrors the epidemic in the human population. It is estimated that 35–40% of adult pets and 50% of pets over age 7 are overweight or obese.[1-4] According to the Association for Pet Obesity Prevention 59% of dogs and 61% of cats in the United States were classified as overweight or having obesity in 2022.[5] Obesity can be defined as an increase in fat tissue mass sufficient to contribute to disease. Dogs and cats weighing 10–19% more than the optimal weight for their breed are considered overweight; those weighing 20% or more above the optimum weight are considered obese.[6-8] Obesity has been associated with several disease conditions, as well as with a reduced lifespan. A combination of excessive caloric intake, decreased physical activity, and genetic susceptibility are associated with most cases of obesity and the primary treatment for obesity is reduced caloric intake and increased physical activity. Obesity is one of the leading preventable causes of illness/death and with the dramatic rise in pet obesity over the past several decades, weight management and obesity prevention should be among the top health issues healthcare team members discuss with every client.

Causes of Obesity

Obesity is a complex polygenic disease involving interactions between multiple genes and the environment. Obesity is caused by an imbalance of energy intake and energy expenditure – it is very simple: too many calories in, not enough calories expended! There are several risk factors that affect energy balance. In today's society, indoor pets (in North America) are typically neutered. While there are many positive health benefits associated with neutering, it is important that metabolic impacts are addressed as well. Studies have demonstrated that neutering may result in decreased metabolic rate and increased food intake, and if energy intake is not adjusted, body weight, body condition score, and amount of body fat will increase resulting in an overweight or obese pet. Other recognized risk factors for obesity include breed, age, decreased physical activity, and type of food and feeding method.[6-9]

Specific breeds of dogs and cats are more likely to become overweight. In dogs, these include Shetland Sheepdogs, Golden retrievers, Dachshunds, Cocker spaniels, Labrador retrievers, Dalmatians, Rottweilers, and mixed breeds. In cats, mixed breeds and Manx cats

Nutrition and Disease Management for Veterinary Technicians and Nurses, Third Edition. Ann Wortinger and Kara M. Burns.
© 2024 John Wiley & Sons, Inc. Published 2024 by John Wiley & Sons, Inc.
Companion Website: www.wiley.com/go/wortinger/3e

have been found more likely to be obese compared to most purebred cats. Veterinary technicians should begin discussions on maintaining appropriate/optimal weight in pets, particularly in at-risk breeds, during the initial puppy/kitten health, and wellness examination.

Health Risks Associated with Obesity

Healthcare teams are aware of the many health conditions associated with obesity in pets including arthritis, diabetes mellitus (DM), cancer, respiratory conditions, cardiovascular disease, skin diseases, lower urinary tract problems, and hepatic lipidosis. Obese pets are also more difficult to manage in terms of sample collection (blood and urine) and catheter placement. Also, obese pets may be more prone to treatment complications including difficulty intubating, respiratory distress, slower recovery time, and delayed wound healing. It is widely believed that obesity affects quality of life and leads to reduced life expectancy. The dramatic impact of excess body weight in dogs and cats has been demonstrated. In cats, it is estimated that 31% of DM and 34% of lameness cases could be eliminated if cats were at optimum body weight. Lifespan was increased by nearly 2 years in dogs that were maintained at an optimal body condition.[10] It is important to recognize and communicate to our clients that fat tissue is not inert, and that obesity is not an aesthetic condition that only affects our pet's ability to interact with us on a physical activity level. Fat tissue is metabolically active and in fact, is the largest endocrine organ in the body and has an unlimited growth potential. Fat tissue is an active producer of hormones and inflammatory cytokines and the chronic low-grade inflammation secondary to obesity contributes to obesity related diseases.[3,10]

The Largest Endocrine Organ

Adipose tissue is more than a storage site for energy; it is now recognized as a multifunctional organ. Adipose tissue plays an active role in a variety of homeostatic and pathologic processes. As an organ, adipose tissue responds to nutrient, neural and hormonal signals, and secretes adipocytokines.[11] Adipocytokines (i.e., leptin and adiponectin) function as hormones to influence energy homeostasis in humans. They also regulate neuroendocrine functions. Adipose tissue secretes a variety of cytokines such as TNF-α, IL-6, resistin, and visfatin that affect immune functions and inflammatory processes throughout the body. Adipocytokines have numerous functions including satiety regulation, carbohydrate and lipid metabolism, and insulin sensitivity as well as many aspects of inflammation and immunity.[12]

Evaluating Weight and Nutrition

Obesity is a difficult disease to talk with owners about because most pet owners do not recognize (or want to admit) that their pet is overweight. All members of the healthcare team need to commit to understanding and communicating the role of weight management in pet health and disease prevention. In particular, the veterinary technician is the primary source for client education; the interface between the client, the doctor, and the rest of the hospital team; and is the key advocate for the patient.

The healthcare team should assess every patient that comes into the hospital, every time they come into the hospital to establish nutritional needs and feeding goals. These goals will vary depending on the pet's physiology, obesity risk factors, and current health status. Designing and implementing a weight management protocol supports the team, the client, and most importantly the patient.[6,8,9]

The first steps in patient evaluation are as follows: a complete history including a detailed nutritional history and a complete physical examination including a complete blood count, serum chemistry, and urinalysis. Signalment data should include species, breed, age, gender, neuter status, weight, activity level, and environment. The nutritional history should determine the type of food (all food) fed, the feeding method (how much and how often), who is responsible for feeding the pet, and any other sources of energy intake (no matter how small or seemingly insignificant).[6,8,9]

The following questions should be part of every nutritional assessment:

- Tell me everything that your pet eats in a day.
- What brand of food do you feed your pet (try to get specific name)?
- Tell me the texture of the food your pet eats.
- Tell me how do you feed your pet – feeding method (how much, how often)?
- Tell me what snacks or treats your pet receives.
- Tell me about any supplements your pet receives.
- What medications, including chewable medications, does your pet receive?
- What type of chew toys does your pet play with?
- What foods or treats not specifically designated for pets (such as human foods) does your pet receive? What and how often?
- Does your pet have ANY access to other sources of food (neighbor, trash, family member, etc.)?

Obtaining a complete nutritional history supports consistency and accuracy of patient information, provides key insights to barriers in client compliance, guides client discussion, and supports the optimal weight management program for the pet. Asking the questions in an open-ended manner allows for more discussion from the pet owner and more detail on what the pet receives each day.

Be sure to weigh the pet and obtain a body condition score and muscle condition score at *every visit* and record the information in the patient's medical record. It is helpful to use the same scale and chart the findings for the client. Body condition scoring (BCS) and muscle condition scoring (MCS) are important tools to assess a patient's fat stores and muscle mass. A healthy and successful weight management program results in loss of fat tissue while maintaining lean body mass and consistent and accurate assessment of weight, BCS, and MCS are important tools to track progress. The use of body condition charts and breed charts are helpful tools in discussing the importance of weight management with clients and help them visualize what an optimal weight would look like on their pet.

Body Condition Scoring (BCS)

The BCS is a subjective assessment of an animal's body fat that takes into account the animal's frame size independent of its weight. A variety of scoring systems with defined criteria have been published. All are useful tools for assessing body condition. In general, dogs and cats in optimal body condition have: (1) normal body contours and silhouettes, (2) bony prominences that can be readily palpated but not seen or felt above skin surfaces, and (3) intra-abdominal fat insufficient to obscure or interfere with abdominal palpation. In addition to body weight, the BCS should always be recorded in the hospital record whenever an animal is examined. Body weight alone does not indicate how appropriate the weight is for an individual animal. A Labrador retriever weighing 30 kg, or a domestic short-hair cat weighing 4 kg, may be underweight, optimal weight, or overweight. The BCS puts body weight in perspective for each individual patient (Table 47.1).

Owners should be taught to perform BCS at home. This is helpful both during a weight loss program and for long-term maintenance. However, it is important to recognize that owners are often reluctant to objectively evaluate

Table 47.1 Body condition and muscle condition scoring system.

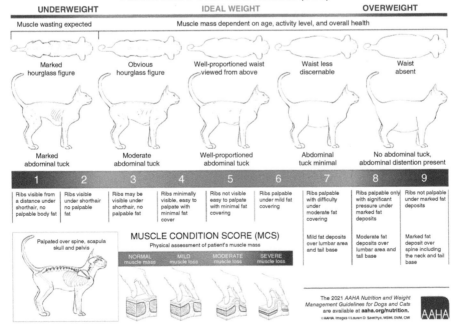

The 2021 AAHA Nutrition and Weight Management Guidelines for Dogs and Cats, aaha.org/nutrition. ©AAHA. Images ©Lauren D. Sawchyn, MSMI, DVM, CMI and AAHA/Sadie Lewandowski.

their pets. Several studies have demonstrated that both dog and cat owners consistently underestimate their pet's body condition scores.[13,14]

However, by reinforcing the health risks associated with obesity and educating owners on performing a BCS on their own pets, we can help pets maintain their ideal body weight. It is important to remind owners to report their pet's BCS monthly and then ensure that this is documented in the medical record.

Body Fat Index Risk Chart Validation

Recent studies by veterinary nutritionists and scientists at the University of Tennessee College of Veterinary Medicine compared a variety of diagnostic methods used to assess body composition with DEXA-scans in dogs and cats presented for weight management programs.[15,16] The primary goal of these studies was to develop practical methods to better diagnose body composition in obese pets. The hypothesis was that a more accurate diagnostic test would promote more effective weight loss in client-owned pets. In addition to current BCS methods, pets were assessed using bioelectric impedance, morphometric measurements, and a newly developed Body Fat Index (BFI) Risk Chart.

Eighty-three client-owned dogs, representing 27 breeds weighing from 11 to 162 lb (5–73.6 kg), and 39 client-owned cats, representing 9 breeds ranging from 6–25 lb (2.7–11.4 kg), were enrolled in these studies. Bioelectric impedance was found to be an unreliable tool for predicting body composition. BCS was inaccurate in 60% of pets.[16] The findings from these studies indicated that when traditional BCS was used to estimate ideal body weight and consequently food dose, over half of the pets received a recommendation to ingest excess calories. By incorporating expanded definitions, using the BFI Risk Chart improved the accuracy of prediction of ideal

for both dogs and cats, particularly those pets with greater than 45% body fat.

Weight Management Program

As with many aspects of healthcare, designing a successful weight management program is not a "one program fits all" for our patients. A successful weight management program includes consistent and accurate weight measurement/patient monitoring, effective and educational client communication, identification of compliance gaps, utilization of tools to reinforce compliance, client and patient support, and program restructure as needed.

Setting a goal for weight loss and calculating the appropriate energy intake starts with determining the pet's ideal body weight. Ideal body weight is a starting goal that is adjusted for appropriate body condition as the pet loses weight. The healthcare team must determine the number of daily calories that will result in weight loss while subsequently providing adequate protein, vitamins, and minerals to meet the pet's daily energy requirement (DER). The DER reflects the pet's activity level and is a calculation based on the pet's resting energy requirement (RER).[7,8]

There are a couple of basic formulas that all technicians should memorize or have on laminated note cards in every exam room (along with a calculator)! The most accurate formula to determine the RER for a cat or a dog is:

RER kcal/day

$$= 70 \left(\text{Ideal Body Weight in Kg} \right)^{0.75}$$

or

$$\text{RER kcal/day} = \left(\text{kg} \times \text{kg} \times \text{kg}, \sqrt{}, \sqrt{} \right) \times 70$$

After RER is determined, DER may be calculated by multiplying RER by "standard" factors related to energy needs. The calculations used to determine energy needs for obese prone pets or for pets needing to lose weight are:[7–9]

Obese prone dogs DER $= 1.4 \times$ RER

Weight loss/dogs DER $= 1.0 \times$ RER

Obese prone cats DER = 1.0 × RER

Weight loss/cats DER = 0.8 × RER

Gathering the above information is crucial to success and only takes a few minutes. This information is the foundation for developing a weight loss program that includes:

1. target weight or weight loss goal,
2. maximum daily caloric intake,
3. specific food, amount of food, and method of feeding.

The weight management program should also include detailed protocols for monitoring the pet's weight (schedule these before the client leaves and send reminder cards), adjusting the pet's energy intake accordingly, and exercise guidelines/suggestions.

Determining Ideal Weight Matters

We have discussed the fact that appropriate calorie reduction is required for successful weight loss. It must be noted that slight inaccuracies can make big differences, especially in smaller pets. For example, a 10 lb (4.5 kg) cat consuming just 10 kcal/day more than RER will gain nearly 1 lb (0.5 kg) or 12% of body weight per year. In other words, eating the equivalent of 10 extra kibbles of a typical dry cat food will cause weight gain in a cat which is equal to a 150 lb (68 kg) person gaining almost 20 lb (9 kg) in a year.[17] Overestimating ideal weight will lead to feeding recommendations that may actually promote weight gain rather than weight loss.

Client/Behavioral Factors

For weight loss programs to be successful, everyone involved in feeding the pet must make a commitment to accomplish that goal. Weight loss will not occur unless the pet owner recognizes the problem and is willing to take corrective steps. Several strategies exist to help owners make this commitment. Careful consideration must be given to the powerful relationship between feeding and the human–animal bond.

Calorie Restriction

Incorporating a detailed food diary is a crucial diagnostic step in developing a weight-loss program. The diary can help in determining how severe caloric restriction will need to be to produce weight loss. Simply calculating estimated energy requirements for cats or dogs will often lead to inaccurate results because of wide variation between individual animals. In practice, individual animals are encountered that need precisely the same, markedly fewer, and occasionally, markedly more calories than calculations suggest. Caloric restriction may be insufficient to produce weight loss or may even produce weight gain in some animals if calculations for caloric restriction are applied without taking into account the calories being eaten to maintain the animal's current weight. There is also a wide range of therapeutic and wellness foods designed for weight control. The caloric density of these products is quite variable. A therapeutic weight loss food should be selected based on the individual needs of each patient.

Exercise

Exercise is the only real-world way to increase energy expenditures. Exercise may also benefit obese patients by lessening the loss of lean body mass and maintaining or improving RER. Additionally, increased physical activity may improve metabolic abnormalities even without significant alterations in body weight. In humans, increased physical activity has been shown to improve insulin sensitivity, partially reverse leptin resistance, and suppress the enhanced proinflammatory response induced by obesity.[18] In some cases, pets fail to lose weight unless exercise is included as part of the weight-reduction plan, regardless of the severity of caloric restriction. One recent study evaluated the effects of environmental enrichment designed to increase physical activity in obese cats. Cats that received enrichments had increased activity and a trend toward increased percentage weight loss. Most importantly, owners of cats that received enrichment had greater satisfaction with the weight loss program.[19]

There are many ways for owners to get their pets active and healthcare team members must discuss these with the client and determine which could work for that specific patient and client. Exercise should start simply – having the owner walk their dog to the end of the driveway for example. Also, starting to play with interactive toys with their cat for a few minutes a day would be a great way to begin to get cats more engaged in exercise. Gradually, you want to educate the owner to build up the distance and time spent exercising.[6] If the owner is excited and takes the dog on a 3-mile walk on the first day, the dog may tire easily and the owner may find this frustrating and not want to walk with their dog again. Remember to advise owners that exercise needs to begin in moderation. By following this, a more successful outcome will result.[14]

Weight Management Guidelines

We have discussed the sensitivity around communicating and implementing a weight management program for dogs and cats. Healthcare teams know how an effective customized weight loss program provides a consistent and healthy rate of weight loss to reduce risk of disease, prevent malnutrition, and improve quality of life. The American Animal Hospital Association (AAHA) produced the AAHA Nutrition and Weight Management Guidelines in 2021 to aid veterinary healthcare teams. These guidelines offer tools for a proper nutritional assessment and the management

of weight loss and long-term maintenance of healthy weight. These guidelines are aimed at raising awareness of the health consequences of pets being overweight or obese. The guidelines also promote the prevention of excess weight and offer suggestions and tools for the management of weight loss and long-term maintenance of healthy weight. The guidelines are downloadable for free to veterinary hospitals.[20]

There are several specific recommendations that support a successful weight loss program including:

1. Emphasizing feeding consistency including feeding the pet from its designated dish only.
2. Be sure the client is using an 8-ounce measuring cup.
3. Recommend the appropriate weight loss food and calculate the initial feeding amount.
4. Discuss the importance of total energy intake (do not feed anything other than the recommended food at the designated amount).
5. If the client wants to "treat" their pet, make appropriate recommendations, and adjust the caloric intake of the base food accordingly.
6. Encourage clients to feed their pets separately if possible.
7. Recommend appropriate exercise for the pet.
8. Offer your client's suggestions on ways other than food to reward or bond with their pet.
9. Evaluate, adjust, communicate, and encourage on a consistent basis.
10. Celebrate success!

Summary

Successful weight management begins with recognition of the disease of overweight and obesity as well as the importance of weight control in our pets. It is essential that the ideal weight of the pet be determined to avoid feeding the fat instead of the pet within. The veterinary healthcare team must communicate the serious effects that even a few excess pounds can have on the health and longevity of their pet's life. Weight management should be a cornerstone wellness program in every hospital and veterinary technicians should be the champion of the program and advocate for the patient.

References

1 Rosenthal M (2007) Obesity in America: Why Brune and Bessie are so heavy and what you can do about it. *Veterinary Forums* **24**: 26–34.

2 Lund E, Armstrong P, Kirk C *et al.* (2005) Prevalence and risk factors for obesity in adult cats from private US veterinary practices. *International Journal of Applied Research in Veterinary Medicine* **3**: 88–96.

3 Lund E, Armstrong PJ, Kirk CA *et al.* (2006) Prevalence and risk factors for obesity in adult dogs from private US veterinary practices. *International Journal of Applied Research in Veterinary Medicine* **4**: 177–86.

4 Armstrong PJ, Lusby AL (2011) Clinical importance of canine and feline obesity. In TL Towell (ed.), *Practical Weight Management in Dogs and Cats*, pp. 3–21, Ames, IA: Wiley Blackwell.

5 Ward E. 2022 State of U.S. pet obesity report. Moving from awareness to treatment. https://www.petobesityprevention .org/state-of-pet-obesity-report. Accessed May, 2023.

6 Burns KM, Towell TL (2011) Owner education and adherence. In TL Towell (ed.), *Practical Weight Management in Dogs and Cats*, pp. 3–21, Ames, IA: Wiley Blackwell.

7 Burns KM (2006) Managing overweight or obese pets. *Veterinary Technician*. June: 385–9.

8 Burns KM (2013) Why is Rocky so stocky? Obesity is a disease! *NAVTA Journal* Convention Issue: 16–9.

9 Toll PW, Yamka RN, Schoenherr WD, Hand MS (2010) Obesity. In MS Hand, CD Thatcher, RL Remillard *et al.* (eds), *Small Animal Clinical Nutrition* (5th edn), pp. 501–42, Marceline, MO: Walsworth Publishing, Mark Morris Institute.

10 Laflamme DP (2006) Understanding and managing obesity in dogs and cats. *Veterinary Clinics: Small Animal Practice* **36**: 1283–95.

11 Ahima RS (2006) Adipose tissue as an endocrine organ. *Obesity* **14**(Suppl 5): 242S–9S.

12 Tilg H, Moschen AR (2006) Adipocytokines: mediators linking adipose tissue, inflammation and immunity. *Nature* **6**: 772–83.

13 Sing R, Laflamme DP, Sidebottom-Nielsen M (2002) Owner perceptions of canine body condition score. *Journal of Veterinary Internal Medicine* **16**(3): 362.

14 Kienzle E, Bergler R (2006) Human–animal relationship of owners of normal and overweight cats. *The Journal of Nutrition* **136**: 1947S–50S.

15 Toll PW, Paetau-Robinson I, Lusby AL *et al.* (2010) Effectiveness of morphometric measurements for predicting body composition in overweight and obese dogs. *Journal of Veterinary Internal Medicine* **24**: 717.

16 Lusby AL, Kirk CA, Toll PW *et al.* (2010) Effectiveness of BCS for estimation of ideal body weight and energy requirements in overweight and obese dogs compared to DXA (abstract). *Journal of Veterinary Internal Medicine* **24**: 717.

17 Michel K, Scherk M (2012) From problem to success: feline weight loss programs that work. *Journal of Feline Medicine and Surgery* **14**: 327–36.

18 Berggren JR, Hulver MW, Houmard JA (2005) Fat as an endocrine organ: influence

of exercise. *Journal of Applied Physiology* **99**: 757–64.

19 Trippany JR, Funk J, Buffinton CA (2003) Effects of environmental enrichments on weight loss in cats. *Journal of Veterinary Internal Medicine* **17**: 430.

20 Cline MG, Burns KM, Coe JB *et al.* (2021) 2021 AAHA nutrition and weight management guidelines for dogs and cats. *Journal of the American Animal Hospital Association* **57**: 153–78.

48

Cachexia

Cachexia is a multifactorial syndrome characterized by severe, chronic, and progressive weight loss and muscle wasting, oftentimes accompanied by anorexia.[1] Cachexia is complex as indicated by severe, chronic, undesired, and progressive weight loss and muscle wasting, with or without loss of fat mass.[2,3] This syndrome is associated with an underlying disease, anorexia, inflammation, insulin resistance, and increased lean muscle breakdown.[4,5] In addition, changes in carbohydrate, lipid, and protein metabolism are seen as a consequence of altered cytokine activity.[2-4]

Unlike weight loss seen with starvation or anorexia, cachexia is distinguished by a loss of adipose tissue with accompanying loss of lean body mass, primarily muscle. Non-muscle protein as found in the organs is preserved in cachexia but not in starvation. Significant loss of mineral content in the bones can also be seen contributing to the overall weakness found in many cachectic patients.[1] This chapter will look at cachexia and the role nutrition plays in managing cachexia.

Sarcopenia

With aging comes a gradual decline of muscle mass, quality, and strength; what is known as sarcopenia. It develops during aging in the absence of disease. Sarcopenia begins early in adult life and progresses – a 30% reduction in lean muscle mass (LMM) is reported from ages 20–80 years,[6-8] although sarcopenic LMM begins during middle age in companion pets. Often the muscle loss is countered by added fat mass (sarcopenic obesity), evident in both humans and companion pets, and increases the challenge of appropriate nutritional management because there is no change in total body weight. Advanced sarcopenia, as with cachexia, is associated with physical disability, poor quality of life (QOL), and increased death risk for pets.[6,9-11]

Starvation versus Cachexia

Weight loss associated with disease differs from that seen with simple starvation. In cachexia, there is an equal loss of muscle and fat characterized by increased catabolism of skeletal muscle. During starvation, fat is mobilized first sparing muscle proteins, resting energy expenditure is decreased and glucose metabolism is reduced. In contrast, cachectic patients have normal or elevated resting energy expenditures and glucose turnover. Adequate nutrition will halt and reverse the metabolic alterations that accompany simple starvation but will not completely reverse the metabolic disturbances associated with cachexia.

This loss of lean body mass has a harmful effect on strength, immune function, and overall survival.[6] Weight loss provides an important prognostic gauge in the overall survival of the patient. Increased weight loss is inversely proportional to survival time.[1,12] Loss of muscle mass is first noticed over the epaxial, gluteal,

Nutrition and Disease Management for Veterinary Technicians and Nurses, Third Edition. Ann Wortinger and Kara M. Burns.
© 2024 John Wiley & Sons, Inc. Published 2024 by John Wiley & Sons, Inc.
Companion Website: www.wiley.com/go/wortinger/3e

scapular, and temporal muscles[13] and is easily detected during a routine physical exam. There does not appear to be a cause-and-effect relationship between anorexia and cachexia, with weight loss exceeding that expected with simply a decrease in caloric intake.[1]

Cachexia has been seen in animals with cancers, cardiac disease, renal disease, and myriad other serious illnesses and injuries. Loss of 25–50% of the lean body mass compromises the immune system and affects muscle strength, with death resulting from infections, pulmonary failure, or both.[14]

Pathophysiology

Cancer-associated starvation occurs as a consequence of an imbalance between the nutritional needs of the patient, the demands of the tumor, and the availability of nutrients in the body.[15,16] The competition for nutrients between the tumor and the host promotes a variety of metabolic disturbances including alterations in carbohydrate, lipid, and protein metabolism. Cytokines play a key role as the main humoral and tumor-derived factors involved in cancer cachexia and may be responsible for the majority of metabolic changes associated with cancer cachexia. Table 48.1 summarizes the effects of cytokines on nutrient metabolism in patients with cancer cachexia.[15]

Phases of Cachexia

There are three phases of cachexia identified in humans; the veterinary profession manages cachexia based on these patterns. Throughout the first phase, the patient does not exhibit any clinical signs; however, the biochemical changes are already occurring. These include elevations seen in lactate levels through the glycolysis process, an increase in insulin levels, causing peripheral insulin resistance, and alterations in amino acid and lipid profiles.[12]

Table 48.1 The effects of cytokines on nutrient metabolism in patients with cancer cachexia.

CHO	Increased resistance to insulin
	Increased glucose synthesis
	Increased Cori cycle activity
Protein	Increased protein breakdown (catabolism)
	Increased liver (acute phase proteins) and tumor protein synthesis
Lipid	Increased lipid mobilization
	Elevated levels of triglycerides

During the second phase of cachexia, clinical signs can become evident presenting as anorexia, weight loss, and lethargy. Often owners attribute these early signs to the pet's aging process and thus do not recognize the clinical significance. The final phase is characterized by marked loss of body fat and protein stores, severe debilitation, weakness, and biochemical evidence of negative nitrogen balance.[3,12] If left untreated, cachexia can be the ultimate cause of death.

Therapeutic Strategies

The optimal therapy is to manage the underlying disease process. In veterinary medicine, therapeutic strategies generally include management of anorexia, nutritional support, nutrient supplementation, and the provision of omega-3 fatty acids.

Managing Anorexia/Hyporexia

Nutritional counseling should be a part of the pretreatment plan for all patients. Veterinary nurses/technicians should help owners understand the importance of measuring caloric intake and should have a sequential plan for maintaining nutritional support throughout the treatment process. This may include simple strategies to increase consumption initially (see Table 48.2) which may progress to assisted feeding if warranted. In a patient with a functional GI tract, enteral feeding is preferred. Strategies for managing anorexia in dogs and cats have been thoroughly reviewed.[17] Table 48.2 is a brief review of those recommendations.

Key Nutritional Factors in the Management of Cachexia

While it is not possible to reverse the wasting process with nutritional supplements alone, our patients do need to be fed, and through manipulation of nutrients, benefits can be seen in some of the changes the body is undergoing.[1] Proper nutrition can be key to managing cachexia with provision of calories, protein, fat, and modulation of cytokine production.[18] Specific dietary recommendations should consider the stage of disease, the patient's energy needs, current and past nutritional status, and ability or willingness to eat.[12]

The caloric distribution in the food should emphasize calories obtained from fats and proteins (rather than carbohydrates) since glucose is the preferred fuel for tumor cells in cancer cachexia patients, and fatty acids and amino acids are not. In cancer cachexia patients, the goal is to feed the patient and starve the tumor cells. Ideally, a food should contain 50–60% of the calories from fat, 30–50% of the calories from protein, and the remaining portion from carbohydrates.[7,12]

Omega-3 fatty acids, especially those found in certain types of cold water fish and fish oil (eicosapentaenoic acid [EPA], docosahexaenoic acid [DHA]), are probably the most important nutraceuticals to consider for animals with cancer.[15,19,20] Studies using animal models have shown that supplementation with EPA and DHA can help to prevent cachexia and metastatic disease processes. These fatty acids obtained from the omega-3 class of fats produce less potent inflammatory mediators than the omega-6 class of fatty acids, which are viewed as pro-inflammatory. When the body uses the omega-3 class of fatty acids to produce cytokines, the inflammatory response produced is decreased in proportion to the level of omega-3 fatty acids in the diet. A recommended dose of 40 mg/kg of EPA, and 25 mg/kg of DHA. Using the common formulation of most fish oil capsules, to achieve this concentration you would need to provide ~1 g capsule/10# body weight.[3,18] Many recovery diets already have this incorporated into the diet and additional supplementation is not recommended.

Dietary protein should be highly digestible and go above levels normally used for maintenance of adult animals, due to the catabolic process. Protein levels of 30–50% are recommended, with dogs around 30–45% and cats around 40–50% DMB. Looking at protein levels another way, the minimum recommended intake is 5.14 g/100 kcal with 6–7 g/100 kcal preferred.[18,20]

As stated previously, tumor cells preferentially use glucose for energy. Selecting a carbohydrate with a lower glycemic index would provide a slower release of carbohydrate-generated glucose into the bloodstream than would those with higher glycemic indexes. Rice is one of the carbohydrates with a highest glycemic index, with barley, sorghum, and corn having much lower glycemic indexes.[12]

Feeding Methods

Enteral feeding is always the preferred delivery method, provided the patient has a functional gastrointestinal tract. Oral feeding of canned or dry pet food would be the first choice with cachexia patients.[12,19,20] When a patient is unwilling or unable to consume the desired amount of food orally, various feeding tubes can be used (See Chapter 38 – Assisted Feeding). The specific tube selected will vary

Table 48.2 Strategies to increase consumption in anorectic/hyporectic patients.

Create ambiance/improve service	Create a quiet comfortable feeding area away from disturbances
Increase palatability	
Increase moisture	Switch to canned food/add water to kibble. **Caution:** some cats may have texture preferences and prefer dry food
Increase fat	Higher fat diets are more energy dense so less food may be required to meet needs.
Increase protein	Dogs may select foods with higher protein level
Sweet and salty	Adding sweet flavor (**No** artificial sweeteners) as top dressing may increase palatability for dogs but not cats. Adding salt (if appropriate) may increase palatability for dogs but not cats.
Freshness, aroma, and food temperature	Provide "fresh" canned/dry foods or home-prepared foods. Warming foods to no greater than body temperature may also release aromas.
Rarity	Uncommon or rare food may entice some dogs and cats to eat. Best to offer foods that are uncommon but not completely novel.
Variety	If a variety of options are provided each should be carefully measured to ensure accurate accounting of food intake/preferences. This approach should not be used if food aversions are likely so that the patient will not develop a learned aversion to all the therapeutic options.
Drug administration	Never top-dress food with medication or use the desired diet to administer medication. Avoid giving medications immediately before/after a meal if possible
Eliminate physical barriers	Be sure food bowls are accessible and account for any limitations in movement (raise bowls, remove E collars, etc.)
Appetite stimulating drugs	No recommended as effects are unpredictable, intermittent, and short-lasting. If above approaches are ineffective assisted feeding is recommended.

based on the patient, the desired length of use, and the owner's willingness to feed at home. Diet selection would also be based on the route selected for feeding. Preparation of home-cooked diets can be used short-term to tempt the patient to eat but should only be used long-term after consultation with a nutritionist. There are also a number of excellent therapeutic diets available that fit the recommended diet profile and can be fed both orally and via tube feeding.

Summary

It is essential that veterinary nurses/technicians recognize and understand cachexia and its effect on patients. Additionally, it is vital for healthcare team members to employ nutritional strategies to help manage anorexia and the imbalance between the nutritional needs of the patient and the availability of nutrients in the body. Feeding strategies should be aimed at alleviating the competition for nutrients between the disease process and the host which results in a variety of metabolic disturbances including alterations in carbohydrate, lipid, and protein metabolism. While cachexia is an obvious sign of biochemical imbalances within the body, these changes have been occurring for a while by the time we see the physical changes. Veterinary healthcare team members need to continue to feed patients through disease and cancer treatment. By recognizing changes these disease processes have caused within the body, a diet recommendation can be used to help the patient instead of the tumor or disease process, thus resulting in more positive outcomes, healthier patients, and happier clients.

References

1 Tisdale M. Mechanisms of cancer cachexia. *Physiology Review.* 2009 vol **89** no. 2 pg. 381-410

2 Hebuterne X, Lemarie E, Michallet M *et al.* (2014) Prevalence of malnutrition and current use of nutrition support in patients with cancer. *Journal of Parenteral and Enteral Nutrition* **38**(2): 196–204.

3 Burns KM (2019) Catabolism in the critical patient. *Today's Veterinary Nurse*: 57–60.

4 Argiles JM, Olivan M, Busquets S, Lopez-Soriano FJ (2010) Optimal management of cancer anorexia-cachexia syndrome. *Cancer Management and Research* **2**: 27–38.

5 Saker KE (2014) Practical approaches to feeding the cancer patient. *Today's Veterinary Practice*: 50–6.

6 Saker KE (2021) Nutritional concerns for cancer, cachexia, frailty, and sarcopenia in canine and feline pets. *Veterinary Clinics of North America Small Animal Practice* **51**: 729–44.

7 Freeman LM (2012) Cachexia ad sarcopenia: emerging syndromes of importance in dogs and cats. *Journal of Veterinary Internal Medicine* **26**: 3–17.

8 Sakuma K, Yamaguchi A (2012) Sarcopenia and cachexia: the adaptations of negative regulators of skeletal muscle mass. *Journal of Cachexia, Sarcopenia and Muscle* **3**: 77–94.

9 Cederholm T, Morley JE (2015) Sarcopenia: the new definition. *Current Opinion in Clinical Nutrition and Metabolic Care* **18**: 18–24.

10 Peterson ME, Little SL (2018) Cachexia, sarcopenia and other forms of muscle wasting: common problems of senior and geriatric cats with endocrine disease. In *Gerontology: An Inside Out Perspective*, pp. 67–75, St Louis, (MO: Purina Institute.

11 Peterson ME, Eirmann L (2014) Dietary management of feline endocrine disease. *Veterinary Clinics of North America Small Animal Practice* **44**: 775–88.

12 Case L, Daristotle L, Hayek M, Raasch M (2011) Nutritional care of cancer patients. In Fascetti, Delaney (eds), *Canine and Feline Nutrition* (3rd edn), pp. 479–86, MO: Mosby Elsevier Maryland Heights.

13 Freeman LM, Rush JE (2006) Cardiovascular diseases: nutritional modulation. In P Pibot, V Biourge, D Elliott (eds), *Encyclopedia of Canine Clinical Nutrition*, pp. 321–36, France EU: Royal Canin Aimargues.

14 Saker K, Remillard RL (2010) Critical care nutrition and enteral-assisted feeding. In MS Hand, CD Thatcher, RL Remillard *et al.* (eds), *Small Animal Clinical Nutrition* (5th edn), pp. 441–2, Topeka KS: Mark Morris Institute.

15 Wortinger A, Burns KM (2015) *Nutrition and Disease Management for Veterinary Technicians and Nurses*, pp. 202–7, Wiley Blackwell.

16 Mauldin GE (2012) Nutritional management of oncological diseases. In AJ Fascetti, SJ Delaney (eds), *Applied Veterinary Clinical Nutrition*, 315–328, Ames, IA: Wiley-Blackwell.

17 Delaney SJ (2006) Management of anorexia in dogs and cats. *Veterinary Clinics of North America - Small Animal Practice* **36**: 1243–9.

18 Freeman LM, Rush JE (2012) Nutritional management of cardiovascular diseases. In AJ Fascetti, SJ Delaney (eds), *Applied Veterinary Clinical Nutrition*, pp. 304–7, Ames, IO: Wiley-Blackwell.

19 Saker KE, Selting KA (2010) Cancer. In MS Hand, CD Thatcher, RL Remillard *et al.* (eds), *Small Animal Clinical Nutrition* (5th edn), pp. 587–607.

20 Forrester SD, Roudebush P, Davenport DJ (2010) Nutritional management of the cancer patient. In CH CJ, ML Higginbotham (eds), *Cancer Management in Small Animal Practice*, pp. 170–6, St. Louis, MO: Elsevier.

49

Dental Health

Pet owners do not always equate oral malodor with periodontal disease. However, the veterinary healthcare team must remind pet owners that a pet cannot truly be healthy if they have periodontal disease. The mouth is constantly inundated by bacteria and provides the perfect environment for microbial growth. As humans need dental care, animals too require dental care to maintain overall health. Dental disease causes pain and discomfort; the associated disease processes may lead to systemic issues. Maintaining oral health depends on professional periodontal management combined with appropriate, effective home care. Dental home care refers to the procedures and products employed by the client to provide plaque and tartar control for their pet. Recommending a home care routine that is effective as well as orally and systemically safe can be a challenge. Optimal results require consistent communication and education between the veterinary healthcare team and the client.

Periodontal Disease

Periodontal disease is a very common and serious disease of adult dogs and cats.[1,2] Understanding the pathophysiology of periodontal disease, particularly the relationship between dental substrates and disease progression is important to successful periodontal management. Periodontal disease is an infection caused by bacteria in the biofilm (dental plaque) that forms on oral surfaces.[1] If treatment is not undertaken, periodontal disease can lead to oral pain, dysfunction, and tooth loss. These changes often lead to behavior changes such as alterations in eating habits to general behavioral changes such as reluctance to groom, decreased socialization, and/or signs of "depression." An association exists between the severity of periodontal disease and pathologic changes in other organ systems. Systemic effects result from both bacteremia and by chronic systemic release of inflammatory mediators and bacterial degradation byproducts.

Periodontal disease refers to gingivitis and periodontitis. It is important for veterinary team members to remember that gingivitis is reversible. Gingivitis can be properly treated and essentially prevented with thorough plaque removal and effective supragingival plaque control. Periodontitis is more severe and primarily irreversible. Periodontitis often requires advanced therapy and meticulous plaque control to prevent progression of the disease. Gingivitis may progress to periodontitis. This progression is unpredictable and heavily dependent on individual animal variability; however, it is known that gingival inflammation is the first step in the development of more severe periodontitis.[2-4]

Risk Factors for Periodontal Disease

There are many risk factors associated with the prevalence and severity of periodontal disease.[5] (Table 49.1)

Bacterial colonization (plaque accumulation) and ensuing inflammation and infection are the leading causes of periodontal disease.[4,6] Several materials accumulate on tooth surfaces and participate in the pathophysiology of periodontal disease. These substances, known as tooth-accumulated materials or dental substrates, are categorized as:

(1) acquired enamel pellicle
(2) microbial plaque
(3) material alba/debris
(4) calculus
(5) stain.

Enamel pellicle is a thin film or cuticle.[7] Early enamel pellicle is composed of protein and glycoproteins deposited from saliva and gingival crevicular fluid and serves to protect and lubricate the tooth. Pellicle and its components provide a framework for initial bacterial colonization and function in dental plaque maturation. Immediately following a dental cleaning pellicle deposition and subsequent bacterial colonization begin again. Studies have demonstrated that within minutes after polishing, approximately one million organisms are deposited per mm^2 of enamel surface.[2,3,7] Bacteria aggregates combine with salivary glycoproteins, extracellular polysaccharides, and epithelial and inflammatory cells to form a soft adherent plaque that covers tooth surfaces. Dental plaque has a specific composition and structure that changes with time. Supragingival dental plaque forms above and along the free gingival margin; subgingival dental plaque is formed entirely within the gingival sulcus. Growth and maturation of supragingival plaque are necessary for subsequent colonization of subgingival surfaces by dental plaque. Supragingival plaque in

Table 49.1 Risk factors for periodontal disease in cats and dogs.

Age
Species
Breed
Chewing Behavior
Genetics
Grooming habits
Patient health status
Home care frequency
Frequency of professional veterinary oral care

dogs with clinically healthy gingivae is primarily composed of gram-positive organisms. As plaque matures, the bacterial composition shifts to a predominantly gram-negative anaerobic flora.

Plaque accumulation along the gingival margin induces inflammation in adjacent gingival tissues. If plaque removal or control is not instituted, gingivitis progresses in severity inducing local changes and allowing subsequent bacterial colonization of subgingival sites. Inflammatory mediators damage the integrity of the gingival margin and sulcular epithelium, allowing further infiltration of bacteria. The immune response of the host attempts to localize the invasion of the periodontal tissues; the result may be further destruction of local tissues due to cytokines released from inflammatory cells. Bacterial plaque is the most important substrate in the development of periodontal disease. Materia alba is a soft mixture of salivary proteins, bacteria, desquamated epithelial cells, and leukocyte fragments. Materia alba and dental plaque are two distinct materials. Materia alba does not have an organized bacterial structure or the adherence properties of dental plaque. The role of material alba in the etiopathogenesis of plaque accumulation and periodontal disease remains unclear. Other debris commonly observed in the oral cavity include food, impacted hair, and miscellaneous foreign materials acquired through chewing behaviors.[7]

Dental calculus is mineralized plaque. Calculus is a hard substrate formed by the interactions of salivary and crevicular calcium and phosphate salts with existing plaque. Calculus accumulates supra- and subgingivally, and calculus deposits thicken with time.[2,3,6,7] It has been demonstrated that calculus control in the absence of plaque control is cosmetic, however, calculus provides a roughened surface that enhances bacterial attachment and plaque development and chronically irritates gingival tissues. Undisturbed calculus is always covered by vital dental plaque.

Acquired dental stain (extrinsic stain) is initially stained pellicle that becomes part of the mineralized, layered laminate of pellicle, plaque, and calculus. Various nutritional, chemical, and bacterial factors affect the presence and intensity of stains. Although nonpathogenic, dental stain is an aesthetic concern to some pet owners and is often a signal to clients to ask questions about their pet's oral health.

Nutrition and Tooth Development

Although puppies and kittens are born without teeth, the nutrition that the bitch or queen receives during gestation and lactation is essential to tooth development in the offspring. Nutrients from the mother must supply the appropriate building blocks for proper development and formation of the teeth before they erupt. Following eruption, nutrient intake continues to impact development and mineralization, enamel strength, and the eruption patterns of remaining teeth. Nutrition influences bacterial composition and dental substrate accumulation. During the life of the pet, nutritional intake and dietary form impact tooth, bone, and mucosal integrity; resistance to infection; and the longevity of the tooth.[1,7]

Nutrition and Dental Health

Nutrition has the potential to influence oral tissues during development, maturation, and maintenance. While mature enamel is a static tissue, nutrition may impact its growth and maturation. The periodontal apparatus is responsible for surrounding, protecting, and supporting teeth. Negative influences involving these structures can result in tooth mobility and exfoliation.[1] Mucosa in the oral cavity has an increased turnover rate, consequently, proper nutrition is essential to maintain tissue integrity (Table 49.2).[1]

Historically, we have not heard a great deal regarding the role of nutrients in periodontal disease.

Specific nutrients that have been investigated, at least in part, include water, protein, soluble carbohydrates, fiber, minerals, and vitamins. Most commercial foods provide adequate levels of nutrients to prevent deficiency diseases provided that the food meets levels recommended by the Association of American Feed Control Officials (AAFCO) and adequate amounts are fed to meet daily energy requirements.

Key Nutritional Factors

The key nutritional factors for oral health should provide an appropriate level of plaque

Table 49.2 Overall nutrient guidelines for foods designed to prevent periodontal disease.

Nutritional Factor	Adult Dogs	Adult Cats
Protein[a]	16%–35%	30%–50%
Digestibility	>80%	>80%
Calcium[a]	0.5%–1.5%	0.5%–1.5%
Phosphorous[a]	0.4%–1.3%	0.4%–1.3%
Texture	Fiber	Fiber
Kibble Size	Increased	Increased

a) Avoid deficiency or excess

control to prevent periodontal disease and gingivitis. Proper food texture and composition can directly affect the environment of the oral cavity through:

(1) maintenance of tissue integrity,
(2) alteration of bacterial plaque metabolism,
(3) stimulation of salivary flow,
(4) cleansing of tooth and oral surfaces by appropriate physical contact,
(5) and chelation of calculus building blocks.

Calculus control is a lesser consideration as calculus control by itself has not been shown to decrease gingivitis and periodontal disease.[7] Calculus, stain, and malodor are considered cosmetic concerns.

Food Texture

The physical consistency (texture) of foods and treats has been assumed to affect the oral health of dogs and cats. Recommendations made about the effect of food texture on oral health are unsubstantiated and even untrue. Food texture can be very efficient in controlling dental plaque and eventually periodontal disease. Studies in dogs and cats have stated that feeding soft foods has increased plaque and calculus accumulation. Additionally, a higher prevalence of periodontal disease has been reported when compared with the same parameters in pets fed dry foods.[1,7] These studies are difficult to compare as different procedures were used to evaluate substrate accumulation and gingival health, and different populations of patients were studied.

Plaque accumulation may be promoted by eating soft foods. However, there is a belief that dry foods provide considerable dental cleansing, but this belief should be regarded with doubt. Canned/moist food may perform like a typical dry food in affecting plaque, stain, and calculus accumulation. Typical commercial dry dog and cat foods do not contribute to dental cleansing.[1,7] As a tooth penetrates a kibble the initial contact causes the food to shatter and crumble with contact only at the tip of the tooth surface. A food should promote chewing and maximize contact with the tooth surface for effective mechanical cleansing. Thus, foods formulated with enhanced textural characteristics promote oral health. Evidence supports foods that possess an appropriate combination of shape, size, and mechanical structure provide considerable plaque, calculus, and stain control in dogs and cats.

Protein

Protein deficiencies cause degenerative changes in the periodontium, specifically the gingivae, periodontal ligament, and alveolar bone in laboratory animals. Reported protein deficiency in dogs resulted in inflammatory and dystrophic changes in the gingivae, periodontal ligament, and alveolar bone. Fortunately, protein deficiency is not seen often in dogs and cats and thus, is not a practical consideration as a standard cause of periodontal disease.

Carbohydrates

Soluble carbohydrates (sugars) and their role in the development of tooth decay (caries) are well recognized. However, dental caries are not seen often in dogs and cats. Most commercial and homemade pet foods do usually contain large quantities of soluble carbohydrates – but in the form of starch.

Fiber

Fiber-containing foods are considered to be "nature's toothbrush" as fibrous foods are considered to:

(1) exercise the gums,
(2) promote gingival keratinization,
(3) and clean the teeth.

Fiber in foods (especially relating to texture), has been shown to alter plaque and calculus accumulation and gingival health in dogs and cats.[8,9] Certain types of fiber combined with specific manufacturing processes can affect a food's texture. The characteristics of fiber which maximize tooth contact time, such as orientation within the kibble matrix, in combination with kibble size and shape that promote chewing, are vital to achieving dental benefits. Classic dry food kibbles do not have the mechanical characteristics for dental cleansing. Simply enlarging the kibble or varying the shape of the product is also not sufficient. If effective plaque control using other measures is not sufficient, or where additional plaque control is needed, daily mechanical reduction of plaque and calculus build-up with a maintenance dental food is a reasonable alternative. One way to gauge whether the texture of a specific dog or cat food is effective in preventing accumulation of dental plaque (or calculus) is whether or not the product's label carries the Veterinary Oral Health Council (VOHC) (http://www.vohc.org) seal of acceptance, specifically stating that the product is effective in controlling plaque.

Periodontal disease in dogs and cats is common, thus, effective home care products which improve owner compliance are not only a valuable addition to an oral health care regimen but are also in the best medical interest of the pet.

Antioxidants

One factor believed to contribute to the cause of periodontal disease is oxidative stress. It has been found that dogs with severe periodontitis had gingival crevicular fluid and serum with lower overall antioxidant capacity versus dogs with gingivitis or mild periodontitis.[10] Cats and dogs can produce some antioxidants but must rely on food for others. Vitamins E and C along with selenium are considered antioxidant key nutritional factors in foods for periodontal disease as:

1) they are biologically important,
2) they act synergistically,
   a) vitamin C and selenium-containing glutathione peroxidase restore vitamin E following reaction with a free radical,
3) and their safety is well documented.

Vitamin E or α-tocopherol is the principal lipid-soluble antioxidant in plasma, erythrocytes, and tissues. Vitamin E is an extremely effective antioxidant protecting cell membrane constituent polyunsaturated fatty acids from oxidation. By scavenging lipid peroxyl radicals faster than the radicals can react with nearby fatty acids or membrane proteins, lipid oxidation is reduced.

Vitamin E levels above the requirement bestow specific biologic benefits.[7] Thus, when looking for improved antioxidant performance for oral health, the food should provide at least 400 IU/kg dry matter (DM) and at least 500 IU/kg DM of vitamin E in dog and cat foods, respectively.[11]

The most effective reducing agent accessible to cells is Vitamin C (ascorbic acid). Ascorbic acid is responsible for:

(1) regenerating oxidized vitamin E, glutathione, and flavonoids,
(2) quenching free radicals intra- and extracellularly,
(3) protecting against free radical-mediated protein inactivation,
(4) quenching free radical intermediates of carcinogen metabolism.

To coincide with recommended levels of vitamin E, and for improved antioxidant performance, foods for adult dogs and cats should contain ≥100 and 100–200 mg vitamin C/kg DM, respectively.

Minerals

A selenium-containing antioxidant enzyme which helps tissues defend against oxidative stress by catalyzing the reduction of H_2O_2 and organic hydroperoxides is glutathione-peroxidase. It also helps to regenerate vitamin E. Thus, for increased antioxidant benefits, the recommended range of selenium for dog and cat foods is 0.5–1.3 mg/kg DM.

Calcium deficiency and phosphorus excess in foods may result in secondary nutritional hyperparathyroidism and significant loss of alveolar bone. It is unlikely that dietary deficiencies in calcium and phosphorus are primary causes of periodontal disease; however, they may contribute to the progression of the disease process and exacerbate bone loss. Calcium deficiency occurs rarely in dogs and cats that consume commercial pet foods that contain calcium levels that meet AAFCO's allowances. Improperly formulated homemade foods are more likely to be deficient in calcium and is yet another reason to encourage owners to utilize a board-certified veterinary nutritionist if they want to pursue a homemade diet for their pet.

A bigger concern is the excessive levels of calcium and phosphorus present in many commercial pet foods is of concern as high levels of calcium and phosphorus have been found to increase calculus in other species. Therefore, the veterinary team should keep in mind the role that calcium and phosphorus have in calculus formation and the amount of calcium and phosphorous in the diet when recommending a specific food as part of an oral care regimen.

Sequestrants that bind salivary calcium are known as polyphosphates (e.g., hexametaphosphate (HMP)). Polyphosphates make salivary calcium unavailable for integration into the plaque biofilm and thus, unable to form calculus.[1] HMP is used as a coating on a variety of treats, dental chews, and foods. Polyphosphates are said to be released during chewing and remain in the oral cavity for longer periods. It has been shown that the addition of HMP to the surface of baked biscuit treats, rawhide chews, and dry foods results in reduced calculus accumulation.[12,13] Additionally, evidence exists to support that there are no significant differences in the accumulation of plaque or calculus in dogs fed dry foods plus HMP-coated biscuits.[1,14] Polyphosphates are not known to directly affect oral microflora populations or plaque accumulation. Veterinary teams should ensure an effective plaque control regimen is always recommended for prevention or post-therapeutic care of periodontal disease.

Zinc ascorbate, zinc gluconate, and other soluble zinc salts reportedly help control plaque accumulation as a result of their antimicrobial activity. These zinc constituents are found in a variety of oral cleansing gels, rinses, and dentifrices.[1]

Vitamins

Additionally, sufficient vitamin content can be an issue in inadequately formulated homemade foods. Vitamins that have been studied in relation to periodontal disease include A, B, C, D, and E. Deficiencies in vitamin A can result in marginal gingivitis, gingival hypoplasia, and resorption of alveolar bone. B-complex vitamin deficiencies (e.g., folic acid, niacin, pantothenic acid, and riboflavin) are correlated with gingival inflammation, epithelial necrosis, and alveolar bone resorption. Vitamin C has an important role as an antioxidant, along with playing a key role in synthesizing collagen. Human literature has reported that ascorbic acid deficiencies adversely affect periodontal tissues, including inflammation of the gingiva.[15] Serum calcium concentrations are controlled with the help of vitamin D. Deficiencies in vitamin D impact calcium homeostasis and negatively affect the gingivae, periodontal ligament, and alveolar bone. Veterinary teams need to be cognizant of the role of these vitamins in oral health, while at the same time realizing deficiencies of these vitamins are highly unlikely to occur in dogs and cats fed commercial foods that contain levels that meet AAFCO allowances.

Dental Home Care

Periodontal disease is a common, chronic infection in dogs and cats and oral health programs should be an integral component of veterinary care. The goal of periodontal therapy is to treat periodontal disease.[6,7] Successful treatment and prevention of periodontal disease in pets requires identification and elimination of exacerbating factors, professional examination and care on a regular basis, and an effective dental home care program. The veterinary team must be proactive in examining the oral cavity and discussing the findings and recommendations with pet owners.

If examination reveals a healthy mouth, the appropriate home care regimen to maintain oral health should be recommended. If examination reveals periodontal disease, appropriate periodontal therapy followed by an effective home care regimen to prevent recurrence should be recommended. It is unreasonable to expect a pet's mouth to stay healthy without appropriate plaque and tartar control between veterinary visits.

Periodontal therapy and home care recommendations rely on both the degree of oral pathology and the degree of owner compliance. To make an effective home care recommendation, veterinarians and veterinary nurses should evaluate the pet's oral pathology to frame the necessary degree of plaque control, be knowledgeable of products that provide proven, effective plaque control, understand the client's willingness and ability to provide oral hygiene and assess the pet's response to oral applications or manipulations.

Dental Home Care Product Categories

There are numerous veterinary exclusive and over-the-counter products available for pet dental care and the effectiveness as well as the evidence supporting claimed efficacy is highly variable. Dental hygiene products are typically divided into the following categories (1) mechanical plaque and calculus control, (2) chemical calculus control, (3) antimicrobial therapy, and (4) barrier agents.[16]

Mechanical plaque and tartar control refer to any means that physically disrupts the accumulation of or removes existing plaque and calculus. The most common methods include tooth brushing, the use of gauze sponges or finger cots, dietary cleansing, and chew aids. The most effective means of mechanical plaque and calculus control when applied correctly and consistently is tooth brushing. The advantages of tooth brushing include effectiveness and affordability. Disadvantages can include difficulty of application and the potential for oral trauma if misused. There are several designs of pet toothbrushes available, and the softness of the bristles combined with the handle and head design make these very desirable for use in pets. It is important to fit the appropriate head size and shape to the pet's mouth to allow for safe and effective oral cleansing. The brush stroke routinely recommended is a modified Bass technique, which involves placing the bristles at a 45° angle to the gingiva and applying gentle circular strokes beginning at the gingival sulcus and continuing coronally. The mechanical action of the brush is adequate to control plaque if used effectively and routinely. Application of flavored dentifrices, gels, or powders to the brush head may increase palatability and acceptability to the pet, as well as compensate somewhat for inadequate brushing technique. Options for the use of a toothbrush include finger cots, gauze applicators, and oral swabs. These may be tolerated better by smaller pets, or in the early phases of oral hygiene training.

Mechanical plaque control can also be provided through dietary cleansing. It is common for veterinarians to recommend a dry dog food as part of an oral care routine. Typical dry pet foods may provide some cleansing benefits, particularly in comparison to moist sticky foods; however, the dental cleansing provided is far from optimal. There are therapeutic dental foods available that effectively reduce plaque and calculus accumulation and gingival inflammation.[17] The advantages of feeding a dental diet include effectiveness, owner convenience, pet acceptance, and optimal nutrition. Dental foods should be assessed for dental efficacy as well as nutrient compatibility appropriate for the animal's life stage and health status.

A history and a nutritional history are extremely important when developing a home care plan, especially if nutrition is going to be part of that plan. It is important to find out any limitations that the pet owner may have in providing home care as this may lead to noncompliance. If an owner is not able to brush their pet's teeth, the veterinary team should consider recommending therapeutic and over-the-counter diets specifically designed to slow the accumulation of plaque and calculus. These diets work by mechanical (abrasion) and/or nonmechanical (chemical) mechanisms.[18] The "kibble" can be larger in size or have a unique texture that mechanically cleans the surface of the tooth or coats it in an "anticalculus" agent.[18,19] Many products may make this claim; however, only those that have been accepted by the VOHC have met preset standards of doing so and can make the claim. The VOHC helps veterinary teams and clients choose effective products which aid in decreasing the accumulation of plaque and/or calculus.[2,3]

The VOHC website (vohc.org) is a research-based tool for guiding clients and veterinary teams to help understand product label claims and select efficacious home care. Veterinary teams can educate and encourage pet owners to select complete and balanced foods for dental health as the lifelong nutritional products for the pet.

Dietary snack foods have long claimed dental benefits for dogs and cats. Unfortunately, most of these claims are unsubstantiated and should be regarded with skepticism. Rawhide chews have demonstrated plaque and calculus reduction when compared to plain cereal biscuits. There are also oral hygiene chews that have reported oral health benefits. Advantages of dental treatments include increased compliance and reinforcement of the human–animal bond. The disadvantages of these products may include pet acceptance, potential for gastrointestinal side-effects, cost, and dietary influences such as caloric excess and nutrient imbalances.

There are numerous chew toys available that claim oral benefits through increased chewing behavior. Most of these claims are unsubstantiated. Inappropriate use or use by aggressive chewers may cause gingival abrasions, fractured teeth, and gastrointestinal disturbances.Veterinary teams understand offering supplemental treats to pets can be an important part of the human–animal bond. However, recommending treats which support oral health is also beneficial. There are a wide variety of treats that have been accepted by the VOHC to decrease plaque and calculus accumulation. Again, it is important for veterinary teams to be familiar with the efficacy of certain treats to aid in making a proper recommendation. Teams should recommend treats that are beneficial to the dental health of a pet, not detrimental. Some treats may be popular but have the potential to do more harm than good. In fact, the AAHA Dental Guidelines Task Force believes that there is no justification for offering hard treats (antlers, synthetic, or natural bones) as these could damage the structural integrity of the tooth, resulting in unnecessary pain and infection for the pet.[18] Chemical agents used for calculus control refer primarily to polyphosphate compounds such as hexametaphosphate and pyrophosphate.[20] These agents act as calcium chelators, binding calcium and decreasing mineralization of plaque into calculus. The purported benefits of polyphosphates are that they are released during chewing and remain for prolonged periods of time in the oral cavity. It has been demonstrated that the addition of hexametaphosphate to the surface of baked biscuit treats, rawhide chews, and dry foods results in reduced calculus accumulation. Polyphosphates have no known direct effect on oral microflora populations or plaque accumulation and an effective plaque control regimen should always be the primary recommendation for prevention or post-therapeutic care of periodontal disease.

Chemical means of plaque control may be applied alone or in conjunction with mechanical procedures. Antimicrobial agents are available for use in veterinary dentistry either topically or systemically. Chlorhexidine is a very effective plaque antimicrobial agent.[21] It has broad-spectrum activity and binds to oral tissues providing some residual antibacterial activity. The effectiveness and safety of chlorhexidine has been well-documented. Potential disadvantages include staining of the teeth and tongue, unpleasant taste, cost, and the potential to increase calculus formation. Chlorhexidine digluconate formulation at 0.1–0.2% is recommended. Fluoride has been reported to decrease tooth hypersensitivity and inhibit bacterial growth and metabolism and is often applied following professional prophylaxis or therapy. Fluoride is potentially toxic and should not be used indiscriminately. Other products available that have reported antiplaque activity include zinc ascorbate and zinc chlorhexidine solutions. Zinc has been demonstrated to exhibit some antiplaque properties and zinc and vitamin C have been associated with wound healing. There are products available that combine anti-microbial and calcium-chelating agents. Caution should be exercised when combining products to avoid negation or potentiation of effects. Augmentation of the salivary peroxidase system is reportedly provided by application of a hydrogen peroxide-producing formula and additional enzymes, glucose oxidase and lactoperoxidase. Systemic antibiotic therapy should not be used indiscriminately but may be appropriate in animals with moderate to severe periodontitis, concurrent systemic disease, or compromise, or in geriatric patients.[7,14]

Another category of plaque and calculus control in pets is the use of a barrier method or dental sealant. Following periodontal therapy, an odorless, tasteless invisible barrier sealant is applied by the veterinarian along the gingival margins of the buccal surface of the dental arcade and is then continued by the animal owner at home on a weekly basis. The inert polymer forms a physical bond to the tooth enamel and creates a barrier that repels attachment of bacterial plaque.

Many oral hygiene aids have varying degrees or claim varying degrees of plaque and calculus control. Caution should be utilized when extrapolating results to individual patients. It is important for the healthcare team to evaluate the evidence that supports the product's efficacy and the product effectiveness. Products that demonstrate efficacy under ideal conditions, for example in a research colony setting, may demonstrate variable effectiveness in the home environment. For example, effectiveness of a dental treatment may vary if the client feeds less than the number of treats tested to deliver the claimed efficacy. An understanding of the product, the evidence that supports the product claims, and the expected client application will support a successful outcome.[14]

Pet Owner Education and Compliance

Dental home care begins with the education of the pet owner on the pathophysiology of periodontal disease in addition to discussing the degree of plaque control appropriate for maintenance of oral health in their pet. Most clients are aware of the importance of oral hygiene for themselves, and this awareness can be utilized to discuss the importance of oral hygiene for their pets. Demonstrating the degree of oral disease present in the pet also effectively stresses the importance of oral care. Discussing oral health as part of systemic health and detailing the client about potential infection to other organ systems reinforces the significance of oral hygiene.

Owner compliance is critical to determining the type of periodontal therapy applied as well as the home care recommendations. Owner compliance is a function of both owner commitment and capability. Some pet owners may lack the commitment required to provide effective plaque control to their pet; some pets may not tolerate oral manipulation. It may take consistent training and handling over time to acclimate a pet to an oral hygiene routine. The client should be instructed in techniques to condition their pet to accept oral manipulations and applications of oral hygiene tools or materials. Another consideration which may affect owner compliance is the lack of ability of the client to apply effective oral hygiene due to lifestyle demands or lack of manual dexterity. Thus, it may be necessary for the pet to be brought to the clinic for routine plaque control by a veterinary team member although this may be inconvenient for some clients. The healthcare team should combine their knowledge of the pet's oral condition and degree of periodontal therapy with an understanding of the level of owner and pet compliance when recommending appropriate home care. Long-term success is largely dependent upon the degree of plaque control administered by the pet owner between professional visits.

Training the pet to accept oral hygiene is best started at a young age. Handling the mouth, introducing a brushing device and application of oral hygiene products should be a routine part of puppy and kitten training. Adult animals may be more difficult to train, however, with consistent behavior modification and positive reinforcement; most pets will learn to tolerate oral manipulations and application of oral hygiene. The training should begin with the animal and the owner in a relaxed and comfortable atmosphere. The owner should begin by simply handling the pet's head and mouth, stroking, and lifting the lips. When the animal is accustomed to oral manipulations the owner can proceed to rubbing the teeth and gingivae with gauze, finger cots, sponge, or cotton-tipped applicators. Following acceptance of these procedures, the use of a pet toothbrush may be introduced. Caution should be used when cleansing the caudal premolar and molar areas to avoid injury to the owner and to the pet. Lingual manipulations

should only be done on very compliant pets as the risk to the owner and the pet, as well as increased avoidance behaviors by the pet are greater.

There are no definitive constraints dictating which method or combination of methods of plaque control is appropriate for all pets. There are a wide variety of oral hygiene aids and the veterinarian and technician should be familiar with their actions and utilize his or her knowledge of the client and the pet to recommend safe and appropriate home care. Remember, a convenient method of recognizing effective products is through identification of the VOHC seal of acceptance. As stated earlier, the VOHC recognizes products with proven efficacy for mechanical control of plaque and/or mechanical and/or chemical control of calculus through a data review system.[2,3,7]

The following basic guidelines are provided for reference and may be used as a starting point to customize home care procedures. In dogs and cats with healthy gingivae or gingivitis, initiation of routine tooth brushing combined with dietary cleansing is appropriate. The rate of brushing necessary for adequate plaque control may vary from daily to weekly depending on the individual animal and the skill of the client. Application of a flavored toothpaste may improve acceptance and concurrent use of a chemical gel or toothpaste may enhance plaque control. Feeding a daily dental diet is an excellent adjunct therapy to reduce plaque accumulation and provides those clients who do not comply with tooth brushing an effective and convenient means of oral hygiene for their pets. The addition of daily dental treats may provide a benefit but should not exceed 10% of the daily energy requirement to avoid caloric excess and nutrient imbalance. Chew toys and devices provide minimal efficacy and have the potential to cause oral trauma. Caution must be taken in using the correct device appropriate for the age, size, and chewing behavior of the pet. Aggressive chewers may demolish a chew toy within minutes while other pets may ignore the toy altogether.

Dogs and cats with severe gingivitis and periodontitis need more vigorous plaque control (following appropriate periodontal therapy) to prevent disease progression. Chemical plaque control agents are very beneficial in pets with moderate to severe periodontitis. Additionally, depending on the extent of oral pathology and periodontal therapy some animals may exhibit oral discomfort following treatment. The use of chemical agents applied gently through swabbing or spraying for several days following therapy will help control plaque accumulation and aid in the healing process. Typically, chemical agents are used for short time periods and then replaced with mechanical control agents for longer-term plaque control.

Regardless of the type of dental home care the veterinary team recommends, plaque control will only be successful if applied effectively by the client and accepted by the pet. It is imperative that healthcare team members be informed about the benefits and the disadvantages of oral hygiene products. The goals of dental home care include control of supragingival plaque consistent with maintenance of periodontal health, prevention of disease progression, and maintenance of oral health between professional visits. When making a home care recommendation, both the owner and the pet must be considered. Idealistic oral hygiene procedures may not be realistic for every case and appropriate home care should be customized to fit the degree of oral pathology and the level of owner compliance.

References

1 Logan EI. Dietary Influences on Periodontal Health in Dogs and Cats. *Vet Clinics of North America*: Dietary Management and Nutrition, Kirk C, Bartges J, eds. 2006. Nov, 2006. **36**(6): 1385–1401.

2 Burns KM (2020) The importance of dental homecare in the management of periodontal disease. *The NAVTA Journal*: December/January, 9–16.

3 Burns KM, Lowery EI (2016) Preventing periodontal disease through homecare. *The NAVTA Journal*: December/January, 40–7.

4 Harvey CE (2005) Management of periodontal disease: understanding the options. *Vet Clin Small Anim* **31**: 819–36.

5 Holmstrom SE. *Veterinary dentistry: A team approach*. 2nd ed. 2013. *Elsevier*. St. Louis.

6 Gorrell C (2013) *Veterinary Dentistry for the General Practitioner* (2nd ed), New York: Saunders Elsevier.

7 Logan EI, Wiggs RB, et al. 2010. Periodontal disease. In: Hand MS, Thatcher CD, Remillard RL, Roudebush P, Novotny B. eds. *Small Animal Clinical Nutrition, 5th ed.* 979–991. Mark Morris Institute, Topeka, KS.

8 Boyce EN, Logan EI (1994) Oral health assessment in dogs: study design and results. *Journal of Veterinary Dentistry* **11**: 64–74.

9 Logan EI (1996) Oral cleansing by dietary means: results of six-month studies. In *Proceedings. Companion Animal Oral Health Conference*, pp. 11–5, Lawrence, KS.

10 Pavlica Z, Petelin M, Nemec A, et al. (2004) Measurement of total antioxidant capacity in gingival crevicular fluid and serum in dogs with periodontal disease. *American Journal of Veterinary Research* **65**(11): 1584–8.

11 Jewell DE, Toll PW, Wedekind KJ, et al. (2000) Effect of increasing dietary antioxidants on concentrations of vitamin E and total alkenals in serum of dogs and cats. *Veterinary Therapeutics* **1**: 264–72.

12 Stookey GK, Warrick JM, Miller LL (1995) Sodium hexametaphosphate reduces calculus formation in dogs. *Am J Vet Res* **56**: 913–8.

13 Warrick JM, Stookey GK, Inskeep GA, et al. Reducing calculus accumulation in dogs

using an innovative rawhide treat system coated with hexametaphosphate. In: *Proc. Am. Vet. Dent. Forum*; 2001. p. 379–82.

14 Roudebush P, Logan EI, Hale FA (2005) Evidence-based veterinary dentistry: a systematic review of homecare for prevention of periodontal disease in dogs and cats. *J Vet Dent* **22**(1): 6–15.

15 Leggott PJ, Robertson PB, Rothman DL, et al. (1986) The effect of controlled ascorbic acid depletion and supplementation on periodontal health. *Journal of Periodontology* **57**(8): 480–5.

16 Burns KM (2006) Oral health in pets: home care and dietary considerations. *Veterinary Technician*: April, 2006, 224–33.

17 Logan EI, Finney O, Hefferren JJ (2002) Effects of a dental food on plaque accumulation and gingival health in dogs. *J Vet Dent* **19**: 15–8.

18 Bellows J, Berg ML, Dennis S, et al. (2019) 2019 AAHA Dental Care Guidelines for Dogs and Cats. *J Am Anim Hosp Assoc* **55**: 1–21.

19 Jensen L, Logan E, Finney O, et al. (1995) Reduction in accumulation of plaque, stain, and calculus in dogs by dietary means. *J Vet Dent* **12**(4): 161–3.

20 Stookey GK, Warrick JM, Miller LL, et al. (1996) Hexametaphosphate-coated snack biscuits significantly reduce calculus formation in dogs. *J Vet Dent* **13**: 27–30.

21 Niemiec B A. Top 5 tools & techniques for oral home care. *Clinician's Brief.* 2015. Pp. 25–27, 90.

50

Nutritional Management of Pancreatitis

One of the leading causes for which pets present to veterinary hospitals is gastrointestinal (GI) problems. However, we know the main challenge to the veterinary healthcare team presented with a pet that has GI dysfunction, is to determine whether this is an emergency or potentially serious problem versus a chronic or intermittent problem. The GI tract is known for its resiliency and the veterinary healthcare team has seen countless pets with clinical signs of acute vomiting and/or diarrhea resolve uneventfully, sometimes without any supportive care. However, this cannot be held to all acute GI events as some may be life-threatening disorders, which if not identified and treated, could lead to poor patient management and/or death of the pet.

Acute pancreatitis is an important differential diagnosis for vomiting and abdominal pain in canines. Pancreatitis is a less common diagnosis in cats because of the challenges in diagnosing pancreatitis in felines. However, over the last 20 years clinical and pathologic reports are finding an increase in the prevalence and subsequent diagnosis of pancreatitis in felines.[1,2]

The Function of the Pancreas

The pancreas' main function is to synthesize and secrete substances which allow for the proper digestion and absorption of food. These substances are digestive enzymes that break down protein, fat, and carbohydrates into their smaller, absorbable components. These enzymes are secreted as inactive zymogens and are kept separate from lysosomes in the pancreatic tissue to prevent premature activation.[1–3] Additional protection mechanisms include pancreatic trypsin inhibitors which are present in pancreatic juice and can inactivate free trypsin, along with antiproteases present in plasma (e.g., alpha-macroglobulin) which are responsible for capturing proteases that escape into circulation.

Bicarbonate is also secreted by the pancreas, to assist in reaching optimal pH in the small intestine for enzyme activity; intrinsic factor allows for the absorption of vitamin B12; and bacteriostatic substances to avoid bacterial proliferation in the small intestine.[1,4,5]

Diet has an important role in pancreatic secretion regulation.[1] A complex system involving the nervous and endocrine systems are responsible for pancreatic secretion regulation. The autonomous nervous system mediates the cephalic phase. Gastrin, a hormone released in response to gastric distention and the presence of nutrients (i.e., protein) mediates the gastric phase. The intestinal phase is mediated by hormones synthesized by the intestinal mucosa. These are known as cholecystokinin (CCK) and secretin. Secretin release is stimulated by the presence of acid in the intestine and intraluminal fatty acids. CCK secretion is stimulated by amino acids, acidic pH, and long-chain fatty acids. CCK stimulates pancreatic secretion.[1,2,5] However, it also leads to delayed gastric emptying and voiding of the

Nutrition and Disease Management for Veterinary Technicians and Nurses, Third Edition. Ann Wortinger and Kara M. Burns.
© 2024 John Wiley & Sons, Inc. Published 2024 by John Wiley & Sons, Inc.
Companion Website: www.wiley.com/go/wortinger/3e

gall bladder. The relative potency of specific nutrients to promote CCK secretion appears to be species-specific. Fatty acids, amino acids, and peptides stimulate CCK release in dogs, but intact proteins do not. Cats secrete CCK in response to long-chain triglycerides and proteins.[1,2,6] Although amino acids also stimulate CCK release, intact protein is more potent in felines.

Pancreatitis

Pancreatitis is defined as inflammation of the pancreas, and this inflammation may be acute or chronic. The difference is mainly histological, not necessarily clinical, though there is some clinical overlap between the two.[1,2] Chronic disease may present initially as an acute-on-chronic episode. Differentiating acute disease from an acute flare-up of chronic disease is not vital for initial management, as initially the cases will be managed the same.

Acute pancreatitis is observed more often in middle-aged dogs and cats, though very young and very old patients may be affected.[1,2] Breed prevalence is noted in Terrier breeds, Miniature Schauzers, and domestic short-haired cats as these tend to be at increased risk for acute pancreatitis. Even so, veterinary team members should remember that any breed or cross-breed can be affected. Breed relationships suggest an underlying genetic tendency. Pancreatitis is believed to be multifactorial with a genetic tendency and superimposed triggering factors (e.g., eating a high-fat meal may be a trigger). Obesity is believed to be a predisposing risk factor. In some feline cases, a recognized association with concurrent cholangitis, inflammatory bowel disease, or renal disease has been found. Cats with acute pancreatitis are also at high risk for hepatic lipidosis.[2,3,6]

History and Physical Examination

Reportedly, 90% of dogs with pancreatitis present to the hospital with acute vomiting.

Vomiting may be sporadic and mild or very severe.[7] Other clinical signs include abdominal pain, depression, anorexia, fever, and diarrhea. Icterus and pale-colored stools may be reported if pancreatic inflammation and edema are severe enough to result in common bile duct obstruction.[5–7] If present, diarrhea is usually of large bowel origin because the transverse colon passes dorsal to the pancreas and is susceptible to local inflammation at that site. Often, an episode of dietary indiscretion has occurred during the 24 hours prior to the onset of vomiting. The owner commonly relates consumption of high-fat human food. Occasionally, the onset of clinical signs is preceded by administration of drugs associated with pancreatitis. Corticosteroids have been linked to pancreatitis in dogs. Cats with pancreatitis have highly variable clinical signs. Cats may present similarly to the canine presentation – acute vomiting, lethargy, anorexia, diarrhea, and abdominal pain. However, in milder but more prolonged cases the presentation is more of a slow, smoldering course. The most common clinical signs in cats are anorexia, lethargy, dehydration, and weight loss.

A complete history is the first step, and a very crucial step, in trying to establish a cause for vomiting and diarrhea.[1,7,8] The signalment and history, as well as a description of the vomiting episodes, are important. First, one must determine whether the animal truly is vomiting. The healthcare team should differentiate the owner's report of vomiting from gagging, coughing, dysphagia, or regurgitation. The description of retching is characteristic of vomiting. Signalment may also be helpful. For example, young, unvaccinated pets are more susceptible to infectious diseases, such as parvovirus. Vaccination status, travel history, previous medical problems, and medication history should be determined. Many drugs can result in vomiting, such as nonsteroidal anti-inflammatory drugs (NSAIDs), which are known to cause GI ulceration and vomiting. The healthcare team member should also explore the possibility of toxin or foreign body ingestion and other concurrent signs that often arise with systemic or metabolic disease.[1,7,8] An example: polydipsia, polyuria, and weight loss are typical of vomiting associated with diabetic ketoacidosis or chronic kidney failure.

The history should then focus on the actual vomiting episodes. The duration, frequency, and relationship of the episodes to eating or drinking should be ascertained. A complete physical description of the vomited material should be documented. A dietary history, including the type of diet or recent dietary changes, is important because vomiting may be associated with an adverse reaction to food. Vomiting of an undigested or a partly digested meal more than 6–8 hours after eating, a time at which the stomach should normally be empty, suggests a gastric outflow obstruction or gastric hypomotility disorder.[1,2] The description of the vomit should include the volume, color, consistency, odor, and the presence or absence of bile or blood. Undigested food suggests a gastric origin, whereas vomit-containing bile makes a gastric outflow obstruction unlikely.[1] Vomit having a fecal odor is suggestive of a low-intestinal obstruction or bacterial overgrowth in the small intestine.[4,6] Hematemesis, (either as fresh, bright-red blood or as digested blood with the appearance of coffee grounds), is indicative of GI erosion or ulceration. Gastric ulceration is caused by metabolic conditions such as hypoadrenocorticism, reaction to certain drugs, clotting abnormalities, gastritis, or neoplasia.

When performing a physical examination, the pancreatitis patients' findings typically include depression, fever, dehydration, and a stance indicative of abdominal pain.[7] Typically, the stance involves the patient in what appears to be a "downward dog" position – the cranial portion is "down" and the caudal portion "up." This is indicative of the patient trying to find a body position that is less painful. Palpation of the abdomen may produce splinting and discomfort which is localized to the right cranial quadrant. Veterinary healthcare team members must be watching for icterus, shock, and coagulopathies, especially in more severe cases.[7] Chronic pancreatitis may result in variable clinical signs. Felines may be limited in the signs they present with, and weight loss and poor body condition may be the only signs.

The laboratory diagnosis of acute and chronic pancreatitis can be very frustrating. Histopathology is considered the gold standard when diagnosing acute and chronic pancreatitis. However, pancreatic biopsies are rarely performed because the procedure is invasive and many patients with pancreatitis are poor anesthetic risks.[1-3] However, laparoscopic techniques for the diagnosis of pancreatic disease in dogs and cats may be a viable alternative as these provide a minimally invasive method for collection of pancreatic biopsy specimens.[5] One of the downsides to laparoscopy is the lack of good visualization of the entire pancreas, which may result in failure to biopsy affected areas of the organ.

Nutritional Evaluation

Every animal that presents to the hospital, every time they present, should be assessed to establish nutritional needs and feeding goals, which depend on the pets physiology and/or disease condition. The role of the veterinary technician is to establish patient history, score the patient's body condition, work with the veterinarian to determine the proper nutritional recommendation for the patient, and communicate this information to the pet owner.

A nutritional history should be taken to determine the quality and adequacy of the food being fed to the pet, the feeding protocol (e.g., whether the pet is fed at designated meals or has free choice, the amount of food given, the family member responsible for feeding the pet), and the type or types of food given to the pet. The technician should ask the owner open-ended questions.[8] This type of questioning helps to uncover more information, as it gets the owner talking; closed-ended questions typically end in a one-word answer thus potentially not uncovering everything the patient eats in a day. It also has the potential to put the pet owner on the defensive, thus sabotaging any relationship veterinary technicians are trying to build with the pet owner – especially when it comes to nutrition.

Nutritional history questions to ask owners:

- Tell me what your pet eats over the course of a day?
- Tell me what other pets and what other family members are in the household?
  - Tell me about your pet's appetite?
  - Tell me about any changes in elimination habits?
- Tell me about any supplements your pet receives?
- Tell me about any medications your pet receives?
- Tell me anything you believe your pet could have obtained without you witnessing it.

The veterinary team member should also ask the owner about the pet's access to foods, supplements, and medications and how much of each the pet consumes each day. Pets also may be fed by more than one family member or receive numerous treats throughout the day. All these factors play a role in proper nutrition of pets.

All members of the health care team should be familiar with taking a nutritional history. Through this mechanism, the team can pinpoint a breakdown in owner compliance (e.g., is more than one person in the household feeding the pet, is the pet getting more calories than is being recommended, etc.) and begin to establish a feeding protocol to insure the pet's proper calorie consumption.

Key Nutritional Factors

Following the veterinarian's diagnosis of pancreatitis, the vomiting and/or diarrhea signs along with the condition of pancreatitis overall, will need to be managed. The healthcare team should be knowledgeable of key nutritional factors and their impact when managing a patient nutritionally.[8] This management of pancreatitis should consider the following nutritional factors:

Begin feeding sooner – Enteral nutrition is the most potent stimulator of intestinal mucosal regeneration. In addition, enteral nutrition may decrease cytokine production, modulate the acute phase response, decrease catabolism, and preserve protein. Experimental models of pancreatitis in dogs have shown the benefit of early enteral nutrition compared with parenteral nutrition in decreasing bacterial translocation and downregulating the severity of inflammation.[1,8] More recent studies in people also suggest that gastric feeding (rather than jejunal) is well tolerated and safe, with no exacerbation of pain. The addition of antiemetics should also aid in instituting enteral feeding as soon as possible.

Water – Water is extremely important when working with patients with acute vomiting and pancreatitis due to the potential for life-threatening dehydration from excess fluid loss and inability of the patient to replace the lost fluid. Patients with persistent nausea and vomiting should be supported with subcutaneous or intravenous rather than oral fluids. Where applicable, moderate to severe dehydration should be corrected with appropriate parenteral fluid therapy.

Electrolytes – Gastric and intestinal secretions differ from extracellular fluids in electrolyte composition, so their loss can result in systemic electrolyte abnormalities. Dogs and cats presenting with vomiting and diarrhea may have abnormal serum potassium, chloride, and sodium concentrations. Serum electrolyte concentrations are useful in tailoring appropriate fluid therapy and nutritional management of these patients. Mild hypokalemia, hypochloremia, and either hypernatremia or hyponatremia are the electrolyte abnormalities most associated with acute vomiting (and diarrhea). Initially, electrolyte disorders should be addressed and corrected with appropriate parenteral fluid and electrolyte therapy. Patients experiencing vomiting and/or diarrhea should begin nutritional therapy ideally containing levels of potassium, chloride, and sodium above the minimum allowances for normal dogs and cats. Recommended levels of these nutrients are 0.8–1.1% potassium (dry matter [DM]), 0.5–1.3% DM chloride, and 0.3–0.5% DM sodium).[1,8]

Digestibility – In managing pancreatitis nutritionally, it is recommended that the diet be highly digestible or ≥85% digestible on a DMB.

Protein – Nutritional therapy for patients with pancreatitis should provide protein at levels of 15–30% DM for dogs and 30–40% DM for cats. In the duodenum, free amino acids (i.e., phenylalanine, tryptophan, and valine) are a strong stimulus for pancreatic secretion – even more than fat.[1,8] Excess dietary protein should be avoided while providing adequate protein for recovery and tissue repair.

Fat – The generalized use of terms such as "low-fat" or "high-fat" is confusing to healthcare team members and clients alike, because there is no established definition of what is a "normal" dietary fat level. This problem is further compounded by the varying ways in which it is possible to express the amount of fat in a diet. The most common expressions are in percentage as is or as fed, percentage of DM, and percentage of metabolizable energy (ME).[1,8] Ideally, the percentage of the ME is the best way to compare foods, as this allows for comparison between foods with varying amounts' of moisture and fiber. It is important to remember that the term "low fat" is relative to the patient's original diet. This is especially important in animals with hyperlipidemia, where fat restriction must be made relative to the current diet that is causing problems. Thus the importance of obtaining a nutritional history.

Solids and liquids higher in fat empty more slowly from the stomach than comparable foods with less fat. Fat in the duodenum stimulates the release of CCK, which delays gastric emptying. Foods with less than 15% DM fat for dogs and less than 25% DM fat for cats are appropriate for dietary management. Obese and hypertriglyceridemic patients recovering from pancreatitis should receive low-fat foods (≤10 and ≤15% DM for dog and cat foods, respectively).[1,8] This will help to reduce fasting serum triglycerides.

Fiber – Foods containing gel-forming soluble fibers should be avoided in vomiting and/or diarrhea patients as these fibers increase the viscosity of ingesta and slow gastric emptying. These fibers include pectins and gums (e.g., gum arabic, guar gum, carrageenan, psyllium gum, xanthan gum, carob gum, gum ghatti, and gum tragacanth). Overall, the crude fiber content should not exceed more than 5% DM.[1,8] Prebiotic fibers such as beet pulp and flax seed help to restore the balance of bacteria in the gut.

Food Form and Temperature – Moist foods are the best form since they reduce gastric retention time. For the same reason, the veterinary healthcare team should educate clients to warm foods between room and body temperature (70–100 °F [21–38 °C]).

Additional Nutritional Factors in Pancreatitis

Ginger – Ginger has been associated with a reduction in nausea and vomiting. The University of Maryland Medical Center website has information discussing ginger and its relation to less vomiting related to motion sickness in humans and may reduce the severity and duration of nausea during chemotherapy (in human patients).[8] The UMMC website also reports preliminary studies suggesting that ginger may lower cholesterol and help prevent blood from clotting. Ginger in nutritional management of canine patients is aimed at soothing and calming the GI tract of these patients.

Omega-3 fatty acids – Omega-3 fatty acids provide the benefit of helping to break the cycle of inflammation associated with pancreatitis.

GI signs are known to be a major reason for which owners bring their pets to the hospital. It is essential for veterinary technicians to identify these clinical signs perform a complete history and evaluation regarding these signs and assist the veterinarian in their diagnosis of pancreatitis based on these signs.

Nutritional management is a crucial part of therapy in the management of pancreatitis. Certain key nutritional factors play a role in managing vomiting and diarrhea in cats and dogs – through enteral and parenteral nutrition – and veterinary technicians should recognize the circumstances and reasoning for the KNFs to ensure a positive outcome for the pancreatitis patient.

References

1 Davenport, D.J., Remilliard, R.L., and Simpson, K.W. (2010). Acute and chronic pancreatitis. In: *Small Animal Clinical Nutrition*, 5the (ed. M.S. Hand, C.D. Thatcher, R.L. Remilliard, et al.), 1143–1153. Topeka, KS: MMI.

2 Hall, E.J. and German, A.J. (2010). Diseases of the small intestine. In: *Textbook of Veterinary Internal Medicine*, 7the (ed. S.J. Ettinger and E.C. Feldman), 1526–1572. St. Loius, MO: Elsevier.

3 Burns, K.M. (2012). Gastrointestinal disorders. In: *Internal Medicine for Veterinary Technicians Wiley-Blackwell* (ed. L. Merrill). 193–261. IA: Ames.

4 Willard, M.D. (2009). Disorders of the Intestinal Tract. In: *Small Animal Internal Medicine*, 4the (eds. R.W. Nelson and C.G. Coumo), 441–476. Mosby: St. Louis, MO.

5 Tams, T.R. (2003). Chronic diseases of the small intestine. In: *Handbook of Small Animal Gastroenterology*, 2nde (ed. T.R. Tams), 211–250. St. Louis, MO: Saunders.

6 Allenspach, K. and Gaschein, F.P. (2008). Small intestinal disease. In: *Small Animal Gastroenterology* (ed. J.M. Steiner), 187–202. Germany: Schlutersche.

7 Burns, K.M. and Poulin, R. (2019). Key nutritional factors in treating pancreatitis. *Today's Veterinary Nurse*, Winter. 10–12.

8 Washabau, R.J. (2013). Pancreas. In: *Canine & Feline Gastroenterology* (ed. R.J. Washabau and M.J. Day), 799–848. St. Louis: Elsevier.

51

Nutrition in Pancreatic Insufficiency

As veterinary healthcare team members, it is important to have an understanding of nutrition and how it relates to and helps in disease management. After all, nutrition is one area of veterinary medicine that affects every pet that comes into the hospital. When the veterinary team is faced with managing a patient suffering from exocrine pancreatic insufficiency (EPI), nutrition overall and certain nutrients specifically, and aid in managing this disease.

Malassimilation occurs when nutrients fail to cross the intestinal wall and the body is unable to maintain weight or ideal body condition, often resulting in patient suffering.[1] The cause may be a result of either maldigestive or malabsorptive diseases. Malabsorption takes place in diseases which alter the structure and function of the mucosa in the small intestinal including the lymphatics. Maldigestion occurs with defects in intraluminal digestion and may result from gastric, pancreatic, or biliary dysfunction. EPI refers to a partial or complete deficiency of pancreatic enzymes. A lack of pancreatic enzymes results in a presumptive diagnosis of EPI. Unlike pancreatitis, EPI is diagnosed on the basis of clinical signs and pancreatic function tests and not primarily the results of pancreatic histopathology, although finding a discernable reduction in pancreatic acinar mass on histology supports a diagnosis of EPI. The pancreas is the only significant source of lipase, so fat maldigestion manifesting as steatorrhea and weight loss is seen.[2]

Pancreatic Acinar Atrophy

In dogs, the principal cause of EPI is understood to be pancreatic acinar atrophy (PAA). Overall, EPI occurs due to a lack of functional pancreatic acinar cells, which in turn may be the result of acinar atrophy or damage from chronic pancreatic inflammation (i.e., chronic pancreatitis).[2–5]

PAA is particularly recognized in young German Shepherd Dogs, in which an autosomal mode of inheritance has been suggested, although a recent study refutes this and suggests that the inheritance is more complex.[6] PAA has also been described in Rough Collies, suspected in English Setters, and sporadically reported in other breeds. Histologic studies in German Shepherd Dogs are suggestive of PAA being an autoimmune disease directed against the acini.[7] Consequently, the islets are spared; thus, dogs with PAA are not usually diabetic. However, affected dogs do not respond to immunosuppressive therapy. The majority of dogs develop the disease during early adulthood. However, some German Shepherd Dogs remain subclinical for a prolonged period and present later in life. Other less common possible causes of EPI in dogs include pancreatic hypoplasia and pancreatic neoplasia. The true incidence and prevalence remain unknown. Approximately 42% of all affected dogs are German shepherds.[3,4]

Nutrition and Disease Management for Veterinary Technicians and Nurses, Third Edition. Ann Wortinger and Kara M. Burns.
© 2024 John Wiley & Sons, Inc. Published 2024 by John Wiley & Sons, Inc.
Companion Website: www.wiley.com/go/wortinger/3e

Exocrine Pancreatic Insufficiency

PAA has not been documented in cats. EPI has traditionally been considered an uncommon disorder in cats with end-stage pancreatitis thought to be the most common cause of EPI in felines.[1,2,8]

The progress of clinical EPI requires approximately a 90% reduction in lipase production and as a result extensive loss of pancreatic acini. Consequently, it is highly unlikely to occur after a severe bout of pancreatitis but rather results from chronic ongoing disease. Nevertheless, the chronic disease may be largely subclinical or only present as occasional clinical acute-on-chronic episodes, so the degree of underlying pancreatic damage may be underestimated.

Veterinary technicians must recognize that patients with an obstructed pancreatic duct or a deficiency in enteropeptidase in the small intestine, exhibit similar clinical signs and are also classified as having EPI – although they do not lack pancreatic enzymes.

Clinical Signs

It is imperative that veterinary technicians and nurses be aware of the clinical signs associated with EPI. If the pancreas is unable to provide sufficient digestive enzymes, bicarbonate, and other substances necessary for proper digestion and absorption; the result is fat, protein, and carbohydrate malassimilation. Dogs and cats with EPI present with a history of chronic small bowel diarrhea (with steatorrhea), weight loss, poor body condition, and failure to thrive. Their appetite is often ravenous, even though the patient is losing weight. Pets with EPI defecate frequently (6–10 bowel movements per day) and stools are typically voluminous, greasy, foul-smelling, and pale in color. Polyphagia, borborygmus, flatulence, pica, and coprophagia are often reported. Vomiting and polydipsia occur less commonly.[1,2,9,10]

Often, canines with EPI have small intestinal bacterial overgrowth (SIBO). This is a result of a deficiency of antibacterial factors present in pancreatic secretions, along with changes in immunity secondary to malnutrition.[1,2,11] Bacterial overgrowth adds to malnutrition in EPI through the destruction of exposed brush border enzymes. In addition, SIBO consumes unabsorbed intraluminal nutrients, thus adding to the malnutrition of the pet. Bacterial hydroxylation of fatty acids may intensify fat malabsorption thus resulting in osmotic and secretory diarrhea.

Overall, dogs and cats suffering from EPI appear normal with the exception of poor body condition (body condition score [BCS] 1/5–2/5) and poor coat quality. Cats with EPI may present having soiled fur in the perineal region.[12] Patients affected with EPI may present with chronic seborrheic skin disease as a result of deficiencies in essential fatty acids and due to the patient becoming cachexic. Veterinary healthcare team members must be mindful of this especially as EPI patients may present to dermatology specialists.[2]

Patients with pancreatic atrophy will be stunted when comparing to unaffected littermates or breed standards. Severely affected patients may have hemorrhages due to a vitamin K-deficient coagulopathy.[1,13]

Laboratory Information

A possible diagnosis of EPI is often made by the veterinarian based on signalment and patient history. Definitive diagnosis is achieved by radioimmunoassay of serum trypsin-like immunoreactivity (TLI). Low fasting TLI values (<2.5 µg/l) indicate EPI in dogs and cats.[1,14]

TLI measures serum levels of pancreatic trypsin and trypsinogen. Trypsinogen leaks out of pancreatic acini in trace amounts in healthy animals (normal canine serum TLI values = 5.0–35.0 µg/l, normal feline serum TLI values = 17.0–50.0 µg/l).[1] In EPI, PAA and fibrosis result in reduced serum TLI values.

When diagnosing EPI due to pancreatic atrophy, serum amylase, isoamylase, and lipase concentrations are not valuable.[1] These tests may be beneficial when EPI occurs concurrently with pancreatitis.[15]

EPI is confirmed by a subnormal feline trypsin-like immunoreactivity (fTLI) concentration. Values less than or equal to 8 μg/l are considered diagnostic (reference range, 12–82 μg/l).[12] The cause of feline EPI is unknown, but EPI is suspected to be secondary to chronic pancreatitis in most patients.[5]

Nutritional Management

It is important for the veterinary healthcare team to understand the role that nutrition plays in managing EPI patients. The main goals of nutritional management are as follows:

1. Provide enough energy and nutrients to maintain an ideal body condition.
2. Avoid nutrient deficiencies.
3. Minimize diarrhea.

Key Nutritional Factors

Treatment of EPI is lifelong and it involves enzyme replacement therapy,[16] typically given with every meal.[17] Pancreatic enzymes are typically provided as dried, powdered extracts of bovine or porcine pancreas. Powder extracts are thought to be more effective than tablets or capsules.[1,4,18] Tablets, capsules, and enteric-coated preparations are not recommended. Veterinary team members must account for the fact that lipase activity of pancreatic enzyme preparations fluctuates significantly. There are several commercial sources of these enzymes, although raw pancreas can also be used. Raw pancreas can be frozen in individual doses for several months without losing enzyme activity. Dogs should receive 30–90 g (1–3 oz.) of freshly thawed, chopped pancreas, whereas cats

should receive 30 g (1 oz.) of chopped pancreas per meal.[1,4] The healthcare team must remind colleagues and clients that the use of raw pancreas carries similar risks associated with feeding any raw meat. This includes the potential to spread zoonotic diseases. Make sure you educate the pet owner and document this conversation in the medical record.

Digestibility

Digestibility is a vital factor in nutritional management of EPI. It is recommended that highly digestible foods have a fat and soluble carbohydrate percentage of ≥90% and protein ≥87% and should be coupled with the addition of pancreatic enzyme preparations to the food.[1]

Highly digestible veterinary therapeutic foods contain meat and carbohydrate sources that have been highly refined to increase digestibility. Ingredients in these therapeutic commercial foods often consist of eggs, cottage cheese, and muscle and organ meats. Highly digestible carbohydrates in pet foods are predominantly starches of corn, rice, barley, and wheat – all of which are readily digested.

Fat

As mentioned, steatorrhea is the most noticeable clinical sign in EPI patients. Feeding a highly digestible food in conjunction with pancreatic enzyme supplementation is more effective than simply decreasing the fat content of the current food. Dietary fat levels for patients with EPI should be in the range of 10–15% dry matter (DM) for dogs and 15–25% DM for cats.[1]

Recently, discussion has centered on the addition of medium-chain triglycerides (MCT) to the EPI patient's food. The addition of MCTs may result in increased total fat assimilation as MCTs are more water soluble and are digested and absorbed by different mechanisms of those used in the digestion and absorption of long-chain triglycerides. One downfall is that supplementation of foods with MCT usually decreases the food's palatability. A decrease in palatability may decrease total food intake and end up being counterproductive. However, when commercial foods that contain MCTs are being used palatability issues are not typically a problem.[1,17]

Fiber

To maximize food digestibility, foods for patients with EPI should be low in fiber ($\leq$5% DM). Even lower amounts are thought to be better. In vitro, dietary fiber impairs pancreatic enzyme activity. A study in humans with EPI showed that decreasing fiber content from 4% to less than 1% reduced fecal weight and fat excretion by one-third and found reduced bloating and flatulence.[1,19] A three-week dietary trial in dogs with EPI, found mild weight loss, increased consumption of food, and increased fecal mass and defecation frequency when fed a low-fat (7% DM), high-fiber (25% DM) food in conjunction with pancreatic enzymes.[20] This is most likely attributable to the low fat and caloric content of the food as well as the effect of high fiber levels on food digestibility.

Vitamins

In patients with malassimilation, micronutrients should also be considered. The lack of pancreatic lipase in EPI results in failed solubilization and absorption of the fat-soluble vitamins A, D, E, and K. If fat absorption remains impaired, Vitamins A and D may be initially administered intramuscularly (0.5–1.0 ml divided into two intramuscular sites every three months).[1] Vitamin A and D supplementation should be given only to those pets with demonstrably low levels of Vitamin A and D, or if fat malabsorption continues, as over supplementation may be harmful.

If vitamin E serum concentrations are low, vitamin E supplementation (400–500 IU, per os, q24h) may be beneficial. Vitamin K deficiency may also occur with severe hemorrhaging the result. Parenteral supplementation of vitamin K1 is recommended (5–20 mg, q12h) in these EPI patients if coagulopathies are detected.[1]

Folate and cobalamin are also of concern in EPI patients. Dogs and cats with EPI often have low serum cobalamin concentrations.[1] Cobalamin deficiency has been linked with poor outcomes in canine EPI as well as treatment failure.[10,21] If the patient is hypocobalaminemic, weekly supplementation by subcutaneous or intramuscular routes is recommended (100–250 µg for cats; 250–1200 µg for dogs) for six weeks or until a normal serum cobalamin concentration is seen.[1,4] To avoid recurrence of hypocobalaminemia, the veterinary team must continue monitoring serum cobalamin levels in the EPI patient. Due to SIBO and bacterial elaboration of folate, in most dogs with EPI serum folate levels are elevated, except in cases of concurrent enteropathies involving the ileum.[1] If this is the case, parenteral folate supplementation (0.5–1 mg, per os q24h) is recommended until the ileal pathology is resolved.

In cats with EPI, there is a high prevalence of concurrent inflammatory bowel disease, therefore, these patients are often best managed nutritionally with a hypoallergenic intestinal type of diet.[2] A study of EPI in cats found 63% of the 16 cases had concurrent diseases. Based on the concurrent disease, the dietary choice of these patients may be affected.[10]

A thorough history, including a nutritional history, should be performed by the veterinary team. Oftentimes the feeding method has been or will need to be changed in EPI patients, thus the nutritional assessment should include open-ended questions aimed at discovering the following:

- the current feeding method
- feeding frequency
- amount fed

- texture of food (canned, dry, etc.)
- how the food is offered
- access to other food
- who feeds the pet
- what other items does the pet receive (treats, snacks, etc.)

Veterinary technicians should educate owners to feed EPI patients multiple small meals per day with pancreatic enzyme supplementation to increase digestibility. Pancreatic enzymes should be added immediately before feeding. Upon discharge, the patient should be fed at least two to three times daily at home to help avoid dietary overload and osmotic diarrhea. The daily energy requirement (DER) of underweight patients should be higher than that for healthy patients ($2 \times$ resting energy requirement for their estimated ideal weight) until ideal body weight and body condition (BCS 3/5 or 4.5/9) are reached. Certain cases may warrant continued feeding above DER in an attempt to offset the persistent degree of malabsorption even after patients reach ideal body weight. It is important to recommend a treat specifically aligned with the nutrient profile described above because we know owners will want to give treats and may sabotage the nutritional management plan by providing high-fat, high-fiber treats.

The veterinary healthcare team should be involved in the dietary management of EPI patients as nutrition is a vital factor in the management of patients with maldigestive diseases. Dietary intake should meet the patient's nutrient needs in a form that promotes nutrient absorption. The organs of the GI tract have very large reserve capacities and the small intestine has a very large and efficient absorptive area. About 90% of the pancreas must be dysfunctional before clinical signs of maldigestion are seen.[22] Consequently, patients with clinical signs of maldigestion have very little digestive capacity remaining.

References

1 Davenport, D.J., Remillard, R.L., and Simpson, K.W. (2010). Exocrine pancreatic insufficiency. In: *Small Animal Clinical Nutrition*, 5the (ed. M. Hand, R.R. Thatcher, P. Roudebush, and B. Novotny), 1135–1142. KS: M.M.I.

2 Watson, P.J. (2014). The exocrine pancreas. In: *Small Animal Internal Medicine*, 5the (ed. R.W. Nelson and C.G. Couto), 598–628. St. Louis, MO: Elsevier Mosby.

3 Parambeth, J.C. and Steiner, J. (2011). Exocrine pancreatic insufficiency in dogs. *Clinician's Brief* May 2011, 55–59.

4 Steiner, J.M. (2008). Exocrine pancreas. In: *Small Animal Gastroenterology* (ed. J.M. Steiner), 294–299. Schlütersche: Hannover, Germany.

5 Kook, P.H., Zerbe, P., and Reusch, C.E. (2011). Exocrine pancreatic insufficiency in the cat. *Schweiz Arch Tierheilkd.* **153** (1): 19–25.

6 Westermarck, E. et al. (2010). Heritability of exocrine pancreatic insufficiency in German Shepherd dogs. *Journal of Veterinary Internal Medicine* **24**: 450.

7 Wiberg, M.E. et al. (2000). Cellular and humoral immune responses in atrophic lymphocytic pancreatitis in German shepherd dogs and rough-coated collies. *Veterinary Immunology and Immunopathology* **76**: 103.

8 Twedt, D.C. (2017). Exocrine pancreatic insufficiency in cats. *Clinician's Brief* June 2027, 48–49.

9 Westermarck, E. et al. (2003). Exocrine pancreatic insufficiency in dogs. *Veterinary Clinics of North America Small Animal Practice* **33**: 1165.

10 Thompson, K.A., Parnell, N.K., Hohenhaus, A.E. et al. (2009). Feline exocrine pancreatic

insufficiency: 16 cases (1992– 2007). *Journal of Feline Medicine and Surgery* **11**: 935–940.

11 Westermarck, E., Myllys, V., and Aho, M. (1993). Effect of treatment on the jejunal and colonic bacterial flora of dogs with exocrine pancreatic insufficiency. *Pancreas* **8**: 559–562.

12 Steiner, J.M. and Williams, D.A. (2000). Serum feline trypsin-like immunoreactivity in cats with exocrine pancreatic insufficiency. *Journal of Veterinary Internal Medicine* **14** (6): 627–629.

13 Perry, L.A., Williams, D.A., and Pidgeon, G.L. (1991). Exocrine pancreatic insufficiency with associated coagulopathy in a cat. *Journal of the American Animal Hospital Association* **27**: 109–114.

14 Williams, D.A. and Batt, R.M. (1988). Sensitivity and specificity of radioimmunoassay of serum trypsin-like immunoreactivity for the diagnosis of canine exocrine pancreatic insufficiency. *Journal of the Veterinary Medical Association* **192**: 195–220.

15 Meyer, D.J. and Williams, D.A. (1992). Diagnosis of hepatic and exocrine pancreatic disorders. *Seminars in Veterinary Medicine and Surgery: Small Animal* **7**: 275–284.

16 Westermarck, E., Wiberg, M., Steiner, J. et al. (2005). Exocrine pancreatic insufficiency in dogs and cats. In: *Textbook of Veterinary Internal Medicine*, 6the, vol. **2** (ed. S.J. Ettinger and E.C. Feldman),

1492–1495. St. Louis, MO: Elsevier Saunders.

17 Villaverde, C. (2012). Nutritional management of exocrine pancreatic diseases. In: *Applied Veterinary Clinical Nutrition* (ed. A.J. Fascetti and S.J. Delaney), 221–233. Ames, IA: Wiley Blackwell.

18 Westermarck, E. (1987). Treatment of pancreatic degenerative atrophy with raw pancreas homogenate and various enzyme preparations. *Journal of the American Veterinary Medical Association* **34**: 728–733.

19 Dutta, S.K. and Hlasko, J. (1985). Dietary fiber in pancreatic disease: effect of high fiber diet on fat malabsorption in pancreatic insufficiency and in vitro study of the interaction of dietary fiber with pancreatic enzymes. *American Journal of Clinical Nutrition* **41** (3): 517–525.

20 Westermarck, E. and Wiberg, M.E. (2006). Effects of diet on clinical signs of exocrine pancreatic insufficiency in dogs. *Journal of the American Veterinary Medical Association* **228**: 225–229.

21 Batchelor, D.J. et al. (2007). Breed associations for canine exocrine pancreatic insufficiency. *Journal of Veterinary Internal Medicine* **21**: 207.

22 Jacobs, R.M., Norris, A.M., Lumsden, J.H. et al. (1989). Laboratory diagnosis of malassimilation. *Veterinary Clinics of North America: Small Animal Practice* **19**: 951–977.

52

Nutritional Management of Hyperlipidemia in Dogs and Cats

A disturbance of lipid metabolism resulting in a higher concentration of blood lipids, (especially triglycerides, cholesterol, or both) is known as hyperlipidemia and/or hyperlipoproteinemia. Hyperlipidemia is an abnormal laboratory finding in fasted patients. It is representative of either accelerated synthesis or slow degradation of lipoproteins.[1] Among dogs and cats, the most common, clinically important type of hyperlipidemia is indicated by higher concentrations of triglycerides in blood, known as hypertriglyceridemia[2,3]. Excess cholesterol in the blood is hypercholesterolemia. We hear a great deal about cholesterol in human medicine and our pet owners are acutely aware of the dangers of high cholesterol. However, unlike humans, most of the cholesterol in dogs is carried on high-density lipoproteins (HDL), the smallest lipoprotein.[4] Veterinary patients with hypercholesterolemia do not have lipemic serum – unless triglycerides are concurrently elevated. This is because HDL particles are small and subsequently do not refract the light.

Plasma and serum of affected animals usually appear milky white and turbid – or lipemic. Extreme hypertriglyceridemia may result in the serum being so lipemic that it is opaque, or lactescent.

Clinically speaking, the importance of hyperlipidemia centers around four facts:[1]

(1) Lipemic serum may interfere with quantitative analyses of other serum analytes.
(2) Hyperlipidemia is abnormal in fasted dogs or cats.

(3) Hyperlipidemic patients are at risk for developing significant clinical illness, including acute pancreatitis.
(4) Dietary management and/or specific medications may reduce or remove the morbidity associated with hyperlipidemia.

Hyperlipidemia Classification

It is important for veterinary teams to understand the classifications of hyperlipidemic states as postprandial, primary, or secondary. The most common in dogs and cats is postprandial hyperlipidemia.[5,6] Postprandial hyperlipidemia is a result of an increase in the number of circulating chylomicrons and can persist anywhere from 7 to 12 hours after a meal (depending upon the diet and amount of fat consumed).[6] Still, serum triglycerides are not expected to >500 mg/dl in a normal animal, even when a high-fat diet is consumed. Circulating chylomicrons carry only a fraction of the body's cholesterol; therefore, consuming a meal has little effect on cholesterol during the 6- to 12-hour postprandial period.

Primary causes of hyperlipidemia are either genetic or familial. In dogs, the principal form is idiopathic hyperlipidemia of Miniature Schnauzers; whereas in cats it is hyperchylomicronemia. The disease in Miniature Schnauzers is characterized by excess concentrations of circulating very-low-density lipoproteins (VLDL) with or without concurrent hyperchylomicronemia.[6–8] In cats, familial

Nutrition and Disease Management for Veterinary Technicians and Nurses, Third Edition. Ann Wortinger and Kara M. Burns.
© 2024 John Wiley & Sons, Inc. Published 2024 by John Wiley & Sons, Inc.
Companion Website: www.wiley.com/go/wortinger/3e

hyperlipidemia is a result of the production of an inactive form of lipoprotein lipase (LPL). Felines with this disease have increased fasting hyperchylomicronemia and elevations in VLDL.[1,6]

Secondary hyperlipidemia is associated with endocrine disorders such as diabetes mellitus, hypothyroidism, hyperadrenocorticism, or pancreatitis. Hypothyroidism can be found concurrently with hypertriglyceridemia and hypercholesterolemia. Hypertriglyceridemia occurs from a decrease in lipid degradation, secondary to a decline in LPL activity. Hypercholesterolemia is seen with impaired low-density lipoprotein (LDL) clearance from circulation.

Clinical Signs

The veterinary healthcare team should understand that signs associated with hyperlipidemia vary in each patient. Patients may present asymptomatically, and diagnosis is typically made on routine blood work. Usually, clinical signs involve the GI tract – vomiting (often intermittent), diarrhea, and/or abdominal discomfort.

It is prudent for veterinary teams to remember that high triglyceride levels (> 1,000 mg/dL) have also been linked with the following:[5,6]

- pancreatitis
- cutaneous xanthomas
- lipemia retinalis
- seizures
- peripheral nerve paralysis
- abnormal behavior.

Dogs with Hyperlipidemia

In canines, GI signs may present, but most often are vague and intermittent. Additionally, there may be non-localizing abdominal discomfort with some occasional pain. However, this is typically accompanied by a brief decrease in appetite. Often, the owner will report sporadic signs, lasting a few hours to a few days that may resolve spontaneously if the dog's food is withheld. Abdominal distention is occasionally reported. There appears to be no gender predilection. It is typically seen in dogs over four years of age; however, younger dogs may be affected. The prevalence of hyperlipidemia in dogs increases with age in predisposed breeds (e.g., Miniature Schnauzers and Yorkshire terriers). Additionally, it can be detected during routine health screening of at-risk patients.[8,9] Dogs may appear lethargic, and abdominal pain may accompany other signs. Often it presents as acute pancreatitis but is ruled out following abdominal radiographs, ultrasound, and laboratory results.[1]

Incidental findings of lipemia retinalis are seen on fundoscopic examination of lipemic dogs and cats. This condition manifests as pale pink retinal arterioles and venules but does not affect the patient's vision. Dogs with acute abdominal pain and vomiting should be evaluated for hyperchylomicronemia at the time of presentation and during the recovery phase when food intake is restored.

Additionally, dogs presenting with a history of seizures should be evaluated for hypertriglyceridemia. A small number of dogs (mainly Miniature Schnauzers), diagnosed with idiopathic epilepsy have been found to have elevated fasting triglyceride concentrations and lipemic serum.[1] Dietary therapy alone has been used successfully to decrease blood triglyceride levels and eliminate seizures. Incidentally, when veterinary nurses are taking a history, owners often remark that the pet's activity level increased as a result of lowering circulating triglyceride levels.

Cats with Hyperlipidemia

Clinical signs in cats with hyperlipidemia differ from those seen in dogs. The most common clinical finding in affected cats is cutaneous xanthoma – a painless, raised lesion caused by accumulation of lipid-laden macrophages or foam cells in the skin.[1] Typically, xanthomas occur over bony prominences and areas of skin exposed to prolonged pressure or direct injury. Additionally, xanthomata may be seen in organs (liver, spleen, kidney, heart, skeletal muscle, and intestines). Lipemia retinalis is more common in cats than dogs.

To confirm hypertriglyceridemia, a blood sample should be obtained following a 12-hour fast of the patient. Clear serum usually has a triglyceride concentration of less than 200 mg/dL. Serum turbidity generally begins to occur between 200 and 300 mg/dL, and lactescent serum is seen around 1,000 mg/dL.[4,6]

Management

Hyperlipidemia occurring secondary to an underlying metabolic disease often improves with correction or treatment of the problem.[4,6] However, veterinary teams must emphasize to pet owners that nutritional management of hyperlipidemia is a lifelong commitment. The current recommendation is to treat triglyceride concentrations greater than 500 mg/dL, even if no signs are present, in an attempt to prevent possible complications.[4,8] Primary hypercholesterolemia is believed to manifest in less severe signs and issues; however, it is recommended that values >750 mg/dL be treated.[5,8]

Nutritional History

Every animal that presents to the hospital should be assessed to establish nutritional needs and feeding goals, which depend on the pet's physiology and/or disease condition. The role of the veterinary technician is to ascertain patient history, score the patient's body condition, work with the veterinarian to determine the proper nutritional recommendation for the patient, and communicate this information to the pet owner.

The first step in evaluating a pet and determining its nutritional status is to obtain a complete history, including signalment (i.e., species, breed, age, gender, reproductive status, activity level, and environment). Next, a nutritional history should be taken to determine the quality and adequacy of the

food being fed to the pet, the feeding protocol (e.g., whether the pet is fed at designated meals or has free choice, the amount of food given, the family member responsible for feeding the pet), and the type or types of food given to the pet. When evaluating a pet, the veterinary technician should ask the owner the following questions in an open-ended manner:

- Tell me what your pet eats in a day.
- What brand and type of snacks or treats do you give your pet?
- Tell me what supplements are given to your pet any supplements.
- Tell me what medications your pet is taking – or has taken.
- Tell me about your pet's play behavior and toys.
- What human foods does your pet consume?
- Does your pet have access to other sources of food?

The owner should also be asked about the pet's access to foods, supplements, and medications and how much of each substance the pet consumes each day. Pets also may be fed by more than one family member or receive numerous treats throughout the day. All these factors play a role in the proper nutrition of pets.

All members of the health care team should be familiar with taking a nutritional history. Through this mechanism, the team can pinpoint a breakdown in owner compliance (e.g., is more than one person in the household feeding the pet, is the pet getting more calories than is being recommended, etc.) and begin to establish a feeding protocol to insure the pet's proper calorie consumption.

Key Nutritional Factors

Fat

It is important for veterinary team members to realize the foundation for the treatment of hypertriglyceridemia is the restriction of dietary fat. Fat of dietary origin produces chylomicrons; therefore, the amount and type of dietary fat are extremely important. A recommendation of feeding less fat than the patient is currently consuming is highly beneficial in the management of hyperlipidemia.[9] Foods comprising <12% dry matter (DM) fat are recommended. Again, a diet history is critical because it helps the veterinary team understand what degree and amount of restriction is indicated in every individual patient.

Caloric intake is very important to monitor in hyperlipidemia patients. If the patient is overweight, calorie restriction is indicated, as excess dietary energy increases VLDL production. Veterinary nurses/technicians should have an in-depth discussion surrounding what constitutes a low-fat diet. A high-fiber diet or a food marketed for weight loss does not necessarily mean that the diet is low fat. Additionally, veterinary technicians need to discuss with owners that a dry and canned product from a pet food company, does not contain the same amount of fat. The healthcare team should contact the pet food manufacturer to ascertain the fat content of the diet and educate the client regarding the exact product recommended.

Fatty Acids

It is well known that marine fish oils are abundant in omega-3 (n-3) fatty acids. N-3 fatty acids effectively decrease production of triglyceride-rich VLDL. Marine fish oils have been recommended as the first line of medical treatment for idiopathic hypertriglyceridemia in dogs. Suggested doses range from 10 to 30 mg/kg to 200 mg/kg body weight.[1] Caution should be taken in the administration of fish oil as fat and calories are increased and must be taken into account when calculating total dietary fat intake.

Vitamins

To reduce triglyceride concentrations, vitamin B3 (niacin) has been used in dogs at a dose of 25–100 mg/day.[10] It is believed to decrease fatty acid release from adipocytes and reduce the production of VLDL particles. It has been reported to reduce serum triglyceride concentrations in dogs for several months without any negative effects.[6,10]

Dietary cholesterol is derived from animal sources; therefore, feeding a diet with lower amounts of animal proteins might help reduce cholesterol concentrations. In dogs, a vegetable-protein-based diet can be fed. However, cats must have animal protein in their diet, so it is recommended to use animal protein sources which are lower in fat and thus potentially lower in cholesterol (e.g., lean fish, chicken, or pork).

Fiber

Many low-fat foods have increased levels of dietary fiber. To date, there have not been studies in animals evaluating the effects of dietary fiber type or amount on reducing serum triglyceride levels. What has been shown is that increasing dietary fiber can lower serum cholesterol levels. Additionally, primarily soluble fibers of differing types have been evaluated. Psyllium, oat bran, guar gum, and pectin are a few that effectively reduce cholesterol in people. Reports have shown cholesterol reductions with fiber range from 3 to 10%, depending on fiber type and amount.[1] Hyperlipemic patients have responded positively to dietary intervention with low-fat, high-fiber foods and substantial decreases in serum triglycerides have been observed.[1] Based on the lipid-lowering effects observed clinically when feeding a low-fat, high-fiber commercial food, and knowing the fiber content of these foods, fiber levels of at least 10% DM are recommended for dogs, and at least 7% DM are recommended for cats.

Treats

Owners will want to treat their pets, so it is best to discuss this behavior upfront. Allow for treats but educate the owner that treats should be restricted to low-fat treats. Give suggestions for using the recommended food – have them take no more than 10% of the daily feeding amount, put this aside, and give it as a treat to the pet. Additionally, offer items such as baby carrots, plain rice cakes, and salt-free nonfat pretzels.

The patient should be reevaluated in four to six weeks to monitor the success of the new, low-fat diet. If triglyceride concentrations have not decreased, a diet history should be performed to ensure the patient is receiving the recommended diet, not receiving additional food sources within the household, and is not accessing food from other sources such as neighbors. The veterinary team must reiterate the importance of disease management through nutrition and empathize with the owner surrounding the need for lifelong management.

References

1 Ford, R.B. and Ludlow, C.L. (2010). Disorders of Lipid Metabolism. In: *Small Animal Clinical Nutrition*, 5the (ed. M. Hand, C. Thatcher, R. Remillard, et al.), 545–557. Topeka, KS: Mark Morris Institute.

2 Ford, R.B. (1993). Idiopathic hyperchylomicronemia in miniature schnauzers. *Journal of Small Animal Practice* **34**: 488–492.

3 Ford, R.B. (1996). Clinical management of lipemic patients. *Compendium on Continuing Education for the Practicing Veterinarian* **18**: 1053–1065.

4 Johnson, M.C. (2005). Hyperlipidemia disorders in dogs. *Compendium on Continuing Education for the Practicing Veterinarian* **27**: 361–364.

5 Schenck, P.A. and Elliott, D.A. (2010). Dietary and medical considerations in hyperlipidemia. In: *Textbook of Veterinary Internal Medicine* (ed. S.J. Ettinger and E.C. Feldman), 710–715. St. Louis, MO: Elsevier Saunders.

6 Fascetti, A.J. and Delaney, S.J. (2012). Nutritional Management of Endocrine Diseases. In: *Applied Veterinary Clinical Nutrition* (ed. A.J. Fascetti and S.J. Delaney), 289–300. Ames, IA: Wiley Blackwell.

7 Whitney, M.S., Boon, G.D., Rebar, A.H. et al. (1996). Ultracentrifugal and electrophoretic characteristics of the plasma lipoproteins of miniature schnauzer dogs with idiopathic hyperlipoproteinemia. *Journal of Veterinary Internal Medicine* **18**: 253–260.

8 Xenoulis, P.G., Suchodolski, J.S., Levinski, M.D. et al. (2007). Investigation of hypertriglyceridemia in healthy Miniature Schnauzers. *Journal of Veterinary Internal Medicine* **21**: 1224.

9 Weeth, L.P. and Morgan, S.K. (2022). Nutritional Management of Hyperlipidemia. *Today's Veterinary Practice. March/April* 22–25.

10 Bauer, J.E. (1995). Evaluation and dietary considerations in idiopathic hyperlipidemia in dogs. *Journal of the American Veterinary Medical Association* **206**: 1684–1688.

53

Brain Aging/Cognitive Dysfunction

Veterinary medicine has seen tremendous advances in medical care and nutrition resulting in pets living longer. In the United States alone, it is estimated that ~48 million dogs are over 7 years of age and ~16 million cats are considered seniors.[1] Consequently, veterinary healthcare team members are seeing many age-related changes and disease conditions such as cancer, renal disease, and cognitive decline, in their canine patients that have been associated with aging in human patients. Cognitive decline in dogs is typically manifested as behavioral changes in one or more of the following areas: disorientation (D), altered interactions with family members (I), disruptions in sleep patterns (S), loss of housetraining (H), and decreased levels of activity(A). Many pet owners attribute behavior changes in their dogs to simply being part of the aging process and believe nothing can be done to help their beloved pet. Unfortunately, some of these behavioral changes lead to owners placing their senior pets in a shelter or electing euthanasia. The combination of these behaviors, known by the acronym DISHA, is diagnosed as cognitive dysfunction syndrome (CDS)[2], and nutrition plays a key role in helping combat this syndrome.

The veterinary healthcare team plays an important role in diagnosing behavioral changes in geriatric patients. These behavioral changes may be noticed by owners but not considered severe enough by the family to warrant a visit to the veterinarian. The effects of aging on the brain are oftentimes subtle and progress slowly; therefore, it is crucial that the healthcare team, specifically the veterinary technician, educate owners about the signs and symptoms associated with cognitive decline so these symptoms can be addressed as soon as possible. In fact, when owners were educated about the behavioral signs of DISHA, 75% stated that they had seen at least one sign. Furthermore, 37% admitted having observed one or more signs several times a week and 32% reported three or more signs. The alarming fact from this study is that only 12% actually talked to their veterinarian about a sign observed in their dog.[3] Behavioral changes may be the first indication of a physical or health problem. If a medical condition is the cause of the changes, early reporting of these changes in the pet by the owners can help lead to early diagnosis and potential medical intervention.

The acronym DISHA, as described above, is used to describe signs often seen in cognitive dysfunction. However, this is not all-inclusive as there are other clinical signs and owner observations that may be associated with brain aging. The healthcare team, especially when presented with a senior pet, should institute a cognitive impairment screening checklist as part of the routine physical examination for senior pets. A checklist, given to the pet owner upon check-in to the hospital, will allow that owner to consider whether or not their pet is exhibiting certain behaviors and is a great way to get clients thinking about their pets' behavior and imply that it may not be simply "old age behavior," but rather a disease condition

Nutrition and Disease Management for Veterinary Technicians and Nurses, Third Edition. Ann Wortinger and Kara M. Burns.
© 2024 John Wiley & Sons, Inc. Published 2024 by John Wiley & Sons, Inc.
Companion Website: www.wiley.com/go/wortinger/3e

Table 53.1 Clinical signs of brain aging.

- Going to wrong side of door
- Decreased awareness
- House-soiling
- Depression or apathy
- Vocalizing at night
- Altered sleep/wake cycle
- Not responding to previously learned commands
- Looking for increased/decreased affection from owner
- Increasing irritability
- No interest in play
- Increase or decrease in appetite
- Pacing/Restless
- Compulsive behaviors (i.e., increased licking)
- Altered relationships with people and other pets

that can be treated. This behavior checklist will also allow the healthcare team to ask more in-depth questions regarding the observations of the client. Oftentimes the client is observing signs in their pet relating to confusion, social relationships, activity level changes, depression/apathy, increased anxiety, sleep-wake cycle alterations, and learning and memory changes and deficits.[4] It is important to note if the patient is going to the wrong side of the door, vocalizing at night, not responding to previously learned commands, searching for an increase or exhibiting a decrease in the amount of affection sought with their owner, increasingly irritable, not wanting to play, having no interest in eating, pacing, and exhibiting compulsive behaviors (increased licking) not previously seen (Table 53.1). This information will assist the healthcare team in a proper diagnosis of CDS. In conjunction with the patient history, a complete physical exam, blood work, urinalysis, and imaging will help to rule out any medical conditions or disease processes that may affect the patient's mental attitude or behavior.

Aging and Its Effect on the Brain

Aging in most species studied to date is accompanied by the progressive accumulation of oxidative damage in many tissues. The brains of older dogs and the brains of older humans have several key features that have been observed. Both have a number of morphologic changes including cortical atrophy, ventricle widening, white matter myelin degeneration, accumulation of degraded proteins, damage to the DNA, and reduction of endogenous antioxidants.[5] The brain in older dogs also accumulates proteins within and around neurons and these proteins may be toxic to the neurons. The result is mitochondrial dysfunction and impaired energy metabolism in cortical neurons. Oxidative damage in older animals' brains may contribute to neuronal dysfunction and accumulation of neuropathologic lesions. The mitochondria use oxygen for normal, aerobic, energy production and one side reaction that may occur is conversion to free radicals within the mitochondria. As mitochondria age, the production of free radicals is increased and subsequently, the mitochondria are less efficient and produce less energy.[4] The brain is especially susceptible to the effects of free radicals due to its' high lipid concentration, demand for oxygen, and limited ability for antioxidant defense and repair. If neurodegenerative processes leading to cognitive dysfunction are influenced by oxidative damage then it is expected that antioxidants would improve learning and memory.

Nutritional Management of Cognitive Dysfunction Syndrome

Physiologic antioxidants act to decrease the effects of free radicals in a biological system. These antioxidants differ from those that are well-known and used as preservatives to keep food fresh. Antioxidants such as vitamins E and C help to neutralize free radicals thus preventing cellular damage. Lipoic acid and L-carnitine increase the efficiency of energy conversion while decreasing the production of free radicals resulting in mitochondrial health.[6] Carotenoids and flavonoids, typically found in fruits and vegetables also aid in reducing cellular damage by inactivating free radicals. Together these create a strong antioxidant bundle which helps to counter cellular alterations resulting from oxidative stress and the neuropathology that comes from aging. Additionally, fatty acids docosahexaenoic acid (DHA) and eicosapentaenoic acid (EPA) contribute to neuronal cell health and are found in the brain in high concentrations.

The addition of DHA and EPA along with the antioxidant package to a food should improve mitochondrial efficiency, decrease free radical production, and absorb free radicals thus resulting in decreased cell damage in the brains of dogs. A series of studies looked at a test food (fortified with antioxidants and mitochondrial cofactors) versus a control food (non-fortified food) to see if the test food would decrease signs of brain aging as manifested by the following: (1) cognitive abilities and (2) improved age-related changes in dogs as observed by owners in their homes. Oddity discrimination tasks (where the dogs had to choose which object was different), discrimination learning (where the dogs had to discriminate between objects, size of objects, and black and white), landmark discrimination tasks (where the dog had to use spatial information to locate objects), and in-home behavioral testing (where owners had to assess changes in their dog's behavior) were studied.[4,5] In addition, behavioral enrichment was studied in conjunction with fortified food in the landmark discrimination study.[6,7] In all studies, it was found that a food fortified with the antioxidant package described above (the test food) will delay or partially reverse age-related deterioration in learning. Environmental enrichment (exercise, novel play toys, and continued testing) was also found to be an important factor in improving the effects of brain aging in dogs and those dogs who participated in the combined group which had fortified food and environmental enrichment both as treatments found their learning ability to be the best preserved.[7]

Cognitive Dysfunction Syndrome Summary

It is necessary that the veterinary healthcare team begin to identify behavioral changes in senior dogs. Dog owners are recognizing changes in their senior dogs but are not discussing these changes with their pet's healthcare team. Utilizing a behavior checklist will open the conversation between the healthcare team and the pet owner and will help to discover certain behaviors that the owner may be seeing in their pet, but ascribe to old age. These behaviors should not be dismissed simply as "old age" especially given the fact that nutritional management has been clinically shown to increase learning ability and attentiveness to solving tasks. Also, antioxidant-fortified nutrition has led to reports of a 74% reduction in house-soiling accidents and a 61% increase in enthusiasm in greeting family members by senior dog owners feeding the antioxidant-fortified food. By pinpointing behaviors consistent with CDS, the healthcare team can provide a nutritional solution to alleviate CDS and strengthen the human–animal bond by improving the quality of life for senior dogs.

Brain Aging

The age at which a pet enters their "senior years" is variable and fluctuates depending on species and breed. Assessing a pet as they reach middle age should be performed more frequently. Additionally, these assessments should be based on breed lifespan, with an appropriate senior wellness workup.[8] The veterinary healthcare team should properly assess a pet to determine whether the feeding plan and nutritional needs of the patient. This includes a complete nutritional assessment, considering any medical conditions (e.g., renal disease, diabetes) that require nutritional modification, and making a nutritional recommendation.[9]

Continued improvements in control of infection and nutrition in recent years have resulted in a gradual increase in the average lifespan of the companion cat and dog. The maximum lifespan of any given species has remained relatively fixed; the average lifespan within a given population can be affected by genetics, health care, and nutrition.[10] It is estimated that more than 40% of the dogs and 30% of the cats in the United States are at least 6 years old, and approximately 30% of these animals are older than 11 years. While we are seeing more and more older animals, it is important to remember that old age is not a disease, and if they are otherwise healthy, old age alone will not kill any animal.[11] Around the world it has been reported that only 1 in 5 owners of older cats and 1 in 4 owners of older dogs are providing age-appropriate nutrition.[12]

Senior or Mature Adult Dogs

The senior, or geriatric, dog is approximately 7 years of age in an animal with an average life expectancy of approximately 13.5 years.[13,14] This range varies widely, however; the figure given here is for medium-sized dogs. Smaller breeds tend to have longer life spans; larger-breed dogs tend to have shorter life spans. The nutritional goals for the senior dog are similar to those for the adult dog – optimize quality of life, increase longevity, and minimize disease. As the animal reaches the age of a senior pet, bodily changes occur. The senior dog has a diminished ability to hear, see, smell, and taste. The animal may not be able to readily adapt to stress, and its organs may not function at a normal level. As animals age, their organs lose the ability to compensate. Many older dogs and cats face chronic renal disease as they age. As the disease progresses, it affects the animal's ability to eliminate waste products. It is important not to feed food that will create additional work for the kidneys or liver. The kidneys must work harder to excrete phosphorus, urea, and other metabolic waste byproducts. The goals of feeding the senior patient are to decrease protein, phosphorus, and sodium. Every animal is an individual; the feeding regimen should take into account each animal's specific needs. Some senior dogs have difficulty maintaining body weight, while others gain weight easily. It is important not to make general recommendations for a subset of animals.

Nutritional management of mature adult dogs is focused upon:

- Maintenance of optimal nutrition
- Risk factor management
- Disease management (i.e., slowing progression of certain chronic diseases)
- Improvement in the quality and length of life.

Older dogs are more susceptible to dehydration especially if they are prescribed diuretics or have chronic renal disease. Access to fresh, clean water must be discussed with pet owners and water intake should be routinely monitored.[14]

As dogs age, they become slower and less active. Thus, it may be appropriate to feed a more energy-dense food to very old dogs. Because of the potential for mature dogs to have different energy needs, energy densities in foods recommended for this age group may vary from 3.0 to 4.0 kcal/g dry matter (DM). Fat levels for the majority of mature dogs should fall between 7 and 15% DMB.[13]

Constipation is a common finding in mature dogs due to reduced water intake, limited activity, and reduced motility in the colon. Fiber helps to combat these findings and normalize the GI tract. Also, fiber added to foods for obese-prone mature dogs dilutes calories. The recommended levels of crude fiber in foods to be fed to mature dogs are at least 2% (DMB).

Healthy mature dogs should receive enough protein to ensure protein–energy malnutrition does not occur. Older pets may begin to lose muscle mass and therefore increasing protein in the diet may be warranted. However, older pets are also at increased risk for renal disease in which case higher levels of protein are not recommended. Improving protein quality, rather than increasing the amount eaten, can provide sufficient protein for the older pet. Dietary protein should not be restricted in healthy mature adult cats. Adequate protein and energy intake are needed to sustain lean body mass, protein synthesis, and immune function. For healthy mature dogs, the protein percentage is recommended to be 15–23% protein DMB.

Senior or Mature Adult Cats

Cats are considered senior at 10–12 years of age.[14,15] Once a cat turns 7, there is an increased risk of age-related diseases. At 7 the cats' nutritional needs are changing. As cats age, they become less active and may lose muscle mass or lean body mass. It is important to feed the older cat to maintain body composition and weight. Remember to discuss fresh-water with senior cat owners. Make yourself aware of the risks older cats may experience and provide food and an environment to decrease those risks, if possible. Many older cats face chronic renal disease as they age. The kidneys must work harder to excrete phosphorus, urea, and other metabolic waste byproducts. Senior cats have an increased requirement for potassium during renal disease. Feeding a food lower in protein and phosphorus but higher in potassium will help meet the nutritional needs of the feline senior renal patient. Always have fresh water available to the pet.

Nutritional management of mature adult cats should be focused on:

- Maintenance of optimal nutrition
- Risk factor management
- Disease management (i.e., slowing progression of certain chronic diseases)
- Improvement in the quality and length of life.

Older cats are more susceptible to dehydration especially if they are prescribed diuretics or have chronic renal disease. In cats, aging impairs thirst sensitivity even further than previously known for cats. Access to fresh, clean water must be discussed with pet owners and water intake should be routinely monitored.

Older pets begin to slow down and are less active. Thus, it may be appropriate to feed a more energy-dense food to senior pets. In mature cats, the energy density of foods should range from 3.5 to 4.5 kcal/g DMB.[14,15]

Fat levels for the majority of mature cats should range between 10% and 25% fat on a DMB.[15] Essential fatty acid requirements should also be met as previously discussed with adult cats.

Constipation is more common in senior pets due to reduced water intake, limited activity, and reduced motility in the colon. Fiber helps to combat these findings and normalize the GI tract. Also, fiber added to foods for obese-prone mature cats dilutes calories. The recommended levels of crude fiber in foods to be fed to mature cats ≤5% DMB.

Healthy mature adult cats should receive enough protein to ensure protein–energy malnutrition does not occur. Older pets may begin to lose muscle mass, and therefore, increasing protein in the diet may be warranted. However, older pets are also at increased risk for renal disease in which case higher levels of protein are not recommended. Improving protein quality, rather than increasing the amount eaten, can provide sufficient protein for the older pet. Dietary protein should not be restricted in healthy mature adult cats. Adequate protein and energy intake are needed to sustain lean body mass, protein synthesis, and immune function. For healthy mature cats, moderate levels of dietary protein – 30–45% DMB are recommended.

Completing a Nutritional Evaluation for Senior Pets

The following are some questions to ask the client when completing a nutritional evaluation:

- ◆ Tell me about the pet's activity level?
  - Have you noticed any changes?
- ◆ Tell me about where your pet spends his/her days and nights.
- ◆ Tell me about any changes in your pets' weight.
  - What's the percentage of change of weight?
  - What's the time frame of the change?
- ◆ How often does your body condition score your pet?
  - Tell me the latest 3 scores that you have done
- ◆ Tell me about your pets' drinking habits?
  - Is water available at all times?
  - How is it offered?
- ◆ What are your pet's exercise habits?
- ◆ Tell me what your pet eats over a 24-hour period
  - What feeding method is used?
  - Does your pet have a good appetite?
  - How much food is offered at each feeding?
  - Have you noticed any difficulties when your pet eats?
  - Tell me of any recent changes in anything your pet eats.
- ◆ What does your pet not like to eat?
- ◆ Does your pet have any adverse reactions to foods or treats?
- ◆ How is the food stored at home?
- ◆ Tell me about the treats your pet receives?
- ◆ Does your pet receive any medications?
  - Supplements
- ◆ Is the pet experiencing any vomiting or diarrhea?
- ◆ Tell me about your pet's sleeping habits
- ◆ Tell me about your pet's toileting habits

Answering these questions will help better identify problems and potential solutions in managing the senior patient, both in wellness and disease.

Scientific Tools

Cutting-edge scientific tools such as Predictive Biology have been utilized to explore the effects of nutrition on cell function. Predictive Biology looks at what is occurring at the gene level. Each gene in the body contains the code to build a specific protein. Nutrients can influence genes to produce more or less of the protein for which they code. This is known as gene expression. It has been found that younger dogs and cats have very different gene expressions than older animals. These gene expression changes affect key metabolic pathways and body functions, including oxidation, inflammation, and the immune system. The next step was to identify nutritional interventions which may positively impact the gene expression alterations in older pets. This, coupled with the scientific knowledge of taste preferences in older pets, resulted in age-appropriate nutrition for older pets which helps to counter the free radicals that lead to aging in every cell.

It is important for veterinary nurses to remember that although pets may not be showing outward signs of aging, every cell in the body does age. As pets age there is an increased risk of impact on the brain; affecting thinking, learning, memory, and social interactions. Ultimately, this may lead to behavioral changes in dogs and cats. Pet owners may notice these changes, but do not attribute the behavior alterations to aging.

References

1 Tyler, J. (2021). More than 50% of US dog and cat population at least 7 years old. Pet. *Food Processing*. https://www.petfoodprocessing.net/articles/14990-more-than-50-of-us-dog-and-cat-population-at-least-7-years-old Accessed April 2023.

2 Ruehl, W.W., Bruyette, D.S., DePaoli, A. et al. (1995). Canine cognitive dysfunction as a model for human age-related cognitive decline, dementia and Alzheimer's disease: clinical presentation, cognitive testing, pathology, and response to L-deprenyl therapy. *Progress in Brain Research* **106**: 217–225.

3 Burns, K.M. (2010). Teaching an old dog new tricks: nutritional management of cognitive dysfunction. *The NAVTA Jl* (convention issue), pp. 17–22.

4 Landsberg, G., Hunthausen, W., and Ackerman (2003). The effects of aging on behavior in senior pets. In: *Handbook of Behavior Problems of the Dog and Cat*, 2nde (ed. G. Landsberg, W. Hunthausen, and L. Ackerman), 269–304. St. Louis: Elsevier.

5 Roudebush, P., Zicker, S.C., Cotman, C.W. et al. (2005). Nutritional management of brain aging in dogs. *Journal of the American Veterinary Medical Association* **227**: 722–728.

6 Dodd, C.E., Zicker, S.C., Jewell, D.E. et al. (2003). Can a fortified food affect behavioral manifestations of age-related cognitive decline in dogs? *Veterinary Medicine* **98**: 396–408.

7 Milgram, N.W., Head, E., Zicker, S.C. et al. (2005). Learning ability in aged beagle dogs is preserved by behavioral enrichment and dietary fortification: a two-year longitudinal study. *Neurobiology of Aging* **26**: 77–90.

8 Linder, D.E. (2017). Diets for each life stage. *Clinician's Brief*, January, 2017. 77–80.

9 Cline, M.G., Burns, K.M., Coe, J.B. et al. (2021). 2021 AAHA nutrition and weight management guidelines for dogs and cats. *J Am Anim Hosp Assoc.* **57**: 153–174.

10 Case, L.P., Carey, D.P., Hirakawa, D.A., and Daristotle, L. (2000). Geriatrics. In: *Canine and Feline Nutrition*, 3rde (eds. Case, L.P., Daristotle, L., Hayek, M.G., Raasch, M.F.), 275–286. St Louis MO: Mosby.

11 Delaney, S. and Fascetti, A. (2012). Feeding the healthy dog and cat. In: *Applied Veterinary Clinical Nutrition* (ed. S. Delaney and A. Fascetti), 85–86. Ames, IA: Wiley-Blackwell.

12 Burns, K.M. (2020). Keeping pets youthful with senior nutrition. *The RVT Journal* **43**(3): 18–23.

13 Debraekeleer, J., Gross, K.L., and Zicker, S. (2010). Feeding mature adult dogs: middle aged and older. In: *Small Animal Clinical Nutrition*, 5e (ed. M.S. Hand, C.D. Thatcher, R.L. Remillard, et al.). Topeka, KS: MMI.

14 Wortinger, A. and Burns, K.M. (ed.) (2015). Feeding the healthy geriatric dog and cat. In: *Nutrition and Disease Management for Veterinary Technicians and Nurses*, 2nde. Ames, IA: Wiley Blackwell.

15 Gross, K.L., Becvarova, I., and Debraekeleer, J. (2010). Feeding mature adult cats: middle aged and older. In: *Small Animal Clinical Nutrition*, 5e (ed. M.S. Hand, C.D. Thatcher, R.L. Remillard, et al.). Topeka, KS: MMI.

54

Kidney Disease

Chronic kidney disease (CKD), aka the "silent killer," affects over one million pets every year. Kidney disease is the second most common cause of death in cats and the third most common cause of death in dogs.[1] The management of kidney disease has evolved with nutrition playing a prominent role in this management. Studies show that dietary therapy should be recommended for cats and dogs with renal insufficiency whenever the serum creatinine values exceed 2.0 mg/dl, so the veterinary healthcare team should no longer wait until the patient becomes uremic.[2,3]

CKD is a disease process wherein there is a loss of functional renal tissue/kidney damage that has existed for at least three months and is a typically progressive process or there is a reduction in glomerular filtration rate (GFR) by more than 50% versus normal, again persisting for at least three months. It has been recommended that the duration of at least three months be used as the benchmark for CKD diagnosis since renal compensatory hypertrophy and improvement in renal function may last for up to three months after the acute loss of nephrons.[4]

Prevalence

The prevalence of CKD has been estimated to be 0.5–1.0% in dogs and 1–3% in cats [5,6] and increases with age, especially in cats. As many as 30–50% of cats 15 years of age or older have CKD.[7,8] CDK is seen most often in older cats,

with a median age of nine years being reported. A rise in diagnosed kidney disease has been observed most likely due to better preventive care resulting in cats living longer. In many cases, the cause cannot be determined. The disease is irreversible, progressive, and carries a poor long-term prognosis. However, with long-term dietary and medical management the cat's quality and quantity of life can be significantly improved.

Clinical Signs

Cats and dogs with early stage kidney disease may be asymptomatic. Typically, polyuria (PU), and polydipsia (PD) may be the first indications of CKD in dogs. In cats, PU/PD is often not recognized in the early stages of CKD, due to cats' capacity to maintain their urine-concentrating ability longer. As the disease progresses this ability is lost, and cat owners notice increased thirst. With disease progression, especially in International Renal Interest Society (IRIS) stages 3 and 4, pets present with nonspecific signs, including poor body condition, weight loss, decreased appetite, lethargy, and dehydration. Other signs that may be seen are nocturia (having to urinate at night), constipation, and diarrhea. Cats may become hypertensive and develop acute blindness. The later stage of the disease may lead to seizures or coma.[1,2]

Azotemia is an excess of urea nitrogen and/or creatinine. The first ability that is lost with the failing kidney is often the kidney's

Nutrition and Disease Management for Veterinary Technicians and Nurses, Third Edition. Ann Wortinger and Kara M. Burns.
© 2024 John Wiley & Sons, Inc. Published 2024 by John Wiley & Sons, Inc.
Companion Website: www.wiley.com/go/wortinger/3e

ability to concentrate the urine. In a cat, the urine becomes both dilute and excessive when 66% of the kidney function has been lost. This change will precede the rise of metabolic waste in the blood (urea – creatinine) which occurs only when approximately 75% of the kidneys are lost. Kidney disease involves a loss of functional renal tissue due to a progressive process that is irreversible.[1]

The kidneys are responsible for maintaining fluid balance, regulating electrolyte balance, acid-base balance, and blood pressure, and maintaining the correct calcium/phosphorus balance. As kidneys fail, their function becomes impaired and the workload on the kidney is increased. Nutritional management of chronic renal failure is directed at improving kidney function and reducing the workload on the kidney. And subsequently, slowing the progression of the disease.

Staging of Chronic Kidney Disease

The IRIS has proposed that the terms chronic renal failure and chronic renal insufficiency be replaced by CKD and that a staging system be used to facilitate the management of feline and canine patients with CKD.[9]

This classification scheme is based on a three-step process:

1. Establish a diagnosis of a chronic (greater than 3 months) disease affecting the kidney.
2. Determine the stage of the disease in an euvolemic patient.
3. Substage the patient based on assessment of proteinuria and blood pressure.

IRIS splits kidney disease into four basic stages according to creatinine levels. Following these four stages are substages of each with respect to proteinuria and the presence of hypertension. IRIS recommends a urine protein creatinine ratio and a blood pressure measurement to evaluate the cat or dog for these substages.

A New Kidney Biomarker

Symmetric dimethylarginine (SDMA) is an innovative kidney function test.

SDMA is a methylated form of arginine, an amino acid. Arginine is released into the circulation during protein degradation and is excreted by the kidneys.

SDMA has three key attributes:

(1) a biomarker for kidney function,
(2) increases earlier than creatinine in dogs and cats with CKD,
(3) and specific for kidney function.

SDMA should be considered complementary to creatinine, and SDMA and creatinine both should be evaluated when assessing kidney function in dogs and cats. The overarching goals of CKD management are to: (1) control clinical signs of uremia; (2) maintain adequate fluid, electrolyte, and acid–base balance; (3) provide adequate nutrition; and (4) minimize progression of kidney disease.[10–13] Nutritional management plays a role in each goal and is the cornerstone of treatment for pets with CKD.

Nutritional Management of CKD

When addressing CKD, the goals of dietary management are to maximize the quality and quantity of life of the pet by ensuring adequate intake of energy, limiting the extent of uremia, and slowing the rate of progression of the disease.[2,14,15] Nutritional therapy is aimed at the following:

1. reduce the workload of the kidney and improve kidney function
2. slow ongoing damage to the kidney
3. reduce the accumulation of toxic waste and signs of illness
4. provide highly palatable and optimally balanced nutrition

To keep as much of the kidney functioning as possible, it is wise to intervene with nutritional therapy as early as possible. Research has shown that cats fed a maintenance food had a significantly greater number of uremic episodes compared with cats fed a therapeutic renal food. There was a significant reduction in renal-related mortality in cats fed a therapeutic renal food [2,3] and a significantly longer median survival time compared with cats that continued eating their regular food.[16] Early detection of renal disease and nutritional intervention can drastically alter the course of CKD, thus giving dogs and cats the opportunity to live longer and with a better quality of life.

Water

Kidney disease causes a progressive decline in urine concentrating ability, and maximal urine osmolality approaches that of plasma (300 mOsm/kg) (i.e., isosthenuria). Patients with CKD should have unlimited access to fresh water for free-choice consumption. If readily consumed by the patient, moist foods are preferred because their consumption generally results in increased total water intake compared with dry food consumption.[14]

Energy

Endogenous protein catabolism resulting in malnutrition and exacerbation of azotemia will occur in the CKD patient unless sufficient amounts of energy are provided. Thus, prevention of malnutrition through adequate energy and nutrient intake is critical in the management of kidney disease. The maintenance energy requirements are a good starting point to determine the amount of calories required each day. Body weight and body condition scores should be performed often to ensure proper energy and nutrient intake. Carbohydrates and fat provide the nonprotein sources of energy in the diet with fat providing approximately twice the energy per gram as compared to carbohydrates. Therefore, fat increases the energy density of the diet, which allows the patient to obtain its nutritional requirements from a smaller volume of food. Providing a smaller volume of food will help to minimize gastric distention; consequently, reducing the incidence of nausea and vomiting.[17]

Protein

Although there is ongoing discussion about the amount of protein needed to manage CKD in cats and dogs, there is consensus that avoiding excessive dietary protein intake is indicated to control clinical signs of uremia in dogs and cats with CKD. Uremic signs most often occur in stage 4 disease but may be observed earlier. Many of the extrarenal clinical and metabolic disturbances associated with uremia are direct results of the accumulated waste products derived from protein catabolism. As mentioned earlier, limiting accumulation of nitrogenous waste products, and achieving nitrogen balance through the proportional decrease of protein intake as renal function declines, is the goal of managing cats and dogs with chronic renal disease. In regard to determining how much protein to recommend for dogs and cats with CKD, all patients should be monitored for signs of protein insufficiency and nutritional management adjusted to maintain ideal body condition. Research shows a controlled protein food increases length and quality of life for dogs and cats with renal failure.[3,18] It is suggested that the protein levels in foods intended for most patients with CKD are 14–20% DMB for dogs and 28–35% DMB for cats. As CKD advances foods with less protein may be needed to control signs of uremia. Additionally, the protein should be highly digestible and of high biological value.

Phosphorus

Decreasing the intake of dietary phosphorus in dogs and cats with CKD has been shown to be beneficial in limiting phosphorus retention, hyperphosphatemia, and secondary renal hyperparathyroidism. Additional beneficial effects of limiting dietary phosphorus intake were shown to significantly prolong survival times compared with patients who were fed a higher phosphorus maintenance food.[3,16,18]

Alkalinizers and Buffers

Alkalinizers and buffers help to counteract the CKD patient's predisposition to metabolic acidosis, a common complication of kidney failure. They also help decrease muscle wasting associated with acidosis. Cats and dogs with chronic renal disease develop metabolic acidosis because of the impaired ability of the failing kidneys to excrete the daily net acid load. Plasma bicarbonate, venous blood pH, and total CO_2 are commonly decreased in cats and dogs with uremia or end-stage chronic renal disease. It is recommended to feed a diet formulated to assist the kidney disease patient with alkalinizing the blood and urine which in turn assists in minimizing acid load.

Sodium and Chloride

Controlled amounts of sodium and chloride help control clinical signs associated with sodium and fluid retention (ascites/edema) and minimize systemic and renal hypertension (primary). Currently, the recommended dietary sodium intake for CKD patients is 0.3% DMB or less for dogs and 0.4% DMB or less for cats. The minimum recommended allowances for chloride for dogs and cats are 1.5 times the recommended sodium levels.[2,14]

Potassium

Hypokalemia is frequently a complication of CKD. Inadequate potassium intake, acidifying diets, or increased urinary losses are all potential reasons for hypokalemia in CKD patients, as are vomiting and inappetence. The proper maintenance of potassium in the body also helps maintain the quality of life. Loss of potassium leads to functional changes in the kidneys, which include reduced GFR and urine concentrating ability. The recommended amounts of potassium in foods for dogs with CKD is 0.4–0.8% DMB and for cats 0.7–1.2% DMB. Oral supplementation may be indicated in cats with CD and hypokalemia.[2,14]

Omega-3 Fatty Acids

The specific dietary fatty acid content of a food may play a role in the progression of CKD by affecting: (1) renal hemodynamics, (2) platelet aggregation, (3) lipid peroxidation, (4) systemic blood pressure, (5) proliferation of glomerular mesangial cells, and (6) plasma lipid concentration. Omega-3 fatty acids (e.g., eicosapentaenoic acid [EPA] and docosahexaenoic acid [DHA]) in foods compete with arachidonic acid to alter eicosanoid production. These alterations are renoprotective. It is suggested that the range for total omega-3 fatty acid content in foods for canine and feline CKD patients is 0.4–2.5% DMB. More research is needed in regard to the omega-6: omega-3 fatty acid ratio. Until then, the recommendation is 1:1–7:1 (omega-6:omega-3 fatty acid).[2,14]

Antioxidants

Antioxidants protect cells from free radical oxidation and promote a healthy immune system. Oxidative damage can promote the progression of renal disease. Antioxidants with omega-3 fatty acids reduce renal oxidant injury. Dietary omega-3 fatty acid supplementation combined with antioxidants can further reduce renal oxidant injury.

B Vitamins

B vitamins help compensate for urinary losses due to kidney disease. B-vitamin deficiency can be caused by decreased appetite, vomiting, diarrhea, and PU. Anorexia associated with renal failure may be exacerbated by thiamin and niacin deficiency.

Soluble Fiber

Growth of bacteria is dependent upon a source of nitrogen. Although dietary protein provides some nitrogen, blood urea is the largest and most available source of nitrogen for bacterial protein synthesis in the colon. Soluble fiber encourages growth of beneficial bacteria in the colon. Urea is the major end product of protein catabolism in mammals. When blood urea diffuses into the large bowel it is broken down by bacterial ureases and used for protein synthesis. The bacterial protein is then excreted in the feces.

Transition

Transitioning to a therapeutic food can be a stressful experience for the healthcare team, the owner, and the patient. Assisting pet owners will help with the success of the transition as well as the treatment of the pet. Veterinary technicians play a vital role in ensuring a smooth transition to the recommended food. A transition can and should take as long as needed – seven days, three to four weeks, or longer – the important point to remember is that the patient needs to be on the food long-term, so it is fine to take a little longer to transition. For most pets, a seven-day transition is recommended. Start on day one feeding 75% of the original food with 25% of the new food. Feed this amount for 1–2 days. If there are any gastrointestinal issues, do not continue with the transition until the signs stop. If the signs continue, the veterinary team will need to assess the transition. If everything is going well and the pet is accepting the new food, continue with 50% of the old diet and 50% of the new diet. Continue for 1–2 days and then

finish with 25% of the old diet and 75% of the new diet for 1–2 days. On the seventh day, feed 100% of the new diet. It is important for the team to remember some pets will take longer to transition. Encourage the owner to keep with the transition, as the recommended nutrition is key in the medical management of the pet.

Palatability

If a pet is not accepting the new food, it is perfectly acceptable to recommend palatability enhancers such as: (1) warming the food (2) adding low-sodium chicken broth, or (3) adding tuna juice (tuna in water only) or clam broth. Due to the concern of concurrent hypertension recommend low salt options. Garlic is not recommended as it has been shown to cause anemia. For cats and brachycephalic dogs, feeding in a wide bowl or flat dish to prevent the whiskers from touching the side of the bowl is advised. Putting the new food and the original food in side-by-side dishes is another tip to get picky patients to eat.

Texture

Cats and dogs are very sensitive to food – the form, the odor, and the taste. The flavor and texture preferences of individual cats are often influenced by early experiences that can affect preferences throughout life. Cats familiar with a certain texture or type of food (i.e., moist, dry, and semimoist) may refuse foods with different textures. Cats do have a preference for certain "flavors" such as animal fat, protein hydrolysates (digests), meat extracts, and certain free amino acids found in animal muscle (i.e., alanine, proline, lysine, histidine, and leucine). Food temperature also plays a role in acceptance of the food by the cat. When feeding canned/moist foods, the preference is for the moist food to be at, or near, body temperature (38.5°C [101.5°F]). These factors are critical to the proper nutrition of a cat, especially if seriously ill.[19]

Taste Aversion

Dogs and Cats can also develop a learned taste aversion. Taste aversions occur when the food is associated with a negative experience. It is important to not feed a hospitalized patient the recommended food while in the hospital. When home, the pet may associate the smells of the food fed in the hospital with the experience in the hospital and be reluctant or refuse to eat it. This is especially true of CKD patients. It is recommended to avoid feeding a patient with kidney disease, during a uremic crisis, with the recommended therapeutic food. Also, the smorgasbord approach where all the available commercial therapeutic foods are given to the pet to see which they like best should be avoided.[20]

Follow Up

The final key to success is providing encouragement and support to the pet owner. Call the owner 2–3 days after starting the food to ensure the transition is going well and to answer any questions the owner may have. Call again in 2 weeks; hopefully, the transition is complete, but if it is not, this is a good time to encourage the pet owner to have patience and to provide an opportunity for questions. Call in 2 months to check in and see how things are going. These calls are a good time to remind pet owners of their next appointment and see if they need any more food or medications. Continue regular calls after the initial start of the food to ensure the cat is doing well on the food, at least every 3–6 months.

Features of Therapeutic Renal Foods

Overall, renal therapeutic foods are formulated to avoid excessive protein, phosphorus, and sodium (relative to maintenance pet foods). Other features of renal foods include increased buffering capacity to help combat metabolic acidosis and additional potassium because of the tendency toward hypokalemia in cats with CKD. Some foods contain antioxidants (vitamins E and C and β-carotene) to minimize oxidative stress, which may contribute to progression of CKD.[21,22] Many foods formulated to manage renal disease also contain increased amounts of omega-3 fatty acids, which have been shown to improve renal function and decrease mortality in dogs with kidney disease.[2,23]

Many healthcare team members have an incorrect perception that renal foods are deficient in protein; however, these foods contain more than adequate amounts of nutrients to maintain body condition of adult dogs and cats. When discussing therapeutic renal foods, it may help team members to avoid using words like "protein-restricted" because pet owners may interpret this to mean deficient or inadequate. Therapeutic renal foods do contain less protein than typical maintenance foods; however, they also have other nutrient differences (as noted above) that contribute to their beneficial effects in managing patients with kidney disease.

Summary

Nutritional management is the single most effective treatment for CKD in cats.[24] Early detection of renal disease and nutritional intervention can drastically alter the course of CKD. As a result, this gives cats the opportunity to live longer and with a better quality of life.

References

1 Chew, D.J., DiBartola, S.P., and Schenk, P.A. (2011). Chronic renal failure. In: *Canine and Feline Nephrology and Urology*, 2nde (eds. Dennis J. Chew, Stephen P. DiBartola and Patricia A. Schenck). 145–196. St. Louis: Elsevier.

2 Ograin, V. and Burns, K.M. (2017). Kidney disease and nutrition: yes, they will eat! *The NAVTA Journal Convention Issue*. 16–21.

3 Ross, S., Osborne, C., Kirk, C. et al. (2006). Clinical evaluation of dietary modification for treatment of spontaneous chronic kidney disease in cats. *Journal of the American Veterinary Medical Association* **229**: 949–957.

4 Polzin, D.J. (2010). Chronic kidney disease. In: *Textbook of Veterinary Internal Medicine*, 7the (ed. S.J. Ettinger and E.C. Feldman), 1991–2020. Saunders/Elsevier: St Louis.

5 Grauer, G. (2015). Laboratory evaluation in dogs & cats with chronic kidney disease. *Clinician's Brief* 65–69.

6 Brown, S.A. (2016). Chronic kidney disease. In: *August's Consultations in Feline Internal Medicine. St* (ed. S. Little), 457–467. Louis: Elsevier Saunders.

7 Polzin, D.J., Osborne, C.A., Adams, L.G., and Lulich, J.P. (1992). Medical management of feline chronic renal failure. In: *Kirk's Current Veterinary Therapy XI* (ed. R.W. Kirk and J.D. Bonagura), 848–853. Philadelphia: Saunders. Ross SJ, Polzin DJ, Osborne CA. Clinical progression of early chronic renal failure and implications for management. In August JR (ed): *Consultations in Feline Internal Medicine*. St Louis: Elsevier Saunders, 2005, pp 389-398.

8 Ross, S.J., Polzin, D.J., Osborne, C.A. (2005). Clinical progression of early chronic renal failure and implications for management. In: *Consultations in Feline Internal Medicine*. (ed. J.R. August), 389–398. St. Louis: Elsevier Saunders.

9 Forrester, S.D., Adams, L.G., and Allen, T.A. (2010). Chronic kidney disease. In: *Small Animal Clinical Nutrition*, 5th (ed. M.S. Hand, C.D. Thatcher, R.L. Remillard, et al.), 765–809. Mark Morris Institute: Topeka, Kansas.

10 Braff, J., Obare, E., Yerramilli, M. et al. (2014). Relationship between serum symmetric dimethylarginine concentration and glomerular filtration rate in cats. *Journal of Veterinary Internal Medicine* **28** (6): 1699–1701.

11 Hall, J.A., Yerramilli, M., Obare, E. et al. (2014). Comparison of serum concentrations of symmetric dimethylarginine and creatinine as kidney function biomarkers in cats with chronic kidney disease. *Journal of Veterinary Internal Medicine* **28** (6): 1676–1683.

12 Yerramilli, M., Yerramilli, M., Obare, E. et al. (2014). Symmetric dimethylarginine (SDMA) increases earlier than serum creatinine in dogs with chronic kidney disease (CKD). [ACVIM Abstract NU-42]. *Journal of Veterinary Internal Medicine* **28** (3): 1084–1085.

13 Hall, J.A., Yerramilli, M., Obare, E. et al. (2014). Comparison of serum concentrations of symmetric dimethylarginine and creatinine as kidney function biomarkers in healthy geriatric cats fed reduced protein foods enriched with fish oil, L-carnitine, and medium-chain triglycerides. *Veterinary Journal*. **202** (3): 588–596.

14 Polzin, D.J. (2007). 11 guidelines for conservatively treating chronic kidney disease. *Veterinary Medicine* **102**: 788–799.

15 Elliott, J. and Watson, A. (2009). Chronic kidney disease: staging and management. In: *Kirk's Current Veterinary Therapy XIV* (ed. J. Bonagura and D. Twedt), 883–892. St Louis: Saunders/Elsevier.

16 Elliott, J., Rawlings, J.M., Markwell, P.J. et al. (2000). Survival of cats with naturally occurring chronic renal failure: effect of dietary management. *Journal of Small Animal Practice* **41**: 235–242.

17 Elliott, D.A. (2012). Nutritional management of kidney disesae. In: *Applied Veterinary Clinical Nutrition* (ed. A.J. Fascetti and S.J. Delaney), 251–268. Ames, IA: Wiley-Blackwell.

18 Jacob, F., Polzin, D.J., Osborne, C.A. et al. (2002). Clinical evaluation of dietary modification for treatment of spontaneous chronic renal failure in dogs. *JAVMA* **220** (8): 1163–1170.

19 Armstrong, P.J., Gross, K.L. et al. (2010). Introduction to feeding normal cats. In: , *Small Animal Clinical Nutrition*, 5th (eds. Hand, Thatcher, Remillard, Roudebush, Novotny), 361–372. Mark Morris Institute, Topeka: Kansas.

20 Delaney, S.J. (2006). Management of anorexia in dogs and cats. In: *Veterinary Clinics Small Animal Practice: Dietary Management and Nutrition*, **36**(6): 1243–1249. St. Louis: Elsevier. doi: 10.1016/j.cvsm.2006.08.001. PMID: 17085232.

21 Yu, S., Gross, K., and Allen, T. (2006). A renal food supplemented with vitamins E, C, and ß-carotene reduces oxidative stress and improves kidney function in client-owned dogs with stages 2 or 3 kidney disease. *ECVIM Congress.*

22 Yu, S. and Paetau-Robinson, I. (2006). Dietary supplements of vitamins E and C and beta-carotene reduce oxidative stress in cats with renal insufficiency. *Veterinary Research Communications* **30**: 403–413.

23 Brown, S.A., Brown, C.A., Crowell, W.A. et al. (1998). Beneficial effects of chronic administration of dietary omega-3 polyunsaturated fatty acids in dogs with renal insufficiency. *Journal of Laboratory and Clinical Medicine* **131**: 447–455.

24 Roudebush, P., Polzin, D.J., Ross, S. et al. (2009). Therapies for feline chronic kidney disease - what's the evidence? *Journal of Feline Medicine and Surgery* **11**: 195–210.

55

Nutritional Management of Digestive Disease in Brachycephalic Dogs

Veterinary hospitals have seen a dramatic increase in the number of dogs affected by brachycephalic airway obstructive syndrome (BAOS). This increase has been seen over the past 20 years, due in large part to the popularity of brachycephalic breeds.[1] These dogs have been bred to accentuate features potential owners look for in brachycephalic breeds. However, the breeding to enhance specific brachycephalic features has had a detrimental repercussion on their health. Veterinary teams are well aware of the respiratory consequences of BAOS; however, many of the dogs also present with alimentary tract signs including[2]

- ptyalism
- excessive swallowing attempts
- regurgitation
- eructation
- vomiting
- changes in appetite.

Veterinary teams need to implement a systematic approach to characterize the nature of the problem as well as the most prudent treatment and follow-up plan.

Brachycephalic Anatomy

Brachycephalic breeds display anatomic and pathophysiologic changes owing to their wide and short skull. However, issues are most commonly reported in French bulldogs, English bulldogs, and pugs.[2] The alterations to skull shape (wide and short) are visible. However,

many also have abnormalities in soft tissue structures, including an elongated soft palate, macroglossia, stenotic nares, undersized nasal chambers, malformed and aberrantly growing nasal conchae, tracheal hypoplasia, and acquired laryngeal complications.[2,3] Common clinical signs relate to the respiratory tract:

- intolerance to exercise and heat
- frequent disruptions in sleep
- syncope.

Today, digestive signs are increasingly reported, with their severity correlating strongly with respiratory signs.[4,5] Clinical improvement and a reduction in postsurgical complications when digestive signs are treated further support the association between digestive and respiratory signs in brachycephalic dogs.[2] Additionally, even in brachycephalic dogs without any alimentary tract sign, lesions of the upper digestive tract are often endoscopically detected.

Increased negative pressure within the upper airways may be responsible for the following[2]:

- secondary respiratory abnormalities
  - everted tonsils
  - laryngeal and tracheal collapse
  - everted laryngeal saccules
- digestive tract lesions
  - hiatal hernia (HH)
  - gastroesophageal reflux.

It is important to note that recent studies highlight the fact that gastroesophageal junction abnormalities and HH have been

Nutrition and Disease Management for Veterinary Technicians and Nurses, Third Edition. Ann Wortinger and Kara M. Burns.
© 2024 John Wiley & Sons, Inc. Published 2024 by John Wiley & Sons, Inc.
Companion Website: www.wiley.com/go/wortinger/3e

underestimated in brachycephalic dogs.[6–8] Additionally, video fluoroscopic swallowing studies have documented the presence of esophageal dysmotility with prolonged esophageal transit time and gastroesophageal reflux in brachycephalic dogs.[9]

Alimentary Tract Signs

Regurgitation and vomiting are the most common digestive signs in brachycephalic dogs. Other digestive signs observed in brachycephalic dogs include the following:

- Ptyalism
- Regurgitation
- Retching
- Vomiting
- Dysphagia
- Aerophagia
- Gastroesophageal reflux
- Pica
- Pain-relieving positioning

Various grading schemes have been published for assessing brachycephalic dogs before and after surgery. These include respiratory (snoring, inspiratory efforts, exercise intolerance, and syncope) and digestive signs (ptyalism, regurgitation, and vomiting). They are graded on frequency and are scaled from 1 (mild) to 3 (marked).[4]

It should be noted that brachycephalic dogs may suffer from chronic enteropathy, with pugs affected by a particularly severe form of protein-losing enteropathy. French bulldogs and English bulldogs may be predisposed to food-responsive diarrhea and chronic flatulence.[2]

Digestive Disease

BAOS is recognized as a progressive disease, with age at presentation ranging from a few months to a few years. After 5 years of age, it is highly unlikely to see BOAS for the first time.[2] A definitive diagnosis includes history, physical examination, detailed clinicopathologic investigations, and diagnostic imaging. Endoscopy examining the upper airways and the digestive tract is also part of the diagnostic approach. The main diseases affecting the digestive system in brachycephalic dogs are as follows[2]:

- Redundant esophagus
- Esophagitis
- Gastroesophageal reflux
- Sliding HH (type 1)
- Delayed gastric emptying
- Gastritis
- Pyloric mucosal fold hypertrophy
- Pyloric stenosis
- Duodenitis

These stomach and swallowing issues correlate to respiratory obstruction. The esophagus experiences backward reflux of stomach contents. This reflux generates pain and inflammation. Intensifying this problem is retention of food in the stomach for prolonged periods. This "pooling" of food in the stomach creates a sensation of nausea and increases the potential for vomiting and/or stomach acid reflux. While this may sound like a separate issue from the respiratory disorder, the reflux, regurgitation, and even herniation of part of the stomach into the chest cavity result due to the extreme inhalation efforts made against the upper airway obstruction that comes from the shape of the brachycephalic head.

History and Physical Examination

A comprehensive history is essential to distinguish the problem, as brachycephalic breeds may present with various combinations of clinical signs. Time should be spent questioning the dog owners as they are unaware that there is a problem due to the fact that owners consider stertor, loud breathing, and regurgitation to be normal for their dog.[8] Clinical signs can be mostly respiratory, or they may involve a mix of respiratory and digestive signs. History taking should focus on ascertaining the presence of digestive signs.[3,4] Physical examination should initially include the following:

- dog's phenotype (e.g., skull dimensions and nares)
- the respiratory cycle (especially the inspiratory effort)
- listen for spontaneous respiratory noises (tachypnea)

This is followed by examination of the head and neck. Remember, it is often difficult to examine the oral cavity as brachycephalic dogs struggle to breathe with their mouth wide open. Thoracic auscultation, albeit potentially challenging due to loud referred upper respiratory tract noises, should be performed. Lastly, the rest of the body should be examined.

Detailed diagnostic investigations are usually required to accurately diagnose alimentary tract disease in brachycephalic dogs. They include clinical pathology, thoracic radiographs, fluoroscopic assessment of swallowing function, and upper airway and gastrointestinal endoscopy.

Brachycephalic dogs with digestive signs are usually medically managed. This management includes dietary modifications and pharmaceutical agents. In cases of HH which remain unresponsive to medical management, surgical management is considered.

Medical Management

Antiemetics, acid-blocking drugs, mucosal "protectants", and prokinetic agents are most often used in brachycephalic dogs with digestive disease.[2] However, it should be noted that clinical trials reviewing the efficacy of these drugs when used in brachycephalic dogs with digestive disease have not yet been performed. Acid-blocking drugs and mucosal protectants (e.g., sucralfate) are indicated with evidence of esophagitis. If there is confirmation of vomiting, antiemetics are suggested.

Nutritional Management

Nutritional management of digestive issues in brachycephalic dogs include modifications, such as the following:

- altering the type of food (e.g., wet food versus dry food)
- altering nutrients within the food (e.g., less fiber and lower fat)
- altering the food's consistency (e.g., adding water)
- meal pattern (e.g., feeding small meals more often through the day).

Modifications such as these are aimed at promoting passage of food through the digestive tract. This in turn decreases the tendency for regurgitation, vomiting, or gastroesophageal reflux.

Body Condition Score

Body condition score (BCS) is a physical assessment of body fat mass. The 9-point BCS scale is validated to correlate with body fat percentage (BF%) using dual-energy X-ray absorptiometry (DEXA).[11] Each incremental increase in the BCS is equivalent to a 5% increase in BF%, while each BCS >5/9 is equivalent to being 10% overweight. Obesity, as quantified using the BCS, is a strong risk factor for BOAS. The impact of obesity on respiratory function incorporates a decrease in minute volume with an increase in respiratory frequency, exercise intolerance, and a decrease in estimated arterial oxygen saturation.[12,13]

It is important for the veterinary team to perform BCS on every brachycephalic patient that visits the hospital and educate owners as to the importance of keeping their dog at an ideal BCS.

Key Nutritional Factors

The veterinary healthcare team should be aware of key nutrients and their impact when managing a brachycephalic patient with digestive disease. It is imperative that these key nutritional factors be understood, implemented, and communicated to the client.

Water

Water is extremely important when working with patients with digestive disease due to the potential for life-threatening dehydration from excess fluid loss and the potential inability of the patient to replace the lost fluid. The brachycephalic dog's hydration status should be monitored and supported with subcutaneous or intravenous fluids if the patient is dehydrated.

Protein

Nutritional therapy for patients exhibiting digestive disease should not provide excess protein. Products of protein digestion increase gastrin and gastric acid secretion.[10,14] Novel ingredient diets or elimination foods have been recommended. Ideal elimination foods should

(1) avoid protein excess
(2) have high protein digestibility (≥87%)
(3) contain a limited number of novel ingredient sources.

Protein quality plays a role in brachycephalic dogs, as the higher the quality the higher the digestibility. Additionally, protein quality helps decrease the fermentation products[15] and results in reduced odor and flatulence in brachycephalic dogs.

A food containing a protein hydrolysate may also be utilized in nutritional management of the brachycephalic patient with digestive disease. Hydrolysis uses water to chemically break proteins into pieces that are so small that the immune system no longer reacts to them. Hydrolyzed protein foods are recommended in dogs with digestive disease.

Fat

Solids and liquids with higher fat content empty more slowly from the stomach than comparable foods with less fat.[14] Fat in the duodenum stimulates the release of cholecystokinin, which delays gastric emptying. Foods lower in fat are recommended for brachycephalic dogs with digestive issues.

Fiber

Foods containing gel-forming soluble fibers should be avoided in dogs with digestive disease as these fibers increase the viscosity of ingesta and slow gastric emptying.[10,14] These fibers include pectins and gums (e.g., gum arabic, guar gum, and carrageenan).

Food Form and Temperature

Moist foods are considered to be the best form since moist foods reduce gastric retention time. For the same reason, the veterinary healthcare team should educate clients to warm foods to between room and body temperature (70–100 °F [21–38 °C]).

Brachycephalic Bowls

A recent suggestion to aid brachycephalic patients with digestive issues concerns the type of the bowl from which they are eating. Veterinary teams should consider discussing certain bowls for their brachycephalic patients with pet owners. Brachycephalic bowls are made at a 45° angled ledge to improve the pet's posture while eating and relieve some of the strain on the cervical vertebrae and spine in breeds that are prone to IVDD. These bowls promote chewing and slower eating, which aids in the pet's digestion. This type of bowl is said to aid in reducing bloating and obesity and aids in providing proper GI motility.[16] This bowl helps the brachycephalic dog lessen the amount of gulping and air swallowed and assists in slowing down the fast brachycephalic eater.

Other Digestive Disease Nutrition Suggestions

Larger meals empty more slowly from the stomach than smaller meals. Therefore, it is recommended to feed small meals more often throughout the day. Additionally, liquids empty more quickly from the stomach as opposed to solid foods. This is due to lower digesta osmolality.[17] Water empties most quickly, while liquids containing nutrients are emptied more slowly. High-osmolality fluids empty more slowly than dilute fluids. Solids are the slowest to be emptied from the stomach. It has been shown in pets that dry foods empty more slowly than moist foods. The ideal food form for patients with GI disorders has a liquid or semi-liquid consistency. Therefore, as mentioned above, using a different consistency of food or adding water to a dry food will help with GI motility.

Summary

Brachycephalic obstructive airway syndrome (BOAS) has increased significantly due to the popularity of brachycephalic breeds. Along with the respiratory signs, the veterinary community is witnessing an increase of signs involving the digestive tract. It is important for the veterinary team to recognize BOAS signs and the accompanying GI signs. Recognition and understanding will help the credentialed veterinary technician and the veterinary team as a whole to work with owners of brachycephalic dogs to ensure the wellbeing of the patient. Veterinary teams need to implement a systematic approach to characterize the respiratory and GI issues, as well as the most practical management and follow-up plan.

References

1 Packer, R.M. and Tivers, M.S. (2015). Strategies for the management and prevention of conformation-related respiratory disorders in brachycephalic dogs. *Veterinary Medicine (Auckl)* **6**: 219–232.

2 Freiche, V. and German, A.J. (2021). Digestive Diseases in Brachycephalic Dogs. *Veterinary Clinics of North America* **51**: 61–78.

3 Kaye, B.M., Rutherford, L., Perridge, D.J. et al. (2018). Relationship between brachycephalic airway syndrome and gastrointestinal signs in three breeds of dog. *Journal of Small Animal Practice* **59**: 670–673.

4 Poncet, C.M., Dupre, G.P., Freiche, V.G. et al. (2005). Prevalence of gastrointestinal tract lesions in 73 brachycephalic dogs with upper respiratory syndrome. *Journal of Small Animal Practice* **46**: 273–279.

5 Poncet, C.M., Dupre, G.P., Freiche, V.G. et al. (2006). Long-term results of upper respiratory syndrome surgery and gastrointestinal tract medical treatment in 51 brachycephalic dogs. *Journal of Small Animal Practice* **47**: 137–142.

6 Reeve, E.J., Sutton, D., Friend, E.J. et al. (2017). Documenting the prevalence of hiatal hernia and oesophageal abnormalities in brachycephalic dogs using fluoroscopy. *Journal of Small Animal Practice* **58**: 703–708.

7 Fenner, J.V.H., Quinn, R.J., and Demetriou, J.L. (2019). Postoperative regurgitation in dogs after upper airway surgery to treat brachycephalic obstructive airway syndrome: 258 cases (2013-2017). *Veterinary Surgery* **49**: 53–60.

8 Dupré, G. and Heidenreich, D. (2016). Brachycephalic syndrome. *Veterinary Clinics of North America Small Animal Practice* **46**: 691–707.

9 Eivers, C., Rueda, R.C., Liuti, T. et al. (2019). Retrospective analysis of esophageal

imaging features in brachycephalic versus non-brachycephalic dogs based on videofluoroscopic swallowing studies. *Journal of Veterinary Internal Medicine* 33: 1740–1746.

10 Burns, K.M. (2015). Gastrointestinal disorders. In: *Nutrition and Disease Management for Veterinary Technicians and Nurses*, 2nde (ed. A. Wortinger and K.M. Burns), 169–174. Wiley Blackwell.

11 Cline, M.G., Burns, K.M., Coe, J.B. et al. (2021). 2021 AAHA nutrition and weight management guidelines for dogs and cats. *Journal of the American Animal Hospital Association* 57: 153–178.

12 Liu, N.-C., Troconis, E.L., Kalmar, L. et al. (2017). Conformational risk factors of brachycephalic obstructive airway syndrome (BOAS) in pugs, French bulldogs, and bulldogs. *PLoS One* 12 (8): e0181928.

13 LiuN-C, A.V., KalmarL, L.J., and Sargan, D. (2016). Whole-body barometric plethysmography characterizes upper airway obstruction in 3 brachycephalic breeds dogs.

Journal of Veterinary Internal Medicine 30 (3): 853–865.

14 Davenport, D.J., Remillard, R.L., and Jenkins, C. (2010, 2010). Gastritis and gastroduodenal ulceration. In: *Small Animal Clinical Nutrition*, 5th (ed. M.S. Hand, C.D. Thatcher, R.L. Remilliard, et al.), 1025–1032. Topeka, KS: MMI.

15 Urrego, M.I.G., de O Matheus, L.F., de Melo Santos, K. et al. (2017). Effects of different protein sources on fermentation metabolites and nutrient digestibility of brachycephalic dogs. *Journal of Nutritional Science.* 6 (e43): 1–5.

16 Burns, K.M. (2022). Do bowls make a difference? In: *Proceedings of the 2022 Veterinary Meeting and Expo*, Orlando, FL.

17 Davenport, D.J., Remillard, R.L., and Jenkins, C. (2010, 2010). Gastric motility and emptying disorders. In: *Small Animal Clinical Nutrition*, 5th (ed. M.S. Hand, C.D. Thatcher, R.L. Remilliard, et al.), 1041–1046. Topeka, KS: MMI.

56

Feline Lower Urinary Tract Disease

Feline lower urinary tract disease (FLUTD) is a term used to describe any condition affecting the urinary bladder or urethra of cats and is a common reason for hospital visits and veterinary evaluation of our feline patients. Regardless of the underlying cause, FLUTD is characterized by the following signs: dysuria, pollakiuria, stranguria, hematuria, and/or periuria (urination in inappropriate places) Table 56.1. Obstructive signs constitute an emergency situation, and the cat should be examined by the veterinary team immediately. It is important that veterinary technicians are aware of signs and symptoms of FLUTD when talking with clients.

Causes of FLUTD

Over the course of the last decade, knowledge of specific causes of FLUTD has increased in the veterinary profession, allowing diagnostic and therapeutic efforts to be directed toward identification and elimination of specific underlying disorders. The most common cause of FLUTD in cats less than 10 years of age is feline idiopathic cystitis (FIC). This is followed by uroliths and urethral plugs. The common causes of FLUTD are divided into two overall categories, established on (1) the presence or (2) the absence of an identifiable cause.[1,2] A diagnosis of FIC is made by excluding all other causes of FLUTD. In older cats (those over 10 years), urinary tract infection and/or uroliths are the most common cause of FLUTD.

In 1981, 78% of feline uroliths were composed of struvite, and only 2% were composed of calcium oxalate. In the mid-to-late-1980s, the occurrence of calcium oxalate uroliths began to increase. Between 1994 and 2002, approximately 55% of uroliths were composed of calcium oxalate, and only 33% were composed of struvite. Since 2001, however, the number of struvite uroliths has continued to increase, while occurrence of calcium oxalate uroliths has decreased. Based on 21,295 feline uroliths analyzed at the Minnesota Urolith Center in 2022, the most common mineral types were struvite (50%) and calcium oxalate (37%), followed by purine (7%). In 2022, 96% of urethral plugs evaluated at the Minnesota Urolith Center were composed of struvite, and 4% were of other mineral compositions.[3]

Diagnostic Evaluation

Urinalysis and diagnostic imaging should be a standard protocol in the evaluation of cats with recurrent or persistent lower urinary tract signs. If there is a history of urinary tract manipulation (e.g., urethral catheterization), evidence of urinary tract infection (e.g., pyuria, bacteriuria, and malodorous urine), or the cat is older (usually over 10 years), a urine culture is warranted. More advanced procedures (e.g., contrast radiography) are appropriate in some cases.

Nutrition and Disease Management for Veterinary Technicians and Nurses, Third Edition. Ann Wortinger and Kara M. Burns.
© 2024 John Wiley & Sons, Inc. Published 2024 by John Wiley & Sons, Inc.
Companion Website: www.wiley.com/go/wortinger/3e

Table 56.1 Clinical signs of FLUTD

Nonobstructive	Obstructive
Pollikiuria	Anuria
Hematuria	Stranguria
Stranguria	Lethargy
Peruria	Vomiting
Licking at the urethral opening	Mentation = Depressed
	Licking at the urethral opening
	Inappetence

As stated, urinalysis is an important part of evaluating patients with signs of lower urinary tract disease. It is ideal to perform the urinalysis in-house since fresh urine samples analyzed within 30 minutes of collection are preferred. Urine specimens evaluated after 30 minutes may form crystals that are not in fact present in the patient. Samples may be refrigerated for up to 8 hours and then evaluated (after the sample has returned to room temperature). However, this method is not the best for evaluating crystalluria and should be avoided.

Although it may be tempting to only perform dipstick analysis, measure urine specific gravity, and omit urine sediment examination, it is very important to perform a complete urinalysis. Sediment examination is the only way to accurately detect pyuria, hematuria, bacteriuria, and crystalluria.[4] Healthcare team members cannot rely solely on urine dipstick analysis since results for detection of pyuria are often false positive in cats, and the occult blood reagent pad on the dipstick is not specific for hematuria (in addition to red blood cells, it also becomes positive with hemoglobin and myoglobin). Pyuria (>5 WBCs/hpf) indicates inflammation, which can be the result of several disorders (urolithiasis, bacterial infection). Pyuria is less commonly observed in cats with FIC.

A number of crystals may be identified on urine sediment examination, but the most commonly identified are struvite (triple phosphate) and calcium oxalate. The presence of crystals indicates that the urine is supersaturated with that substance and the patient is at risk for forming uroliths. It is worth noting that cats also may have crystals and never develop uroliths. Without other findings such as uroliths or urethral plugs, the presence of crystals alone is not diagnostic of urolithiasis or struvite disease. Struvite crystals may be present in normal cats and cats with struvite uroliths (sterile or infection-induced), nonstruvite uroliths (including some cats with calcium oxalate uroliths), urethral plugs, as well as other urinary disorders such as FIC.

Survey radiographs are helpful for identifying radiopaque uroliths and crystalline-matrix urethral plugs. Positioning should also include the caudal abdomen (urethra) in the radiograph, or there may be risk of missing potentially important information. Normal survey radiographs do not exclude FIC, radiolucent uroliths (urate/purine), small uroliths (<2 mm), neoplasia, blood clots, or anatomic defects. In these cases, abdominal ultrasonography and/or contrast urethrocystography are useful. After thorough diagnostic evaluation if no cause is found, a diagnosis of FIC is very likely.

When managing cats with FLUTD, it is recommended that a multimodal approach be used to attain the best results. This approach includes identifying and treating underlying medical conditions, modifying the home environment, addressing behavioral issues, and managing nutritional factors.

It has been determined that the most common cause of FLUTD in cats less than 10 years of age is feline idiopathic cystitis (FIC). Diagnosis of FIC is through exclusion of other FLUTD causes. In older cats (over 10 years), urinary tract infection and/or uroliths are the most common cause of FLUTD.

Factors that have been found to be significantly associated with FIC development are classified into the following categories:[4–6]

- psychogenic (e.g., anxiety, fearfulness, and nervousness)
- physiologic (e.g., sedentary, decreased water intake, and increased BCS)
- environmental (e.g., indoor versus outdoor, less hunting activities, and using a litterbox).

Pathogenesis of FIC

Although FIC is suspected when all other causes are ruled out, the following steps have been theorized to play a major role in the pathogenesis of FIC,[6–9]

1 The stress response system (SRS) is activated when a cat perceives stress in its environment.
2 The SRS heightens activity in the sympathetic nervous system and increases outflow down the spinal cord to the urinary bladder. In otherwise healthy cats, this response is regulated/dampened by activity of the hypothalamic/pituitary/adrenal input.
3 Increased sympathetic input to the bladder is believed to cause neurogenic "inflammation," which leads to
   o increased permeability of the urinary bladder mucosa
   o greater access of substances in the urine to sensory neurons in the bladder wall
   o increased pain receptors/fibers in the bladder
   o release of inflammatory cytokines from cells in the bladder wall and increased sensitivity of afferent nerves.
4 Sensory input via afferent input from the bladder is transmitted back to the brain and perceived as pain, which causes additional stress

The result is a vicious cycle affecting the brain and the urinary bladder. Therefore, to increase success of managing cats with FIC, treatment approaches should be aimed at both the brain and the bladder.

Nutritionally Managing Cats with FIC

The goals of managing cats with FIC are as follows:

1 reduce stress
2 provide pain relief
3 decrease severity of clinical signs
4 increase the interval between episodes.

Feeding moist food (>60% moisture) has been associated with a decreased recurrence of clinical signs in cats with FIC. During a 1-year study, clinical signs recurred less often in cats with FIC when fed a moist food compared with cats fed the dry formulation of the same food.[6,10] Beneficial effects have been observed in cats with FIC when urine specific gravity values decreased from 1.050 to values between 1.032 and 1.041. Additional methods for increasing water intake (e.g., adding broth to foods, placing ice cubes in the cat's water, and providing water fountains) also may be helpful for some cats.

A recent study shows that consistently feeding a therapeutic urinary food was associated with a reduction in recurrent episodes of FIC signs. This is the first study to definitively show that foods of different nutritional profiles impact the expression of acute episodes of FIC signs in cats. Additionally, the addition of L-tryptophan, a precursor of serotonin that inhibits neurotransmitters in the brain to balance mood, as well as hydrolyzed casein, a bioactive peptide that helps relieve anxiety in cats, have been presented as nutrients that will aid in managing the stress component of FIC.

Increasing salt content of food is an effective method of causing urine dilution in cats, but the potential for adverse effects should be considered. At this time, there are differing opinions regarding the role of sodium in cats with kidney disease. In a recent study, the effects of high-salt (1.2% sodium, dry matter basis (DMB)) intake for 3 months were evaluated in six cats with mild azotemia due to naturally occurring chronic kidney disease. These cats had progressive increases in BUN, serum creatinine, and serum phosphorus compared with consumption of food with 0.4% sodium (DMB). Based on all findings to date, further study is needed to better determine the role of sodium in healthy cats fed long term as well as cats with hypertension, chronic kidney disease, and calcium oxalate uroliths. In pending further studies, it is sensible to avoid high-salt foods in cats with chronic kidney disease and monitor kidney function when high-salt foods are fed to cats at risk for kidney disease.

Inflammation plays a role in many causes of FLUTD, especially FIC and urolithiasis. Therefore, a key nutritional factor for managing cats with FLUTD includes omega-3 fatty acids, specifically EPA and DHA, which are known to have potent anti-inflammatory effects. Additionally, vitamin E and beta carotene are helpful for counteracting oxidative stress and reducing free radical damage, conditions that often accompany inflammation.

Managing stress and anxiety nutritionally involves foods that contain specific nutrients with proven anti-anxiety benefits and offers an innovative approach for management of FIC. Nutritional management with L-tryptophan and alpha-casozepine is supported by clinical studies in dogs and cats.[11,12] Additionally, a nutritional approach is beneficial for cats as the owner may no longer need to administer daily treatments causing stress to the owner and the cat. Through nutrition, cats can receive the necessary nutrients to decrease anxiety and stress. This will strengthen the human–animal bond and subsequently increase compliance.

Serotonin, a major neurotransmitter in the brain, is responsible for regulating mood and emotion in animals and human beings. Tryptophan is an amino acid that serves as a precursor for the synthesis of serotonin. Serotonin is not able to cross the blood–brain barrier (BBB) to enter the central nervous system. However, tryptophan and 5-hydroxytryptophan are able to cross the BBB by way of a carrier protein. Pro-inflammatory cytokines are linked to many behavioral or psychiatric diseases in animals and human beings.[11] Feline stressors (i.e., those associated with unusual events) can increase the level of pro-inflammatory cytokines.[12] As a result, chronic stress can lead to anxious pathological states, and this could be linked with a shift in tryptophan metabolism.

Historically, milk from cows has been considered to have tranquilizing effects in humans.[12,13] This calming effect was hypothesized to be from a natural component in the cow's milk created via digestion (tryptic hydrolysis) in human babies. Researchers first identified a decapeptide, obtained via tryptic hydrolysis, responsible for the anxiolytic activity.[6,12] This milk protein is known as alpha-S1 casein. It is converted to a bioactive peptide via hydrolysis (with trypsin) to form hydrolyzed casein. Hydrolyzed casein has a natural affinity for the benzodiazepine site of the GABA receptor and has been shown to regulate anxious and stressful behavior in multiple species. In felines, a study associated alpha-casozepine with a significant decrease in fearfulness and an increase in contact with people.[14]

Nutritional management aimed at addressing FLUTD, specifically FIC, will lead to improved compliance, overall better healthcare for cats, and fewer painful FIC recurrences. Nutritional management will help reduce pain associated with FLUTD and strengthen the human–animal bond between pets and their owners. The healthcare team must educate owners about the impact of stress in cats and how nutritional management allows the owner to participate in the long-term management of urinary health for their feline family member.

Managing Cats with Feline Idiopathic Cystitis

The goals of managing cats with FIC are to decrease severity of clinical signs and increase the interval between episodes of lower urinary tract disease. Over the past 40 years, many different treatments have been recommended to control signs in cats with FIC, yet only a few have been evaluated in clinical trials of cats with FIC.

Environmental Enrichment

In addition to nutritional management, the currently recommended treatment for cats with FIC also includes environmental enrichment and stress reduction. Environmental enrichment is also an important adjunct to therapy in all types of FLUTD.[3,6,14] The veterinary healthcare team plays a crucial role in educating cat owners about the importance of environmental enrichment, stress reduction, and litter box management. Cats with FIC should avoid stressful situations (e.g., conflict with other cats in the home). Owners should be educated to provide opportunities for play/resting (horizontal and vertical surfaces for scratching, hiding places, and climbing platforms). Any changes (e.g., switching to a new food) should be made *gradually* so the cat has adequate time to adapt and avoid becoming stressed.

A recent prospective study evaluating effects of multimodal environmental modification was reported in 46 client-owned cats with FIC. The findings showed significant reductions in lower urinary tract signs, fearfulness, and nervousness after treatment for 10 months. With cats that are suffering with FIC, stressful situations (e.g., conflict with other cats in the home) should be avoided or minimized. Owners should provide opportunities for play/resting (horizontal and vertical surfaces for scratching, hiding places, and climbing platforms). Any changes (e.g., switching to a new food) should be made gradually so the cat has adequate time to adapt and avoid becoming stressed.

Another critical component of managing cats with FLUTD, especially FIC, involves appropriate use and maintenance of litter boxes in the home. The majority of cats prefer clumping, unscented litter; however, it may be necessary to give cats several choices and let them select their preference. It may be possible to have cats within the home that prefer different types of litter or litter boxes. In general, uncovered litter boxes are recommended because they are less likely to trap odors inside. For older cats with mobility issues, the owner should select a litter box with low sides to facilitate the cat getting in and out of the box. Litter boxes should be scooped daily and washed every few weeks with warm, soapy water. Because plastic can absorb odors over time (months to years), owners should consider replacing litter boxes with new ones periodically. Finally, there should be an adequate number of litter boxes (the 1 + 1 rule = 1 more than the number of cats) in the home, and they should be located on multiple floors where cats can enter and exit readily. More detailed information about environmental enrichment and litter box management is available in the suggested reading. It may be helpful to encourage owners to read this additional information as well because their involvement is critical for a successful outcome. Finally, healthcare team members, especially technicians, play a crucial role in educating cat owners about the importance of environmental enrichment and litter box management.

Managing Cats with Struvite Uroliths or Urethral Plugs

Treatment options for cats with struvite uroliths include physical removal of uroliths or dissolution via nutritional management. Mean time required for dissolution of sterile struvite uroliths using these foods is approximately 1 month. For cats with suspected struvite uroliths, it is appropriate to transition to feeding a canned calculolytic food over a 7-day period. Cats should be re-evaluated every 2–4 weeks (urinalysis and abdominal radiographs). Urine pH should remain <6.1 and specific gravity should be <1.040 if canned food is being fed exclusively. Nutritional management (dissolution) should be continued 1 month beyond radiographic resolution of the urolith.

After dissolution or removal of struvite uroliths or urethral plugs, nutritional management should be continued to prevent recurrence. There are several commercially available foods for struvite prevention; however, only one (Prescription Diet® s/d® Feline, Hill's Pet Nutrition) has been evaluated in cats with struvite disease. Several other foods formulated for struvite prevention have been evaluated in healthy cats by measuring urine saturation values of struvite. A dissolution (calculolytic) food is appropriate for initial management after relieving urethral obstruction; this should be followed by feeding a struvite-preventive food indefinitely, with the cat being evaluated routinely by the veterinary healthcare team.

Managing Cats with Calcium Oxalate Uroliths

The treatment of choice for calcium oxalate urolithiasis is urolith removal, followed by methods to prevent recurrence. At present, the standard of care for preventing calcium oxalate urolith recurrence is to feed moist therapeutic food and encourage water intake. There are several commercially available therapeutic foods for prevention of calcium oxalate uroliths in cats.

All cats should be monitored for recurrence including urinalysis every 3 months to detect calcium oxalate crystalluria and diagnostic imaging every 6 months to detect uroliths. If uroliths recur, less invasive procedures such as voiding urohydropropulsion are more likely to be effective when uroliths are smaller.

Summary

Increased understanding of specific causes of FLUTD has allowed diagnostic and therapeutic efforts to be directed toward identification and elimination of specific underlying disorders. The most common cause of FLUTD in cats <10 years of age is feline idiopathic cystitis (FIC), followed by uroliths, and urethral plugs. A diagnosis of FIC is made by excluding all other causes of FLUTD. In older cats (>10 years), urinary tract infection and/or uroliths are the most common cause of FLUTD. It is imperative that veterinary technicians have a thorough understanding of FLUTD and then how the various treatments affect the different types of FLUTD. Veterinary technicians play a very important role in the treatment of FLUTD. The history obtained from discussions with the pet owner aids in the diagnosis of FLUTD. The technicians' discussion of the treatment plan with the client is key to the client's understanding and compliance with the veterinarian's recommendation and ultimately the health of the pet.

References

1 Grauer, G. (2013). Current thoughts on pathophysiology and treatment of feline idiopathic cystitis. *Today's Veterinary Practice*. Nov/Dec. 38–41.

2 Lulich, J.P., Kruger, J.M., Macleay, J.M. et al. Efficacy of two commercially available, low-magnesium, urine-acidifying dry foods for the dissolution of struvite uroliths in cats. *J Am Vet Med Assoc* 2013;243: 1147–1153.

3 Minnesota Urolith Center – University of Minnesota. 2022 Minnesota Urolith Center Global Data. March 2023, z.umn.edu/2022GlobalUrolith Accessed 7/17/2023

4 Burns, K.M. (2014). *FLUTD – using nutrition to go with the flow*, (Convention issue). 7–12. *NAVTA Journal*.

5 Lulich, J.P. (2007). FLUTD: Are you missing the correct diagnosis? In: *Proc 2007 Hill's FLUTD Symposium 2007:* 12–19 (http://www.hillsvet.com/conferenceproceedings).

6 Burns, K.M. (2015). FIC: Why all the stress? *The NAVTA Journal Convention issue*. 8–13.

7 Defauw, P.A., Van de Maele, I., Duchateau, L. et al. (2011). Risk factors and clinical presentation of cats with feline idiopathic cystitis. *Journal of Feline Medicine and Surgery* **13**: 967–975.

8 Westropp, J.L., Kass, P.H., and Buffington, C.A. (2006). Evaluation of the effects of stress in cats with idiopathic cystitis. *American Journal of Veterinary Research* **67**: 731–736.

9 Westropp, J.L., Welk, K.A., and Buffington, C.A. (2003). Small adrenal glands in cats with feline interstitial cystitis. *Journal of Urology* **170**: 2494–2497.

10 Markwell, P.J., Buffington, C.A., Chew, D.J. et al. (1999). Clinical evaluation of commercially available urinary acidification diets in the management of idiopathic cystitis in cats. *Journal of the American Veterinary Medical Association* **214**: 361.

11 Pereira, G.G., Fragoso, S., and Pires, E. (2010). Effect of dietary intake of L-tryptophan supplementation on multi-housed cats presenting stress related behaviors, April, BSAVA congress proceedings.

12 Beata, C., Beaumont, G., Coll, V. et al. (2007). Effect of alpha-casozepine (Zylkene) on anxiety in cats. *Journal of Veterinary Behavior* **2**: 40–46.

13 Beata, C. (2014). L-tryptophan and alpha-casozepine: What is the evidence? In: *Hill's Global Symposium on Feline Lower Urinary Tract Health Proceedings*, April, Prague.

14 Stella, J.L., Lord, L.K., and Buffington, C.A. (2011). Sickness behaviors in response to unusual external events in healthy cats and cats with feline interstitial cystitis. *Journal of the American Veterinary Medical Association* **238**: 67–73.

Further Reading

Cameron, M.E., Casey, R.A., Bradshaw, J.W. et al. (2004). A study of environmental and behavioural factors that may be associated with feline idiopathic cystitis. *Journal of Small Animal Practice* **45**: 144–147.

Buffington, C.A., Westropp, J.L., Chew, D.J. et al. (2006). Clinical evaluation of multimodal environmental modification (MEMO) in the management of cats with idiopathic cystitis. *Journal of Feline Medicine and Surgery* **8**: 261–268.

Lulich, J., Kruger, J. et al. (2013). Efficacy of two commercially available, low-magnesium, urine-acidifying dry foods for the dissolution of struvite uroliths in cats. *Journal of the American Veterinary Medical Association* **243** (8): 1147–1153.

Section V

Feeding Management for other Companion Animals

57

Avian

One area of veterinary medicine that affects every pet that comes into the hospital, including companion birds, is nutrition. Every bird that presents to the hospital should have a nutritional assessment every time they present. Many of the problems for which birds present to veterinary hospitals are nutrition-related. Psittacine and passerine species have unique nutritional requirements, and if owners are not familiar with the proper care and feeding of the particular species owned, the bird is at risk for disease or malnutrition.[1-3] Each avian species has differing nutritional demands, and it is important to review the needs of the particular breed of bird with the owner.

Nutritional Overview

Nutritional deficiencies and excesses may result in immune dysfunction, increased susceptibility to infectious diseases, and metabolic and biochemical derangements. Clinically, veterinary teams may see the following result: nutritional secondary hyperparathyroidism, thyroid hyperplasia (dysplasia), hemochromatosis, and the potential for many other issues. Healthcare teams must familiarize themselves with the reasons for the development of nutritionally induced illnesses occurring in companion psittacine and passerine birds. Until recently, specific nutritional requirements for these birds were unidentified. Consequently, veterinary team members would compare the well-known nutrient needs

of poultry to those of other avian species. Today, the profession is aware of nutritional differences between poultry and other avian species and has commercially prepared foods specific to the individual physiologic and nutrient needs of the companion bird species. Another reason for nutrition-induced problems is the perception that all seed diets, especially those comprised on only one seed type (e.g., millet or sunflower) as well as diets made up of fruits, vegetables, and other human foods, are complete and provide all the nutrients birds need. This is a misperception, as the majority of seeds available commercially are deficient in specific nutrients (e.g., specific amino acids, vitamins, trace minerals, and macrominerals such as calcium and sodium). Therefore, owners must be educated that seeds are not and should not be the main diet for most species of companion birds.

Additionally, it is suggested that the most common cause of dietary-induced diseases in companion birds occurs when fruits and vegetables are added to commercially prepared foods or supplemented seed mixtures. The most readily available fruits and vegetables are comprised mainly of water, carbohydrates, and fiber and are deficient in protein, vitamins, and minerals – especially when compared to the nutrient recommendations for psittacine and passerine birds.[4] As a result, fruits and vegetables mainly dilute vital nutrients present in nutritionally balanced commercially prepared foods. Because of the high moisture content, most birds prefer fruits and vegetables

Nutrition and Disease Management for Veterinary Technicians and Nurses, Third Edition. Ann Wortinger and Kara M. Burns.
© 2024 John Wiley & Sons, Inc. Published 2024 by John Wiley & Sons, Inc.
Companion Website: www.wiley.com/go/wortinger/3e

as opposed to dry extruded or pelleted foods and seed mixtures. Birds will often select food items based on water content, texture, color, or taste, instead of nutrient content.[2,4] This selection process can lead to imbalanced nutrient intake and is another reason companion birds develop nutritional deficiencies. Again, this leads to another myth – that birds are able to balance their diets. The end result oftentimes is that a bird may become habituated to or fixated on a particular food item (e.g., sunflower, safflower, millet seeds, grapes, and oranges) and refuse to eat other food items which provide a complete and balanced array of nutrients.

Nutritional Assessment

As with other species presenting to the veterinary hospital, one of the most important steps is to obtain a detailed history from the owner (Table 57.1). We have discussed the fact that nutrition and husbandry-related problems are very common findings and can lead to various medical conditions. The patient history should include a list of foods offered daily. In addition, clients should be encouraged to provide a sample of any commercially prepared foods they feed. A good idea is to ask the owners to take a picture of the birds' home environment, including all items that are offered to their bird to eat and/or drink. If the typical food fed is a commercially prepared food, observe the label for nutrient information or guarantees. The key nutrients of concern are protein and calcium. Many foods commonly fed to companion birds are composed primarily of carbohydrates and fat. When reviewing the label of an acceptable commercially prepared food, the guaranteed amount of protein should be at least 12%. Additionally, the healthcare team should be able to determine the source of calcium included in the food by the ingredients listed on the label. It is important to note that seeds ordinarily contain more phosphorus than calcium.

If the food label does not contain nutrient information or is just a list of ingredients such as seeds or dried fruit, it is recommended to not use this particular food long term. It is essential for all birds that their foods be appropriately balanced with carbohydrates, proteins, fats, vitamins, minerals, and water. Good nutrition is important for companion birds to ensure

- the health of the bird
- proper growth and maturation
- defense against disease
- reproductive health.

Three methods of providing nutrients and achieving these objectives are as follows: (1) commercially prepared foods, (2) seeds and seed mixtures, and (3) homemade mixed foods.

Commercially Prepared Diets

The benefits of using commercially prepared, nutritionally complete foods are similar in birds as in other companion animals. Ninety percent or more of the nutrients for companion dogs and cats in North America can be supplied through commercially prepared foods and has been determined to contribute markedly to the health of these animals. The same is true of companion birds. Nutrient balance and owner convenience are benefits offered by commercially prepared foods. Most manufacturers follow established nutrient recommendations[4] (Table 57.2) to formulate foods for companion birds. Extruded or pelleted diets are recommended as they tend to supply all the nutrients in a pellet. Pelleted diets help prevent the variation of nutrients. Well-meaning owners may feed imbalanced seeds or human foods. Also, some birds may consume various quantities of imbalanced foods fed separately.

Healthcare team members should encourage owners to bring the bird food package in with their bird and compare the nutrient levels of the food to those recommended in Table 57.2. By reviewing the package of the bird food, this

Table 57.1 Avian history questionnaire.

- Signalment – gender, age, and species
- Chief complaint – reason for bringing the bird to the hospital
- From where did you acquire the bird? Breeder? Prior owners?
- Living environment–
  - Type of cage
  - What is the cage lined with: newspapers, shavings, etc.?
  - Perches – number and type
  - Toys in the cage – what kind and what are they made from? How are they attached to the cage?
  - Where in the house is the bird kept?
  - Any cleaners or other household supplies used near the bird cage?
  - Is the bird allowed out of cage? Flight? Supervised? Interactive playthings?
  - How often is the bird handled?
- Diet
  - What is the bird being fed?
  - How often is the bird fed?
  - How is the birds' appetite?
  - How much is fed?
  - What types of bowls are used?
  - Where is the water bowl?
  - What is the source of the birds' water?
  - How often is water changed?
  - Any supplements added to food or water?
  - Is food commercially prepared or homemade?
  - How is food stored?
- Cage mates
  - Are there other birds in the cage? If so, what species?
  - Are there other birds in the house? If so, what species?
- Behavior
  - Overall attitude?
  - Does the bird vocalize?
  - Any changes to vocalizations?
  - Past behavior-related problems?
- Medical History
  - Any prior illness?
  - Has the bird ever been prescribed medications? What was the reason? What was the medication?
  - Any illness in other birds in the house, or other pets in the house?
  - Has this bird been to a veterinary hospital prior?

Table 57.2 Nutrition recommendations for avian foods[4]

Nutrient	Psittacine minimum	Maximum	Minimum	Passerine maximum
Gross energy (kcal/kg)**	3200	4200	3500	4500
Total protein (%)	12.0	–	14.0	–
Linoleic acid (%) Amino acids	1.0	–	1.0	–
Lysine (%)	0.65	–	0.75	–
Methionine (%)	0.30	–	0.35	–
Methionine + cystine (%)	0.50	–	0.58	–
Arginine (%)	0.65	–	0.75	–
Threonine (%)	0.40	–	0.46	–
Vitamins (fat-soluble)				
Vitamin A activity (total) IU/kg	8000	–	8000	–
Vitamin D3 (IU/kg)	500	2000	1000	2500
Vitamin E (ppm)	50	–	50	–
Vitamin K (ppm)	1.0	–	1.0	–
Vitamins (water-soluble)				
Thiamin (ppm)	4.0	–	4.0	–
Riboflavin (ppm)	6.0	–	6.0	–
Niacin (ppm)	50.0	–	50.0	–
Pyridoxine (ppm)	6.0	–	6.0	–
Pantothenic acid (ppm)	20.0	–	20.0	–
Biotin (ppm)	0.25	–	0.25	–
Folic acid (ppm)	1.50	–	1.50	–
Vitamin B12 (ppm)	0.01	–	0.01	–
Choline (ppm)	1500	–	1500	–
Minerals				
Calcium (%)	0.30	1.20	0.50	1.20
Phosphorus (%)	0.30	–	0.50	–
Calcium–phosphorus ratio	1.0–1.0	2.0–1.0	1.0–1.0	2.0–1.0
Potassium (%)	0.40	–	0.40	–
Sodium (%)	0.12	–	0.12	–
Chloride (%)	0.12	–	0.12	–
Magnesium (ppm)	600	–	600	–
Trace minerals				
Manganese (ppm) 6	5.0	–	65.0	–
Iron (ppm)	80.0	–	80.0	–
Zinc (ppm)	50.0	–	50.0	–
Selenium (ppm)	0.10	–	0.10	–

Source: Kollias and Kollias [4].

will help decide if there are any incongruities in the nutrient profile.

As mentioned earlier, it is suggested that a formulated diet be provided to best achieve the balance of nutrients required for companion birds. These formulated foods come in a variety of forms with the most popular being[5]

1 pellets
2 extruded diets with a pellet appearance
3 whole grains and/or seeds with added pelleted material.

A seed-based food with a vitamin/mineral mix coating on the outside of the seed is another option. However, typically, the seed is not hulled. When the bird dehulls the coated seed, necessary vitamins and minerals are removed, thus creating a nutritional imbalance, putting the bird's health at risk.

Two processes are used when pelleted diets are manufactured – bound and extruded. Bound pellet manufacturing involves the grinding of grains such as corn, soybean, and oat groats (oat berries). Following the grinding process, vitamins, minerals, and other components are added to produce a balanced food (per the manufacturer's recommendation). The grinding process produces a consistent pellet, which makes it difficult for birds to pick out their favorite part of the diet. With bound pellets in general, the food material is not cooked, and the diet will have a longer fiber chain length. Bound pelleted diets may not be as palatable as the extruded diet.[2,5,6]

Extruded pellets utilize finely ground grains which are mixed with vitamins, minerals, etc., until a balanced formulation is reached. This pellet mixture is then forced through an extruder, under pressure and high temperatures. The mixture will take on the shape of the "die" in the extrusion process. This allows for extruded pellets to be made into different shapes and colors.[6]

Extruded pelleted diets come in a variety of sizes and should be selected based on the species and size of the bird. Owners must be instructed to monitor their bird to prevent picking out certain colored pellets and ignoring others. Owners should not choose colors or shapes because their bird "likes these" as this can be expensive and wasteful. Companion birds are healthier when they are psychologically stimulated, and this can occur by presenting multi-colored pellets in an assortment of shapes (Figure 57.1).

Historically, providing diets for birds has included seed-based diets. Although pelleted diets have allowed bird owners to provide a better balanced diet without vitamin and mineral supplementation, not every bird will eat them.[7] Also, as discussed earlier, each species has different nutritional requirements. For example, certain passerine species (e.g., canary and finch) require seed in their base diet. However, for the psittacine species (e.g., budgerigar, cockatiel, and lovebird), seed is not the recommended diet, and a balanced pelleted food is advised as the appropriate base diet. Overall,

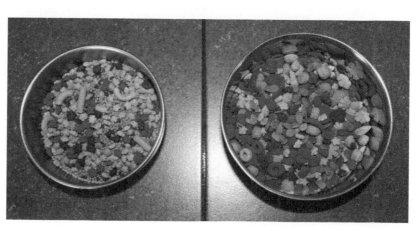

Figure 57.1 Smaller pellets: Left (cockatiels) and the larger; right (small parrots). (© Kara M. Burns.)

many seed diets are high in fat and lower in other essential nutrients and therefore should be considered a treat. As with any species, treats should be offered in small quantities, or the bird will be at risk for malnutrition – most likely obesity.

Transition from a seed diet to a pellet is believed to be difficult. However, this is not the case even in older birds. Healthcare team members must educate owners on what to look for when transitioning a bird from seed to pellets. Owners should ensure that their pet is ingesting the food, not simply crushing the pellet in the hopes of finding a kernel inside. Two signs that indicate that the bird is actually eating the pellets are seen in the production of fecal material and a color change of the fecal material associated with the pellet color being ingested.[6]

To aid owners in transitioning their birds from seed to pellet, formed seed products have been manufactured (i.e., Nutriberries® Lafeber Co., Cornell, IL) (Figure 57.2). These products comprise whole grains and seeds which are mixed with additional components and are affixed together. This is similar to pellets, but this product is not ground. The bird must pick off the seed to eat.

Owners can also learn to transition their birds from seed to pellets through the slow introduction of increased pellets in the seed mixture over a period of time. The transition is recommended to take 7–14 days, with the final diet consisting of 100% pellets.

Avian Key Nutritional Factors

Water

Water is the most critical nutrient, and all birds should have access to fresh, clean water at all times (Figure 57.3). Water should be changed on a daily basis, and the healthcare team is responsible for reviewing this important piece of husbandry with owners. Water is important for birds as it acts as a food carrier and aids in digestion. As we have seen in other species of companion animals, some foods have higher water content than others. Some avian species are more physiologically proficient at extracting water from their foods. Birds should never go for more than a few hours without access to fresh clean water. More than 50% of a bird's

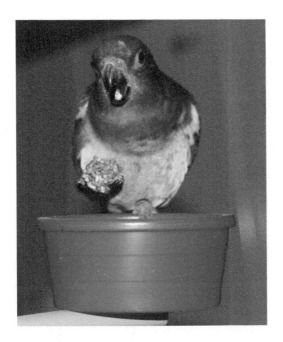

Figure 57.2 Meyer's parrot with Seed Ball/Nutriberries® Lafeber Co., Cornell, IL. (© Kara M. Burns.)

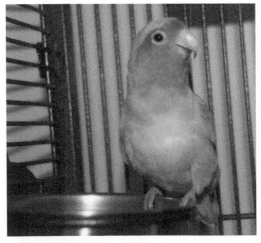

Figure 57.3 Lovebird with a water bowl. (© Kara M. Burns.)

body weight is made up of water and in young birds, the percentage may be even higher.[2] Water intake plays an important role in avian thermoregulation. It is important to note that reproducing females may require more water for egg production and for heat regulation while incubating eggs. Water should be provided in bowls or dishes that the bird can reach easily. They should not be located in a place that collects feces, feathers, food, etc. Healthcare team members should educate owners to attach water bowls to the wall of enclosures, near or above food bowls. Water bowls should not be placed directly under the favorite perching area to cut down on excrement in the water. Separate bowls should be provided specifically for bathing.

Birds typically accept municipal tap water, but it is recommended that well water be boiled before allowing the bird to drink freely. If owners are hesitant to boil water, the healthcare team should recommend providing bottled water to their birds. This recommendation is made due to the fact that well water can be contaminated easily by bacteria colonies in the pipes leading to the faucet.[8]

Protein and Amino Acids

Protein requirements differ among species. The minimum recommended protein allowance for maintenance in psittacine companion birds is 12%, and in the passerine species it is 14%.[4,9]

As with all foods, the quality of the protein is dependent on bioavailability and essential amino acid content. Bird food formulations must avoid excess and deficiency of proteins and amino acids. For the majority of companion birds, the following amino acids are considered essential: arginine, isoleucine, lysine, methionine, phenylalanine, valine, tryptophan, and threonine. Budgies also require glycine.[9] Too much protein in the diet of birds has been associated with renal disease, behavioral changes (biting, feather picking, nervousness, and rejection of food), and regurgitation. Poor weight gain, poor feathering, stress lines on feathers, plumage color changes, and poor reproductive performance are clinical signs associated with protein and amino acid deficiencies.[2,9]

Fats and Essential Fatty Acids

Fats are a more concentrated source of energy in a diet. Essential fatty acids (linoleic and arachidonic) are required in birds for the following: the formation of membranes and cell organelles, hormone precursors, and the basis for psittacofulvins (i.e., feather pigments found in psittacine species). The typical recommended linoleic allowance for psittacine and passerine companion bird diets is approximately 1%.[4] It is important for healthcare team members to note that in birds, lipogenesis takes place primarily in the liver. Pet birds fed high energy diets may develop illness associated with hepatic lipidosis. This is heightened if exercise is restricted in the bird.

As with other companion animals and humans, too much fat in the diet of a bird may result in obesity, hepatic lipidosis, congestive heart failure, diarrhea, and oily feather texture. Increased fat levels may also interfere with the absorption of other nutrients such as calcium. Low amounts of fat in the diet may lead to weight loss, reduced disease resistance, and overall poor growth, especially when coupled with restriction of other energy-producing nutrients.[4,8,10]

Carbohydrates

Carbohydrates are another energy source which can be converted into fat in the liver in birds and vice versa. Glucagon is the major component of carbohydrate metabolism in birds. The result of inadequate carbohydrates in the diet is the utilization of glucogenic amino acids to manufacture carbohydrates. The process involves amino acids being shifted away from growth and production and instead utilized in glucose synthesis.[10] Carbohydrates are the only source of energy utilizable by the nervous system; therefore, neurological abnormalities may indicate deficiency in a diet that is otherwise adequate in kilojoule content.[8,10]

Calcium

Calcium is an important dietary element for companion and caged birds. Calcium is essential for bone and eggshell formation. Calcium is also necessary for blood coagulation and nerve and muscle function. Remember to review the list of ingredients on the bird food label, as this will help determine if a source of calcium is included in the food. Seeds commonly contain more phosphorus than calcium. Thus, an added calcium source such as calcium carbonate, dicalcium phosphate, bone meal, ground limestone, or ground oyster shells helps balance the calcium–phosphorus ratio of bird foods.

It is recommended that all birds' nutritional regimen be reviewed to ensure proper amount of calcium is being fed. This is especially true for birds fed a seed diet. Calcium supplementation can be provided in the form of a cuttlebone, mineral block, crushed oyster shell, or baked crushed eggshell. Birds will eat the calcium if provided and when needed to meet physiologic demands. Cuttlebones should be placed in the cage, with the soft side facing the bird. Cuttlebones are strictly a calcium source and are not beak-sharpening devices.[6] It should also be noted that high phosphorus in the diet can negate adequate amounts of calcium in the diet. High phosphorus levels will interfere with calcium absorption from the intestinal tract. The calcium-to-phosphorus ratio for psittacine and passerine companion birds should range from 1 : 1 to 2 : 1.[6,10] This is another reason to provide a nutritionally balanced diet as seeds, fruit, vegetables, and meat are extremely calcium-deficient but do have higher amounts of phosphorus. For example,

corn has a 1 : 37 ratio and muscle meat has a 1 : 20 ratio.[6]

Vitamins and Minerals

Vitamin requirements for companion birds are similar to those of companion mammals. The major exception is that the active form of vitamin D required by birds is vitamin D3 (cholecalciferol) as opposed to vitamin D2 (ergocalciferol). Vitamin C is important in specific fruit-eating species, but for the majority of passerine and psittacine species, a complete and balanced diet will provide the necessary amounts of vitamin C. However, vitamin C supplementation has been suggested to assist debilitated birds as the ability to create vitamin C is reduced and the patients' requirements are greater.[8,10]

If the bird is prescribed antibiotics, the healthcare team should monitor the patient closely as vitamin deficiencies may result from the antibiotics interfering with normal intestinal microflora. Intestinal infections (e.g., giardiasis) may block vitamin absorption from the intestine (e.g., vitamin E and vitamin A). Hypervitaminosis has become an increasing problem, as clients may over-supplement formulated food or multivitamin preparations, thereby causing renal failure due to hypervitaminosis D.[2] Hypervitaminosis A can also result in disease, especially in nectarivorous (those birds that eat the sugar-rich nectar of flowering plants or the juices of fruits) birds.[6,8,10]

Fruits and Vegetables

Fruits and vegetables are typically presented as supplementation to the pet birds' commercial diet. Fruits are made up of mainly sugars and water and thus should not be offered in excess. Fruit is a necessary part of the diet for some psittacine species such as eclectus and lories, but these are exceptions. Fruit should not be fed more than a couple of times in a 7-day period.

Companion birds receive greater nutritional benefit from vegetables as opposed to fruits. As much as possible, fresh or cooked dark green, red, and orange vegetables should be offered on a daily basis. One vegetable that should *not* be offered is comfrey. Comfrey is a green leaf herb especially popular in canary aviaries, which may lead to liver damage. Proper husbandry suggests the healthcare team educate owners to place fruit and vegetables in a separate container and leave in the cage no longer than 30 minutes. Time restriction will help decrease the likelihood of microorganism growth.[6]

Poultry Nutrition for Backyard Flocks

Raising poultry has fast become a popular hobby for many individuals, and the responsible chicken owner wants information about proper nutrition for their flock. Providing the right nutrition for your chickens means ensuring that what they eat provides the six basic nutrients: proteins (essential amino acids), fats (fatty acids), carbohydrates, vitamins, minerals, and water, which they will need to grow up healthy. Deficiency of even one nutrient can lead to serious health consequences for poultry.[11] Thus, when formulating a diet for poultry, the main concern is that the bird's nutrient requirements are met.

Water

Water is an essential nutrient and is required in greater amounts than any other nutrient. A general guide for poultry is that they will drink approximately twice as much water as the amount of feed.[11] Although, many factors influence water intake, including environmental temperature, relative humidity, salt, and protein levels of the diet, birds' productivity (rate of growth or egg production), and the individual bird's ability to resorb water in the kidney. Water softens feed and helps move it through the digestive tract. Water is a component of blood (90% of blood content) and is responsible for transporting nutrients from

the digestive tract to cells and finally, carries away waste products. Water also helps cool the bird through evaporation. Consequently, specific water requirements cannot be given for all circumstances. A baby chick comprises ~80% water. Even though this percentage decreases as a bird gets older, the need for water remains.[11] Inadequate water supply for >12 hours has a harmful effect on growth of young poultry and egg production of layers; water deprivation for >36 hours results in a significant increase in death of both young and older poultry. Cool, clean water must be available at all times.

Energy

To meet their daily energy needs, poultry can adjust their feed intake. Energy needs and, consequently, feed intake also vary considerably with level of productivity, environmental temperature, and amount of physical activity.[11] However, an individual bird's daily need for amino acids, vitamins, and minerals is predominantly independent of these factors.

Poultry eating a diet with a higher energy content will decrease its feed intake; thus, their diet must contain a correspondingly higher amount of amino acids, vitamins, and minerals. Nutrient density of the feed should be modified in proportion to energy to provide appropriate nutrient intake based on requirements and the actual feed intake.[11,12]

Carbohydrates

Carbohydrates provide energy for poultry and comprise the largest portion of a poultry diet. Carbohydrates are typically consumed in the form of starch, sugar, cellulose, and other non-starch compounds. Poultry typically do not digest cellulose and the non-starch compounds (crude fiber) well. Conversely, poultry can utilize most starches and sugars.[12] Important sources of carbohydrates in poultry diets include corn, wheat, barley, and other grains.

Fats

Dietary fats come in the form of triglycerides – a glycerol backbone with three fatty acids attached. Fatty acids are a long chain of carbon and hydrogen which have a high energy density. Fatty acids are responsible for cell membrane integrity and hormone synthesis. Linoleic acid is considered an essential fatty acid because poultry cannot generate it from other nutrients.[12] Therefore, linoleic acid must be included in the poultry diet.

As mentioned in Chapter 4, fat (e.g., animal fats or vegetable oils) is used as a concentrated source of energy/calories in a diet. Fats also assist in the absorption of fat-soluble vitamins, in addition to improving the handling qualities, palatability, and pellet quality of a feed. Poultry physiology can absorb fats without expending energy; therefore, substituting carbohydrate calories with fat calories is occasionally done in the warmer weather months to alleviate poultry from feeling over-heated.

Fatty acids in the diet of a laying hen can impact the fatty acid content in the yolk of an egg.[12] High levels of omega-3 fatty acids can be found in flaxseed, camelina, and fish meal; if these are in the diet, they can be packaged into the egg by the laying hen.

Saturated fats are solids, and unsaturated fats are liquid when at room temperature. Table 57.3 lists the types of fats that can be used in poultry diets. It is important to note that vegetable oils are not cost-efficient, so including these in poultry diets is not economical.

Poultry must have fat in their diet to absorb the fat-soluble vitamins A, D, E, and

K. Additionally, fat is added to poultry feed to reduce grain dust. The addition of fat also improves feed palatability.

It is important for veterinary team members to remember that fats, including those in feed, may become rancid. Although veterinary teams can see this occur any time of the year, the risk of feed going rancid is even greater in the warmer months. To prevent this from occurring, antioxidants are added to poultry diets containing added fat.

Proteins

Protein is important to the overall health of poultry. Protein consumed by poultry is broken down into protein-building blocks (amino acids) through the digestive process. Next, amino acids are absorbed by the blood and transported to cells that convert the individual amino acids into the specific proteins required by the animal. Proteins are used in the formation of body tissues such as muscles, nerves, cartilage, skin, feathers, and beak. Egg white is also high in protein.

There are 22 amino acids commonly found in feed ingredients.[11,12] Eleven of the amino acids are considered essential and must be supplied in the feed. Poultry diets typically contain a variety of feedstuffs to ensure the necessary amino acids are being supplied at the right levels.

Most feed packages show the crude protein percentage in that feed. No information is provided regarding the quality of the protein. Protein quality is based on the presence of the essential amino acids. Methionine and lysine are the two most critical amino acids in poultry. Deficiencies will manifest in a substantial decrease in productivity and the overall health of the flock. Most commercial poultry diets contain methionine and lysine supplements. Due to the supplementation, the feed can contain less total protein; without methionine and lysine supplementation, the feed would need to contain excessive amounts of the other

Table 57.3 Fats used in poultry diets

Saturated fats	Unsaturated fats (usable)	Supplemental fats
Tallow	Corn oil	Animal fat
Lard	Soy oil	Poultry fat
Poultry fat	Canola oil	Yellow fat
Choice white grease		

amino acids to meet the methionine and lysine requirements.

Protein sources in poultry diets are mainly plant proteins: soybean meal, canola meal, corn gluten meal, etc. Animal proteins include fishmeal, meat meal, and bone meal.

Minerals

Minerals are needed in the body for

- bone formation
- formation of blood cells
- blood clotting
- enzyme activation
- energy metabolism
- proper muscle function.

It is necessary for poultry to have higher levels of macrominerals and lower levels of microminerals in their diets. Microminerals include copper, iodine, iron, manganese, selenium, and zinc, and these minerals perform essential roles in the body's metabolism. Macrominerals are calcium, phosphorus, chlorine, magnesium, potassium, and sodium. Calcium is important for proper bone formation and eggshell quality along with blood clot formation and muscle contraction. Phosphorus is important in bone development, cell membrane composition, and aids in numerous metabolic functions.

Poultry feed grains are low in minerals, so mineral supplements are needed. Examples include limestone or oyster shells for calcium and dicalcium phosphate for phosphorus and calcium. Typically, microminerals are provided in a mineral premix.

Vitamins

Vitamins are essential for normal body function, growth, and reproduction. Although poultry require vitamins in small quantities, a deficiency of one or more vitamins can result in various diseases or syndromes. Vitamins are divided into two categories: fat-soluble and water-soluble. The fat-soluble vitamins are A, D, E, and K. The water-soluble vitamins include vitamin C and B vitamins. No dietary requirement exists for vitamin C as poultry can synthesize vitamin C.[12] However, if an individual bird or a flock is stressed, vitamin C supplementation has been shown to be of benefit.

Some vitamins are produced by microorganisms in the digestive tract. When sunlight hits the bird's skin, Vitamin D is produced. Other vitamins must be supplied in the diet because poultry cannot synthesize them. Many essential vitamins are partially supplied by feed ingredients (e.g., alfalfa meal). To offset any fluctuation of vitamin levels found naturally in food and to assure adequate levels of all vitamins, a vitamin premix is recommended.

References

1 Rupley, A.E. (1997). *Manual of Avian Practice*. Philadelphia, PA: Saunders.

2 Burns, K.M. (2021). Avian nutrition: it's for the birds. *Today's Veterinary Nurse* 14–17.

3 Burns, K.M. (2022). Avian, exotics, and rodents. In: *Textbook for the Veterinary Assistant*. 2nd (eds. K.M. Burns and L. Renda-Francis) Ames, IA: Wiley Blackwell.

4 Kollias, G.V. and Kollias, H.W. (2010). Feeding passerine and psittacine birds. In: *Small Animal Clinical Nutrition*, 5th (ed.

M.S. Hand, C.D. Thatcher, R.L. Remillard, et al.), 1255–1269. Mark Morris Institute. Topeka, KS.

5 Orosz SE (2007) Formulated diets in avian nutrition. September 2007. http://lafebervet .com/avian-medicine-2/avian-nutrition (last accessed 5/03/2023).

6 Tully, T. (2009). Birds. In: *Manual of Exotic Pet Practice* (ed. M. Mitchell and T. Tully), 250–298. St Louis MO: Saunders Elsevier.

7 Hess L (2009) The nutritional content of pet bird diets. October. http://lafebervet.com/avian-medicine-2/avian-nutrition (last accessed 5/03/2023).

8 Macwhirter, P. (2009). Basic anatomy, physiology, and nutrition. In: *Handbook of Avian Medicine*, 2nd (ed. T. Tully, G.M. Dorrestein, and A.K. Jones), 25–55. St Louis MO: Saunders Elsevier.

9 Brue, R.N. (1994). Nutrition. In: *Avian Medicine: Principles and Application* (ed. B. Ritchie, G. Harrison, and L. Harrison), 70–85. Lake Worth, FL: Wingers.

10 McDonald, D. (2006). Nutritional considerations: Section I: nutrition and dietary supplementation. In: *Clinical Avian Medicine*, vol. **1** (ed. G.J. Harrison and T.L. Lightfoot), 85–107. Palm Beach, FL: Spix Publishing.

11 Korver, D. (2023). Nutritional requirements of poultry. *Merck Veterinary Manual.* https://www.merckvetmanual.com/poultry/nutrition-and-management-poultry/nutritional-requirements-of-poultry accessed June 2023.

12 Jacob J. Basic Poultry Nutrition. Small and Backyard Poultry. https://poultry.extension.org/articles/feeds-and-feeding-of-poultry/basic-poultry-nutrition/ Accessed May 22, 2023.

58

Small Pet Mammals and Reptiles

Small mammals are extremely popular pets that are brought to veterinary hospitals for advice about proper care, including nutritional management, husbandry, and treatment of medical disorders. As with the other species we have discussed in this book, each species of small mammals presents its own unique nutritional challenges. Nutritional management of ferrets, rabbits, guinea pigs, and other small mammals should be dependent upon lifestage, level of physical activity, and state of health. Pet parents of small mammals will need information about proper feeding to meet the needs of maintenance, growth, reproduction, or stress. Disorders may result in these mammals due to an improper diet or poor husbandry.

Nutritional Assessment

Nutritional management begins with assessment of the pet, the animal's food, and the method of feeding. From this assessment, the healthcare team can begin to formulate a feeding plan. The nutritional assessment is similar to that performed in other species. It begins with a detailed history of the animal, a nutritional history, husbandry practices, and the animal's environment. A systematic physical examination should be performed and the body condition score (BCS) and pets' weight recorded. The five-point BCS system appears to be most useful in assessing the BCS in small mammals. BCS is a qualitative assessment of body fat and muscle. BCS should be performed at every visit and documented in the medical record. With small mammals, husbandry, diet, and/or disease may lead to loss of body fat and is suggestive of starvation. Excessive loss of muscle is indicative of advanced starvation, forced inactivity, or altered metabolic states.

Ferrets

Ferrets are popular pets because of their low maintenance needs, their relatively small size, and their fun inquisitive nature. Ferrets are strict carnivores that have a very short, simple gastrointestinal (GI) tract. Ferrets' GI tract lacks a cecum and ileocolic valve. Because of their shorter GI tract, ferrets' GI transit time is rapid – approximately 3–6 hours. Highly digestible foods containing large amounts of protein and fat should be offered. Also, the nutritional make-up should include minimal digestible (soluble) carbohydrate and fiber.[1,2]

Ferrets are obligate carnivores, and as with other carnivorous species, young ferrets imprint on food by smell and develop strong food preferences by the time they are a few months old. Consequently, ferrets should be exposed to a variety of food tastes, textures, and smells. Also, providing exposure to various protein sources as juveniles will assist in diet flexibility as an adult. This can be extremely helpful when ferrets experience medical conditions that may require restricted or altered diets at an older age.[3]

Nutrition and Disease Management for Veterinary Technicians and Nurses, Third Edition. Ann Wortinger and Kara M. Burns.
© 2024 John Wiley & Sons, Inc. Published 2024 by John Wiley & Sons, Inc.
Companion Website: www.wiley.com/go/wortinger/3e

Foods with higher animal fat for energy, higher amounts of good-quality meat (not plant) protein, and minimal carbohydrate and fiber are recommended for ferrets. Whole-prey diets are appropriate, but owners typically do not want to feed a whole prey diet. In the United States, dry kibble is commonly the diet fed to ferrets. Usually, dry foods are recommended for ferrets because they are more energy-efficient, cost less, and are easier to store and feed than moist foods or whole prey diets. Healthcare team members should familiarize themselves with the ingredients listed on the package and be prepared to educate owners. The crude protein should be 30–35% DMB and composed primarily of high-quality meat sources, and the fat content should be 15–20% DMB. Growing kits need 35% protein DMB and 20% fat DMB, and lactating females require 20% DMB fat and twice the calories of the nonpregnant ferret.[2]

Ferrets find commercial grocery store cat foods very palatable due to the coating on the kibble. This coating is made from animal fat and digest. However, these foods may not be nutritionally adequate for the various life stages. Minimally stressed ferrets may live on these foods for years, but nutritional deficiencies may occur, especially in breeding animals.[2] Pelleted ferret food is the preferred diet, although premium dry kitten food is generally acceptable for meeting the ferret's nutritional requirements for growth and reproduction. Moist/canned food as the major part of the diet should be avoided as ferrets most likely are not able to consume enough protein and fat on a dry matter basis (DMB).[1]

The specific amino acid requirements for ferrets are not known, but the assumption is that the requirements are similar to those of cats. It should be noted that strict carnivores need high biologic value proteins. Therefore, nutritional protein for ferrets should come from animal-based ingredients.

As discussed, ferrets do well when eating commercial foods containing 15–20% DMB fat.[2,3] Ferrets are assumed to require linoleic and arachidonic acids in their diets. Linoleic acid is abundant in vegetable oils. Arachidonic acids are found in animal-based ingredients. Fatty acid requirements should be met by providing meat-based commercial cat or mink foods.

It is believed that ferrets do not have dietary requirement for carbohydrates, including fiber, as is seen in other obligate carnivores. Glucose is provided by hepatic gluconeogenesis, using amino acids. Dietary fiber is considered to be a factor in weight control and reduction. It is also considered to play a role in certain specific GI disorders. The short digestive tract of ferrets dictates hydrolysis of most dietary fuels, with little or no hindgut fermentation of fiber. The intestinal tract of ferrets is relatively deficient in brush-border enzymes, therefore creating an inability to absorb calories from carbohydrates.[1,2] As a rule, foods with additional fiber should not be fed to healthy or lactating ferrets or young kits. Additional fiber may be considered in ferrets with fiber-responsive disorders.

It is highly recommended to offer a ferret a variety of food items throughout life. This may include a minimum of weekly whole-prey foods, daily high-quality ferret kibble, and small amounts of high-quality canned cat food or other meat-based treats fed two to three times a week. This variety would be mentally enriching for the ferret. Ferrets are intelligent animals and will need environmental enrichment to keep them stimulated.

This feeding strategy would also increase the variety of the ferret's diet preferences.

Starving a ferret for longer than 3 hours should not be recommended due to their short GI tract and the short GI transit time. In the United States, many ferrets over 2 years of age are likely to develop insulinoma. Fasting a ferret with an insulinoma for more than 3 hours could result in a serious hypoglycemic condition.[1,3,4]

Clean, fresh water should always be available. The best method for watering ferrets is with a sipper bottle or a heavy crock-type bowl. Ferrets are fun-loving animals, and they especially love to play in the water, so the healthcare team must educate owners to provide bowls that are not easy to tip over.

Rabbits

Rabbits are popular pets because they are small, relatively easy to care for, fastidious, quiet-mannered, and can be litter-box trained. Two pair of upper incisor teeth differentiates lagomorphs from rodents. The smaller, second upper incisors (peg teeth) are found behind the first. These peg teeth lack a cutting edge. Rabbit teeth are hypsodont. Malocclusion and overgrowth commonly occur with the incisor teeth as these can grow 10–12 cm a year during the course of the rabbits' life. Rabbit teeth are developed for a high-fiber, herbivorous diet.[1,5] Rabbits are herbivorous hindgut fermenters and have a GI system similar to that in horses.[6] The rabbits' GI tract consists of a noncompartmentalized stomach and a large cecum. The simple stomach has thin walls and indistinctly separated glandular and nonglandular areas. It is important to note with owners that rabbits are unable to vomit due to a well-developed cardiac sphincter.

Nutritional management of a rabbit should provide sufficient fiber to support normal GI motility as well as to ensure sufficient amounts and types of digestible nutrients are available to the cecal microflora for fermentation. Rabbits also need enrichment, and thus the diet should stimulate normal foraging behavior throughout the day (Figure 58.1).

Rabbits derive amino acids directly from the foods they ingest, as well as from cecotrophs. Essential amino acids in the rabbit include arginine, glycine, histidine, isoleucine, leucine, lysine, methionine, phenylalanine, threonine, tryptophan, and valine. Grasses tend to contain limited amounts of methionine and isoleucine; however, they are abundant in arginine, glutamine, and lysine. Synthetic amino acids are regularly added to commercial mixes for

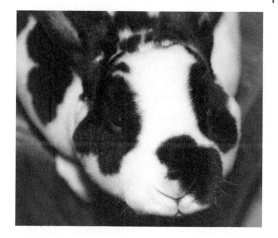

Figure 58.1 Rex rabbit (exhibiting Broken Rex color pattern). (Reproduced with permission from Kara M. Burns, LVT, VTS (Nutrition).)

rabbits as these cereals are often low in methionine and lysine. Conversely, legumes are high in lysine and may be used to balance low lysine levels in cereal-based diets. Rabbits have the ability to digest forage-based protein because of the increase in protein digestibility that occurs as a result of cecotrophy. An appropriate protein level for pet rabbits is 12–16% DMB. For lactating does, the level may increase to 18–19% protein DMB.

Although simple sugars and starches can be used for providing energy, excessive levels of these should not be fed. Lagomorphs have a rapid gut transit time, resulting in starch and simple sugars not being completely digested in the small intestine. These are then directed into the cecum, where they may be used for fermentation by the cecal microorganisms. Carbohydrate overload in the cecum predisposes to enterotoxemia, especially in young animals. Low-energy grains such as oats are recommended for the rabbits' diet as opposed to corn or wheat. Care should be taken to not process the grains too finely.

Fiber is an essential nutrient for the maintenance of GI health. Fiber also helps promote normal dental attrition and encourages normal foraging behavior, thus decreasing the potential for behavioral issues. The digestion of fiber in rabbits overall is poor; however, indigestible fiber is essential for stimulating gut motility and helping control gut transit time. Manufacturing processes play a role in the digestibility of commercial rabbit foods. For example, the finer the grinding, the longer the gut transit and cecal retention times, which lead to greater potential for cecal dysbiosis.[5,7]

In the dietary management of rabbits, balance must be established between providing enough indigestible fiber to maintain normal motility, cell regeneration, secretion, absorption, and excretion, while simultaneously providing enough digestible fiber for sufficient bacterial fermentation in the gut. The total dietary fiber levels recommended for pet rabbits is 20–25% DMB. Healthcare team members should educate owners to provide an ad libitum source of indigestible fiber (e.g., grass and/or hay). Also, owners should ensure the amounts of other dietary components are limited. This will ensure that the rabbit eats the primary fiber source. Commercial foods used as a portion of the diet should preferably have a crude fiber content of >18% DMB, with indigestible fiber at >12.5% DMB.

Fat provides another source of energy and increases palatability. Fat also decreases dustiness and crumbling of commercially manufactured pellets. As with other species, rabbits are prone to obesity. Rabbits are also at risk for hepatic lipidosis. Consequently, high-fat diets must be avoided. The recommended level of fat for rabbits is 2.5–4% DMB.

In the nutritional management of rabbits, vitamins A, D, and E are important and should be part of the dietary make-up. Gut bacteria synthesize B vitamins in sufficient quantities. So, adding B vitamins to commercial foods may be unnecessary. Vitamin K synthesis in the gut is not as efficient. Therefore, vitamin K is often added to the commercial formulation by the rabbit food manufacturer. Vitamins A and E are readily destroyed by oxidation, so it is imperative that food preparation and storage methods prevent losses from excess light or heat. The recommendation is to store rabbit feed at 15°C (60°F) and feed within 90 days of milling.[8] If the food comprises more than 30% alfalfa meal, there should be sufficient vitamin A in the form of the precursor b-carotene. However, if the alfalfa is over a year post harvest, vitamin A deficiency can occur. Vitamin recommendations for pet rabbits include[1,9]

- 7000 to 18,000 IU vitamin A/kg food
- 40–70 mg vitamin E/kg food
- 2 mg vitamin K/kg food.

The role of calcium regulation and vitamin D differs in rabbits than in other species. The presence of vitamin D is not required for the intestinal absorption of calcium. Vitamin D is important for the metabolism of phosphorus. Vitamin D deficiencies can lead to hypophosphatemia and osteomalacia[1,5,9]. Husbandry education should include cage placement as sunlight is necessary for endogenous synthesis of vitamin D in rabbits. Commercially prepared rabbit pellets are supplemented with vitamin D. For pet rabbits, a level of 800 to 1200 IU/kg is recommended.[1,9]

Guinea Pigs

Guinea pigs are herbivores with simple stomachs. The teeth of guinea pigs are open-rooted and erupt continuously. Unlike other rodents which typically have yellow incisors, a distinguishing factor of guinea pigs is white incisors. The guinea pig's digestive tract is long and has a gastric emptying time of roughly 2 hours. The total GI transit time ranges from 8 to 20 hours. The normal flora found in the GI tract includes mainly lactobacillus and occasionally *Streptococcus spp.*, yeast, and soil bacteria. The majority of the digestive process happens in the cecum. The cecum of a guinea pig is a thin-walled sac divided into several lateral pouches by smooth muscle bands (taenia coli). The cecum is normally found on the central and left side of the abdomen and may contain as much as 65% of the GI contents.[1,10]

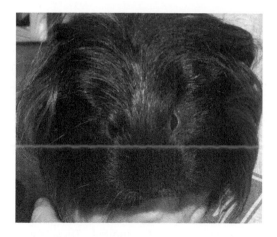

Figure 58.2 Silkie breed of Cavy. (Reproduced with permission from Kara M. Burns, LVT, VTS (Nutrition).)

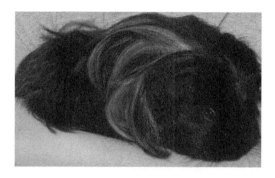

Figure 58.3 Silkie breed of Cavy – young adult. (Reproduced with permission from Kara M. Burns, LVT, VTS (Nutrition).)

Guinea pigs exhibit coprophagous behavior, a fact which is important to educate owners (Figures 58.2 and 58.3).

Guinea pigs do not like change. Guinea pigs develop dietary preferences early in life and do not adjust readily to changes in type, appearance, or presentation of their food or water. Guinea pig owners are encouraged to expose their pets to small amounts of different foods and vegetables while they are young. This will help the guinea pig accept variety in their feedstuffs. This reluctance to change can be a dangerous characteristic of guinea pigs; thus, it is important to educate owners to be cognizant of this fact and to gradually transition guinea pigs if introducing something new in the diet. Client education will hopefully prevent a self-imposed fast by a pet guinea pig that is fed new food.

A crude protein level of 18–20% DMB is sufficient for growth and lactation. The recommended minimum level of the crude fiber is 10% DMB.

Guinea pigs require a dietary source of vitamin C (ascorbic acid) because they lack the enzyme involved in synthesizing glucose to ascorbic acid. This enzyme is l-gulonolactone oxidase. Nonbreeding adult guinea pigs require 10 mg/kg daily of ascorbic acid with higher levels needed for growing and pregnant animals; 30 mg/kg daily is recommended during pregnancy.

The recommended diet for pet guinea pigs consists of guinea pig pellets and grass hay, supplemented with fresh vegetables.[11] Good-quality grass hay should be available at all times. A variety of leafy greens can be offered in handfuls, as guinea pigs like greens. Remember to advise owners to wash and prepare fresh food. Also, it is important to advise owners that fresh foods should not be left in the cage and should be removed after a few hours if not eaten. Fruits, rolled oats, and dry cereals should be offered only in very small quantities, if at all, as treats.[1,10,11] Any additions or changes to the diet should be made gradually.

Commercially prepared guinea pig foods typically contain 18–20% DMB crude protein and 10–16% DMB fiber. Pellets are fortified with ascorbic acid; but almost half of the initial vitamin C content may be oxidized and lost 90 days after the diet has been mixed and stored at 22 °C. Many commercially prepared guinea pig diets are now available with stabilized vitamin C, and these diets should be stored in a cool, dry area (<70 °F (22 °C)). Foods can be refrigerated or frozen but should be protected from condensation and increased storage temperature and humidity in vegetables and fruits or in the drinking water. Foods with higher levels of ascorbic acid are

- red and green peppers
- broccoli
- tomatoes
- kiwi fruit
- oranges.

Many types of leafy greens (kale, parsley, beet greens, chicory, and spinach) are high in vitamin C, but many contain high levels of calcium or oxalates; these should be offered in only small amounts. Vitamin C can be added to the water at 1 g/l. In an open container, water with added vitamin C loses more than 50% of its vitamin C content in 24 hours. Water must be changed daily to ensure adequate activity of the vitamin.

Other Small Mammals

Hamsters, gerbils, mice, and rats naturally hoard food items. Therefore, it is difficult to determine truly how much food is actually being ingested. Education of owners must include information on the natural hoarding tendencies of rodents. Although owners need to be aware when the food dish of these small mammals is empty, consistently filling the bowl may result in obese small mammals.

Most rodents are omnivorous, often eating grasses, seeds, grain, and occasionally invertebrates in the wild.[12,13] Dietary requirements of species in laboratory settings are well-established. However, for pet small mammals, needs are best met with a formulated diet supplemented with small amounts of fresh foods and seeds for variety and interest. Seed mixtures are popular choices for small mammals; however, seed mixtures regularly lead to selective feeding. A nutritional imbalance can result from small mammals eating high-calorie seeds (sunflower) while ignoring the formulated pellets. Many rodents have a short life span, so determining a nutritional deficiency is rare. The most common form of malnutrition in rats is obesity. Studies show an increase in length of life as well as a decrease in certain disease conditions in rats fed a calorie-restricted diet.[14] Gerbils exhibit sensitivity to high-fat, high-cholesterol diets, resulting in changes in the gerbils' levels of blood cholesterol.

Formulated pelleted diets for laboratory rodents are convenient and nutritionally balanced diets for early life and reproduction. However, laboratory rodent diets are relatively high in fat and low in fiber, and when provided ad libitum, they cause obesity. Consequently, the amount of pelleted diet owners provide daily should be limited. Diets formulated specifically for pet rodents are now commercially available. Owners should supplement their pet's diet with feeds high in fiber such as vegetables, limited amounts of fruit, and occasional treats.

Protein requirements for rodents range from 14% to 17% DMB in hamsters, from 14% to 16% DMB in rats and mice, and up to 22% DMB in gerbils.[12,13] Nutritional management of hamsters, rats, mice, and gerbils should ensure these ranges are followed. Nutritional management of reproducing small mammals should contain higher levels of protein.

Hedgehogs are primarily insectivorous. Insects frequently eaten by free-ranging animals include beetles, caterpillars, earwigs, flies, and centipedes. However, hedgehogs can be more omnivorous and somewhat opportunistic in their feeding behavior; thus, the diet may also include snails and slugs, earthworms, woodlice, mollusks, and sometimes small vertebrates like frogs, toads, snakes, birds, and their eggs, as well as small mammals in the form of carrion.

Most captive adult diets consist of a protein source such as meat-based dry or canned cat or dog/puppy food, which should be free of gravy, and/or a formulated hedgehog food. Some rehabilitators add a commercially available diet for insect-eating songbirds. Some rehabilitators also mix the protein source with a small amount of crushed, unsweetened cereal (oat, bran, moistened muesli, or whole grain wheat). The diet may also be supplemented with a multivitamin and/or even a pancreatic enzyme supplement to aid digestion and promote a more rapid build-up of body reserves, particularly in underweight juveniles. It is recommended to offer food once or twice a day to most adults. It is suggested that a once a day feeding, offered in the evening to these nocturnal animals, may reduce the risk of obesity in healthy animals.

Treats can include fresh fruit such as banana, raisins and sultanas, dry cat, or hedgehog kibble, unsweetened crushed "digestive biscuits" (hard, cereal-based treats), or small amounts of cooked chicken. Hedgehogs cannot digest lactose and therefore should never be offered cow's milk.

The ideal diet is a commercially prepared hedgehog food. If hedgehog food is not used, premium food for less active cats or dog food are alternatives. Food should be rationed to prevent obesity. In addition to the main diet, ~1–2 tsp (5–10 ml) of varied moist foods and/or invertebrate prey (e.g., canned cat or dog food, cooked meat or egg, low-fat cottage cheese, mealworms, earthworms, waxworms, and gut-loaded crickets) and ~1 tsp (5 ml) of vegetable/fruit mix (e.g., beans, cooked carrots, squash, peas, tomatoes, leafy greens, banana, grape, apple, pear, and berries) should also be provided daily.

Sugar gliders are highly social and are best housed in pairs or small groups. Sugar gliders have a great sense of smell to locate food. Free-ranging gliders feed on insects, larvae, arachnids, and small vertebrates during the spring and summer. Additionally, they will eat invertebrates as a source of protein. Plant products such as sap, blossoms, and nectar make up the bulk of the diet during the autumn and the winter wet season. They are hindgut fermenters and retain a well-developed cecum that uses bacterial fermentation to break down complex polysaccharides contained in gum. There are a number of captive diets recommended for gliders. Additionally, there are recipes for sugar gliders if the owner would like to make the food for their pet.

Chinchillas' natural diet consists of grasses, cactus fruits, dry roots and tubers, as well as the bark and leaves of small shrubs and bushes. Chinchillas' food items are high in dietary fiber, with minor amounts of fat, sugar, or protein. The digestive system of chinchillas is perfectly adapted to these nourishments, and the long intestine guarantees an optimal utilization of the sparse food.[15]

Chinchillas have a high requirement for dietary fiber; thus, captive chinchillas should be fed a high-fiber diet, but low in protein, sugar, and fat. The bulk of the diet should consist of high-quality grass hay. The hay must always be freely available, dry, and free of odor, mold, or dust.[16,17] High-fiber chinchilla food or rabbit pellets, ~15–30 ml (1–2 tsp) per animal per day, can be offered along with dried herbs. Small quantities of fresh vegetables can also be fed.

The digestive system of the chinchilla is perfectly adapted to extract energy and nutrients from a barren food supply, thus leaving captive chinchillas at risk for obesity and hepatic lipidosis.[17] Educate clients to **not** feed high-fat foods, like nuts and seeds, or foods rich in sugar, like fruits (e.g., raisins). Like rabbits and guinea pigs, chinchillas produce two types of fecal pellets: one nitrogen-rich intended for cecotrophy and one nitrogen-poor delivered as fecal pellets.

Water has to be freely available. In the wild, chinchillas nibble rain drops from leaves or stones, either water bowls or water bottles are suitable and have different advantages. While water intake is larger from bowls, which may reduce the risk for urolithiasis,[18] water in bottles stays clean longer.

As with other species, water is extremely important and should be discussed with small mammal owners. Fresh, clean water should be provided. Typically, water bottles are used as these help prevent bedding from getting wet and are often preferred by small mammals. However, with time, water bottles may become clogged or start to leak. It is best for the healthcare team to educate owners to change water and test water bottles every day.

Reptiles

It is recommended that the healthcare team always consult a comprehensive reference for feeding guidelines in specific species, as species variations are considerable when speaking of reptiles. Species specific inadequacies in diet and nutrition can cause a multitude of disease conditions in reptiles. Owner education regarding the proper diet needed to provide for a healthy long life is a must when dealing with a reptile patient. Husbandry plays a huge role in the health and prevention of nutrition-related disorders. Dietary deficiencies are not commonly seen in snakes, which eat a whole animal diet; however, a variety of dietary deficiencies are commonly seen in lizards, turtles, and crocodiles. One of the most common is metabolic bone disease, which is caused by inappropriately low calcium intake, low vitamin D3 intake, or excessive phosphorus intake. This disease may be prevented by feeding a suitable diet and by exposing the animal to ultraviolet (UV) light, either naturally or artificially. It is essential that reptiles, especially lizards, have full spectrum lighting available during normal daylight hours. Animals with metabolic bone disease must be treated very gently because their bones are subject to pathologic fracture. Vitamin A deficiency is commonly seen in turtles and tortoises and usually manifests as an overgrown beak, palpebral edema, and conjunctivitis (Figure 58.4).

The feeding of lizards is dependent upon the species. Herbivores should be fed a variety of dark leafy greens and vegetables. Insectivores will eat meal worms, crickets, etc. Carnivorous lizard species should be fed prey consisting of the bones, contents of the GI tract, muscle, and fur. Lizards that fall into the omnivore family should be fed dark leafy greens and insects. It is important to remind reptile owners not

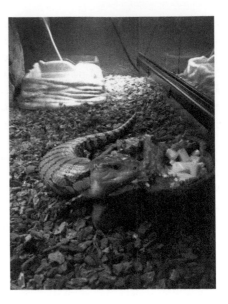

Figure 58.4 Blue tongue skink cage and nutrition example. (© Kara M. Burns.)

to feed the same foods every day – reptiles prefer variety. Many captive lizards are omnivores and will eat mealworms, crickets, grasshoppers, and waxworms. Most insects are calcium-deficient; so, to improve nutritional composition, lizards should be fed a nutritionally supplemented diet. Lizards in the wild are primarily carnivores, eating invertebrate or vertebrate prey. In general, captive lizards require vitamin and mineral supplementation with an emphasis on a variety of food. Juvenile lizards should be fed 1 to 2 times a day, with adults requiring feeding 2 to 3 times per week. Most lizards are diurnal and require day feedings and time to bask in natural or ultraviolet light.

Herbivorous lizards, such as the green iguana, require a varied diet to ensure adequate nutritional balance. Recommended diets for herbivores include leafy greens (e.g., romaine lettuce and collard greens), mustard greens, and clover. Vegetables, including green beans, okra, carrots, and squash, are also adequate dietary substances. It is important to note that certain vegetables, such as spinach, cabbage, peas, and potatoes, contain substances that bind calcium and other trace minerals, inhibiting their absorption.

Commercial iguana food is available to provide a base diet for these animals. Commercial diets do not require additional supplementation if the captive lizard is fed a diet based primarily on such purchased food. Homemade diets of vegetables and fruit should always be supplemented with appropriate vitamins and minerals. Technicians can advise lizard owners to purchase a quality reptile vitamin, containing vitamin D3, to be administered 1 to 2 times a week if a good diet is provided. Common iguanas also require protein for normal growth and development. Juvenile iguanas in captivity generally need more protein and calcium than do adults. Common protein sources include dark green leafy vegetables such as collards, turnip greens, kale, bok choy, and broccoli with leaves. Iguanas should never be fed a meat-based diet or any commercial food other than iguana food. Do not feed commercial dog or cat food, as this will cause renal disease and death.

Snakes are carnivores, and they feed on whole prey. Eating the entire prey allows for added nutrients such as calcium. Snakes will defecate the parts of the prey they do not use. As mentioned, supplementation is typically not necessary when feeding whole prey such as rats and mice.

Water should be provided in a bowl for bathing and drinking. Note that some lizards (e.g., chameleons) will drink water only if it is in the form of droplets on plant leaves, similar to dew. Therefore, it is important to spray or mist the animal's enclosure several times a day. In addition, most lizards should be sprayed with water or allowed to bathe to prevent skin problems associated with low humidity.

Aquatic turtles are omnivorous and will eat fish, algae, leafy greens, etc. There are commercial foods available for aquatic turtles and should be fed in moderation. Educate turtle owners to ensure these commercial foods have essential nutrients needed for aquatic turtles. Any food items with animal proteins should **NOT** be fed to aquatic turtles.

References

1 James, W., Carpenter, J.W., Wolf, K.N., and Kolmstetter, C. (2010). Feeding small pet mammals. In: *Small Animal Clinical Nutrition*, 5th (ed. M.S. Hand, C.D. Thatcher, R.L. Remillard, et al.), 1215–1236. Mark Morris Institute., Topeka, KS.

2 Bell, J.A. (1999). Ferret nutrition. *Veterinary Clinics of North America: Exotic Animal Practice* 2: 169–192.

3 Powers, L.V. and Brown, S.A. (2012). Basic anatomy, physiology, and husbandry. In: *Ferrets, Rabbits, and Rodents*, 3e (ed. K. Quesenberry and J. Carpenter), 340–353. St Louis, MO: Saunders.

4 Wolf, T.M. (2008). Ferrets. In: *Manual of Exotic Pet Practice* (ed. M. Mitchell and T. Tully), 346–375. St Louis, MO: W.B. Saunders.

5 Campbell-Ward, M.L. (2012). Gastrointestinal physiology and nutrition. In: *Ferrets, Rabbits, and Rodents*, 3e (ed. K. Quesenberry and J. Carpenter), 232–244. St Louis, MO; Saunders.

6 Cheeke, P.R. (1994). Nutrition and nutritional diseases. In: *The Biology of the Laboratory Rabbit*, 2e (ed. P.J. Manning, D.H. Ringler, and C.E. Newcomer), 321–335. New York: Academic Press.

7 Pinheiro, V., Guedes, C.M., Outor-Monteiro, D. et al. (2009). Effects of fibre level and dietary mannanoligosaccharides on digestibility, caecal volatile fatty acids and performances of growing rabbits. *Animal Feed Science and Technology* 148: 288–300.

8 Brooks, D.L. (2004). Nutrition and gastrointestinal physiology. In: *Ferrets, Rabbits and Rodents: Clinical Medicine and Surgery*, 2e

(ed. K.E. Quesenberry and J.W. Carpenter), 155–160. St Louis, MO: W.B. Saunders.

9 Harcourt-Brown, F.M. (2002). *Textbook of Rabbit Medicine*. Edinburgh: Butterworth-Heinemann.

10 Quesenberry, K.E., Donnelly, T.M., and Mans, C. (2012). Biology, husbandry, and clinical techniques of guinea pigs and chinchillas. In: *Ferrets, Rabbits, and Rodents*, 3e (ed. K. Quesenberry and J. Carpenter), 280–294. St Louis, MO; Saunders.

11 Riggs, S.M. (2008). Guinea pigs. In: *Manual of Exotic Pet Practice* (ed. M. Mitchell and T. Tully), 457–474. St Louis, MO: W.B. Saunders.

12 Lennox, A.M. and Bauck, L. (2012). Basic anatomy, physiology, husbandry, and clinical techniques. In: *Ferrets, Rabbits, and Rodents*, 3e (ed. K. Quesenberry and J. Carpenter), 340–353. St Louis, MO; Saunders.

13 Keeble, E. (2009). Rodents: biology and husbandry. In: *BSAVA Manual of Rodents and Ferrets* (ed. E. Keeble and A. Meredith), 1–17. Gloucester, UK: British Small Animal Veterinary Association.

14 Masoro, E.J. (2009). Caloric restriction-induced life extension of rats and mice: a critique of proposed mechanisms. *Biochimica et Biophysica Acta* **1790** (10): 1040–1048.

15 Kohles, M. (2014). Gastrointestinal anatomy and physiology of select exotic companion mammals. *Veterinary Clinics of North America: Exotic Animal Practice* **17** (2): 165–178.

16 Wolf, P., Schröder, A., Wenger, A., and Kamphues, J. (2003). The nutrition of the chinchilla as a companion animal – basic data, influences and dependences. *Journal of Animal Physiology and Animal Nutrition (Berl)* **87** (3, 4): 129–133.

17 Pollock C, Parmentier S. Basic information sheet: Chinchilla. January 24, 2019. LafeberVet Web site. https://lafeber.com/vet/basic-information-for-chinchillas/ Accessed 5/2023.

18 Hagen, K., Clauss, M., and Hatt, J.M. (2014). Drinking preferences in chinchillas (*Chinchilla laniger*), degus (*Octodon degu*) and guinea pigs (*Cavia porcellus*). *Journal of Animal Physiology and Animal Nutrition (Berl)* **98** (5): 942–947.

59

Equine

Feeding the precise amount and finding the correct balance of nutrients is important to the overall health and wellbeing of horses. Today, horses are domesticated and considered companion animals. Companion horses today consume a variety of feeds ranging in physical form from forage with a high content of moisture to cereals with a high amount of starch; and from hay in the form of physically long fibrous stems to salt licks and water. Horses are nonruminant herbivores that naturally spend 60–75% of their day grazing. Typically, they ingest approximately 2% of their body weight (dry matter basis) per day while grazing (Figure 59.1).[1-7]

Domesticating horses has resulted in adaptations in feed, feeding times, and feeding methods – similar to domesticated cats and dogs – where the horse is "meal-fed" and materials such as starchy cereals, protein concentrates, and dried forages have been introduced. Companion horses are confined more of the time in stalls or smaller pastures, are typically fed only 1–2 times per day, and spend less time of the day (approximately 40%) eating.

The diets formulated for horses contain on average 5% fat and 7–12% protein, with carbohydrate being the major source of energy (~80%). This is a result of the evolution of horses to eating grass and other forages. Grasses and hays provide a strong foundation for the feeding of horses. Protein is essential to the maintenance and replacement of tissues but is sometimes considered to be an expensive source of energy; however, dietary protein and fat can contribute to meeting the physiological energy demands of the horse. Protein converts the carbon chain of amino acids to intermediary acids and some of the carbon chains to glucose. Fat can aid in meeting energy demands following its hydrolysis to glycerol and fatty acids. Subsequently, the glycerol can be converted to glucose, and the fatty acid chain can be broken down by a stepwise process called ß oxidation in the mitochondria which yields adenosine triphosphate (ATP) and acetate or acetyl coenzyme A and requiring tissue oxygen.[1-7]

Carbohydrate digestion and fermentation yield mostly glucose and acetic, propionic, and butyric volatile fatty acids. The portal venous system collects these nutrients, and a proportion of them are removed from the blood as they pass through the liver. Both propionate and glucose contribute to glycogen (liver starch) reserves, and acetate and butyrate bolster the fat pool and comprise primary energy sources for many tissues.

Nutritional Physiology

Multiple compartments make up the digestive tract of the horse and therefore, the nutritional physiology of cats and dogs differs significantly from that of the horse. Each compartment has

Nutrition and Disease Management for Veterinary Technicians and Nurses, Third Edition. Ann Wortinger and Kara M. Burns.
© 2024 John Wiley & Sons, Inc. Published 2024 by John Wiley & Sons, Inc.
Companion Website: www.wiley.com/go/wortinger/3e

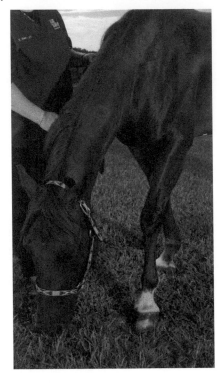

Figure 59.1 American quarter horse grazing.

its own function in terms of utilizing ingested feed. The oral cavity is responsible for physically processing foods into smaller particles (~1.6 mm). This allows for passage through the esophagus and increases the surface area for the small intestine enzymatic action. The oral cavity also breaks down structural carbohydrate for bacterial fermentation in the large intestine. Horses chew an average of 60,000 times per day. It is only during chewing that the salivation process is activated. Given the increased chewing in the equine species, a horse will average 5–10 l per day of saliva, which in turn acts as a lubricant for passage into the esophagus.[3-5]

The stomach is responsible for ~8% of the total capacity of the equine GI tract. The stomach's retention time can range from 2 to 18 hours. The fundus and the pylorus are the two main regions making up the stomach. The pyloric region secretes 10–30 l of gastric juice per day. The small intestine of the horse is 50–70 ft long and has a volume of 40–50 l. The transit time of the small intestine averages 2–8 hours. Toward the anterior end of the small intestine, pancreatic juice aids in the digestion of lipids, protein, and nonstructural carbohydrates. Microvilli line the small intestine, thus increasing the surface area of the gut. As mentioned earlier, digestion in the small intestine is dependent upon oral processing and types of feed (e.g., forage is less digested than processed feed). The large intestine can hold a large volume (100 l) and has a very slow transit time of approximately 50 hours.[1,2] The large intestine is responsible for the fermentation of structural carbohydrates to volatile fatty acids which are responsible for 50% of the metabolizable energy. Additionally, the large intestine absorbs roughly 80 liters of water per day. B vitamins are produced by the bacteria absorbed in the large intestine. Nonprotein nitrogen is not utilized well in the large intestine.

Key Nutritional Factors for Horses

Water, energy, protein, minerals, and vitamins are the main nutrients with which veterinary healthcare teams should be concerned. Water is the most important nutrient in all mammalian species. Fresh, abundant water should always be available. Horses drink an average of 25 L of water per day. In conditions of extreme heat or stress, the number of liters a horse will drink per day increases to 100.[2] In addition, healthcare team members should remind owners that the more grain their horse ingests, the more water intake the horse will need.

Energy is measured in terms of digestible energy (DE) and fed in kilocalories. The amount of DE horses' need will be dependent upon various factors: physiologic state, activity level, environment, and the size of the individual horse. Most of the energy utilized by the horse is from carbohydrates that are ingested through the horses' natural feed. The amount of kcal/kg in various carbohydrate feeds is shown as follows:

Feed	kcal/kg
Oats	3000
Alfalfa (early bloom)	2100
Bermuda grass hay	1800
Corn cobs	1250

As with other species, fat in the diet provides the horse with high density energy. Nevertheless, fat should not exceed 20% of the total equine diet or 30% of the concentrate. Surpassing these levels puts the horse at risk for loose stools and most likely will result in decreased palatability.

The amount of protein in the diet is generally expressed as "crude protein (CP)" and is communicated as % dry matter (DM). Again, the amount of protein needed by an individual horse is dependent upon many factors, including physiologic state, type of diet, age, and quality of diet. The protein quality increases the closer the proportions of each of the various indispensable amino acids in the dietary protein conform to the proportions in the mixture required by the tissues.[3-5]

Calcium and phosphorus are considered together because of their interdependent role as the main elements of the crystal apatite, which provides the building blocks for the skeletal system. The physiologic state of the horse will aid in predicting the calcium requirement of the individual horse. The average adult horse weighing approximately 500 kg will need ~20 g of calcium and 14 g of phosphorus per day. It is important to balance the ratio of calcium to phosphorus, with a mature horse needing a ratio of 1.1 : 1 to 6 : 1. The ratio for a growing horse is recommended to be 1.1 : 1 to 3 : 1.

Sodium is the principal determinant of the osmolarity of extracellular fluid and as a result, the volume of that fluid. Chloride concentration in the extracellular fluid is directly related to that of sodium. Rarely do companion animals have an excess or deficiency of sodium or chloride; however, these are both conditions of which to be watchful. Daily sodium requirements are recommended to be approximately 0.18–0.36% DM. If the requirements for sodium are met, chloride deficiency is rare. Good sources of sodium and chloride can be found in grains with premixture and salt blocks.

Potassium is the main intracellular cation. Deficiencies in equines are rare; excess potassium is not a common problem. However, excess potassium can lead to hyperkalemic periodic paralysis, a syndrome of intermittent weakness in horses accompanied by elevated serum potassium concentration. This syndrome appears to be confined to descendants of the American Quarter Horse. Forages are approximately 1–4% potassium. Cereals are relatively poor sources of potassium.

A trace element needed to aid in antioxidant defense in horses is known as selenium. Selenium forms an integral part of the GSH-Px molecule and catalyzes peroxide detoxification in body tissues at which time reduced glutathione (GSH) is oxidized. It is closely involved with the activity of α-tocopherol (vitamin E), which protects polyunsaturated fatty acids from peroxidation. The requirement is 1–2 mg/day for a 500 kg horse or 0.1–2 ppm. Selenium deficiencies produce pale, weak muscles in foals and a yellowing of the depot fat, known as "White Muscle Disease." It is imperative that pregnant mares receive adequate amounts of selenium in their diet. Selenium is highly toxic to animals, with the minimum toxic dose through continuous intake being 2–5 mg/kg feed. Too much selenium results in skin, coat, and hoof abnormalities.[3-5]

Grazing horses derive their vitamin A from the carotenoid pigments present in herbage. The principal one is β-carotene with 1 mg of β-carotene equating to approximately 400 IU of vitamin A. Horses that graze for 4–6 weeks build up a 3–6 months supply of vitamin A in the liver.

Carotene levels (mg/kg DM) amounts	
Pasture grass/alfalfa	300–600
Good hay	20–40
Poor hay	4–5

Requirements for vitamin A during certain life stages are as follows:

- Mature horses require 30 IU/kg body weight.
- Gestation/lactation stage requires 60 IU/kg body weight.
- Growth stage requires ~50 IU/kg body weight.

Vitamin E functions as a cellular antioxidant in conjunction with vitamin A and is required for normal immune function. Fresh green forage and the germ of cereal grains are rich sources of vitamin E. Adult horses require 80–100 IU/kg DM. Although deficiencies are rare, two neurological disorders of horses have been recognized to involve α-tocopherol status: equine degenerative myeloencephalopathy and equine motor neuron disease. These diseases typically are seen in horses that do not have access to pastures, with the consumption of poor-quality hay, and in horses with low concentrations of circulating levels of α-tocopherol.

Types of Feed

There are three types of feed that are commonly used in the feeding of horses: roughages, concentrates, and complete feeds. Roughages include grasses and forage legumes cut for hay. Most common species of grass are suitable, but the preferred are the more popular and productive grasses such as rye grasses, fescues, timothy, and cocksfoot. Other grasses found in permanent pastures are acceptable as well and include meadow grasses, brome, bent grass, and foxtails. Legumes utilized are as follows: red, white, alsike, and crimson clovers and trefoils; lucerne; and sainfoin. Roughages

are relatively low in energy and have >18% crude fiber. Roughages are considered to be the foundation of an equine feeding program. Quality hay can provide energy for the maintenance requirements of the horse. Legumes and nonlegume grasses that are well-managed and fertilized (proteinaceous roughages) provide >10% CP as opposed to carbonaceous grasses (those that are not well-maintained or fertilized) provide <10% CP. It is important that the healthcare team educate clients on the features of satisfactory roughage including the following:

- mold-free
- tactile softness and flexibility
- leafy with fine stems (2/3E, ¾ protein)
- pleasing, fragrant aroma
- bright green with no brown or yellow.

It is also important to educate owners that additional handling of roughages can result in loss of:

- ¼ of the leaves
- ¼ to 1/3 energy and protein
- 90% of β-carotene.

(See Figure 59.2.)

Concentrates are typically a cereal grain that may or may not have supplemented protein, minerals, and vitamins. Concentrates are high in energy (typically 50% greater than forage)

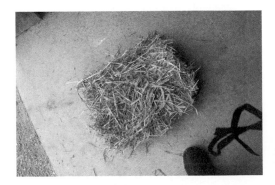

Figure 59.2 Roughage that meets quality criteria. (Reprinted with permission from S. Loly, H. Hopkinson (eds), *Large Animal Medicine for Veterinary Technicians* (2022). John Wiley & Sons, Inc.)

and are less than 18% crude fiber. Oftentimes, concentrates are used as a supplement if forage is insufficient in nutrients – especially energy and protein. Concentrates are needed more often in certain life stages such as gestation (especially later in the gestation period), lactation, growth, and in work horses. As a rule, it is best to not exceed 50 : 50 (wt: wt) concentrate to roughage. Anything new should be introduced and transitioned slowly. It is important for healthcare team members and owners alike to remember that concentrates are energy-dense, especially compared to roughages; therefore, excess concentrate may lead to laminitis, rhabdomyolysis, developmental orthopedic disease, and obesity.

Complete feeds are normally a mixture of roughage and concentrate – regularly an 80% roughage to 20% concentrate mixture. Complete feeds are manufactured by completely grinding the food and formulating it into a pellet, thus making it easier (all in one) for the owner. However, there is a potential increase in cost for this convenience. Because the complete feed is pelleted or wafered, care must be given to the potential risks associated with inadequate particle size, including colic, choking risk, wood chewing, and coprophagy (Figure 59.3).

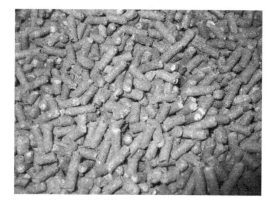

Figure 59.3 A complete feed. (Reprinted with permission from S. Loly, H. Hopkinson (eds), *Large Animal Medicine for Veterinary Technicians* (2022). John Wiley & Sons, Inc.)

Healthcare team members must discuss the need for fresh, clean water to be always available when discussing nutritional management of horses with clients. Energy for maintenance can be met completely with quality hay. However, owners may supplement with the concentrate if necessary. It is imperative that the horse is not supplemented in excess of 50% by weight with the concentrate. Adequate amounts of vitamins A and E are supplied through good-quality green roughage. Nutrition is the foundation for good health and affects every horse; thus, nutrition should be discussed with every visit.

Pediatric Equine Nutrition and Care

The objective of a feeding plan for foals and young horses is to create a healthy animal which will lead to a healthy adult horse. The specific objectives of a feeding plan for a young horse are to achieve healthy growth, optimize trainability and immune function, and minimize obesity and developmental orthopedic disease. Growth is a complex process involving interactions between genetics, nutrition, and other environmental influences. Nutrition plays a role in the health and development of growing horses and directly affects the immune system body composition, growth rate, and skeletal development.

Foals should be assessed for risk factors before weaning to allow implementation of recommendations for appropriate nutrition. A thorough history and physical evaluation are necessary. Additionally, body condition scores (BCS) provide valuable information about nutritional risks. Growth rates of young horses are affected by the energy density of the food and the amount of food fed. It is important that horses be fed to grow at an optimal rate for physiologic development and body condition rather than at a maximal rate.[2,8]

Nutritional requirements and dietary composition of the foal change markedly from the time they are transitioned from neonate to weanling. The foal transitions from a continuous supply of nutrients from the dam in utero to sporadic absorption of ingested nutrients post birth. Concurrently, the neonate's metabolism no longer is dependent upon the maternal glucose concentration to maintain normal glucose levels, and the pancreas initiates the regulation of glucose homeostasis. This alteration in energy metabolism is dramatic and does not always occur smoothly, leading to limited energy reserves (glycogen and fat) in the neonatal foal. Even in the "normal" neonatal foal, hypoglycemia occurs frequently and veterinary healthcare teams must be aware of this fact. In the sick foal, severe hypoglycemia will result if the foal is deprived of energy for even a short period of time.[1,9,10]

The neonatal foal has a high metabolic rate, and thus frequent ingestion of high volumes of milk to meet its energy requirements for maintenance and growth is needed. During the first week to months of foals' life, calorie needs are as follows:

- First week ~150 kcal/kg/day
- Three weeks ~120 kcal/kg/day
- One to two months ~80–100 kcal/kg/day

Healthy foals less than 7 days old will nurse approximately seven times per hour for approximately 1–2 minutes a time. After 7 days, there is a decrease in the number of times a foal will nurse, but conversely there is an increase in the duration of time nursing. The mare's milk averages about 64% sugar (as lactose), 22% protein, and 13% fat. Thus, the main energy source of energy for the foal is glucose.[9–12]

After the first 24 hours, foals will start to eat small amounts of hay, grass, and grain along with the mare's feces. It is understood that the feces provide the initial microbial flora needed by the foal to aid in the digestion of the hay, grass, and grain. Until several weeks of age, the roughage and grain are not well-digested by the foal. It is at this time that transitioning from weaning (milk-based diet)

to a forage-based diet is gradually occurring. The milk amount produced by the mare peaks after approximately 2 months of lactation, and then the amount of milk produced begins to decline. Shortly thereafter, the foal will be weaned from the mare and rely on solid feed for an increasing proportion of its nutritional requirements. Maturation of hindgut function is complete around 3 or 4 months of age.

Energy Requirement

The energy requirement of growing horses is determined through calculating the total energy required for maintenance in addition to the energy required for growth or gain. The daily energy requirement (DER) is dependent upon a number of factors; the environment, the foal's age, the desired average daily gain (ADG), and individual characteristics with the specific foal. The individual characteristics healthcare team members must take into account when calculating the daily energy requirement include metabolic and health characteristics. The optimal growth rate for horses has yet to have been determined; therefore it is difficult to determine the exact energy requirement. If horses grow too quickly and too much weight is added, skeletal integrity and longevity may be adversely affected. On the other hand, inadequate energy intake will result in poor and slower growth rates, and young horses will look unhealthy. Most nutritionists and equine specialists will follow the formula recommended by the National Research Council (NRC). This formula calculates the daily energy requirement of growing horses in the following manner:

$$DE \text{ (Mcal/day)} = (56.5x - 0.145) \times BW$$
$$+ (1.99 + 1.21x - 0.021 \times 2) \times ADG$$

(x is age in months; ADG is average daily gain; BW is body weight in kilograms).

Most horse owners will feed to achieve an ADG of 1.1–1.4 kg/day and with some owners aiming slightly higher. Veterinary healthcare teams and owners must be aware of what feed is being fed, how much is being fed, other feedstuffs that are being added to the diet, etc., as well as the energy concentration for total diets consumed. The team must perform a nutritional assessment prior to beginning a feeding plan and on every subsequent patient visit (whether farm visit or hospital visit). The average energy concentration for the total amount of feed (on an as-fed basis) given to a growing horse can range from 2.5 Mcal/kg with diets consisting of 70% concentrate to 30% hay ratio to 0.72 Mcal/kg for certain pasture-fed growing horses. Young horses have been found to gain enough energy from pasture feeding to sustain adequate growth. Many factors must be taken into consideration whether the horse is pasture-fed or concentrate- and roughage-fed. These factors would include the forage type and quality (if pasture fed), training level of the young horse, environmental conditions, body condition, and health of the growing horse. Again, the feed or pasture will also need to be evaluated for protein level, protein quality, vitamin and mineral level, etc. Any and all of these factors will influence the desired rate of growth in young horses. Restrictions in protein have a direct correlation to restrictions in the growth rate of a young horse.

Crude protein requirements for the growing horse can be calculated using the following equation:

$$\text{CP requirement} = \left(\text{BW} \times 1.44\,\text{g CP/kg BW}\right)$$
$$+ \left((\text{ADG} \times 0.20)\,/\text{E}\right)/0.79$$

The E in the equation represents the efficiency of the use of dietary protein. Estimates from the NRC for the efficiency of use of dietary protein in the young horse are as follows:

- ~50% for 4–6-month-old horses
- ~45% for 7–8-month-old horses
- ~40% for 9–10-month-old horses
- ~35% for 11-month-old horses
- ~30% for 12 month and older horses.

It is important also to remember that the quality of protein, as defined by amino acid composition, also plays a huge role in the growing horse; and poor-quality protein sources can have significant effects on growing horses. Also, inadequate amounts of dietary energy will be consumed if the feed is too low in either digestible energy or protein, even though plenty of feed may be available. Thus, growth rate in the young horse will decrease if inadequate intake of dietary energy or protein occurs. A slower growth rate has the potential to mask other nutritional deficiencies and if slowed significantly may reduce the body size of the horse at maturation. At a fast growth rate, a deficiency in minerals may result. If a deficiency of calcium, phosphorus, zinc, or copper occurs, developmental orthopedic disease may result. Conversely, if the young horse has too high dietary protein and energy intake, a rapid growth rate may occur, increasing the risk of developmental orthopedic disease and obesity.[6,7,9,10]

When feeding the young horse from nursing to maturity, fresh, clean water should be available at all times. Oftentimes, busy veterinary healthcare team members forget to mention the importance of this key nutrient.

The weight of growing horses should be obtained by owners as often as possible (bi-weekly is recommended). This can be accomplished through the use of a weight tape if scales are not available. Additionally, the healthcare team and the owner should record body weight and food intake. A BCS should be obtained at least every 2 weeks. This level of attention to BCS is important to the development of a healthy growing horse. Also, routinely assessing body condition delivers immediate feedback about optimal nutrition. This will prepare the owner to continue these observations throughout the life of the horse. Routine BCS will monitor horses throughout their lifespan and should result in fewer skeletal diseases, overweight or obesity, and many other related problems. Veterinary healthcare team members should reassess growing horses during farm calls and work in conjunction with the owners' observations to detect the potential or occurrence of under- or overnutrition. Reexamination should include body weight and body condition scoring, nutritional assessment, and determination of correct feed amount calculations.

Critical Care Nutrition

Nutritional support is becoming the standard of care in critically ill horses. Nutrition in critically ill horses can be administered orally. When this is not possible, horses can be fed intravenously or parenterally. It is imperative that nutrition be assessed and administered throughout the entire hospitalization of the critically ill equine patient. Enteral nutrition is considered less expensive and more physiologic, or more natural, for the patient. Enteral nutrition is also believed to provide enhanced immunity to the horse and is somewhat easier to administer. Remember the adage, "if the gut works, use it." This adage is a result of studies in a variety of species which show enteral nutrition helps support organ function, improves organ blood flow, improves immune function, and helps the patient gain weight. Current guidelines suggest the use of enteral nutrition whenever it is tolerated by the horse over the use of/or in combination with parenteral nutrition. Veterinary technicians play a large role in the management of nutrition in critically ill horses and should understand that early enteral nutrition with parenteral supplementation (if necessary) is the standard operating procedure for critically ill horses.

Nutritional support should be considered in patients that have, or are at risk for, increased metabolic rate. This would include equines that are growing; have experienced a history of malnutrition or hypophagia; have underlying metabolic abnormality that has the potential to worsen if food is withheld; have experienced trauma or sepsis; have an increased energy demand. The healthy adult horse can withstand food deprivation (simple starvation) for 24–72 hours with little systemic effects.

However, in stressed and injured animals, food deprivation has a greater effect. [6,11–14]

Stressed or injured horses have an increased resting metabolic rate and use their own protein as the chief energy source. This is known as catabolism. Increased metabolic rate and catabolism in the equine patient leads to accelerated body wasting. Total body protein synthesis is reduced since the body is using amino acids for energy. Subsequently, the horse has increased metabolic demands, uses protein for energy, develops insulin resistance and glucose intolerance, exhibits poor wound healing, and decreased immune function, and becomes extremely weak. Despite protein supplementation, the critically ill horse will continue to experience protein catabolism. Therefore, simply providing protein is not the answer, rather nutritional supplementation will help minimize protein loss; provide essential and conditionally essential amino acids, vitamins, and minerals; and subsequently decrease morbidity due to illness.

Enteral Nutrition

Enteral nutrition (EN) can comprise normal feed, slurry diets made primarily from the patients' normal feed, and liquid diets containing micro and macro minerals. Typically, normal feed is not tolerated by the horse because the appetite has decreased significantly, and nutrition must be given through a nasogastric (NG) tube. When implementing the use of an NG tube, making slurry from a complete pelleted feed is advantageous because it is relatively inexpensive and is well-balanced for an adult horse. Also, these formulations contain fiber, which aids in gastrointestinal activity, colonic blood flow, and colonic mucosal cell growth and absorption. However, making slurry out of the feed may not easily pass through the NG tube. If slurry is to be made, one kilogram of pelleted complete feed should be soaked with 6 l of water. Administer slurry through a large bore

NG tube using a marine supply bilge pump or if the pump is not available, pulverize the pellets before water is added. Take great care and caution when administering the slurry and be cognizant of the horses' reaction as you do so. Administer the slurry very slowly. Since an adult horses' (~450 kg) stomach volume ranges from 9 to 12 L, each feeding should not exceed 6–8 L.[2] If prolonged feeding is required (i.e., dysphagia; head, neck oral trauma; prolonger anorexia with functional GI tract), an indwelling esophagostomy tube is considered a better option for enteral feeding. Longer-term intubation with use of a smaller bore tube will not be conducive to the aforementioned slurry diets. Liquid enteral formulations (human and equine) have been recommended in enteral feedings through an esophagostomy tube. Enteral feeding should be introduced gradually over a period of days, with the goal being to feed the specific calculated Daily Energy Requirement (DER) or Daily Energy Expenditure (DEE) for that patient.[6,11,14] Energy requirements are dependent upon the weight, age, body condition, and metabolic stress of the horse. Maintenance requirements for adult, healthy horses, on average are 33–40 kcal/kg/24 hours or ~18,000 kcal/day. When attempting to meet the nutritional requirement in a critically ill horse, using the DEE/DER is an acceptable goal.[11] To calculate use the following equation:

Horses ≤600 kg: DEE (Mcal/day) = 1.4 + (BW × 0.03)

Horses ≥600 kg: DEE (Mcal/day) = 1.82 + (BW × 0.0383) − [0.000015 × BW]

(BW = Body Weight in kilograms)

The patient should be evaluated daily (and in some instances multiple times a day) to determine nutritional status and changes. Body condition scoring and weight tapes are recommended. When utilizing the weight tape, technicians should measure the girth just behind the elbow. The circumference determined will correlate with pounds or kilograms. Technicians need to be aware that with critically ill horses, body weight can fluctuate dramatically with changes in fluid balance. Diet and hydration status can vary the weight of a horse by 5–10%.

Parenteral Nutrition

Whenever the gastrointestinal tract is obstructed, dysfunctional, damaged, or painful, parenteral nutrition (PN) is indicated. Parenteral nutrition is also indicated if there is an alteration in plasma electrolytes or acid–base status to the extent that clinical signs are evident. The healthcare team should be aware that if dehydration and/or shock are evident clinically, mesenteric blood flow is commonly inadequate for the intestines to sufficiently absorb fluids for correction of dehydration or shock. Therefore, the healthcare team must get nutrition into the horse as soon as possible – waiting is not an option. Studies suggest that in patients who cannot tolerate oral nutrition, parenteral nutrition improves wound healing, minimizes muscle loss, decreases the weight loss seen in catabolic patients, and improves immune function. As was stated above, using the GI tract is the gold standard, but in times when enteral nutrition is not tolerated, parenteral feeding must begin as soon as possible.

Parenteral nutrition formulations are made up of protein in the form of amino acids, carbohydrates in the form of dextrose, and lipids in the form of long-chain fatty acids. Also, electrolytes, minerals, and vitamins can be added to the formulation. The carbohydrates and lipids meet the energy needs of the horse, break down the autologous protein for energy, and work synergistically with the protein for wound healing and increased immune function.

Parenteral nutrition is administered for short periods of time, multiple times a day. Total parenteral nutrition is a misnomer in veterinary medicine versus human medicine. Human medicine has a greater ability to prepare nutritional supplementation per individual patient and includes a wider range of microminerals, compared to what is available in veterinary medicine. When calculating parenteral nutrition volumes for adult horses, resting energy requirements should be used. However, protein requirements should be determined using maintenance requirements or estimated using the formula: 0.5–1.5 g protein/kg BW/d. The higher end of this formula is recommended in sick, compromised patients. The ratio of nonprotein calories/nitrogen should be at least 100 : 1 in the final solution. To begin, the goal is to provide 30–40% of the solution's calories with lipids and 60–70% with protein. Lipid supplementation may be increased to ~60% in those equine cases that need prolonged parenteral nutrition feeding.[6,11,14]

The addition of lipids to parenteral nutrition is beneficial in patients with persistent hyperglycemia or hypercapnia, reducing the dependency on glucose as the principal energy source. The amount of fat used will depend on the amount of carbohydrate provided; with fat storage occurring in the presence of excess carbohydrate calories.[11]

When administering parenteral nutrition, veterinary technicians should be aware of the risk of thrombophlebitis. Administration of PN solutions should be through a dedicated catheter placed in an aseptic manner. To minimize this risk, nonthrombogenic catheters such as polyurethane catheters should be used. Parenteral nutrition can be administered through an 18-g portal, while fluids and medications can be administered through a 14-g portal.

Whether the solution can be administered via a peripheral catheter or central line is directly related to the osmolarity of the solution (Figure 59.4).

PN solutions are typically administered as a constant rate infusion over a 24-hour period. Once the solution is warmed to room temperature, it is recommended to utilize the entire solution in this time frame to prevent contamination and lipid particle

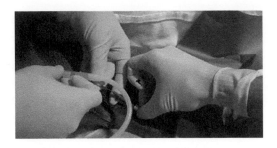

Figure 59.4 Aseptic technique is used for placement of a bilumen catheter that will be used to administered PN. (Reprinted with permission from S. Loly, and H. Hopkinson (eds), *Large Animal Medicine for Veterinary Technicians* (2022). John Wiley & Sons, Inc.)

destabilization. The team should begin administering 25–30% of the calculated nutritional requirements per hour. Subsequently, the administration rate should be increased by 25% every 6–8 hours, until 100% of the horse's basal metabolic requirement is being provided.[11] Monitor urine and blood glucose every 4–6 hours and serum triglycerides and blood urea nitrogen (BUN) daily. If the renal threshold of glucose (200–220 mg/dl with normal renal function) is exceeded, glucosuria and osmotic diuresis may develop. The rate of infusion should then be decreased to a tolerated level.[11] Once the equine patient is able to tolerate enteral feeding, the rate of parenteral nutrition administration should be decreased slowly (by half every 6–8 hours), to avoid hypoglycemia due to elevated insulin levels.

It is imperative that the healthcare team reevaluate the nutritional plan every day while administering PN. If the patient is not improving with this modality over several days and remains anorectic, options to institute enteral nutrition should be considered.

The parenteral nutrition line should not be removed. If the horse needs to be walked or removed from the stall for any reason, take the bag of parenteral nutrition with the horse. Keeping the PN bag with the horse decreases the risk of contamination and sepsis at the catheter site. It also helps avoid potential hypoglycemia due to sudden discontinuation of a glucose infusion. The veterinary team should change fluid lines used for PN every 24 hours.

Monitoring serum triglycerides is important to prevent hyperlipemia, especially in miniature horses and ponies. Electrolytes should be monitored at least once daily, and the horse should be weighed, if possible, each day. At the minimum, veterinary technicians should perform daily nutritional assessments to guide any needed adjustments to the nutritional plan of the hospitalized patient. At times, a critically ill patient may require more frequent assessments.

Potential complications with PN administration can be classified into three main categories, namely, mechanical, metabolic, and septic. Mechanical complications usually involve catheter-related problems. Examples include occlusion, premature removal, line disconnection/ breakage, and/or thrombophlebitis. These problems can be avoided by the technician's strict adherence to aseptic techniques and careful monitoring of patients. Metabolic complications are more likely to occur with PN solutions formulated to deliver total caloric requirements. The most common metabolic complication in equines is hyperglycemia and decreases in plasma electrolyte concentrations – especially potassium. Other complications include hypertriglyceridemia, hyperammonemia, or electrolyte changes consistent with refeeding syndrome (e.g., hypokalemia, hypophosphatemia, and hypomagnesemia). Reformulation of the PN solution is required if any of these problems occur. The most serious and potential life-threatening complication is sepsis. Technicians need to use strict aseptic techniques when placing a catheter. Nursing management of catheters carrying hyperosmolar solutions containing amino acids requires special focus because the solution type is an excellent medium for colonization of bacteria. Aseptic technique and focused nursing care should be the same for all types of fluid administration but is especially important in patients receiving PN. If signs of sepsis develop without an identifiable source, contamination of the solution and/or intravenous catheter should be suspected. A culture and sensitivity of both should be considered, due to the potential complication that many veterinary hospitals have the PN solution compounded at an outside facility.

In summary, EN and PN are viable nutritional choices for critically ill equine patients. When applicable, combined enteral and parenteral feeding is recommended to prevent intestinal hypertrophy and to facilitate healing by promoting intestinal growth. Proper nursing care and aseptic technique are also crucial to a positive patient outcome in both EN and PN. Nutritional requirements of hospitalized patients should be carefully monitored by the veterinary technician. Understanding some of the potential complications that can occur should enhance the effectiveness of EN and PN.

References

1 Burns, K.M. (2022). Nutrition. In: *Large Animal Internal Medicine for Veterinary Technicians* (ed. S. Loly and H. Hopkinson), 104–141. Ames, IA: Wiley Blackwell.

2 Burns, K.M. (2022). Animal nutrition. In: *McCurnin's Clinical Textbook for Veterinary Technicians and Nurses*, 10the (ed. J.M. Bassert, A.D. Beal, and O.M. Samples), 271–319. Elsevier, St Louis: MO.

3 Frape, D. (2010). *Equine Nutrition and Feeding*, 4the. Ames, IA: Wiley-Blackwell.

4 Geor, R. (2009). *Equine Nutrition, Veterinary Clinics of North America: Equine Practice*. St Louis, MO: Elsevier/Saunders.

5 Pilliner, S. (2009). *Horse Nutrition and Feeding*, 2e. Ames, IA: Wiley-Blackwell.

6 Geor, R.J. (2018). Internal medicine and clinical nutrition. In: *Equine Internal*

Medicine, 4the (ed. S. Reed, W.M. Bayly, and D.C. Sellon). 205–232. St Louis, MO: Elsevier/Saunders.

7 Gordon, M.B., Young, J.K., Davison, K. et al. (2023). Equine nutrition. In: *AAEVT's Equine Manual for Veterinary Technicians*, 2nde (ed. S. Denotta, M. Mallicote, S. Miller, and D. Reeder). 12–55. Ames, IA: Wiley-Blackwell.

8 Burns, K.M. (2017). Equine nutrition. The *NAVTA Journal*. April/May. 30–35.

9 Lewis, L.D. (1996). Growing horse feeding and care. In: *Feeding and Care of the Horse*, 2e (ed. L.D. Lewis), 264–276. Media, PA: Williams & Wilkins.

10 Lewis, L.D. (1995). Growing horse feeding and care. In: *Equine Clinical Nutrition: Feeding and Care*, (ed. L.D. Lewis). 334–352. Baltimore: Williams & Wilkins.

11 Carr, E.A. and Holcombe, S.J. (2009). Nutrition of critically ill horses. *Veterinary Clinics of North America: Equine Practice, Clinical Nutrition.* **25** (1): 93–108.

12 Dunkel, B.M. and Wilkins, P.A. (2004). Nutrition and the critically ill horse. *Veterinary Clinics of North America: Equine Practice* **20** (1): 107–126.

13 Lewis, L.D. (1996). Feeding and care of horses with health problems. In: *Feeding and Care of the Horse*, 2nde (ed. L.D. Lewis). Media, PA: Williams and Wilkins.

14 Lewis, L.D. (1995). Sick horse feeding and nutritional support. In: *Equine Clinical Nutrition: Feeding and Care.* (ed. L.D. Lewis). Baltimore: Williams and Wilkins.

Index

Note: *italic* page numbers refer to *figure* and **Bold** page numbers reference to **tables**.

Nutrition and Disease Management for Veterinary Technicians and Nurses, Third Edition. Ann Wortinger and Kara M. Burns.
© 2024 John Wiley & Sons, Inc. Published 2024 by John Wiley & Sons, Inc.
Companion Website: www.wiley.com/go/wortinger/3e